# CONNECTIONS FOR HEALTH

# CONNECTIONS FOR HEALTH

Kathleen D. Mullen
*University of North Carolina—Greensboro*

Robert S. Gold
*Southern Illinois University*

Philip A. Belcastro
*Manhattan Community College*

Robert J. McDermott
*Southern Illinois University*

wcb

Wm. C. Brown Publishers
Dubuque, Iowa

**Book Team**

Edward G. Jaffe
*Executive Editor*

Brenda Fleming Roesch
*Editor*

Raphael Kadushin
*Developmental Editor*

Julie E. Anderson
*Designer*

David A. Welsh
*Senior Production Editor*

Carol M. Schiessl
*Photo Research Editor*

Mavis M. Oeth
*Permissions Editor*

Kathy R. Loewenberg
*Art Production Assistant*

**wcb group**

Wm. C. Brown *Chairman of the Board*

Mark C. Falb *President and Chief Executive Officer*

**wcb**

**Wm. C. Brown Publishers, College Division**

G. Franklin Lewis *Executive Vice-President, General Manager*

E. F. Jogerst *Vice-President, Cost Analyst*

Chris C. Guzzardo *Vice-President, Director of Marketing*

George Wm. Bergquist *Editor in Chief*

Beverly Kolz *Director of Production*

Bob McLaughlin *National Sales Manager*

Craig S. Marty *Director of Marketing Research*

Eugenia M. Collins *Production Editorial Manager*

Marilyn A. Phelps *Manager of Design*

Faye M. Schilling *Photo Research Manager*

Cover © Brian Lanker for *Sports Illustrated.* Photograph of rhythmic gymnast Stacy Oversier.



ISBN 0-697-00063-X

Library of Congress Catalog Card Number: 85-071845



Printed in the United States of America
10 9 8 7 6 5 4 3 2

*To those who seek to live life to the fullest, exploring the connections along the way.*

# Contents

*CHAPTER TWENTY*

## Aging: Adaptations for Wellness 496

# Preface

In 1979, a landmark document *Healthy People: The Surgeon General's Report on Health Promotion and Disease Prevention* set the stage for what is often called the second public health revolution. The first was represented by the struggle to overcome the pandemic infectious diseases that lasted through the middle of the twentieth century. The major weapons in this revolution included improved sanitation, development of effective vaccines and immunization programs spanning not only the U.S., but most of the world. In the U.S. today, only 1 percent of the people who die before their 75th birthday die from infectious diseases. This is an indication of the effectiveness of this first revolution.

The major killers today are heart disease, stroke, cancer and accidents. The second public health revolution is targeted at these causes of death and disability. And to some extent substantial progress is being made. Life expectancy at birth for Americans is now 74.7 years, an increase of 27.4 years since the beginning of this century. While much of this increase can be linked to our efforts early in this century, life expectancy increased more between 1970 and 1983 than it did in the 20 years prior to 1970. Although we often point to our efforts among the young as the principal reason for this increase in life expectancy, most of the increase between 1970 and 1983 was due to decreases in mortality among the middle aged (45–64) and elderly populations (65–84). These changes, however, are not without their costs. In 1983, health care expenditures in the U.S. totaled $355.4 billion, an average of $1,459 per person. This represents 10.8 percent of the U.S. gross national product.

These changes notwithstanding, another public health revolution has begun to gain momentum in part because of these dramatic increases in life expectancy, but more so because of the growing concern for quality of life. That revolution has taken several shapes and been called by various labels, but has been most identified with the term WELLNESS. Unfortunately, the term wellness has been used by many to describe different things. There have, in fact, been several personal health books that have claimed to take a wellness approach, but we feel that *Connections for Health* is the first book that truly integrates a wellness approach throughout. We also feel that this is the first personal health book that not only integrates wellness concepts throughout, but is also thoroughly documented.

There are some additional characteristics of *Connections* that distinguish it from other books currently available. We recognize that health issues are not only matters of individual choice, but that there are also social and cultural factors over which we may have little control—yet they influence our health. It is because of this that we have included in each chapter some recognition of these factors. In addition, we have included in each chapter boxed highlights called exhibits to supplement the text and wellness activities to improve understanding of the major concepts. *Connections* is structured in a way that we think will improve understanding and allow for effective learning. Discussion questions, thorough documentation, wellness activities, chapter summaries and supplementary reading lists are all designed with this in mind.

There are many people who contributed support and guidance to this book. Among those we want to thank in particular is Mr. Ed Jaffe, Executive Editor, who worked with us on the early development and structuring of the book. We would also like to thank our reviewers, whose feedback was important to the completion of the project: Richard St. Pierre, Penn State University, University Park; William B. Hemmer, State University of New York, Brockport; Linda Sue King, University of New Mexico, Albuquerque; Hollis N. Matson, San Francisco State University; Susan Z. Newton, Central Washington University; Phillip J. Marty, University of Arkansas, Fayetteville; Sharon E. Schwindt, Central Washington University; James G. Paulat, DeAnza College; Charlene Agne-Traub, George Mason University; Carol J. Teske, Kutztown State College; Sidney Young, City University of New York at Lehman College; James H. Rothenberger, University of Minnesota, Minneapolis; Keith Howell, University of North Carolina, Greensboro. We are excited about *Connections* and feel that it brings focus to the meaning of wellness and personal health.

# CONNECTIONS FOR HEALTH

# UNIT ONE

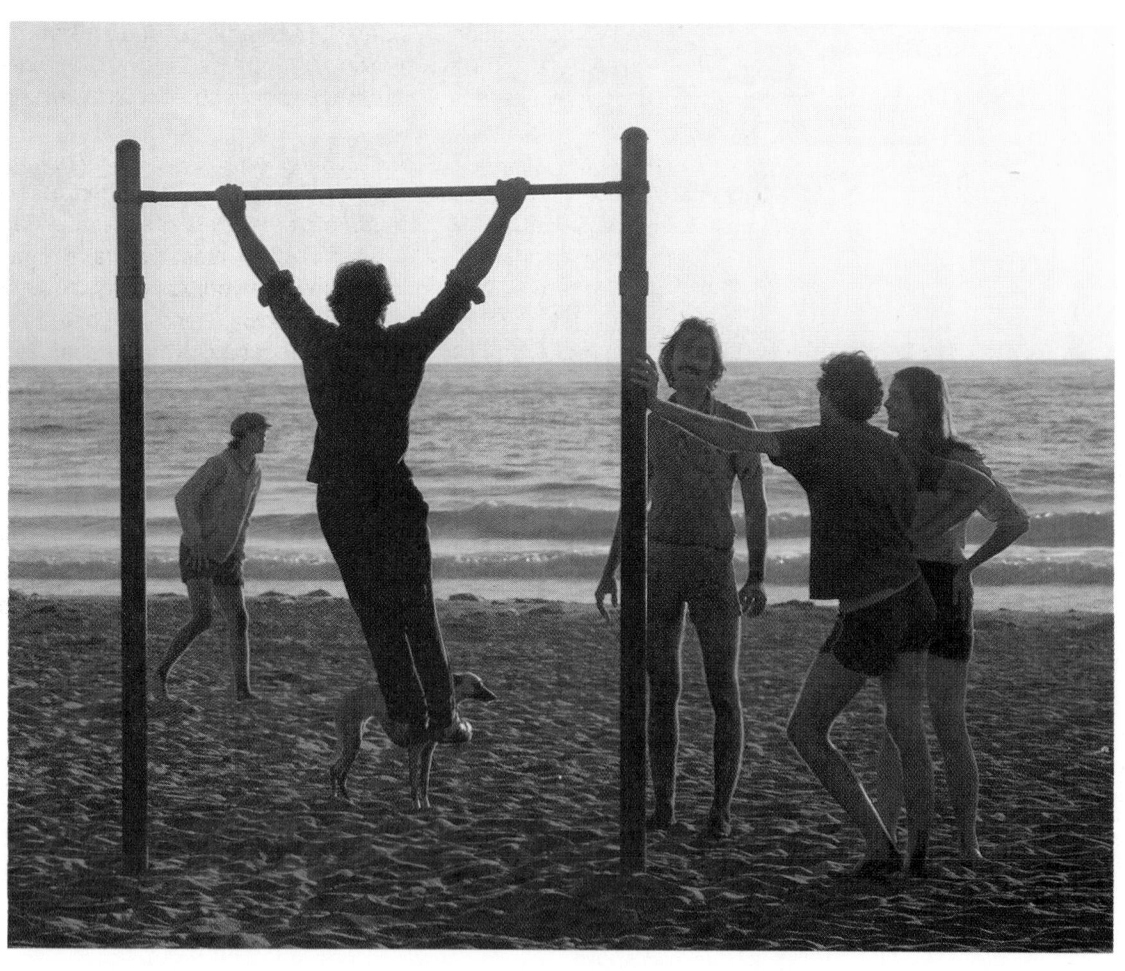

# Baselines of Health and Well-Being

Health has traditionally been defined as the freedom from disease. Maximum well-being, though, involves much more than that. In Unit One we will introduce a fresh approach to personal health called "wellness."

Wellness is a self-designed and dynamic style of living. It aims at optimal physical functioning, a positive emotional attitude, and a capacity to live life to the fullest. The real key to wellness, though, lies in self-initiative and self-responsibility. Unless you take an active role in your own well-being and recognize your capacity to set and achieve personal goals, high-level wellness is inconceivable.

Chapters 1 through 6 will help you establish those goals by exploring the basics of personal well-being and by offering practical guidelines on how to implement a wellness life-style. We will consider how "mental wellness" and a positive approach to life's stress can improve your well-being. We will also discuss how nutrition, weight control, and physical fitness affect wellness.

We can't force you to maximize your own health. That is the kind of decision you must make for yourself. Our overview of the wellness perspective should, though, suggest just how crucial that decision can be—and how life-enhancing your own wellness program can become.

CHAPTER ONE

# Wellness: A Quality of Living



Wellness is a term that has gained widespread popularity in recent years. Community wellness programs are springing up around the country; local bookstores are stocking up on wellness literature. People in general are becoming more aware of and interested in their own health and wellness: witness the unprecedented number of fitness and health-food enthusiasts alone. Wellness has gained so much attention that the popular press has come to label it a "wellness movement" or "wellness revolution."[1]

What is this "wellness movement" and what can it mean for you? Is wellness different from health? This chapter will introduce you to the concepts of health and wellness and the role they can play in your life. In addition to describing wellness and health, the issues surrounding what motivates people to choose a life-style of high-level wellness will be presented. Reading this chapter may begin to motivate you to choose a lifetime of wellness.

# DESCRIPTIONS OF HEALTH

Traditionally, health has been viewed as freedom from disease. If you had no signs or symptoms of illness, you were well. In 1947 the World Health Organization defined health in broader terms: "Health is a state of complete physical, mental, and social well-being, and not merely the absence of disease and infirmity."[2] While this definition started health professionals and the general public in thinking of health as a state of well-being, the process has been slow. Many of us still tend to believe the false notion that if we are not sick we must be well. Personal health care is viewed by many solely in terms of the yearly physical. We have standard employee-benefit packages of "disease insurance" and "sick days." We measure our nation's health status by **morbidity** (disease) and **mortality** (death) rates. In general, we are part of a "disease care" not a "health care" system.

**Health promotion** programming is a relatively new and innovative approach to health care. This approach relies on **disease prevention** in addition to the treatment of disease[3]. Too many Americans are dying young. Prevention of premature chronic disease is an important goal of health promotion programs.

The following analogy dramatically portrays the vastly understated fact of premature death in the United States.

> Beginning this October 1, two jumbo jets crash everyday of the year, killing 501 people per day (359 men, 142 women). The average age is 58, with a range of 30 to 65. At the end of the year 183,000 citizens have died prematurely. That same year, another four jumbo jets crash daily, extensively injuring 1,562 people per crash and, after six months of intensive care, these crash victims are restored to one-half of their pre-accident health and mobility.[4]

If this air-travel situation actually existed, Americans would be up in arms, demanding some immediate remedy. Additionally, most Americans would be unwilling to take the risks involved in air travel. Although most Americans are unaware of it, they are currently facing this problem of premature death and disability. This airplane analogy is equivalent to the number of deaths and disabilities that occur in the population under age sixty-five from heart disease and stroke alone.

What are the causes and risk factors associated with premature death in the United States? How can this situation be remedied? The first step is to determine the basic elements associated with health.

Advocates of health promotion and disease prevention have delineated four major determinants of health: environment (prenatal, physical, social, cultural, educational, and economic); behavior (life-style); heredity (genetic predisposition); and health-care services (availability and accessibility of medical personnel, technology, and facilities). (See figure 1.1.) Henrick Blum, a health planner who devised the Environment of Health Model, designed the model so that the width of the arrows of each determinant indicate his view of the importance each element plays in health promotion and disease prevention. Other health planners,[5] however, make the assumption that all four determinants have an equal impact on health.[6] The elements in the circle surrounding the arrows are factors which are believed to influence the determinants of health. These include population, culture, mental health, ecological balance, and natural resources.

Health planners, using an environmental model of health, have estimated the role of each determinant in the leading causes of death in the United States. On the average, 43 percent of the leading causes of death in the United States are related to **life-style factors,** that is, individual practices and habits such as exercise, nutrition, and stress management. (See table 1.1.) When environmental factors are added to this, it can be seen that Americans could have some personal measure of control over approximately 62 percent of the current leading causes of death.

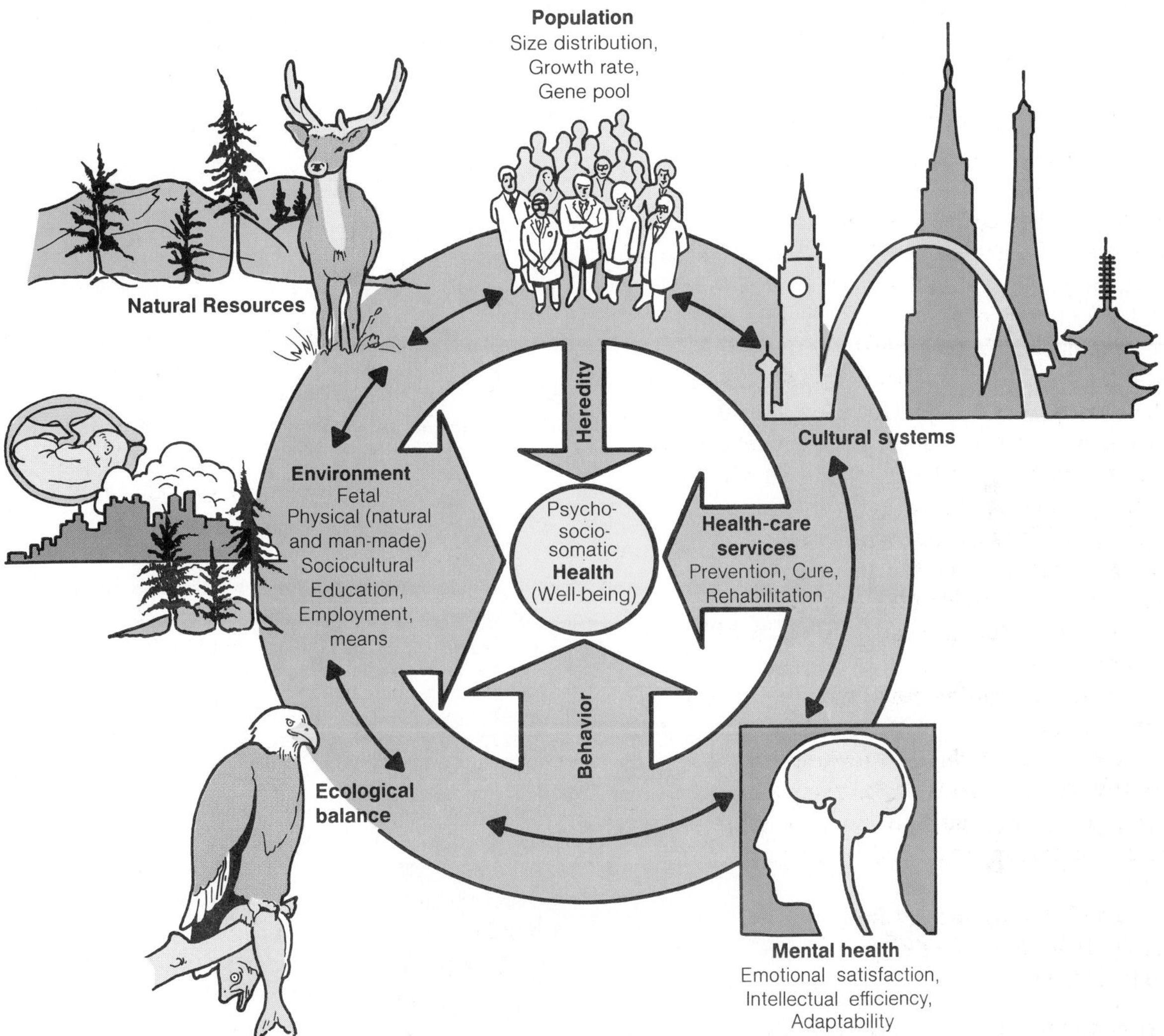


**Figure 1.1**
The environment of health model. *Source:* From Blum, H. L., *Planning for Health—Development Application of Social Change Theory.* © 1974 Human Sciences Press, Inc., New York. Reprinted by permission.

Health-promotion and disease-prevention programs aim at these known behavioral and environmental risk factors. In 1979 the Surgeon General's Office issued a report entitled *Healthy People* which delineated health goals for each age group in the United States. These goals are based on known risk factors for five age groups.

Here is the major goal cited for young adults: "Goal: To improve the health and health habits of adolescents and young adults, and, by 1990, to reduce deaths among people ages 15 to 24 by at least 20 percent, to fewer than 93 per 100,000."[7] Subgoals for young adults include developing safe driving habits; avoiding the use of firearms; adopting good health habits (dental care, nutrition, exercise, not smoking, using alcohol moderately if at all, and

**Table 1.1 Estimates of Percentage of Mortality for an Environmental Model of Health**

| Cause of Mortality | Percentage Allocation of Mortality to the Epidemiological Model | | | |
|---|---|---|---|---|
| | *Health-care Organization* | *Life-style* | *Environment* | *Human Biology* |
| Diseases of the heart | 12 | 54 | 9 | 28 |
| Cancer | 10 | 37 | 24 | 29 |
| Cerebrovascular disease | 7 | 50 | 22 | 21 |
| Motor-vehicle accidents | 12 | 69 | 18 | 0.6 |
| All other accidents | 14 | 51 | 31 | 4 |
| Influenza and pneumonia | 18 | 23 | 20 | 39 |
| Diseases of the respiratory system | 13 | 40 | 24 | 24 |
| Diseases of the arteries, veins, and capillaries | 18 | 49 | 8 | 26 |
| Homicides | 0 | 66 | 41 | 5 |
| Birth injuries and other diseases peculiar to early infancy | 27 | 30 | 15 | 28 |
| Diabetes mellitus | 6 | 26 | 0 | 68 |
| Suicides | 3 | 60 | 35 | 2 |
| Congenital anomalies | 6 | 9 | 6 | 79 |
| Percent allocation—average | 11 | 43 | 19 | 27 |

Source: G. E. Alan Dever, *Community Health Analysis: An Holistic Approach* © 1980 Aspen Systems Corporation, Rockville, Md. Reprinted by permission.

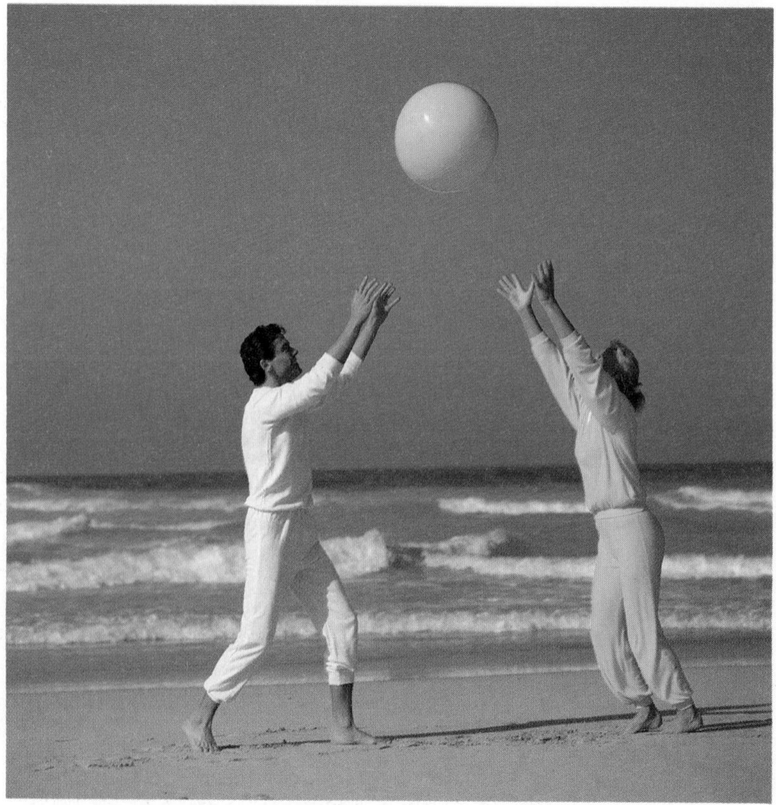

**Figure 1.2**
Both personal behaviors and the environment affect an individual's health status.

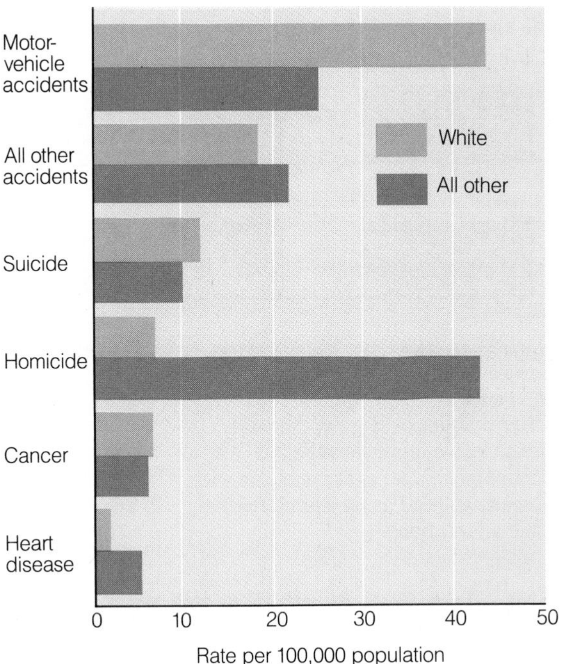


**Figure 1.3**
Major causes of death for ages fifteen to twenty-four: United States, 1976. *Source:* Based on data from the National Center for Health Statistics, Division of Vital Statistics.

Favorable
Supports
Wellness
Low
High
Individual
Initiative and action
Toward
Sociocultural
Unfavorable

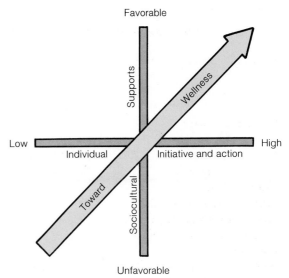

**Figure 1.4**
Direction and progress toward wellness. Wellness involves both personal initiative and action, and the availability of social support networks. Improvements in both dimensions will be necessary for achieving higher levels of wellness.

avoiding drug abuse); developing a responsible attitude toward sexuality; and talking about problems or stressful situations.[8]

Although disease prevention and health promotion are necessary components of an improved health-care system, they continue to place a major emphasis on disease and lead us to rely on the medical-care system as our primary means to health.[9] Is there more to well-being than health as it is currently depicted? Advocates of a new concept—wellness—believe so.

## THE WELLNESS CONCEPT

**Wellness** has been described as a process involving a zest for living,[10] a self-designed style of living that allows you to live your life to the fullest.[11] Because the wellness concept has recently become popular, many believe it to be a phenomenon of a 1970s health consciousness. Actually, the concept of high-level wellness was first proposed by Halbert Dunn during the 1950s. Dunn was a well-known physician and statistician who served from 1935 to 1960 as Chief of the National Office of Vital Statistics. Dunn's idea of high-level wellness was based on the World Health Organization's definition of health.[12] Dunn saw WHO's definition of health as a positive statement of well-being with implications for the existence of multiple levels of wellness. Dunn was careful to point out, however, that the "state" of health was different from the "process" of wellness. He saw health as a relatively passive state of homeostasis or balance; he viewed wellness as a dynamic concept or a process of continuously moving toward one's potential for optimal functioning.

Dunn believed that a person's level of wellness was dependent on three criteria: (1) direction and progress, (2) the total individual, and (3) how the individual functions.[13] The first criterion—direction and progress—implies that wellness is not a static state, but rather a movement toward ever-higher potentials of functioning. (See figure 1.4.) You cannot attain a "state" of wellness and then stop. If

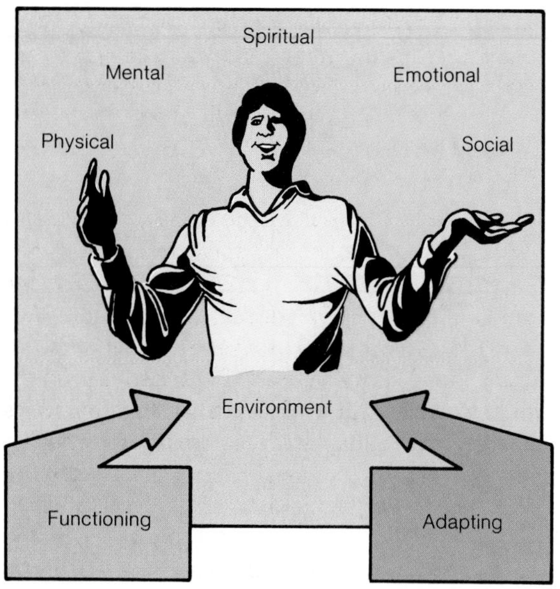


**Figure 1.5**
A model of well-being. A well person is one who, within a given environment, is constantly moving toward wellness in all dimensions of being (physical, mental, emotional, social, and spiritual) both during daily functioning and during times of challenge when adaptation is necessary. *Source:* Adapted courtesy of Dr. Robert Russell, Southern Illinois University at Carbondale, Carbondale, Ill.

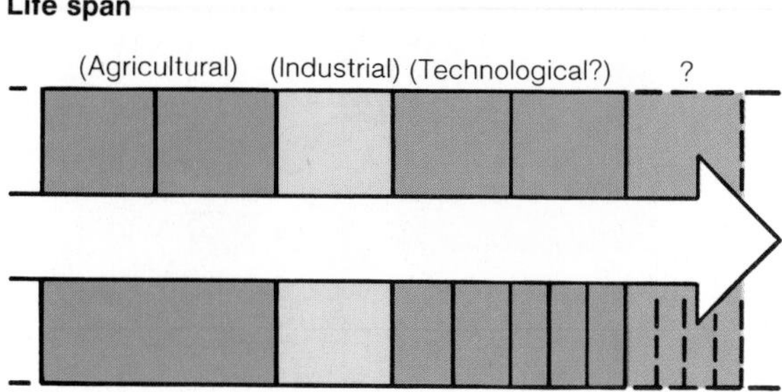


**Figure 1.6**
Value changes over time and life spans. As we move into the technological age, changes occur with increasing speed as do associated value adaptations.

you are not moving forward and upward toward high-level wellness, then you must be moving backward, away from your wellness potential. Wellness is active and requires individual initiative.

Dunn's second criterion for wellness maintains that we must be concerned with the total person, including the physical, mental (intellectual), emotional (feeling), social, and spiritual dimensions. Robert Russell, professor of health education, has developed a model which unites this total-person concept with Dunn's third criterion of functioning.[14] (See figure 1.5.)

Russell's model depicts an individual surrounded by the five dimensions of the total person. In Russell's view, the spiritual dimension unites all other dimensions—mental, physical, emotional, and social. Spiritual well-being may be, but is not necessarily, of a religious nature. It is also considered to encompass your philosophy of life, your values, or what gives meaning and purpose to your life. Individuals, in their many-faceted dimensions, function daily in the environment that surrounds them. Functioning implies skills or activities of daily living (life-style) that impact on the five dimensions. These daily activities include life-style choices such as what we eat, how and when we exercise, the ways we choose to relax and cope with stress, how we communicate with other people, the types and quantity of products we consume, and how we treat the environment.

Adaptation is an essential element of wellness. Daily life brings sudden, unexpected opportunities or challenges that call for adaptation. Our world is changing at an increasingly rapid pace, and such change requires creative and frequent adaptation. The number of complete value changes taking place in the world during a typical life span (see figure 1.6) has increased steadily.[15] In the past, the values of one generation had meaning and application for the next. There was little change in the world from generation to generation. If you were raised on a farm chances are you would be a farmer, and the skills and values you attained during your formative years would be relevant to your survival and well-being. With the industrial revolution the pace of world change increased; a person could have a complete change of world values within a single life span.

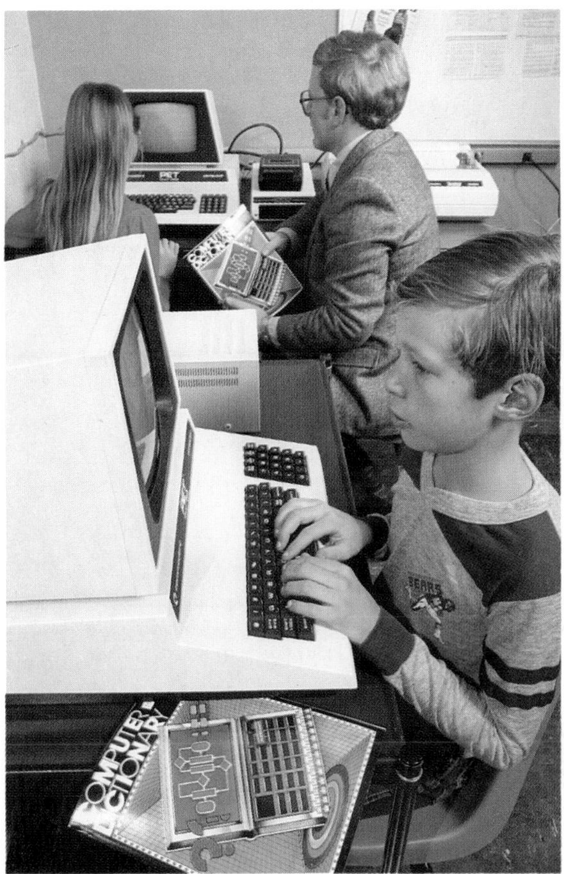


**Figure 1.7**
New technologies trigger rapid changes in society as a whole.

Today, with the advent of the technological revolution, the pace continues to increase. How many changes will we have to make during this life span? How many changes will our children be expected to make? How can we be well with such constant change and adaptation required of us?

In 1970, Alvin Toffler documented the problems inherent in rapid change and labeled the syndrome "Future Shock."[16] Such rapid change continues (see figure 1.7). Ten years before Toffler's work, however, Halbert Dunn spoke to the same concern:

> In today's world . . . the spurts of change are becoming a turbulent, racing torrent. There seem to be no quiet pools in this flood of change which permit one to slow down and rest for a bit, to become accustomed to an altered situation before facing the next disturbance. Can we, as individuals and families, attain and maintain wellness while riding the crest of a social millrace? This is the problem that we must face up to, because we cannot slow down the social changes now in process.[17]

Dunn believed that wellness and change could coexist. This would require that we be willing to face inconsistencies in our thinking, and reexamine our beliefs and practices in light of contradictions that come to our attention as a result of changes in our world. Knowing how and when to question is an essential wellness skill we must cultivate in ourselves and others. Such adaptation requires creative coping and greater energy output. When it is successful, adaptation returns us to a balanced level of functioning.

A well person then is one who, within a given environment, is constantly moving toward wellness in all dimensions of being (physical, mental, emotional, social, and spiritual), both during daily functions and during times of challenge when adaptation is necessary. Wellness is not based on a concern for disease and its prevention, but rather on optimal functioning and creative adapting.

Wellness is not simply a concept to be applied at an individual level. Dunn believed that wellness could be expanded to include the family, the community, and eventually the world.[18] Just as the ripples on a pond expand outward when a stone is thrown in, so does individual wellness expand and ripple outward to affect the family, the community, and the world. It is easier to seek high-level wellness for yourself if you are a member of a well family, community, and world.

Donald B. Ardell, author of the book *Fourteen Days to a Wellness Lifestyle,* has proposed a Worseness/Wellness Life-Style Continuum that depicts four major life-style choices on the road to high-level wellness. As Ardell's continuum (see figure 1.8) illustrates, sporadic efforts toward health do not lead you to high-level wellness. Wellness requires self-direction, self-esteem, and self-responsibility.

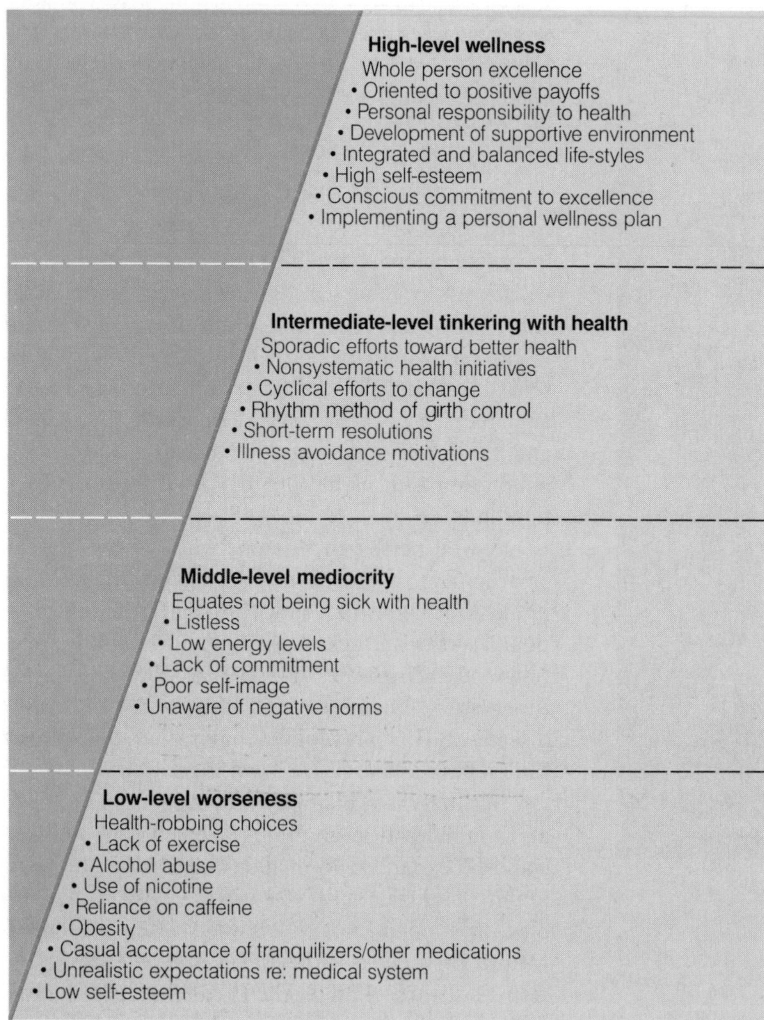


**Figure 1.8**
A worseness/wellness life-style continuum. *Source: From 14 Days to a Wellness Lifestyle,* by Donald Ardell. Copyright © 1982 by Donald Ardell. Reprinted by permission of Whatever Publishing, Inc., Mill Valley, Calif.

## SELF-RESPONSIBILITY FOR HEALTH AND WELLNESS

Americans have, in recent years, grown increasingly vocal about their "rights." Articles and books on such topics as the "right to health care" and the "right to health" abound. But what of a balance between rights and responsibilities? In 1975 John Knowles, physician and president of the Rockefeller Foundation, convened a group of physicians, philosophers, social scientists, and medical administrators to study health as a means for influencing the quality of American life. The proceedings of this meeting, "Doing Better and Feeling Worse: Health in the United States," contained strong statements regarding health as a right and a responsibility. To quote Dr. Knowles:

> The cost of sloth, gluttony, alcoholic intemperance, reckless driving, sexual frenzy, and smoking is now a national, and not an individual, responsibility. This is justified as individual freedom—but one man's freedom in health is another man's shackle in taxes and insurance premiums. I believe the idea of a 'right' to health should be replaced by the idea of an individual moral obligation to preserve one's own health—a public duty if you will. The individual then has the 'right' to expect help with information, accessible services of good quality, and minimal financial barriers.[19]

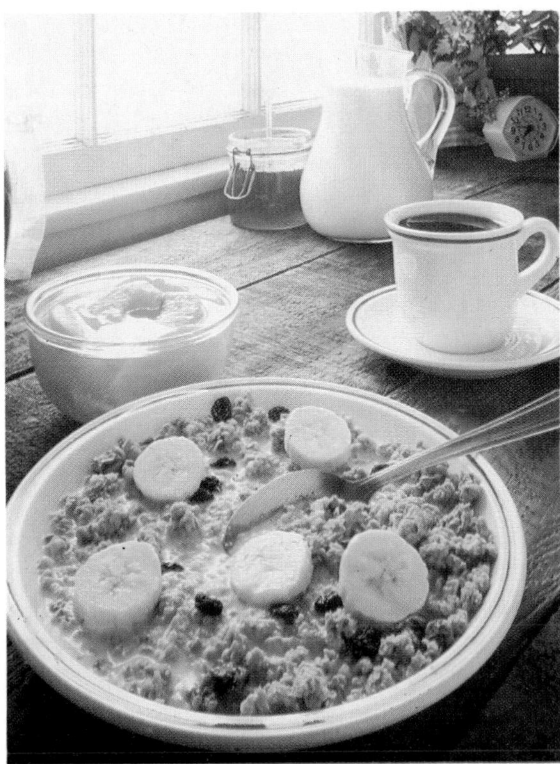

**Figure 1.9**
Even such simple, daily habits as eating a balanced breakfast can significantly improve your health status.

Another private foundation that supports wellness programs has taken the stance that responsibility for health and wellness has probably been more overlooked than the topic of rights. In their 1978 annual report the Victoria Foundation makes the following statement:

> Recently, attention has been given to the idea that in certain key ways the citizen bears first responsibility for his own health. This applies for all citizens, whether they reside in suburbia or the ghetto. An irony of American life is that even the poor suffer primarily from outlooks and indulgences spawned by affluence. Advances in transportation reduce the exercise which comes from walking. Television fosters sedentary routines. A plethora of fast cars kills more of us than most of the dread diseases kill in any emerging nation. It is probably true that more Americans suffer from abdicated responsibility than from denied rights."[20]

A prime example of individual involvement in achieving a state of health was demonstrated by Nedra Belloc and Lester Breslow.[21] Their research findings indicate that a number of simple health habits (see figure 1.9) significantly affect health and life expectancy. These health habits include: (1) three meals a day at regular times instead of snacking, (2) breakfast every day, (3) moderate exercise (long walks, bicycling, swimming, gardening) two or three times a week, (4) seven or eight hours sleep a night, (5) no smoking, (6) moderate weight, and (7) no alcohol or moderate use. This study of nearly 7,000 adults, who were followed for five and one-half years, found that the physical health status of adults reporting they practiced all seven health habits was consistently the same as those thirty years younger who practiced few or none of the positive health habits.

The key to high-level wellness also lies in **self-responsibility,** or an active sense of accountability for your own well-being. The first step in becoming responsible for your personal level of wellness is to recognize that you make choices that impact on your total being—physically, mentally, emotionally, socially, and spiritually. This realization should result in a freeing experience. If you are experiencing high-level wellness through your daily life-style choices you have good reason to celebrate. However, just as important, if you find yourself falling somewhat short of your wellness potential, you have the power, the right, and the responsibility to choose differently. While health educators, physicians, hospitals, YMCA/YWCAs, and the like can provide valuable knowledge and assistance in carrying out your wellness plan, the initiative and action must come from you. As Halbert Dunn once commented "We cannot take high-level wellness like a pill out of a bottle. It will come only to those who work at following its precepts."[22]

## PERSONAL AND SOCIAL INFLUENCES

Your life-style is not completely a result of individual behavior, as many would have you believe. Rather, life-styles are a combination of personal behavior modified and influenced by a lifelong process of socialization.[23] Socialization is carried on by the institutions with which we interact, such as families,

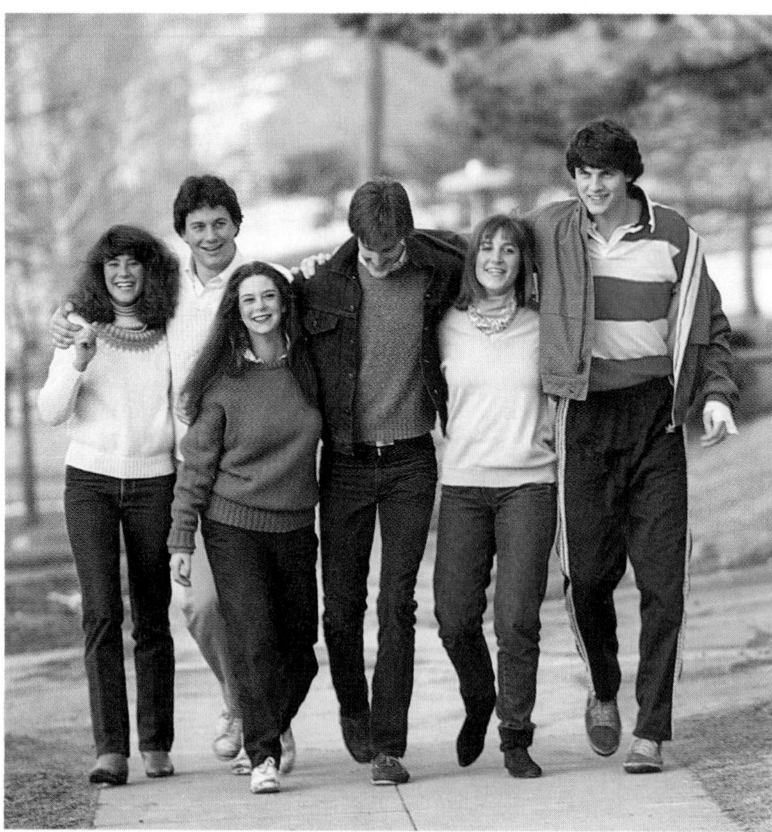

**Figure 1.10**
A strong social support network can encourage and compliment your wellness life-style.

churches, schools, unions, businesses, and clubs.[24] Robert Allen, author of the book *Lifegain,* believes that we live in an anti-health and anti-wellness culture: one that actually encourages us to be "overweight, underexercised, improperly nourished, tense, accident prone and unfit."[25] We are encouraged in these anti-wellness life-styles through the social norms exhibited by our culture. **Social norms** are the behaviors expected, exhibited, and rewarded by a given culture. Our western culture seems to set up barriers to wellness at every turn. Many Americans, for instance, would enjoy a nutritious snack on their daily work breaks. When they go to the refreshment area, however, they find the snack machines loaded with candy bars, potato chips, and cookies—no fresh fruit or other nutritious alternative is readily available.

Allen suggests that a combination of self-responsibility and building supportive environments is one way to circumvent the anti-wellness social norms bombarding us daily. You are responsible for assessing social traps which may impede your wellness planning. You must choose which social norms you will maintain and which you wish to change. When you choose to change, include in your planning the creation of a social support network (see figure 1.10) that expects and encourages you to move toward higher levels of wellness. Join a group that exercises together. Share your wellness plan with a friend or two. Ask your friends for emotional support or other forms of assistance that would be helpful. Encourage your family and friends to join in your wellness program. And provide strokes and encouragement for those around you who may also be seeking high-level wellness. (See Activity for Wellness 1.1.)

1.1 ACTIVITY FOR WELLNESS 1.1

# Healthstyle: A Self-Test

All of us want good health. But many of us do not know how to be as healthy as possible. Health experts now describe *life-style* as one of the most important factors affecting health. In fact, it is estimated that as many as seven of the ten leading causes of death could be reduced through common-sense changes in life-style. That's what this brief test, developed by the Public Health Service, is all about. Its purpose is simply to tell you how well you are doing to stay healthy. The behaviors covered in the test are recommended for most Americans. Some of them may not apply to persons with certain chronic diseases or handicaps, or to pregnant women. Such persons may require special instructions from their physicians.

Key:

A Almost Always
S Sometimes
N Almost Never

***Cigarette Smoking***

If you never smoke, enter a score of 10 for this section and go to the next section on *Alcohol and Drugs*.

| | A | S | N |
|---|---|---|---|
| 1. I avoid smoking cigarettes. | 2 | 1 | 0 |
| 2. I smoke only low-tar and low-nicotine cigarettes *or* I smoke a pipe or cigars. | 2 | 1 | 0 |

**Smoking Score:** ________

***Alcohol and Drugs***

| | A | S | N |
|---|---|---|---|
| 1. I avoid drinking alcoholic beverages *or* I drink no more than one or two drinks a day. | 4 | 1 | 0 |
| 2. I avoid using alcohol or other drugs (especially illegal drugs) as a way of handling stressful situations or the problems in my life. | 2 | 1 | 0 |
| 3. I am careful not to drink alcohol when taking certain medicines (for example, medicine for sleeping, pain, colds, and allergies), or when pregnant. | 2 | 1 | 0 |
| 4. I read and follow the label directions when using prescribed and over-the-counter drugs. | 2 | 1 | 0 |

**Alcohol and Drugs Score:** ________

***Eating Habits***

| | A | S | N |
|---|---|---|---|
| 1. I eat a variety of foods each day, such as fruits and vegetables, whole-grain breads and cereals, lean meats, dairy products, dry peas and beans, and nuts and seeds. | 4 | 1 | 0 |
| 2. I limit the amount of fat, saturated fat, and cholesterol I eat (including fat on meats, eggs, butter, cream, shortenings, and organ meats such as liver). | 2 | 1 | 0 |
| 3. I limit the amount of salt I eat by cooking with only small amounts, not adding salt at the table, and avoiding salty snacks. | 2 | 1 | 0 |
| 4. I avoid eating too much sugar (especially frequent snacks of sticky candy or soft drinks). | 2 | 1 | 0 |

**Eating Habits Score:** ________

1.1 *continued* ACTIVITY FOR

# WELLNESS

| | A | S | N |
|---|---|---|---|
| ***Exercise/Fitness*** | | | |
| 1. I maintain a desired weight, avoiding overweight and underweight. | 3 | 1 | 0 |
| 2. I do vigorous exercises for fifteen to thirty minutes at least three times a week (examples include running, swimming, brisk walking). | 3 | 1 | 0 |
| 3. I do exercises that enhance my muscle tone for fifteen to thirty minutes at least three times a week (examples include yoga and calisthenics). | 2 | 1 | 0 |
| 4. I use part of my leisure time participating in individual, family, or team activities that increase my level of fitness (such as gardening, bowling, golf, and baseball). | 2 | 1 | 0 |

**Exercise/Fitness Score:** ________

| | A | S | N |
|---|---|---|---|
| ***Stress Control*** | | | |
| 1. I have a job or do other work that I enjoy. | 2 | 1 | 0 |
| 2. I find it easy to relax and express my feelings freely. | 2 | 1 | 0 |
| 3. I recognize early, and prepare for, events or situations likely to be stressful for me. | 2 | 1 | 0 |
| 4. I have close friends, relatives, or others whom I can talk to about personal matters and call on for help when needed. | 2 | 1 | 0 |
| 5. I participate in group activities (such as church and community organizations) or hobbies that I enjoy. | 2 | 1 | 0 |

**Stress Control Score:** ________

| | A | S | N |
|---|---|---|---|
| ***Safety*** | | | |
| 1. I wear a seat belt while riding in a car. | 2 | 1 | 0 |
| 2. I avoid driving while under the influence of alcohol and other drugs. | 2 | 1 | 0 |
| 3. I obey traffic rules and the speed limit when driving. | 2 | 1 | 0 |
| 4. I am careful when using potentially harmful products or substances (such as household cleaners, poisons, and electrical devices). | 2 | 1 | 0 |
| 5. I avoid smoking in bed. | 2 | 1 | 0 |

**Safety Score:** ________

**WHAT YOUR SCORES MEAN TO YOU**

***Scores of 9 and 10***

Excellent! Your answers show that you are aware of the importance of this area to your health. More important, you are putting your knowledge to work for you by practicing good health habits. As long as you continue to do so, this area should not pose a serious health risk. It's likely that you are setting an example for your family and friends to follow. Since you got a very high test score on this part of the test, you may want to consider other areas where your scores indicate room for improvement.

***Scores of 6 to 8***

Your health practices in this area are good, but there is room for improvement. Look again at the items you answered with a "Sometimes" or "Almost Never." What changes can you make to improve your score? Even a small change can often help you achieve better health.

***Scores of 3 to 5***

Your health risks are showing! Would you like more information about the risks you are facing

ACTIVITY FOR 1.1
# WELLNESS

and about why it is important for you to change these behaviors? Perhaps you need help in deciding how to successfully make the changes you desire. In either case, help is available.

***Scores of 0 to 2***

Obviously, you were concerned enough about your health to take the test, but your answers show that you may be taking serious and unnecessary risks with your health. Perhaps you are not aware of the risks and what to do about them. You can easily get the information and help you need to improve, if you wish. The next step is up to you.

## YOU CAN START RIGHT NOW

In the test you just completed were numerous suggestions to help you reduce your risk of disease and premature death. Here are some of the most significant:

***Avoid Cigarettes***

Cigarette smoking is the single most important preventable cause of illness and early death. It is especially risky for pregnant women and their unborn babies. Persons who stop smoking reduce their risk of getting heart disease and cancer. So if you're a cigarette smoker, think twice about lighting that next cigarette. If you choose to continue smoking, try decreasing the number of cigarettes you smoke and switching to a low-tar and nicotine brand.

***Follow Sensible Drinking Habits***

Alcohol produces changes in mood and behavior. Most people who drink are able to control their intake of alcohol and to avoid undesired, and often harmful, effects. Heavy, regular use of alcohol can lead to cirrhosis of the liver, a leading cause of death. Also, statistics clearly show that mixing drinking and driving is often the cause of fatal or crippling accidents. So if you drink, do it wisely and in moderation. *Use care in taking drugs.* Today's greater use of drugs—both legal and illegal—is one of our most serious health risks. Even some drugs prescribed by your doctor can be dangerous if taken when drinking alcohol or before driving. Excessive or continued use of tranquilizers (or "pep pills") can cause physical and mental problems. Using or experimenting with illicit drugs such as marijuana, heroin, cocaine, and PCP may lead to a number of damaging effects or even death.

***Eat Sensibly***

Overweight individuals are at greater risk for diabetes, gallbladder disease, and high blood pressure. So it makes good sense to maintain proper weight. But good eating habits also mean holding down the amount of fat (especially saturated fat), cholesterol, sugar, and salt in your diet. If you must snack, try nibbling on fresh fruits and vegetables. You'll feel better—and look better, too.

***Exercise Regularly***

Almost everyone can benefit from exercise—and there's some form of exercise almost everyone can do. (If you have any doubt, check first with your doctor.) Usually, as little as fifteen to thirty minutes of vigorous exercise three times a week will help you have a healthier heart, eliminate excess weight, tone up sagging muscles, and sleep better. Think how much difference all these improvements could make in the way you feel!

***Learn to Handle Stress***

Stress is a normal part of living; everyone faces it to some degree. The causes of stress can be good or bad, desirable or undesirable (such as a promotion on the job or the loss of a spouse). Properly handled, stress need not be a problem. But unhealthy responses to stress—such as driving too fast or erratically, drinking too much, or prolonged anger or grief—can cause a variety of physical and mental problems. Even on a very busy day, find a few minutes to slow down and relax. Talking over a problem with someone you trust can often help you find a

1.1 *continued* ACTIVITY FOR WELLNESS 1.1

satisfactory solution. Learn to distinguish between things that are "worth fighting about" and things that are less important.

***Be Safety Conscious***

Think "safety first" at home, at work, at school, at play, and on the highway. Buckle seat belts and obey traffic rules. Keep poisons and weapons out of the reach of children, and keep emergency numbers by your telephone. When the unexpected happens, you'll be prepared.

**WHERE DO YOU GO FROM HERE**

Start by asking yourself a few frank questions: *Am I really doing all I can to be as healthy as possible? What steps can I take to feel better? Am I willing to begin now?* If you scored low in one or more *sections* of the test, decide what changes you want to make for improvement. You might pick that aspect of your life-style where you feel you have the best chance for success and tackle that one first. Once you have improved your score there, go on to other areas.

If you already have tried to change your health habits (to stop smoking or exercise regularly, for example), don't be discouraged if you haven't yet succeeded. The difficulty you have encountered may be due to influences you've never really thought about—such as advertising—or to a lack of support and encouragement. Understanding these influences is an important step toward changing the way they affect you.

***There's Help Available***

In addition to personal actions you can take on your own, there are community programs and groups (such as the YMCA or the local chapter of the American Heart Association) that can assist you and your family to make the changes you want to make. If you want to know more about these groups or about health risks, contact your local health department or the National Health Information Clearinghouse. There's a lot you can do to stay healthy or to improve your health—and there are organizations that can help you. Start a new HEALTHSTYLE today!

For assistance in locating specific information on these and other health topics, write to the National Health Information Clearinghouse.

Source: *Healthstyle: A Self-Test.* Office of Disease Prevention and Health Promotion, Department of Health and Human Services, Washington, D.C., 1980.

# HEALTH AND WELLNESS BEHAVIOR

A great deal of research has been conducted in the area of health behavior in an attempt to discover why we do what we do concerning our health and wellness. This body of research makes one point quite clearly. Human behavior is a complex and not easily understood phenomenon.

One contemporary theory of health behavior suggests three major determinants: predisposing, enabling, and reinforcing factors.[26] (See figure 1.11.)

## Predisposing Factors

All individuals accumulate a number of health beliefs, attitudes, and values during their life span, along with a wide variety of health knowledge. Together, these personal preferences and motivations toward health and wellness accumulate and interact to help shape our health and wellness behaviors. Some of the health knowledge, beliefs, and habits we pick up along the way come from accurate and reliable sources, and tend to serve us well. Others, however, are picked up through advertisements, articles in popular magazines, conversations with well-meaning relatives and friends, and the like.[27] These

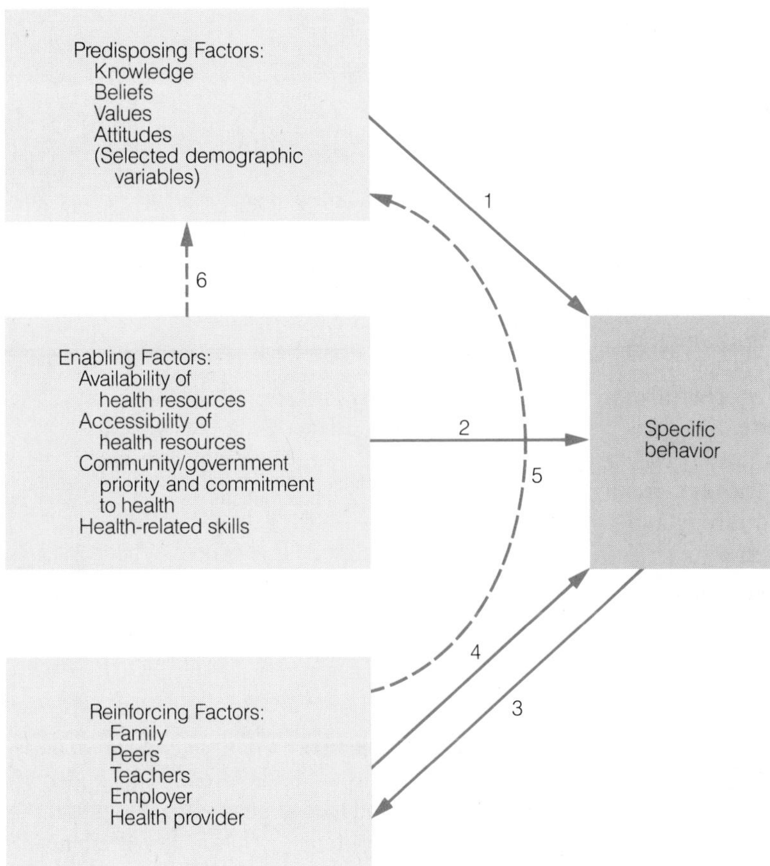


**Figure 1.11**
Three categories of factors contributing to health behavior. *Source:* From Greene, Lawrence W. et al., *Health Education Planning: A Diagnostic Approach.* © 1980 Mayfield Publishing Company, Palo Alto, Calif. Reprinted by permission.

beliefs, many of which may have no scientific basis, often become intertwined with our more reliable health beliefs and values.

**KNOWLEDGE** An accurate and reliable health-knowledge base is a sound foundation on which to build a wellness life-style.[28] Most of us, however, can think of numerous personal instances where our health behavior was in direct conflict with our knowledge. How many of us, for instance, continue to drive our automobiles without fastening our seat belts, or even after consuming several alcoholic drinks too many? Knowledge must be combined with other motivating factors if we are to move toward high-level wellness.

**PLEASURE AND PAIN** Pleasure and pain can be viewed as flip sides of the same coin. Both are strong human motivators. Basically, people tend to seek pleasurable sensations and to avoid painful ones. Sometimes, however, pleasure is delayed and comes to us at some expense of pain. To better understand this pleasure/pain dichotomy let's analyze three bicyclers, Tom, Bill, and Rita, all of whom meet three mornings a week to exercise together.

Tom took up the sport of long-distance cycling after his doctor prescribed it in order to help increase his work capacity, which was slowly decreasing as a result of heart disease. Bicycling isn't an especially thrilling experience for Tom. However, because he now bicycles, Tom has increased the amount of activity he can do before having signs of chest pain. The consequences of his bicycling—being able to play with his children, keep up with his friends and colleagues on the tennis courts, and so forth—bring Tom his greatest pleasurable motivation.

Bill has always been athletically inclined; he played football and track in both high school and college. Bill enjoys the pleasure of pushing his physical self to the limits of his endurance. He finds that long-distance cycling is one means to the pleasurable state of knowing he has done his best. The pleasure of the moment is an essential motivator for Bill.

Rita was a jogger throughout her college years and had enjoyed the challenge, but after a while she became bored and decided to try long-distance cycling as an alternative. Rita has found that she enjoys the pleasurable company of Bill and Tom, and is constantly amazed by the beauty of nature on these early morning jaunts. In addition to the pleasures of the moment, Rita finds that her bicycling pleasures carry over into all dimensions of her life. She feels mentally and emotionally refreshed on the days she cycles, and enjoys her work, family, and friends more. Rita's motivation appears to be spread throughout her life-style. All three bicyclers are moving in a positive direction toward creative adaptation and optimal functioning within their environment and circumstances.

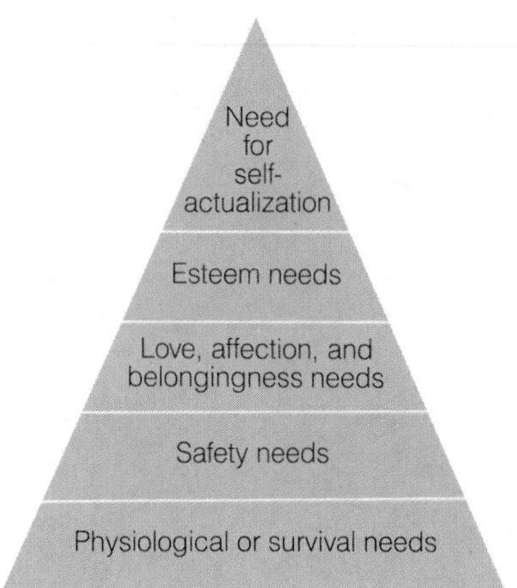


**Figure 1.12**
Maslow's hierarchy of human needs.
*Source:* Data (for diagram) based on Hierarchy of Needs, in "A Theory of Human Motivation," in *Motivation and Personality,* 2d ed. by Abraham H. Maslow. Copyright © 1970 by Abraham H. Maslow.

**FULFILLMENT OF NEEDS** Another strong motivator of our health and wellness behavior is the fulfillment of needs. Maslow has developed a model (see figure 1.12) that depicts our basic human needs as a triangular hierarchy, placing basic survival needs at the base.[29] As our physical and psychological survival needs are met we move upward in the triangle to safety, love, esteem, and finally self-actualization needs. Maslow's theory is based on the belief that we must satisfy lower-level needs before we can attempt the higher levels. Ultimately, a healthy person will be motivated by a need for self-actualization, or a striving to become everything one is capable of becoming. Self-esteem and love/belongingness needs are also strong wellness motivators. Most of our daily life-style activities are tied into how we see ourselves and how we view others' perceptions of us.

Although we are often motivated by the desire to fulfill our various needs, these actions are not always healthy or socially acceptable. We have a very basic need for food, which we satisfy by eating. If we choose to satisfy this need with Twinkies and soft drinks much of the time, however, we will not be meeting our nutritional needs adequately. We must combine our motivations with a reliable knowledge base.

**THE CREATED NEED** Our industrial society, based on principles of mass production and consumption, has produced a new category of human need. We must contend with the "created need" daily. Madison Avenue advertising executives are masters of the "created need." Americans have become convinced that they need everything from electric toothbrushes to automatic garage-door openers. Every time we open a magazine, turn on the television, or walk down the street, we are bombarded with messages trying to convince us of another "need" to add to our list. A sound knowledge base does not seem adequate in helping us to avoid such unnecessary, and often harmful, creation of needs. We must be consciously aware of our environment and begin to question ourselves about our personal values, beliefs, attitudes, and knowledge regarding these "created needs" and their possible impact on our levels of well-being.

## Enabling and Reinforcing Factors

Once we have the personal initiative to attempt a wellness life-style, implementation and maintenance become the important focus. Skills and resources are the **enabling factors** which help us

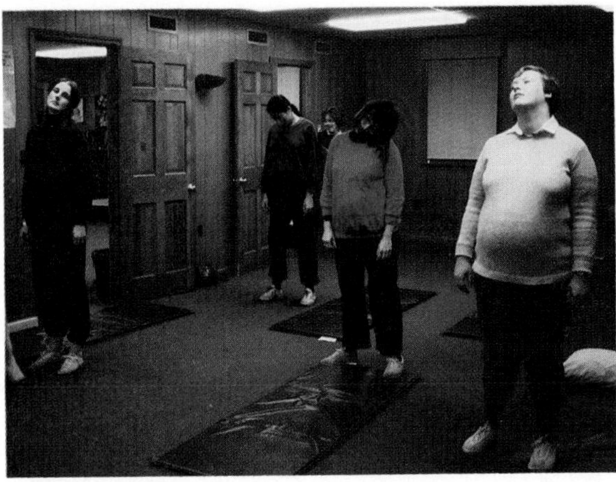

**Figure 1.13**
American social support for easily accessible wellness resources, such as this exercise class for pregnant women, is growing.

implement our wellness plan. Fred, a college sophomore, has noticed that he is under a good deal of stress lately, and he believes that relaxation would be helpful. Fred has tried to relax on his own but it doesn't seem to be helping. In order to "relax," Fred needs to learn the skills involved in deep muscle relaxation. While reading the local paper Fred discovers that there are several stress-management classes offered on campus that teach such skills and allow time and facilities for practice. He decides to sign up for one of the free evening workshops to enhance his wellness life-style.

The availability and accessibility of wellness resources is an important concern. Factors such as cost, distance, transportation, hours open for use, and so forth must all be considered. Many options for wellness are impractical because the recreation center's swimming pool closes too early, the wellness center's cooking class is all the way across town, or we cannot afford to take three hours a week to attend the relaxation-training class. American social support for readily available and easily accessible wellness resources is growing slowly. (See figure 1.13.) In the meantime, we must learn to be more flexible and creative in our personal life-styling efforts.

Once we have the necessary skills and resources we are back, once again, to the motivation issue—how do we maintain our initiative? **Reinforcing factors** are especially important during this phase. We do not live in a vacuum. Others react, both positively and negatively, to our various behaviors. Some of the more common sources of feedback and reinforcement include our family, peers, instructors, employers, and physicians. At different points in our life the reinforcement and support of certain individuals will carry more weight than others. Studies have shown, for instance, that children are significantly influenced by the beliefs and behaviors of their peer groups.[30]

Let's check in on Fred's stress-management efforts and see how he has been reinforced. Fred is really excited by the new skills he has learned in his stress-management workshop. These skills give him a new sense of mastery over his life. Through the evening workshop he has also met several new friends who have interests similar to his own. These new friends offer each other positive support and feedback. In addition to their daily relaxation sessions, they decide to try jogging a mile several times a week, both for the social outlet and the reduction of stress.

Fred needs his new support group, however, because his roommates are not equally accepting of his new activities. They don't understand why Fred wants to take a good twenty minutes to relax when he could be partying with them. Fred will undoubtedly have setbacks in his stress management program. Having some friends who will support his desire to improve in managing stress, however, will increase his chances for success.

As we have seen, predisposing, enabling, and reinforcing factors work together in a cyclical manner to influence our wellness life-styles. As we interact with others and the environment we receive feedback that cycles into our health and wellness decision-making process.

## WELLNESS: WHERE DO YOU START?

Wellness, that process of optimal functioning and creative adapting, doesn't just happen. You must supply the initiative and action for the journey toward high-level wellness. Below are three basic steps that should help you on your way.[31]

1.2

ACTIVITY FOR

WELLNESS

## Personal Wellness Contract

Area ____________

***Goal***

______________________________________________

***Current Status***

______________________________________________

______________________________________________

***Objectives***

The following are the specific steps I will take to accomplish the above goal, which I will record in a daily journal, and which will be used as the standards for judging the success of my project.

______________________________________________

______________________________________________

______________________________________________

***Plans***

This is how I plan to carry out the above objectives on a day-to-day basis.

______________________________________________

______________________________________________

______________________________________________

### Step 1: Commitment

Begin your wellness life-style by making a commitment. This doesn't mean that you have to become a vegetarian or a marathon runner. It does mean accepting responsibility for your own well-being. Wellness begins with an attitude of self-responsibility and self-respect.

### Step 2: Assessment

Assess your current life-style, including your social/cultural support networks. What areas of your life need special attention for cultivating better functioning, adaptation, and growth? Pay special attention to your motivations for wellness and any reinforcements you give and receive.

ACTIVITY FOR 1.2

# WELLNESS

***Resources***

These are the up-to-date, professional sources that I am using as guidelines and that verify my objectives and plans.

______________________________

______________________________

______________________________

______________________________

______________________________

***Special Considerations and Reinforcers***

______________________________

______________________________

______________________________

______________________________

I will complete this action between ____________ and ____________

______________________________ ______________________________

My Signature Supporter's Signature

Source: Mullen, Kathleen D. and Gerald D. Costello, *Health Awareness through Self-Discovery: A Workbook.* © 1981 Burgess Publishing Co., Minneapolis, Minn. Adapted by permission.

## Step 3: Action

Act. Develop your personal plan for wellness taking into account possible motivators and barriers. Seek out reliable information that is supported by professional research. Find out what opportunities are available for learning and practicing the various skills you may need. Locate or build a support network that will give you the positive feedback you will need. Ask someone in your support network to contract with you for improvements in your wellness life-style. A sample wellness contract is shown in Activity for Wellness 1.2.

Start slowly—you have spent a number of years building your current life-style. Don't attempt a complete overhaul immediately. Explore options and opportunities, and take the time to develop a sound life-style of high-level wellness. (See "News from Health Research.")

1.1 EXHIBIT

# News From Health Research: Toward a Better Understanding

Picture yourself in front of your home television, watching the early evening news. A medical graphic of some kind flashes onto the background screen as the newscaster reports, "Today at X University, Drs. Y and Z announced the results of a scientific study which shows that. . . ."

When the thirty-to-ninety-second "spot" about the research study is over, what will happen to that piece of information relayed to millions of people? Will it prompt responses like, "One more thing is bad for my health? I'm going to just tune out all of those studies and live my life"; or, "Now they're saying that's OK for you? A month ago some other scientist said it was harmful for my health. When those researchers get their act together, I'll start listening." Will it prompt a simpler reply of "Oh," then be forgotten? Or will it spark an instant controversy, with headlines for days and discussions everywhere?

Assuming that health decisions are based partially on available "facts" about the impact of various choices, it becomes very important to be able to evaluate new facts and sort out conflicting ones, both now and throughout life. Even attitudes are involved here, because the lack of these evaluation skills promotes a "tuned-out" attitude toward research news and health recommendations. If it seems as if "Everything causes cancer" or "Even the experts don't know how what I eat affects my health," youngsters and adults easily can decide to ignore all health news.

## UNDERSTANDING BASIC CONCEPTS ABOUT RESEARCH AND THE RESEARCH PROCESS

Scientific expertise is not necessary to understand the research process and its results. Basically, health research involves testing, one at a time, the parts of an educated guess (hypothesis) about how living beings function. Because nature is so complex and involves so many variables, a single experiment rarely has "complete" or "perfectly clear" results. Therefore, many experiments must be completed to address the same question. These variations add different pieces to the puzzle. When a single experiment can be repeated by several different scientists with the same results, its conclusions become more and more accepted.

Public confusion about health-research findings understandably results when many complex experiments are conducted and simultaneously, while an independent, aggressive media industry seeks "headline news." Because health is a subject highly relevant to the public, and because mass changes in health habits often have large economic and political implications, research findings often are newsworthy. Indisputable cause-and-effect research findings about possible cancer-causing substances, for example, would be information everyone would like to know and information that conceivably could wipe out entire commercial markets. Lacking indisputable results but having a large field of "expert scientific researchers" available, the various forms of news media legitimately report on whatever pieces of the puzzle are available. As in any other business, the reporters' skills in relating that information and putting it in perspective vary greatly. Readers' or listeners' abilities to understand the information and put it into perspective varies even more; especially when most of them are not specifically trained for that kind of skill.

Much of the time there is incomplete information available for our decisions in life, especially the most important ones. Our decisions need the best information available at the time and our best judgment. Part of judging new health information is having an understanding of how health research is conducted and what is reasonable and realistic to expect from it. The following basic concepts provide a strong foundation for that understanding:

### Research yields new knowledge, but also uncovers new questions.

In most health areas, a body of knowledge is regarded as "currently accepted fact" and a set of questions outlines what we don't know and are trying to find out. High-quality studies yield both new information about the facts and revised versions of the remaining questions.

## EXHIBIT 1.1

**Legitimate scientific controversies exist.**

Different scientists give conflicting or seemingly conflicting messages about certain topics because they are interpreting "current facts" differently; because they are willing to differing degrees to extend the usually incomplete facts into life-style recommendations; and/or because they are conducting studies that explore different variations of complex questions.

**Most research questions take a long time to investigate.**

There are very few sudden, astonishing results. "Long" usually means years and can stretch into decades. This is because there are many, very strict requirements for research to yield supportable conclusions; because the effectiveness of a treatment or preventive action may take years to become measurable; and because basic research often goes through several further stages of testing, into clinical research and demonstration projects. In addition, results must be replicated and agreed on by other scientists.

**Health messages based on research can change as scientists discover new knowledge. Meanwhile, people make health decisions daily.**

As scientists learn more about the mechanisms of health and disease, they must refine or revise their own ideas and advice to the public. Thus, youngsters must learn to deal with change and to adapt health decisions to new information, instead of "turning off" when new information conflicts with previous "truths." Because knowledge and uncertainty are mixed in all health areas and legitimate controversies exist, there are not as many "absolute answers" to health questions as we would like to have. While health knowledge is constantly evolving, however, youngsters must realize that they face daily health decisions now, including choices about eating, sleeping, exercising, smoking, and taking medication. Informed health decisions, therefore, use the best information available at the time.

**Researchers draw conclusions from studies of large groups of people. Conclusions about "risk factors" are guides to individuals, not guarantees.**

Research results draw conclusions from differences in large groups of subjects. The results do not necessarily apply to every individual, and individual exceptions do not invalidate the conclusions for others. Science can help us make choices by identifying actions that probably will enhance health or increase the risk of disease.

Understanding the concept of a risk factor can allow students to see how research results bring information to health decision-making. It's extremely important, though, that "risk" be understood in its appropriate context. Psychological and social development, especially during teen years, requires that youngsters learn how to take risks. Teenagers frequently do not discriminate among risks, often seeing risk-taking as a way of demonstrating "bravado" rather than selecting some reasonable risks as a constructive way for learning how to meet new challenges in life. The concept of "risk factors" is different. It involves increasing or decreasing the probability of disease and/or death by engaging in or avoiding a disease-related behavior over time.

Some students point out that there are health risks all around us, and say that heeding health messages would make life overprotected and dull. In response to this, a discussion about driving can provide a helpful parallel. There is some risk of injury or death associated with stepping into a car to go somewhere. That doesn't mean we should stop using cars. However, certain reasonable and prudent actions can be taken to lower the risk of death and disability from auto accidents. These include wearing seat belts, keeping the car in good mechanical condition, not exceeding the speed limit and not drinking alcohol before driving. Even doing all of these won't guarantee that a driver will never be injured or killed in a car accident; but they will significantly lower the risk. It's also possible that a drunk driver without a seat belt in a mechanically faulty car could speed from one place to another and not necessarily be injured or killed; but the risk is much higher. If the driver does avoid an accident, that doesn't mean all auto safety precautions are useless and should be ignored.

Similarly, there are reasonable and prudent actions to take to lower disease risks. In the cardiovascular area, these actions include not

## 1.1 *continued* EXHIBIT

smoking, getting blood pressure checked and keeping it under control if it's high, controlling weight and being physically active. Doing these things won't guarantee avoiding cardiovascular disease, but they lower the risk. Some who ignore this advice may not develop cardiovascular disease, but their risk of disease is higher. Even if they "escape," that doesn't invalidate the value of preventive actions.

**Research can't answer some questions expeditiously because there are ethical considerations. Because scientists don't put people into experimental extremes that would harm them, it's difficult to get clear-cut answers to many research questions.**

Epidemiological research collects information about large populations over time, usually without "experimenting" on them, and makes statistical connections between certain factors. For obvious reasons, much research on humans is epidemiological; our society doesn't condone using masses of people as "guinea pigs." Research involving experiments on humans is very carefully regulated and uses procedures which minimize danger to participants.

Because we don't put human subjects into experimental extremes, however, it's more difficult to get clear-cut answers to many scientific questions. The scientific methods used are humane, but are often less direct and take longer. A major challenge to researchers is to develop research designs that are humane yet scientifically "tight" enough to yield meaningful results. Elements like sample size and composition, duration of the study and controls for other variables are important.

### APPLYING CRITICAL THINKING APPROACHES TO REPORTS OF HEALTH NEWS

A youngster who understands the foregoing basic concepts about research will be more likely to avoid the trap of an "extreme" reaction to health news—i.e., either ignoring it totally or basing a life-style decision on a single report. This is especially important in relation to television and radio news reports (which are very brief and are over before they can be reread or studied), and news heard "secondhand" from peers or adults.

Television and radio reports can trigger further investigation and critical analysis. If a scientific study is newsworthy, written reports usually appear in newspapers and magazines the same day or week it is covered by the electronic media. Gathering a variety of news reports on a particular study or set of research results is one helpful way to work toward conclusions because comparing the reports may point out gaps and controversies.

The following is a sample "Critical Thinking Checklist" to help assess media reports about research results. Students will discover that most news reports answer only some of these questions. Teachers should then encourage students to analyze what information is given and what information is missing from particular news reports, and how new health information can contribute to their personal health decision-making.

#### *Credibility of the Source*

A. What is the source of the research results?

B. Who paid for the study? Do the funders have any economic or other stakes in the research results? What is the probability for objectivity or bias?

C. Has any agency or organization responded to the announcement of research results? Do they have any economic or other stakes in the results? What are the probabilities for objectivity or bias?

D. Is the reporter known for prior experience in reporting on scientific research?

#### *Factors in the Study Design*

A. What type of research was done? Was the research at the "test-tube" stage, animal-testing stage, or human-testing stage?

B. Over what period of time did the study take place?

C. How many subjects were in the study?

D. Did the subjects have particular characteristics (age range, male or female, past disease history, etc.)?

E. Was there a control group for the study?

F. Have all relevant variables been considered?

#### *Interpretation of the Results*

A. How are the results being stated? Are there "qualifying" words that limit the applicability of the results (such as "in animals," "some," "may," "probably")?

## EXHIBIT 1.1

B. Do the results depend on a measurement of change? If so, is there an indication of the significance of the change (either statistically or biologically)?

C. Has the study been repeated by other researchers, with similar results?

D. Does the article differentiate between "fact" and "opinion"?

E. Does the study deal with a "risk factor"? If yes, do the results identify actions which will probably enhance health or probably increase the risk of disease?

F. Are the results part of an ongoing scientific controversy? If so, what side of the controversy has been given added weight by this study?

***Application of the News***

A. Does the article make clear what is known and what is not known about the research topic?

B. Does the article note what questions remain after the study and/or what new questions it generates?

C. Are the research results reported in this article relevant to one of my personal health decisions? If so, is there enough information in the article to make me consider changing one of my decisions? Do I need to obtain additional information?

**LOCATING ADDITIONAL HEALTH INFORMATION RESOURCES**

Usually one news report about a research result will not give sufficient information for a person to make or change a health decision. It then becomes important to know where to look for other "pieces of the puzzle."

There are several possibilities for obtaining further health information, and the helpfulness of different resources will vary from locale to locale. General categories include:

- health professionals (health educators, nurses or physicians, or other health professionals);
- state and local health agencies;
- state and local education agencies (health-related components);
- local chapters of voluntary health organizations;
- local chapters of professional medical associations;
- hospitals, especially university medical centers;
- community health-education centers;
- libraries, especially for both lay and professional journal articles, and other references; and
- telephone "yellow pages."

Consider again the brief television news report scene at the beginning of this article. Students who have learned the concepts and skills outlined here will be able to put such a report into a general context of how research operates, locate written news pieces about the topic, ask analytical questions about the report, and know where to go for further information. The information they use in their health decision-making can be more accurate and more meaningful. It's even possible that the ability to begin to understand "the experts," to ask knowledgeable questions and to find useful answers could in itself help motivate students to give more thought to their health decisions and life-style habits. These are all exciting potentials.

Source: *Journal of School Health* 52.10 (December 1982):614–18. Copyright 1982 American School Health Association, Kent, Ohio 44240.

## DISCUSSION QUESTIONS

1. Do you have a "tuned out" attitude toward health and wellness research news or recommendations?

2. What are some of the ethical concerns of using human subjects in health research? Can you think of three specific examples?

3. What is your major source of health information? Television? Newspaper? Magazines? Friends? How carefully do you analyze the health information presented?

4. What are some local sources of professional health information? Try and think of at least five.

# SUMMARY

1. Traditionally, health has been viewed as freedom from disease. Current health promotion efforts typically involve prevention of chronic disease by helping people change factors that put them at risk for such diseases. This may lead to an overreliance on the medical-care system as the primary means to health.

2. Life-style factors are an important cause of death in the United States. The U.S. Surgeon General's Office has issued a report entitled *Healthy People,* which delineates the leading causes of death and related risk factors in the United States. The *Healthy People* report emphasizes five life-style factors for young adults: developing safe driving habits; avoiding the use of firearms; adopting good health habits; developing a responsible attitude toward sexuality; and talking about problems or stressful situations.

3. Wellness is a self-designed style of living that allows people to live life to the fullest. Wellness is not a static state that one can achieve; wellness is an active process that requires individual initiative. Wellness is not concerned with disease and its prevention, but rather with optimal functioning and creative adapting.

4. One of the keys to both health and wellness is self-responsibility. One study of self-responsibility for life-style factors has indicated that the physical health status of people who practiced seven common good health habits was the same as the physical health status of people thirty years younger who practiced few such good health habits.

5. Another important key to health and wellness is a social support network. American society is presently constructed with many barriers to health and wellness. Creating a social support group is an important motivator and reinforcer in our attempt to live a wellness life-style.

6. Human behavior is a complex phenomenon. One behavior model suggests that there are three major determinants of health behavior—predisposing, enabling, and reinforcing factors. These factors work together in a cyclical manner to influence our wellness life-styles.

7. To begin a wellness life-style follow three important steps: (1) make a commitment to yourself; (2) assess your current life-style; and (3) take action—investigate information, locate resources for skill development, build a support network—and have fun.

### Recommended Readings

Allen, Robert. *Lifegain.* New York: Appleton-Century-Crofts, 1981.

Sheehy, Gail. *Pathfinders.* New York: Bantam Books, 1981.

Yankelovich, Daniel. *New Rules: Searching for Self-Fulfillment in a World Turned Upside Down.* New York: Random House, 1981.

### References

1. J. Grossman, "Inside the Wellness Movement," *Health* 13 (1981): 10–12, 14–15.

2. World Health Organization, "Constitution of the World Health Organization," *Chronicle of the World Health Organization* 1 (1947), 29–43.

3. U.S. Department of Health and Human Services, *Healthy People,* Public Health Service, 1979.

4. John W. Farquar, M.D. *The American Way of Life Need Not Be Hazardous to Your Health* (New York: W. W. Norton, 1978).

5. G. E. Alan Dever, *Community Health Analysis: An Holistic Approach* (Georgetown, Md.: Aspen Systems Corp., 1980).

6. Marc Lalonde, *A New Perspective on the Health of Canadians—A Working Document,* April 1974 (Ottawa: Office of the Canadian Minister of National Health and Welfare).

7. U.S. Department of Health and Human Services, *Healthy People* (Washington, D.C.: Public Health Service, 1979).

8. U.S. Department of Health, Education, and Welfare, *Living Well* (Washington, D.C.: Public Health Service, 1980).

9. Dever, *Community Health Analysis.*

10. Halbert L. Dunn, *High Level Wellness* (Arlington, Va.: R. W. Beatty, 1961), 4.

11. Donald B. Ardell, *Fourteen Days to a Wellness Lifestyle* (Mill Valley, Calif.: Whatever Publishing, 1982).

12. Dunn, *High Level Wellness,* 4.

13. Halbert L. Dunn, "High-Level Wellness in the World of Today," *Journal of the American Osteopathic Association* 61 (1962): 9.

14. Robert Russell, unpublished paper (Carbondale, Ill.: Southern Illinois University, Health Education Department).

15. Dunn, "High-Level Wellness in the World of Today."

16. Alvin Toffler, *Future Shock* (New York: Bantam Books, 1970).

17. Dunn, "High-Level Wellness in the World of Today."

18. Dunn, *High-Level Wellness.*

19. John Knowles, M.D., "Doing Better and Feeling Worse: Health in the United States," *Daedalus,* Winter 1977, 59.

20. Victoria Foundation, 1978 Annual Report (Montclair, N.J.), 11.

21. Nedra Belloc and Lester Breslow, "Relationship of Physical Health Status and Health Practices," *Preventive Medicine* 1 (1972): 409–21.

22. Dunn, "High-Level Wellness in the World of Today."

23. Trevor Hancock, "Beyond Health Care: Creating a Healthy Future," *The Futurist* 16 (August 1982): 6.

24. Robert Allen, *Lifegain* (New York: Appleton-Century-Crofts, 1981).

25. Allen, *Lifegain.*

26. Lawrence Green, et al., *Health Education Planning: A Diagnostic Approach* (Palo Alto, Calif.: Mayfield Publishing Company, 1980).

27. Godfrey Hochbaum, *Health Behavior* (Belmont, Calif.: Wadsworth Publishing Co., 1970), 34.

28. Green, et al., *Health Education Planning,* 72.

29. Abraham Maslow, *Toward a Psychology of Being,* 2nd ed. (Princeton, N.J.: Van Nostrand, 1968).

30. Godfrey M. Hochbaum, *Health Behavior* (Belmont, Calif.: Wadsworth, 1970), 51–53.

31. "Wellness: Getting into the Health Habit," *Hamot Happenings* 20.3 (1982): 5–6. Monthly publication of the Hamot Medical Center, Erie, Penn.

CHAPTER TWO

# Mental Wellness: Beyond Mental Health



Wellness affects the quality of our lives. In many ways, wellness is more mental than it is physical. Wellness programs that ignore the mental dimension of wellness disregard not only a major part of the person but the very part that makes us a person.

Mental wellness may be the heart of wellness in general. Self-concept, self-responsibility, competence, and realism are among the major keys to wellness. Life-style factors such as smoking are obviously important determinants of health, but whether we will live longer, healthier, happier lives if we jog and eat a balanced diet is strictly a matter of speculation. But we do know that social supports, such as a network of friends we can count on in good times and bad, are the best predictor of longevity. Kathleen Mullen[1], in fact, found that experts on wellness considered the mental/emotional aspects of health to be in many ways the key elements of wellness.

In everyday usage, however, the term "mental health" often means mental illness. A community mental health center, for instance, is a place where the mentally ill can receive treatment close to home. In most states a department of mental health or department of mental hygiene operates state hospitals and other facilities for treatment of the mentally ill. The National Association for Mental Health provides services and advocacy for the mentally ill and their families, and educates the public about mental illness. The National Institute of Mental Health conducts a wide-ranging program of research and training, virtually all of which is focused on mental illness.

In this chapter we shall examine a wellness rather than an illness concept of mental health. Although we may seem to be introducing a new idea, such a concept is not without precedent in the field of mental health. Efforts to define a positive concept of mental health extend at least as far back as the 1930s and William Henry Burnham's[2] examination of "the wholesome personality."

## WHAT MENTAL WELLNESS IS NOT

Marie Jahoda[3] argued that we cannot define mental wellness or "positive mental health" in terms of normality, nor of absence of symptoms, nor of happiness. Normality, she points out, is a statistical concept—not an ideal. **Normal** is whatever state is shared by most of the people in a population at a given time. As H. G. Wells pointed out, in the land of the blind the sighted man may be thought insane with his "ravings" about "seeing" things.

Nor can we define mental wellness on the basis of a lack of symptoms alone. Unhealthy people may not show any symptoms. In mental health as in physical health, wellness must be seen as something more than the mere absence of symptoms of illness. We cannot expect the mentally healthy individual to be happy all the time. Everyone has emotional ups and downs. And we all must at times face experiences to which happiness would be an abnormal response.

Moreover, mental wellness cannot be defined in terms of "adjustment," "functioning," or "never having needed help." The problem with adjustment as a criterion is much the same as with normality. Joining the SS and murdering Jews, for instance, was a very successful adjustment to society in Nazi Germany, but we would not point to it as an example of mental health. Those who refused to adjust to society in Nazi Germany were more likely to have been the mentally well members of that society.

Our society is certainly not so pathological as was Germany under Hitler but is it necessarily healthy to adjust to a society still plagued by widespread poverty, racism, and sexism? Or, on the other hand, hasn't the healthiest adjustment been made by those who are actively rebelling against such elements in our society?

Ability to function is no better criterion. Mentally healthy people are able to function in all areas of their lives (family, work, play). But ability to function is not exclusive to healthy individuals. Even some individuals with a variety of mental illnesses may be able not only to function well, but may excel in many roles.

Finally, we cannot define mental wellness in terms of never having needed help with an emotional problem. We wouldn't say that someone who has never been treated by a physician will necessarily remain physically well. There are many people who have never had any kind of treatment but may be in need of such help.

## MAJOR CONTRIBUTIONS TO THE CONCEPT OF MENTAL WELLNESS

Although the term wellness is of relatively recent origin, essentially the same concept has been explored under other names by a number of theorists. We will discuss the contributions of a few of the most important.

### Burnham and the Wholesome Personality

In Burnham's view the **wholesome personality** was characterized by integration, self-respect, purposive activity, objectivity, persistence, democracy, and what he called the genetic point of view—the ability to see the problems of the present as learning experiences and to turn what might have been destructive pressures into the means of achieving higher levels of integration. In addition to these traits, the wholesome personality slept and relaxed well, had a sense of humor, and faced the world with a good humor composed of serenity, hope, and happiness.

The key trait of the wholesome personality was integration or wholeness. In Burnham's words, "It is represented at a low level by the absorbed attention of the unspoiled child performing his own little task, and shown at a high level by the scientist and the artist doing some great work for its own sake."[4] Integration refers to the full commitment of the personality to the task at hand. Being fully involved in whatever you are doing here and now, not worrying "in the back of your mind" about something else or daydreaming of being somewhere else. This does not mean rigidly fixing your attention on one thing and being oblivious to all else surrounding you. But it does mean the ability to attend to the principal task

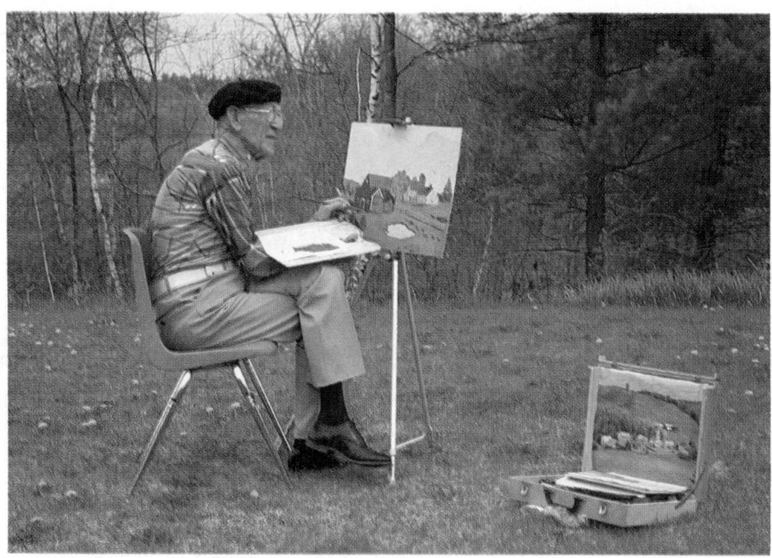

**Figure 2.1**
The wholesome personality is able to concentrate fully on the task at hand.

at hand and not being easily distracted by unimportant stimuli. For people with an integrated personality there are no internal struggles or conflicts, because they are able to concentrate on what needs to be done at the moment. (See figure 2.1.)

Such integration comes naturally to a young child in its self-directed activities. All too often, however, adults disrupt a child's integrated behavior, wanting the child to pay attention to them instead of to his or her own tasks. Rigid schedules and unrewarding tasks soon teach the growing child inattention and divided consciousness. If instead the child is given worthwhile and rewarding tasks to be completed at the child's own pace, the natural integration of childhood can be preserved and developed into mature adult integration. While such tasks may be given, it is even more important that the child be left free of adult interference much of the time to choose appealing tasks. Children grow more through freedom than through direction.

To grow in integration children must not only have meaningful tasks to perform but those tasks must require concentration and effort. Adult-assigned tasks must be added to, rather than replace, the self-selected tasks of the younger child. These tasks should be achievable with effort in a fairly short period of time with no ambiguity about when the task is completed. In the early tasks, success should be assured if the child applies reasonable effort.

Ability to persist in a task despite obstacles is yet another element in the development of a wholesome, integrated personality. Fortunately, Burnham says, the best training in meeting difficulties comes naturally if one is carrying out meaningful tasks. The same can be said for the necessary experience of coping with hardships and danger. A person who has always been sheltered from hardships, who has never taken any risks nor faced any dangers, will not develop the self-reliance and persistence necessary for integration and self-respect.

Integration of the personality means that there must be no conflict between the intellect and the emotions. One must not dominate or repress the other. Emotion should provide the stimulus for intellectual activity in the performance of a task rather than providing a distraction from it.

## Fromm and the Productive Character

Psychoanalyst Eric Fromm has described what he termed **productive character** in contrast to the "nonproductive orientations" typical of most people.[5] By productiveness Fromm meant our human ability to use our natural powers and to achieve our potentials. Productiveness implies that a person is guided by reason in the use of those powers. A productive person sees himself or herself as the "actor" rather than the acted upon. Productive characters feel at one with their powers and not alienated from them.

According to Fromm, there are two ways in which the world outside yourself can be experienced. The first is "reproductively," by recording an

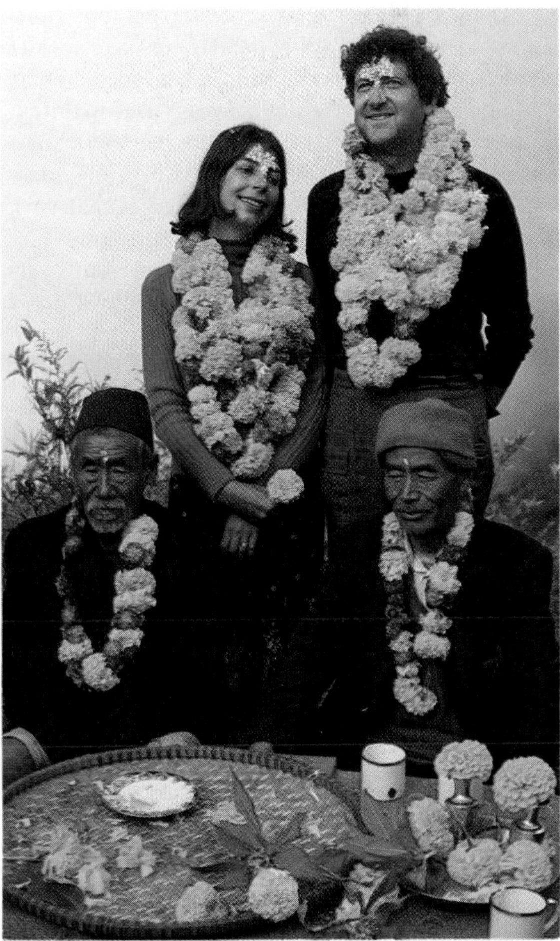

**Figure 2.2**
Fully functioning personalities are flexible and open-minded. These two Americans, visitors in Nepal, are experiencing a Hindu wedding ceremony.

experience passively like a camera. The other is "generatively," by conceptualizing reality, by enlivening and recreating the new material of experience through the action of your own mind. The productive character has this type of active rather than passive relationship with external reality.

## Rogers and the Fully Functioning Person

Psychologist Carl Rogers, originator of client-centered therapy and one of the founders of the human-potential movement, has described what he termed the **fully functioning person.**[6] In Rogers's view most people do not function at their full potential. Most people only maintain life, whereas fully functioning people enhance life. According to Rogers the fully functioning person can be recognized by five characteristics:

1. An openness to experience that is clearly the opposite of the defensiveness characteristic of the partially functioning majority. Every stimulus is freely attended to without distortion by any defense mechanism. New experiences are welcomed and sought out. Different perspectives are examined and accepted on their own merits. The fully functioning person can disagree with others without disliking them and can find friends on both sides of a conflict without feeling disloyal.

   This openness is internal as well as external. The fully functioning person is aware of his or her own feelings, needs, and weaknesses. These too are seen without defensiveness and are accepted for what they are. Whatever deficiencies the fully functioning person may have, he is aware of them and seeks to cope with them rather than deny them.
2. The fully functioning person experiences life to its fullest every moment, rather than according to some fixed preconceived script. Living in this way lends itself to the possibility of experiencing many new things. This is consistent with the first characteristic, as well as with Burnham's concept of integration. (See figure 2.2.)

   The fully functioning person is able to adapt to new situations. Instead of trying to impose some preconceived structure on experience, the fully functioning person finds structure in experience. A flowing, continuously changing reorganization of self and personality emerges from experience. This concept of existential living might be described as living flexibly, adaptably, and spontaneously.
3. **Organismic trusting** is Rogers's name for the third characteristic. By trusting your own organism, Rogers means a willingness to accept answers, decisions, and other feelings that come from within but without conscious

process. It can be called intuition, gut reaction, or a hunch, but whatever you call it, the fully functioning person, according to Rogers, learns to trust and rely on the organism.

The fully functioning person, who is open to all experience, brings to bear on any problem all the data from sense impressions, memory, previous learning, and internal visceral states without distortion by any defense mechanisms. With this data store to draw on, the fully functioning person can often arrive at correct decisions immediately and without conscious thought. Knowing that this decision is not merely projection or rationalization imposed on experience, the fully functioning person can trust these intuitions or gut reactions.

4. The fourth characteristic is **experimental freedom**—the freedom to make choices between alternate courses of action. Like Fromm's productive character, Rogers' fully functioning person feels in control, acting and not just being acted upon. The fully functioning person adjusts to experience through a series of choices, not through a series of simple reactions.

   Like everyone else, the fully functioning person's ability to choose may be limited by prior experience, the environment, or bodily limitations. The fully functioning person feels in control and experiences an exhilarating sense of personal power in which all things seem possible. Openness to experience, existential living, and organismic trusting probably make the fully functioning person far freer from any conditioning or other constraints of the past than any other person can possibly be.

5. The fifth characteristic, which flows out of the four preceding characteristics, is **creativity.** Rogers does not confine his definition of creativity to artistic endeavors such as painting or composing music. Creativity refers more broadly to the production of new and effective thoughts, actions, or things. All of that external and internal experience, channeled by a person of flexibility, organismic trust, and decisiveness, could scarcely fail to produce something new and useful.

These five characteristics describe a fully functioning person, who leads a life that "involves a wider range, a greater richness, than the constricted living in which most of us find ourselves."[7] But with that greater range, greater variety, and greater richness come challenge and uncertainty. The fully functioning person has given up the defenses that most of us cling to for fear of what we would surely face if we were open, flexible, and in control. As Rogers put it: "This process of living the full life is not, I am convinced, a life for the faint-hearted. It involves the stretching and growing of becoming more and more of one's potentialities."[8]

## Maslow and the Self-Actualizing Person

Abraham Maslow is a major contributor to modern motivation theory, one of the founders of humanistic psychology, and may come to be regarded as second only to Halbert Dunn in shaping the wellness movement. Maslow's contributions to the concept of mental wellness flowed out of his theory of human motivation.[9]

Other psychologists had described human needs as a conglomerate, with all needs present at once and competing for gratification. Maslow described a hierarchy of needs motivating human behavior. You will remember from chapter 1 that at the primary level are the physiological needs—for food, water, oxygen, protection from extreme temperature, and so on. Only when these needs have been met do the second level of needs become felt—the need for safety and security. Only when a basic level of safety and security has been achieved does the third level of need become felt—the need to feel loved and accepted. When this need is minimally satisified it is succeeded by the fourth level—the need for self-esteem. (See figure 2.3.)

Finally, when all the more basic levels of needs, from the physiological through self-esteem, have been satisfied, the highest level of need emerges. This is the need for **self-actualization**—a drive to achieve your full potential, to be all that you can possibly be. It is the need to do that "stretching and growing" that Rogers also mentioned.

Not everyone, however, reaches this highest level of need. Poverty and deprivation keep many at the first and second level of needs, struggling to meet their basic physiological needs and to achieve some security that those needs will be met in the future.

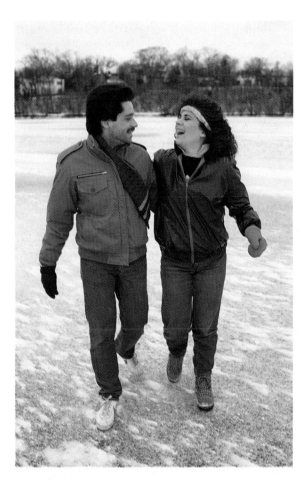

**Figure 2.3**
According to Maslow, the human need for acceptance and love becomes vital once physiological and safety needs have been satisfied.

Others, less economically fortunate, may never achieve self-esteem or a sense of being loved and accepted and thus remain trapped at those need levels. Others may never overcome insecurity and fear learned early in life and may spend their entire life desperately and compulsively building up wealth as a bulwark against their fears. Only a few people ever reach the level of the need for self-actualization.

Maslow set out to identify persons—both among his own acquaintances and among historical figures—who had lived rich, fulfilling lives and seemed to be motivated by the need for self-actualization. Maslow could not definitely identify anyone as being purely motivated by self-actualization, but he compiled a list of forty-eight persons he believed might be self-actualizers. Among those he listed were Albert Einstein, Abraham Lincoln, Eleanor Roosevelt, Franklin Roosevelt, and five-time presidential candidate Eugene V. Debs. Both the listing and his description of the individuals were inevitably subject to Maslow's own biases and preconceptions.

Despite any such biases, Maslow seems to have made a very sincere attempt at objectivity in developing his list. The similarities to the descriptions given by Rogers, Fromm, and Burnham give further support to the validity of Maslow's conclusions. The sixteen common characteristics of self-actualizing individuals include:

1. Self-actualizers perceive reality accurately and without distortion, even when reality is unpleasant or painful. This is clearly similar to the openness described by Rogers and the objectivity noted by Burnham.
2. Self-actualizers show a high level of self-acceptance and of acceptance of others as they really are. Such self-acceptance is to be expected in a person whose need for self-esteem has been satisfied. It is also consistent with the other personality descriptions we have previously examined.
3. Self-actualizers have loving intimate relationships with one or several people. Although many of Maslow's subjects were unpopular people, they all had at least one loving intimate relationship. Again, this seems self-evident in persons who had already satisified their needs for love and acceptance.
4. Self-actualizers possess a high degree of autonomy or independence. They judge for themselves what is right or wrong and stick by their judgments even if this makes them unpopular. They have the strength to stand alone when necessary. This does not mean that they are rebellious or loners but that they have the courage to stand up for what they believe.
5. Self-actualizers show a natural, effortless, and highly individual spontaneity in thought and in emotion. They respond in fresh and different ways to the events of the day instead of becoming trapped in a limited repertoire of responses.
6. Self-actualizers are task-oriented rather than preoccupied with self. They are genuinely concerned with the tasks they perform and see them as more than a means to personal

gratification. To them a job is not just a way to make money or achieve status—it is a meaningful and important activity in itself. They are likely to have a commitment to some larger cause or purpose toward which their work is directed.

7. Unlike so many people who are only comfortable with the familiar and who resist change, self-actualizers are attracted to the new, the different, and the unexpected.
8. Not only are they attracted by new experiences, self-actualizers possess a continued freshness of appreciation that enables them to approach familiar experiences from a fresh perspective. They see something new each day in the familiar. They avoid lumping experiences into categories and dismissing each new instance as merely one more instance of a familiar category. Instead, each time the familiar is reexperienced it is seen as though it were the first time.
9. Self-actualizers possess a sense of spirituality which may or may not be religious in a formal sense. Maslow found that this spirituality is typically centered on a sense of unity with nature or with the universe, and is shaped by one or more "peak experiences." This spiritual sense of oneness is related to a sense of belonging to all humankind. Peak experiences, sometimes called "mystical" or "oceanic" experiences, involve a sense of exhilaration and feelings that your boundaries as a person have suddenly dissolved and that you have become part of all nature. Such experiences are sometimes achieved through, or caused by meditation, prayer, drugs, or stress. They may also occur spontaneously with no specific trigger phenomenon.
10. Related to these characteristics, self-actualizers have a sense of belonging to all humankind—Maslow uses the German word *gemeinschaftsgefuhl,* meaning brotherly feeling, to describe this feeling. For them the brotherhood of humankind is a felt reality, not a platitude. Their view of humankind does not divide into "us" versus "them"; they see everyone as a part of "us". Possessing this sense of belonging allows them to feel empathy for the situations of persons in other cultures with the same acuteness of empathy that they feel for their own family and close friends.
11. Self-actualizers have a tendency to relate to others as unique individuals rather than as types or group members. The self-actualizing person is essentially uninfluenced by prejudice or bias. This characteristic is logically related to traits 8 and 9.
12. Self-actualizers have a firm sense of right and wrong. Their ethical views usually are not wholly conventional, but they are consistently applied. Their behavior is guided by their own ethical principles, which they place above convention, peer pressure, or even the law.
13. Self-actualizers exhibit a resistance to acculturation. Although they usually seem outwardly to accept the norms of their society, privately they are casual and detached about them. They show a rather calm and good-humored rejection of the stupidities and imperfections of their culture. They are a part of their culture without being dominated or limited by it, seeming to select from their culture what they judge to be good about it and to reject what they find to be bad. This may bring them into conflict with institutions of their culture. When it does, they are able to fight vigorously against social pressures that persons still struggling for acceptance or not yet confident of their self-esteem would be unable to resist.
14. Although self-actualizers enjoy being with people, they are also able to tolerate and even enjoy solitude. They seek solitude on occasion and use it for meditation or for periods of intense concentration.
15. Self-actualizers are creative and inventive in some areas of their life. They are not necessarily artistically creative, but they have their own unique ways of doing and thinking rather than being followers of the usual. This is identical to Rogers's use of the concept of creativity.
16. Self-actualizers possess a benign sense of humor. They laugh at common human failings, pretensions, and foolishness rather than more hostile subjects. (See Exhibit 2.1.)

2.1 EXHIBIT 2.1

## Laugh a Little, Live a Lot

If someone were to ask me, "To what do you attribute your good health," I would answer: I exercise, keep active, and watch my diet (if I don't, Delores does).

But of equal importance are two other elements that contribute to my happiness and health—involvement with people and being able to laugh.

It has been said that laughter is an "instant vacation" and I couldn't agree more. Fun is not only pleasurable, it's good for us; laughter and fun are the most wonderful tonics in the world. I think that the more pressures and problems a person faces, the greater the need for humor to keep things in perspective.

I've found that humor is an excellent antidote for tension and anger. Instead of dwelling on the point of irritation, share a joke or two with someone or share a funny incident from a similar situation. After a few good laughs, the feelings of resentment diminish.

Having fun, laughing, comes naturally to children; it does not have to be taught. But somewhere along the way many adults lose the knack of applying humor to their daily lives. This is regrettable, since humor—laughing or creating laughter—is as important as any medicine on any drug shelf. And it costs absolutely nothing.

Entertaining GI's in three wars, I have seen the healing power of laughter. Now, science has confirmed that having fun—just feeling happy or joyous—has a measurable effect on our health, well-being, and even how long we live.

I remember once entertaining at a mental hospital here in the States. "I'd like to sing a little song for you," I said, "but I need music. Is there anyone in the audience who can play 'Buttons and Bows'?"

"Yes," the patients yelled. "Charlie can!"

Charlie came up to the piano and played with one finger while I sang. About a month later, I got a letter from a doctor at the hospital. It said: "I thought you'd like to know that Charlie was one of the worst cases we've ever had. But from the day you brought him up on the stage and made him smile, he has improved. We think now he'll eventually lead a normal life."

But you don't have to be Bob Hope to have fun bringing fun to others. I remember a Massachusetts truck driver who became an amateur clown in his spare time to combine a hobby with doing good. It helped him to get out of himself, he said and to make people happy. "There's no money in the world," he said, "that can buy a smile on a child's face."

Nearly everyone has a talent or ability he or she can share. We all have the "gland" of helpfulness and enjoy doing something for others once we see a need. I've noticed when you do, it comes back to you in carloads.

I've been dealing in humor most of my life, trying to spread a little cheer and, incidentally, being cheered myself in the process. And I've found that for me and so many others, the benefits of laughter are no laughing matter.

Source: *The HOPE Newsletter,* published by the Bob Hope Heart Research Institute, Seattle, Wash. Reprinted with permission.

### DISCUSSION QUESTIONS

1. How do you feel after having a good laugh?
2. Do you laugh often?
3. Have you ever considered the effect you have on others when you share your good humor and pleasurable activities?

## AN ATTEMPT AT SYNTHESIS: WHAT MENTAL WELLNESS IS

Based on these points and others in the literature, there are ten characteristics of mental wellness that seem to be constant. This synthesis is still incomplete, but these important elements stand out. The mentally well are:

1. Real. Mentally well people respond in a genuine, spontaneous way to events. The mentally well aren't pretentious or phony; they say what they mean and feel no need to censor their words or actions to get approval or to make an impression. They are unselfconsciously themselves in the here and now. This quality of being real is sometimes called authenticity.
2. Realistic. Realism means knowing the difference between what is and what ought to be; between what we can change and what we cannot change. The realistic person is capable of modifying beliefs in light of new evidence. The mentally well person possesses what Saint Francis prayed for—the strength to accept the things that cannot be changed, the courage to change those that can be, and the wisdom to tell the difference.
3. Able to satisfy their needs. Mentally well people recognize their own needs and do what they must to satisfy them. They are not hung up at a primitive level of their need hierarchy, wasting energy on neurotic needs that do not promote personal growth. They are competent—that is, they know how to satisfy their needs. They are not helpless, nor do they pretend to be.
4. Free and responsible. Mentally well people are autonomous. They feel that they are in control of their own lives. They are inner-directed, accepting responsibility for their own actions or feelings.
5. Open to experience. Mentally well individuals experience both their internal and external realities accurately and fully. They welcome new experiences and often seek them out, but are not compulsive thrill-seekers. Even experiences that brought pain, grief, or other unpleasantness are seen by the mentally well person as having potential for personal growth; the unpleasantness can often be defused by humor.
6. Capable of intimate relationships. In many ways this is an extension of an openness to experience. The healthy person is open to the risks and the satisfactions of both physical and emotional intimacy. The ability to give and receive love is basic to healthy human development. Equally basic is the ability to trust in another and to be open in sharing one's feelings. The healthy person's awareness of and pleasure in bodily feelings is not blocked by any neurotic anxieties or phobias. Physical intimacy with romantic partners is a natural and fully enjoyed extension of emotional intimacy for the mentally well person.
7. Tolerant and accepting of others: Mental wellness is not compatible with racism, sexism, or ageism. A healthy person judges people on their individual merits and does not expect them to fit within a narrow limit of belief and behavior. A mentally well person is able to like a person while rejecting some part of that person's behavior.
8. Capable of reacting in a wide variety of ways. The mentally well person does not react in a stereotyped fashion. The ability to lead is balanced by the ability to follow; the ability to judge, by the ability to empathize; the ability to act, by the ability to yield.
9. Capable of *joie de vivre.* Enjoying life is a major characteristic of mental wellness. The healthy person enjoys the major elements of life—family, community, and job. These elements don't have to be perfect; the mentally well enjoy the pleasures of ordinary life. They notice the flowers in the field. On the other hand, the mentally well individual is not a "Pollyanna" (i.e., someone who is unflinchingly optimistic, and only sees the good side of everything). (See Activity for Wellness 2.1.)

2.1 ACTIVITY FOR WELLNESS 2.1

## What's Your "Fun Level"?

Having fun is good for your health. If you find that surprising, you probably could benefit from the following "pleasure assessment" profile.

**Step 1.** Just for the fun of it, place yourself on the Fun and Pleasure Scale below. Zero (0) is neutral: you don't think much about fun, one way or the other. Plus 5 means that your life is filled with pleasant activities. Minus 5 means that you never have fun, that you get no pleasure out of life.

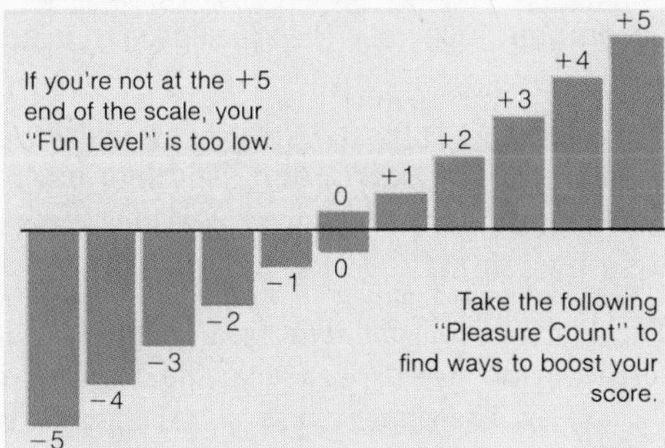

If you're not at the +5 end of the scale, your "Fun Level" is too low.
Take the following "Pleasure Count" to find ways to boost your score.
+5
+4
+3
+2
+1
0
0
−1
−2
−3
−4
−5


**Step 2.** List your top ten favorite activities, and the number of times you have done them this week:

| | Activity | Times Done |
|---|---|---|
| 1. | | |
| 2. | | |
| 3. | | |
| 4. | | |
| 5. | | |
| 6. | | |
| 7. | | |
| 8. | | |
| 9. | | |
| 10. | | |

What is the total number of times you've had fun this week?

If your weekly "fun count" was less than ten, you're not doing pleasurable things as often as you should. Make time for at least one of these activities every day. If anyone asks why you're having so much fun, explain it's for your health!

**Warning:** Serious, prolonged bouts of depression should be dealt with by a mental-health professional. Contact your mental-health agencies for assistance.

Source: Courtesy of Dr. Arthur Ulene, Feeling Fine Productions, Inc., Los Angeles, Calif.

10. Self-accepting. Probably the most crucial characteristic of the mentally well personality is a positive self-concept. A deep and confident sense of liking oneself and feeling worthwhile is one of the most universally recognized characteristics of mental wellness. Most of characteristics 1 through 9 are predicated on accepting and liking oneself and all are facilitated by a positive self-concept.

# SOCIAL INFLUENCES AND MENTAL WELLNESS

High-level wellness is not easily achieved. This is partly due to the many barriers to wellness that are erected by our culture. Among the barriers to mental wellness are poverty, stereotypes and prejudices, age segregation and ageism, the "traditional" nuclear family, and our schools.

## Poverty

As we have seen, Maslow's concept of a hierarchy of needs[10] indicates that we cannot move to higher motivational levels until our more basic needs have been met. A starving man only feels a need for food. Many Americans are living at the two lower levels of human needs. If they are not struggling to get enough to eat or to keep a roof over their heads, they are struggling to achieve some degree of security for their ability to continue to meet those needs in the future.

## Stereotypes and Prejudices

A regrettably large part of our cultural learning includes stereotypes and prejudices. It is hard to grow up in our society without becoming tainted with some elements of racism, sexism, ageism, and the whole mass of stereotypes and prejudices that are a part of our culture. Prejudices render us intolerant and unable to accept the differentness of others; they also keep us from seeing things as they are. We cannot be realistic or open to experience in areas in which we are prejudiced and influenced by stereotypes.

In the words of Halbert Dunn:

> The human brain is required to solve problems as they arise in daily life. The brain is so constructed that it will come up with correct solutions if it can. It does its work well to the degree that it has access to the information it needs for the solution of the problem in hand. But erroneous beliefs fixed in the mind, hate and prejudices, and the lack of essential information keep the brain from doing its job and, in the course of time, bring about mental and physical illness.[11]

To whatever extent we accept a stereotype as applying to us and try to live up to it, we are abandoning our authenticity—our realness. By living in a stereotyped fashion we abandon our ability to react in a variety of ways and deny our freedom and responsibility. Our ability to meet our own needs may be vitally impaired by accepting a stereotype for ourselves.

## Age Segregation and Ageism

Childhood and adolescence are modern inventions. This doesn't mean that people in past ages were born as fully grown adults, but until relatively recent history, there was no social-role distinction between infancy and adulthood. In primitive societies, once a child was weaned, that child was then ready to take up some productive role.

Uril Bronfenbrenner warns that our society is becoming "a society that is segregated not only by race and class, but also by age."[12] This growing segregation, he argues, is the cause of the increasing influence of the peer group. Children have turned to their age-mates as a source of values "less by choice than by default."

> The isolation of children from adults simultaneously threatens the growth of the individual and the survival of the society. The young cannot pull themselves up by their own bootstraps. It is primarily through observing, playing, and working with others older and younger than himself that a child discovers both what he can do and who he can become—that he develops both his ability and his identity. It is primarily through exposure and interaction with adults and children of different ages that a child acquires new interests and skills and learns the meaning of tolerance, cooperation and compassion. Hence to relegate children to a world of their own is to deprive them of their humanity.[13]

Along with their segregation from adults, the young are given no meaningful role to play in society. Being a student may be a vital role for the young, but the young rarely perceive it that way. Furthermore, society doesn't respect or reward the young's performance in that role to the extent that a truly meaningful role would seem to merit. The lack of a meaningful role makes the development of a positive self-concept more difficult.

The young are not the only victims of isolation and meaninglessness. Age segregation has also meant that the elderly are increasingly excluded from the mainstream of our society. They too are

2.2 EXHIBIT 2.2

## An Unfortunate Side of the Nuclear Family

A drunken father was less a psychological disaster to a boy who had a stalwart uncle to lean on and look up to than he is today for the boy with no other adult male figure close at hand. A neurotic, overly critical mother was often balanced for the child of the past by a warmhearted grandmother or aunt. A "nuclear" family leaves only a very small margin for error. One bad parent is a serious problem for a child; two constitute a catastrophe.

### DISCUSSION QUESTIONS

How can the implied problems of the nuclear family be exaggerated by:

1. single-parent families?
2. households with latchkey children (i.e., a household where both parents work full time and children may be forced to care for themselves during the day after school)?

often denied any meaningful role; all too many are forced to retire and ghettoized in retirement communities or institutionalized in nursing homes. These conditions constitute major barriers to continued mental wellness for those individuals who have had the longest to strive for its achievement.

## The "Traditional" Nuclear Family

Most of us continue to believe that the typical, "normal" American family is composed of mom and dad and the kids—the "traditional" nuclear family. In fact, such a family pattern is not truly traditional in our society. Prior to World War II, most American families were extended families with several generations of adults and their children living together. Only on the frontiers were two-generation families common; the pioneers reared their children alone in their new home. As time passed and the pioneer families became established they too became multigenerational, extended families. The increasing mobility of the postwar era broke up extended families and the nuclear family became the new norm.

The child raised in an extended family had an assortment of adults to look to for guidance, sympathy, support, and example. There were grandparents, aunts, uncles, and grown-up cousins as well as parents of other children. Such a diversity of role models offered a degree of protection against any bad examples. The normal development of children has always been threatened by disturbed, indifferent, or brutal parents, but in the nuclear family, the harmful influence is undiluted by equally close contact with other adults. (See Exhibit 2.2.)

In addition to diluting the effect of bad role models, the extended family exposed children to an array of role models. A diversity of role models does not guarantee that the child will grow up to be tolerant of differences and capable of reacting in a variety of ways, but it does make such elements of mental wellness more likely to be learned.

Today, the nuclear family is once again a minority among American families. Unfortunately, much of the shift away from the nuclear family is due to the growing numbers of single-parent families. The barriers to wellness are thus heightened rather than diminished. Day-care, Big Brother and Big Sister programs, and other arrangements can help give children broader exposure to adult models but they aren't adequate substitutes for family. (See figure 2.4.)

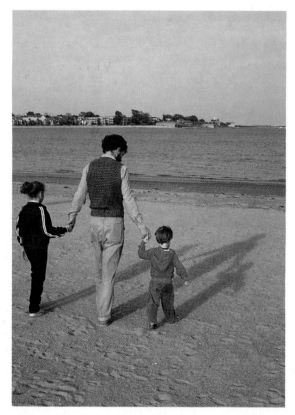

**Figure 2.4**
Single-parent homes are becoming increasingly common in the United States.

## Our Schools

Schools ought to be places for growing, for expanding horizons, for discovering connections. Instead, it may well be, as Marilyn Ferguson says, that "as the greatest single social influence during the formative years, schools have been the instruments of our greatest denial, unconsciousness, conformity, and broken connection."[14] Widespread concern has been expressed about the apparent failure of many of our schools to teach students how to read, write, or do basic math. But there is not enough awareness that part of the reason for these failures may be what the schools far too often do succeed in teaching—conformity, inactivity, anxiety, and negative self-concept. Maybe students can't read, but they can sit quietly (most of the time) in assigned seats, line up for recess, hold up their hands to speak, and control their bladders until the scheduled opportunity for a visit to the restroom. They may not know how laws are made to govern society but they know how a hall pass works.

In fact, Ferguson speaks of "pedogenic illness."[15] By this she means learning disabilities that are caused by the teacher or the school. "The child who may have come to school intact, with budding courage to risk and explore, finds stress enough to permanently diminish that adventure. . . . Dis-ease, not feeling comfortable about ourselves, probably begins for many of us in the classroom."[16] (See Exhibit 2.3.)

For a good discussion of how some American schools may make it harder for children to learn, see John Holt's *How Children Fail.*[17] That schools need not operate in this manner is clearly illustrated in Holt's *How Children Learn,*[18] and in Joseph Featherstone's *Schools Where Children Learn.*[19]

Illustrating the stressfulness of school, not just for some children but for most children, Ferguson notes that: when biofeedback subjects think about their school experiences an alarm reaction is registered; when a group of adults in a PTA workshop were asked to write about one of their school experiences every single one described a negative or traumatic experience; and school is a common theme of adult nightmares.

In longitudinal studies of normal adolescent boys, it has been found that school was ranked by the boys as the greatest area of conflict in their lives.[20] These students, who were not rebellious, had no serious emotional difficulties, experienced harmonious relations with their parents, and had good self-concepts, nevertheless saw school as a negative experience. These boys had adapted successfully to school and most did well in their studies, but they still felt restricted in the school environment.

Many of our schools seem obsessed with rules and conformity, often at the expense of learning. An amusing illustration of the type of learning that is really promoted by our control-obsessed schools is provided by an account of a segment of the TV show "Candid Camera" which is recounted by Eda LeShan: "A Candid Camera crew asked a group of first grade children what they had learned in the first few months of going to school. One child said, 'I learned to hold up my hand,' another said, 'To control yourself,' another, 'how to be quiet,' and another, 'My teacher yells even louder than my mother.' "[21] This is not an atmosphere in which growth toward mental wellness is likely to occur.

2.3 EXHIBIT 2.3

# He Always

He always wanted to explain things,
But no one cared.
So he drew.
Sometimes he would draw and it wasn't anything.
He wanted to carve it in stone or write it in the sky.
He would lie out on the grass and look up at the sky;
And it would be only the sky and him and the things inside him that needed saying.
And it was after that, he drew the picture.
It was a beautiful picture.
He kept it under his pillow, and would let no one see it.
And when it was dark, and his eyes were closed, he could see it.
And it was all of him,
And he loved it.
When he started school he brought it with him.
Not to show anyone, but just to have it with him like a friend.
It was funny about school,
He sat in a square, brown desk
Like all the other square, brown desks,
And he thought it should be red.
And his room was a square, brown room
Like all the other rooms.
And it was tight and close
And stiff.
He hated to hold the pencil and chalk,
With his arm stiff and his feet flat on the floor,
Stiff.
With the teacher watching and watching.
The teacher came and spoke to him.
She told him to wear a tie like all the other boys.
He said he didn't like them,
And she said it didn't matter.
After that they drew.
And he drew all yellow and it was the way he felt about morning;
And it was beautiful.
The teacher came and smiled at him.
"What's this?" she said, "Why don't you draw something like Ken's drawing?"
"Isn't that beautiful?"
After that his mother bought him a tie.
And he always drew airplanes and rocketships like everyone else.
And he threw the old picture away.
And when he lay out alone looking at the sky,
It was big and blue and all of everything.
But he wasn't anymore.
He was square inside and brown
And his hands were stiff,
And he was like everything else.
And the things inside him that needed saying didn't need it anymore.
It has stopped pushing;
It was crushed,
Stiff,
Like everything else.

Source: The source of this poem is unknown. It was supposed to have been given to a twelfth-grade English teacher by a student who committed suicide two weeks later.

## DISCUSSION QUESTIONS

1. What should the teacher have done with this poem initially?

2. Is there any way this tragedy could have been prevented?

# PROMOTING YOUR OWN MENTAL WELLNESS

There is no easy path to wellness. In striving for mental wellness, we must try to practice the elements of mental wellness such as being real, being open to experience, and accepting others without prejudice. Those are not easy tasks, nor is there any single path to wellness. For each of us the right path will be different. We must each find our own way to wellness.

There are a number of guides which you may find helpful in developing your own program of growth toward wellness. Oscar Ichaza's *Psychocalisthentics* describes a thirty-day program of mental exercises aimed at increasing insight, breaking free from rigidity and programming, increasing awareness, and achieving one's personal goals.[22] A unique approach is taken by Daniel Shapiro in his book *Precision Nirvana,* which attempts to combine Zen with behavioral psychology and succeeds to a remarkable degree.[23]

Here are a few activities that you may find helpful in seeking mental wellness.

1. Keep a private journal. Make a daily record of what you do, what you think, and what you feel. Review your diary or journal once each week at a regular time. Look for patterns in how you react and in how you feel. You may learn a lot about yourself in this way. As you try other activities for wellness, record them in your journal. Look to see what changes, if any, they have stimulated.

   As you identify problem areas, set goals for behavior change. Then record the frequency of the goal behavior in your journal and record the consequences that follow the behavior. Changing the consequences is one of the best ways to change the behavior.
2. Relax or meditate. Practice some form of meditation or relaxation technique. Such practice will help relieve any stresses or pressures you are under. There is also evidence that meditation tends to improve your self-concept, enhance awareness of yourself and your environment, and increase your openness to trying new behaviors.

   There are numerous types of meditation and relaxation. Most evidence seems to show that one is about equivalent to another. If you choose one that appeals to you it will probably be a good technique for you. Chapter 3 discusses relaxation skills in greater detail.
3. Make affirmations: An **affirmation** is a verbal description of a desired condition stated as if it were present reality. It is something you repeat to yourself over and over again until you become convinced of its reality and your conviction then helps to make it become objectively true.

   This approach was introduced by Émile Coué, a French physician, as part of his method of autosuggestion. Coué recommended repeating the phrase, "Every day, in every way, I'm getting better and better." It appears that repetition of this phrase or others like it can have an impact on self-concept and self-confidence.

   Write your own affirmation and practice repeating it to yourself five times just before going to bed every night and the next morning when you get up. Think through your affirmation—"I am always on time," may not be as good as "I am easily on time"—and make it a simple statement of what you hope to achieve. Start with just one affirmation. Later, you may want to develop several.

   There are a number of other ways you may want to try using affirmations:

   A. Type or write your affirmation on a slip of paper and paste it to your mirror, your telephone, or anywhere you will see it often during the day.
   B. Sing or chant your affirmations aloud while you are driving or some other time when you are alone—or maybe even if you are not alone.
   C. Write your affirmation ten times in the first person—"I, David, feel relaxed and confident in front of a group." Then write it ten times in the second person—"You, David, feel relaxed and confident in front of a group." Then write it ten times in the third person—"David feels relaxed and confident in front of a group."
   D. Tape-record yourself reciting your affirmations and listen to them while you are working, driving, or going to sleep.

E. Visualize the desired end result happening right now with yourself in the picture enjoying it.

F. Draw or paint a picture of yourself living out your affirmation and put it up where you will see it often.

4. Expand your awareness. Mental wellness incorporates an openness to experience and a joy in the large and the small things in life. It requires a level of awareness that is greater than that of most people. Here are a few activities that may help you to achieve an expanded awareness:

   A. Think of some place you have been recently. Write down a detailed description of that place. Then go back and compare your description to the actual place. Try it again. You should get better.

   B. Watch a sunrise or sunset without thinking about anything else. Such undivided attention is far from ordinary.

   C. Put together an assortment of foods with contrasting tastes, textures, and temperatures—hot and cold; smooth, crisp, crumbly, and crunchy; sweet, sour, salty, and bitter; and so on. Then try them one after another. Contrast the tastes and try different combinations. Better still, wear a blindfold while a friend feeds bites of the different foods to you; this works best if you haven't seen the foods first.

   D. Remember times that you enjoyed touching or being touched by someone (don't just think about sexual touching). Make a point of touching friends—a hug, a pat on the back, squeezing a hand, and so on. This may involve overcoming some anxieties and expanding your behavior options. (See Activity for Wellness 2.2.)

   E. Exchange massages with a friend. Or massage your own head and neck or your feet. (See figure 2.5.)

2.2 ACTIVITY FOR WELLNESS 2.2

## Spend More Quality Time Together

Quality time (QT) is a precious commodity. It is to relationships what clean air is to the environment—that is, integral.

It is not really true that familiarity breeds contempt; it merely begets forgetfulness of the importance of QT. We are confident that at some point in your life, you have enjoyed quality time with somebody. There is no need to dwell on what QT is, except to note that it includes a sense of being in the moment, free from the preoccupations of future expectations, plans, and dreams, and past regrets, accomplishments, and delights. We think that QT is evident in relationships marked by:

- shared recreational activities
- holding hands
- writing and receiving a love letter
- giving and receiving a massage
- meditating together before or after making love
- sharing a meal in joy and appreciation
- reading a meaningful statement aloud
- music, art, dance

These are a few thoughts. How might you put some more QT into your relationships? What examples occur to you?

1. ____________________
2. ____________________
3. ____________________
4. ____________________
5. ____________________

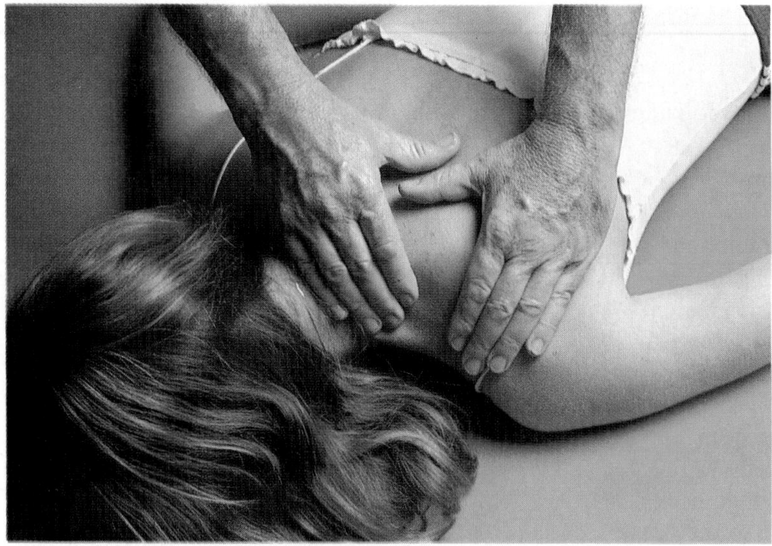

**Figure 2.5**
Giving and receiving massages can expand your awareness of the small pleasures of life.

5. Expand your experience. It is important for you to be open to experiences and to be able to try new behavior options if you are to achieve mental wellness. The following activities may help you make a start at increasing your openness:
   A. When you have choices to make, try brainstorming. Make a list of all the alternatives you can think of without weighing or evaluating any of them until you can't think of any more alternatives. Then consider them all seriously.
   B. For the next three weeks, make a point each week of doing something you never did before. Don't cheat—only significant new somethings count.
   C. Do something (legal and not really dangerous) that you never had the nerve to do before. Enter a talent contest, learn to ski, go skydiving, or do something else that's daring for you.
   D. Explore another culture or life-style by living it for a while. You could do this at home or by traveling somewhere.
   E. Live a day backwards. Start your day with supper and end it with breakfast. Relax, watch TV during the morning; do your work in the evening. Try to think of other things you can reverse for one day. For many of you, this may be impractical but it can be a fascinating experience if you try it.

## SUMMARY

1. Mental wellness may be the heart of wellness in general.

2. Often the term mental health is confused with mental illness.

3. Mental health cannot be defined in terms of absence of symptoms, or by ability to function.

4. A number of theorists have contributed to our concept of mental wellness including Burnham's view of "the wholesome personality," Fromm's "productive character," Rogers's "fully functioning person," and Maslow's "self-actualizing person."

5. Any attempt at fully describing mental wellness is still incomplete at this point, but an effort is made to provide such a synthesis.

6. Potential social barriers to mental wellness include poverty, stereotypes and prejudices, age segregation and ageism, the "traditional" nuclear family, and our schools.

7. Important elements that can promote mental wellness include keeping a journal, relaxation or meditation, making affirmations, expanding your awareness, and expanding your experience.

## Recommended Readings

Ardell, Donald B., and Tager, Mark J. *Planning for Wellness.* Portland, Oreg.: Wellness Media Ltd., 1981.

Burns, David D. *Feeling Good: The New Mood Therapy.* New York: Morrow, 1980.

Coan, Richard W. *The Optimal Personality: An Empirical and Theoretical Analysis.* New York: Columbia Univ. Press, 1974.

Duncan, David F. "Wellness: The Concept and the Movement—Relevance for Mental Health and Vice Versa." Paper presented at the annual meeting of the American Public Health Association, Los Angeles, 1981.

Dunn, Halbert, *High Level Wellness.* Thorofare, N.J.: Slack, 1961.

## References

1. Kathleen D. Mullen, "Wellness Constructs: A Decision Theoretic Study" (Ph.D. diss., Southern Illinois Univ., 1983).

2. William H. Burnham, *The Wholesome Personality* (New York: Appleton-Century, 1932).

3. Marie Jahoda, *Current Concepts of Positive Mental Health* (New York: Basic Books, 1958).

4. Burnham, *Wholesome Personality,* p. 35.

5. Eric Fromm, *Man for Himself* (New York: Holt, Rinehart & Winston, 1947).

6. Carl Rogers, *On Becoming a Person* (Boston: Houghton Mifflin, 1961).

7. Rogers, *On Becoming a Person,* 195.

8. Rogers, *On Becoming a Person,* 196.

9. Abraham Maslow, *Motivation and Personality* (New York: Harper and Rowe, 1954); "Deficiency Motivation and Growth Motivation," in *Nebraska Symposium on Motivation,* edited by M. R. Jones (Lincoln, Nebr.: Univ. of Nebraska Press, 1955); and *Toward a Psychology of Being,* 2nd ed. (New York: Van Nostrand, 1968).

10. Maslow, *Motivation and Personality* and *Toward a Psychology of Being.*

11. Halbert Dunn, *Your World and Mine* (New York: Exposition Press, 1956), 91.

12. Urie Bronfenbrenner, *Two Worlds of Childhood: United States and USSR* (New York: Russell Sage Foundation, 1970).

13. White House Conference on Children, working papers and final reports of the forums (Washington, D.C., 1970). Mimeographed.

14. Marilyn Ferguson, *The Aquarian Conspiracy: Personal and Social Transformation in the 1980's* (New York: St. Martin's Press, 1980), 282.

15. Ferguson, *Aquarian Conspiracy,* 282–85.

16. Ferguson, *Aquarian Conspiracy,* 283.

17. John Holt, *How Children Fail* (New York: Dell, 1964).

18. John Holt, *How Children Learn* (New York: Dell, 1967).

19. Joseph Featherstone, *Schools Where Children Learn* (New York: Avon, 1971).

20. Daniel Offer, *The Psychological World of the Teenager* (New York: Basic Books, 1969).

21. Eda LeShan, *Conspiracy Against Childhood* (New York: Atheneum, 1967), 252.

22. Oscar Ichaza, *Psychocalisthenics* (New York: Simon & Schuster, 1967).

23. Deane H. Shapiro, Jr., *Precision Nirvana: Care & Maintenance of the Mind* (Englewood Cliffs, N.J.: Prentice-Hall, 1978).

CHAPTER THREE

# Stress: Coping Positively



Everyone experiences stress; the college student's life abounds with stress. Making the transition from high school to college is a stressful major life event. High school is a relatively secure environment; college is designed to be stressful. This new environment means a new type of independence, rigorous academic standards, roommate and peer pressures, and, initially, a different support system. As if these pressures aren't enough, there are the uncertainties of choosing a major field of study, worrying about the future job market, worrying about financing four or five years of higher education, and fears of failure. Individually and collectively, these pressures can often seem overwhelming.

More and more, we are realizing that one of the "hidden" aspects of our advancing technological age is that of stress—its challenges, its consequences, and its opportunities. Stress, and learning how to manage it, has become so important that one can hardly avoid reading about it as a cause of illness and disease. Across the country there are many stress-management programs designed to prevent or ameliorate stress, or enhance coping skills.

This chapter will first clarify the terminology associated with stress, then illustrate the physiological pathways of the stress response, then discuss the relationship of stress to disease. The second focus will be on the challenges of managing stress for personal growth. The third focus will be on personal and social considerations that can foster or hinder effective coping with stress.

# A WELLNESS PERSPECTIVE ON STRESS

In chapter 1, you read that wellness includes direction and progress during your attempt to adapt and function within the environment. Wellness is a conscious process of being more committed to and involved with your life. Wellness approaches to stress management include three major phases: (1) regular assessment, (2) intervention, and (3) reinforcement. These phases help one move toward personal growth, development, and realization of potentials.[1]

## Assessment

**Assessment** is a "tuning in" and "taking stock" of your life. It is important to be sensitive to stress, to recognize the source of stress, and to examine and choose the appropriate stress-management strategy. Assessment is the art of determining what's happening now and comparing that to what you would like to have happen in the future. Once you have made an assessment, you can consciously proceed to make changes if you choose to do so.

## Intervention

The phase of **intervention** involves "doing." The doing is usually accomplished via habits, practices, or skills, which are used either to improve the status quo, or to reduce the frequency and intensity of the stress response. When used, these actions keep stress from accumulating and serve to enhance levels of wellness.

## Reinforcement

**Reinforcement** is both the development of payoffs and a support system for being more involved with your health and well-being. The payoffs are the observable benefits of trying to manage your life more effectively. Payoffs range from sleeping better at night following regular practice of relaxation exercises, to the positive feelings received from employing time-management strategies in order to organize better study habits. Your support system is composed of the links between you and others who support you and your efforts. Both payoffs and a support system are motivators for continued success in managing stress.

When you are involved consciously and regularly in the processes of assessment, intervention, and reinforcement, you are moving toward your wellness potentials. From a wellness perspective, even failures can lead to growth if they are used as an assessment to begin anew.

# COMPONENTS AND TERMINOLOGY OF STRESS

The terminology used to describe stress is often overwhelming, sometimes contradictory, and usually confusing. A recent survey asked college students to respond to the open-ended statement "Stress is ______." The results revealed that stress has different meanings for different students. The most common adjective, used by 40 percent of the students to describe stress, was pressure. Other common descriptions of stress included tension, frustration, and strain. The survey's author noted two startling conclusions from these responses. First, the responses denoted stress as undesirable, with little or no positive effects. Second, most responses tended to focus on the source of the stress rather than the condition itself.[2] There appears to be confusion and misunderstanding with the concept of stress and the terminology used to describe it.

## The Meaning of Stress

Hans Selye, pioneer researcher on stress, has described **stress** as the "nonspecific response of the body to any demand made upon it."[3] Although each demand is unique or specific, according to Selye, each event calls for adaptation by the body. It is this demand for readjustment that is referred to as nonspecific. Selye further states that, whether we consider a demand or situation to be pleasant or unpleasant, each demand will require us to readjust or adapt, thus creating the stress response.

This description of stress depicts three key points. First, stress is the "reaction" or mobilization of bodily resources in response to a stimulus. Second, there is mobilization of resources for adaptive or adjustment purposes. Third, the stimulus can be pleasant and desirable, or unpleasant and undesirable. For now, keep in mind that "stress is a state that one is in, and this should not be confused with any agent that produces such a state."[4]

## Stressors

The agent or stimulus that elicits the stress reaction is referred to as the **stressor.** Each day you encounter a variety of stressors with a range of intensity. Types of stressors include social stressors, such as noise and crowding; psychological stressors, such as anxiety and worry; psychosocial stressors, such as an unreasonable teacher, a new girlfriend or boyfriend, or a new job; biochemical or physical stressors, such as injury or intoxicants (alcohol and drugs); and philosophical stressors, which result from a value-system conflict or an inability to decipher direction and/or purpose to your life.[5] These categories are not exhaustive, but they do illustrate that in each of our lives there are numerous potential triggers for eliciting stress. (See figure 3.1.)

**INTENSITY OF STRESSORS** In addition to a variety of stressors, there is also a range in the strength of the response the stressor elicits. This is referred to as intensity and can be viewed as a continuum with **micro-stressors** on the one end and **macro-stressors** on the other. Most of the stressors encountered daily are micro-stressors, such as getting up, running to class, and exhilaration over an unexpectedly high grade on a test. They are encountered and adapted to with varying degrees of regularity. More intense stressors, such as the death of a friend or family member, pregnancy or fathering a pregnancy, or transferring to another school, can be macro-stressors.[6] It is a mistake, however, to assume that macro-stressors are harmful and micro-stressors are not harmful. All stressors elicit the stress response to some degree, and require that we adapt or cope.

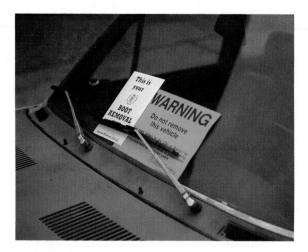


**Figure 3.1**
Stressors come in many forms.

The assessment phase of stress management suggests that we "tune in" to our bodies and learn to recognize when we are experiencing the stress response. Table 3.1 presents some of the more common signs and symptoms of the stress response. Take a moment to assess which of these symptoms you usually notice while experiencing stress.

**PRIMARY VERSUS SECONDARY STRESSORS**
A **primary stressor** is a demand or event that initiates the stress response. **Secondary stressors** are events that result from the primary stressor and keep the stress response activated. Together, they can create a vicious cycle and prolong the stress response.

Consider Pam, a college senior who decided to take twenty credits during her final semester. Pam has too much to do and not enough time to accomplish it. In her stimulus overload, Pam frantically flip-flops from one assignment to another without finishing any of them. Pam has become so preoccupied with trying to juggle projects that she has lost sight of her goals for doing the projects. Her sense of urgency and competitive urge to achieve has lead Pam to "doubling her effort." Pam now finds her doubled effort is interfering with her leisure-time pursuits which are her prime source of relaxation. After receiving lower grades than she had expected on her first few projects, Pam becomes frustrated and questions her ability to succeed. Depressed and worried about her performance, Pam loses motivation at a time when she should be considering her next assignment.

Table 3.1 **Some of the More Common Signs and Symptoms of Stress**

| Emotional | Muscular |
|---|---|
| Forgetfulness | Shaky hands |
| Nervousness | Back pain |
| Worrying | Tension headaches |
| Difficulty sleeping | Stiff muscles |
| **Cardiorespiratory** | Twitches |
| Heart pounding | **Gastrointestinal** |
| Cold, sweaty hands | Upset stomach |
| Headaches (throbbing pain) | Constipation |
| Shortness of breath | Diarrhea |
| Rapid breathing | |

Pam is not unlike many college students. Stimulus overload, or too many commitments, would appear to be the primary stressor in this example. Increased effort, less than expected results, frustration, and worry are secondary stressors. The interrelationship of primary and secondary stressors serves to keep alive the stress response. It is not any one "micro-stressor," but a combination, that generates continued effort by the body to adapt. This interrelationship of primary-secondary stressors is unique to each person, as it is based on personality and on individual perceptions of events in the world around us.

**PERCEPTION OF STRESSORS** According to Hans Selye, it is not the stressor that is important, but "how you take it." One interpretation of "how you take it" is how you perceive the event and the kind of meaning attached to it. This partially explains why people do not respond to the same stimulus with the same intensity or duration. What is a stressor for your friends, roommates, or family may not be a stressor for you. Each person's unique combination of personality, behavior patterns, life experiences, socialization experiences, and set of beliefs is involved. The kind and amount of stress, as well as how one copes with stress, are directly related to perception.

A different scenario could be created for Pam, for example. The second scenario has Pam accepting the challenge of twenty credits, a challenge that stimulates Pam's desire to learn and motivates her to use the available time wisely. As Pam is

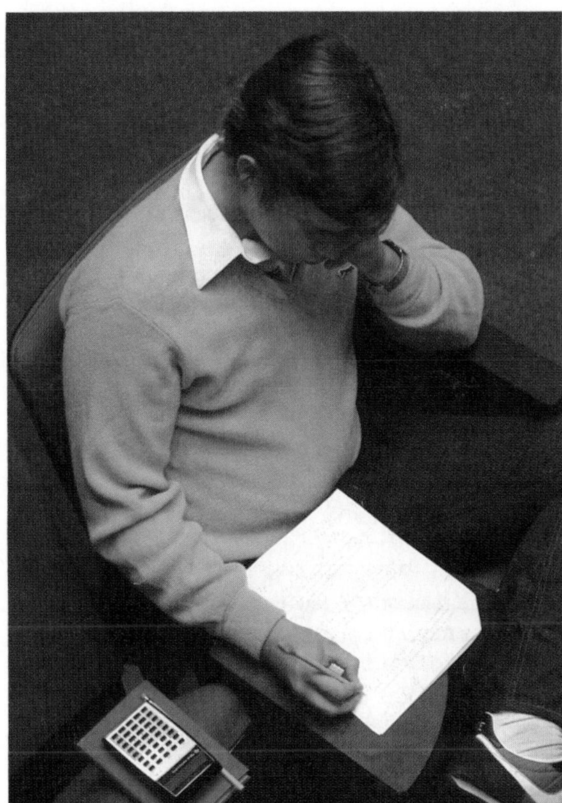

**Figure 3.2**
Exams can seem less of a stressor if you view them as an opportunity to learn or demonstrate what you know.

"stretched" in this endeavor she feels positive about trying new experiences. Success is not equated with performance, but measured by experiences gained. There is a difference in using stress to one's advantage rather than letting stress control the person. (See figure 3.2.)

**DESIRABILITY: EUSTRESS AND DISTRESS**
Into every person's life some stress must fall; to be alive is to experience stress. It is our mind's and body's way of adapting. In this context, the only way you can be totally free of stress is to be dead. Selye coined the term **eustress** to designate desirable stress. Eustress is that stress which is experienced to maintain life, such as through cardiovascular regulation, digestion, and hormonal secretions. Desirable stress

3.1 EXHIBIT

# Video Games: Hazardous to Your Health?

Think a quarter is all you stand to lose to the alien invaders? Think again. Those death rays can backfire. In some people, the stress of video play sends blood pressures and heart rates soaring.

For the past five years, cardiologist Robert S. Eliot, M.D., has been watching to learn how his patients respond to stress. After tests on more than 1,000 subjects, Dr. Eliot believes that one-third of the population has an unsuspected physiological overreactivity to mental stress—a reactivity that may make them particularly susceptible to heart disease.

To locate these "hot reactors," Eliot's laboratory at the University of Nebraska Medical Center has more than $300,000 in computerized equipment: machines that automatically monitor blood pressure, heart rate, stroke volume and the amount of resistance the heart must counteract to move blood through the vessels. Eliot even has blood-analysis machines to monitor secretions of the adrenal glands. But the heart of Eliot's stress lab, the machine that produces the stress, is cheap. It's a popular video game designed for arcade or home.

To find out if you are a hot reactor, you could have someone record your blood pressure while you play a video game. It can be that simple. But if you are in an age bracket where you have to worry about heart disease, don't do it, warns Eliot. Video games pack quite a punch. "We've seen such dramatic changes in video-game players' physiology that I feel a doctor should be around in case something happens." His demonstration speaks for itself.

**Hot, Cold, and Running Reactions**
The solid black and colored lines show the systolic pressures of two bankers playing video games. Banker Jones is a hot reactor. Banker Smith is cool. (On the surface, Smith is an aggressive Type-A, and Jones a passive Type-B.) To compare mental and physical stress responses, the broken line is another banker exercising on a treadmill.

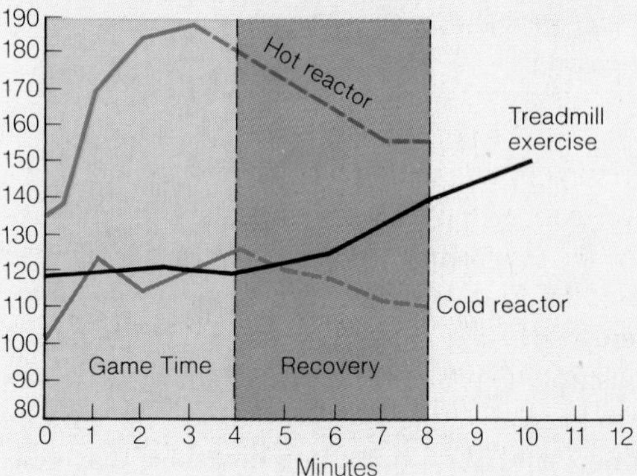


One of Eliot's patients, a middle-aged administrator, has a baseline blood pressure of 134/89 when he sits down to play the game. He appears calm. But within seconds, though he doesn't feel any different, his body responds with signs similar to those of an athlete in action. His systolic pressure jumps to 207, while his diastolic pressure falls to 66. Meanwhile his pulse rate increases from 80 to 109 beats per minute, and his cardiac output doubles from 4.4 liters of blood per minute to 8.4.

also includes life events in which the individual is taxed, challenged, and perceives a potential for personal growth. How one takes a stressor is a prime determinant of eustress. College athletes, for instance, commonly experience stress, both before and during their competition. Most athletes perceive this stress as eustress. Before the competition the stress response helps them "get up for the game." During competition, controlled and channeled stress helps bring out the athlete's best effort.

The flip side of eustress is **distress.** Generally, distress is taken to mean too much stress. But how much stress is too much? Broadly speaking, distress is experiencing too many stressors in a short time. It may also be too many stressors over the long haul, exceeding your ability to cope effectively and remain in control. Intense, prolonged, and unrelenting stress carries with it the potential to wear the mind and body down, affect system and organ functioning, and upset physical and psychological balance. How much is too much varies from person to person.

## EXHIBIT 3.1

Peripheral resistance, the amount of force the heart must push against to move blood through the vessels, has decreased by more than half; his blood vessels have dilated to allow blood to flow more easily.

So far the patient's body has reacted dramatically but in ways nature intended. Stress has triggered an outpouring of catecholamines, substances produced by the adrenal glands to stoke up the body to fight or flee. The response is immediate. To achieve the same elevated heart rate and blood pressure by running on a treadmill—or track—would take eight or nine minutes rather than the same number of seconds.

Nature also intended, though, that such powerful stimulation be vented by physical action. Activity uses up the catecholamines as they are excreted into the blood stream, damping the physiological increases. But instead of springing to action, the patient continues to play the video game. His physiological responses soon take an ominous turn.

Suddenly the little blips on the colored screen get smaller and start moving faster. The patient still feels much the same, but his body is no longer behaving like an athlete's; instead, he has symptoms like those that can lead to a stroke. Stress is squeezing his blood vessels like a clamp on a garden hose. His peripheral resistance triples, cutting his heart output back to 4.4 liters per minute. His blood pressure goes from 207/66 to 183/125. Eliot stops the game. "What you are doing," he tells his patient, "is like drag racing a car with the brakes on. Your heart is pumping against dramatically increased pressure. There is a limit to what that organ can do."

Ironically, public concern over video games has been directed at the kids who play them—not the adults, who may run a greater health risk from these physiological changes. In Marlborough, a town outside Boston, the machines have been banned to kids during school hours. The ordinance may help keep kids in class, but it may also lessen the arcade congestion during lunch so their parents can play. From the looks of things, it's the parents, not the kids, who can't afford the stress.

Work with laboratory animals has shown that excess catecholamines can rupture small muscle fibers in the heart within five minutes. Autopsies of young men who suffered stress-related heart attacks showed that their heart muscles had ruptured in seconds from stress-induced outpouring of catecholamines. The patient on the computer game protests that he should be allowed to keep playing. He thinks he is winning.

In another test, a subject is thought to be a "cold reactor." His pulse remains at 110/70 as he plays the game, but on a hunch the cardiologist sends in a woman to compete with him. Now his blood pressure rises to 140/102; though it should be observed that the woman's blood pressure is going off the chart at 188/120.

Fortunately, most people are cold reactors. When playing video games, their pulses rise only eight to sixteen beats per minute and their blood pressure rises 10mm to 20mm. But you can't tell whether you are a hot or a cold reactor by the way you feel. "We have had heart rate increases of sixty beats per minute and blood pressure as high as 220mm within one minute of starting a computer game. It happens quite a lot, but the patients have no awareness."

## THE PHYSIOLOGY OF STRESS

Stress is a response to a stimulus—a response involving interaction between the brain and subsequent reactions throughout varying organs of the body. These complex reactions maintain the **homeostasis,** or balanced state, of the body. Homeostasis involves coordinated processes that keep the body from deviating so far from the norm that illness, disease, or death might result. The physiology of the stress response is essential for homeostasis.

The stress response occurs through two major pathways in the body: the **central nervous system** and the **endocrine system.** The manifestations each person recognizes when under stress include increased heart rate, increased breathing rate, increased perspiration, increased muscle tension, a dry mouth, and a general overall increase in body metabolism. Central nervous system stimulation and endocrine secretions are responsible for these manifestations.

3.1 *continued* EXHIBIT 3.1

Most women are icy reactors to video games. "They think the games are foolish and don't respond at all," explains Eliot. But the same women are often hot reactors in other situations. To find these hot reactors, Eliot uses a competitive interview with another woman.

Video games are just one way to simulate the stresses we face in everyday life, adds Mark McKinney, Ph.D., assistant professor of preventive and stress medicine at the University of Nebraska and a colleague of Eliot's. There are other stress producers used in the laboratory—interviews, arithmetic tests or holding a hand in ice water—that can create much the same physiological response. The difference between those tests and video games is that people don't go out of their way to engage in them, let alone spend countless hours and quarters for the experience.

No one has yet taken a random sample of players from an arcade and tested them for physiological reactivity, but it may be that the people who play the games are those who get the biggest physiological kick. No one knows whether video games cause endorphin secretions—the stuff that is thought to create runner's high—but the researchers think it's not unlikely. According to Eliot, we do know that the games can cause dramatic increases in cortisol, another product of the adrenal glands, which is secreted during vigilance and long-term physical activity.

In any case, it may be no accident that video-game players call themselves both jocks and addicts: jocks because what they are playing is the mental side of sports, and addicts because for at least one-third of them the payoff is the powerful internal kick from playing.

For hot reactors, the games give "all the excitement of competition without the physical component," says Eliot. "But if you don't take it out on a playing field, you take it out on yourself." Video games are not likely to go away. They are too much fun. But unless we find a way to avoid or work off the powerful physiological stimulation of the games, Eliot fears "we may be heading toward a generation of hypertensives in this country where young people play video games instead of more sporting activities which condition the body."

Source: Reprinted from *American Health: Fitness of Body.* © 1982 American Health Partners, New York.

## DISCUSSION QUESTIONS

1. What is the difference between a "hot reactor" and a "cold reactor"?

2. What activities do you participate in regularly that, like video games, would be considered mental stressors? Try to think of at least three.

3. Would you categorize the activities you just listed as eustress or distress? Explain your response.

## The Nervous System Pathway

The Central Nervous System (CNS) consists of the brain and spinal cord. Brain function is divided into two parts; a voluntary system, and an autonomic system. The **Autonomic Nervous System** (ANS) regulates bodily functions not normally controlled voluntarily, such as heart rate, breathing rate, and glandular secretions.

Nervous system involvement begins immediately when a stressor is encountered. As soon as a stressor is perceived, the outer layer of the brain transmits certain chemical messages to the **hypothalamus.** The hypothalamus is then responsible for stimulation of the autonomic nervous system. Since energy expenditure is required to meet a stressor, the ANS stimulates body metabolism, affecting various bodily functions (see figure 3.3). One of the major targets of the ANS stimulation are the **adrenal glands** which, when stimulated, release the hormones **adrenalin** and **noradrenalin.** Adrenalin and noradrenalin are the action-preparation hormones of the body and are often responsible for the remarkable feats accomplished during emergencies.

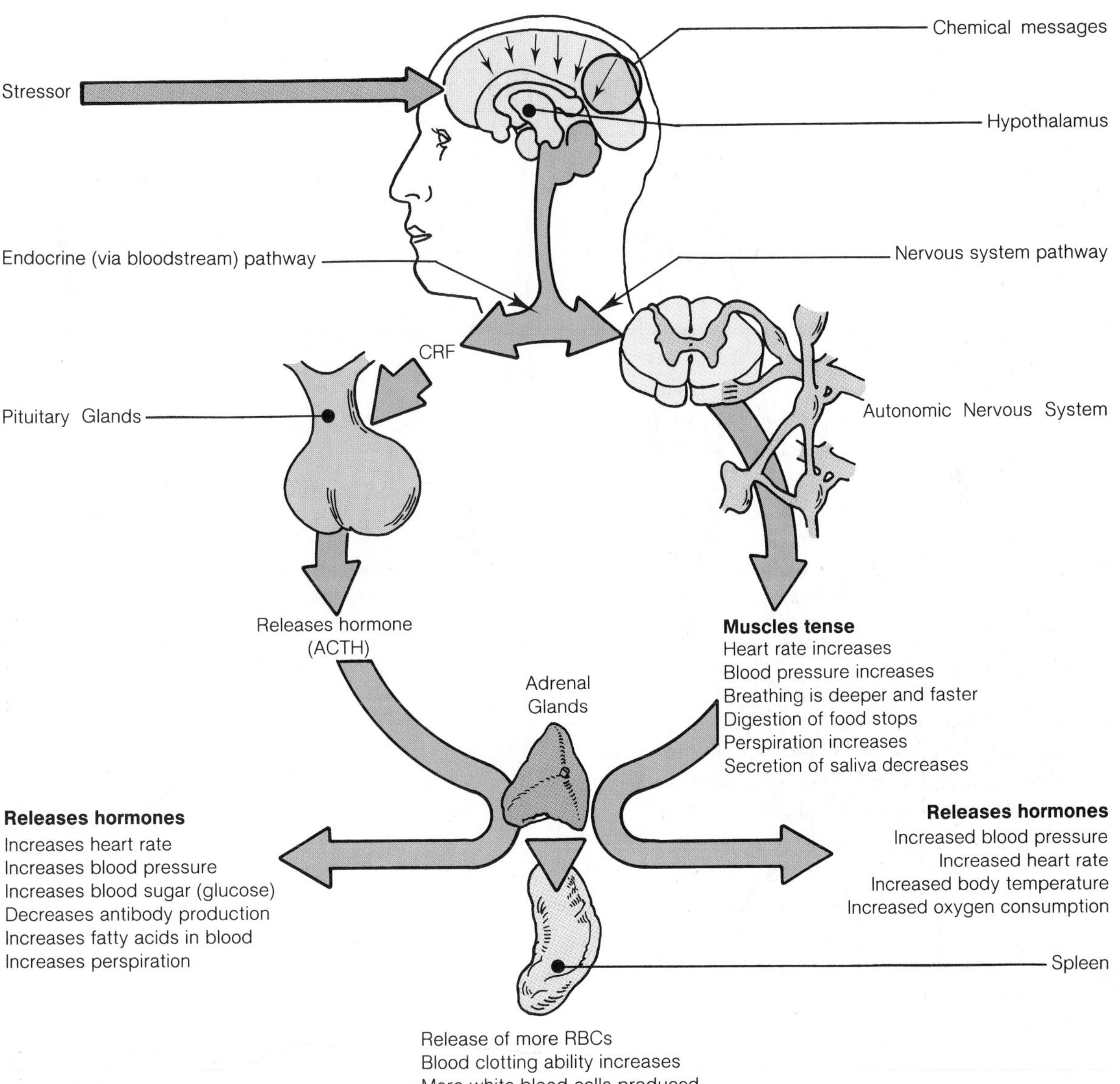


**Figure 3.3**
Stressors affect various bodily functions.

The demands most likely to trigger the ANS, with subsequent release of the action-preparation hormones, are fear, severe pain, anger, and any situation that threatens physical harm.

## The Endocrine System Pathway

Simultaneously with nervous-system stimulation, the hypothalamus releases a hormone called corticotropin releasing factor (CRF) whose function is to activate the pituitary glands. The pituitary glands, when stimulated by CRF, secrete another hormone, called adrenocorticotrophic hormone (ACTH), into the general body circulation. Once in the bloodstream, the ACTH circulates to its target, the adrenal glands. The adrenal glands then secrete hormones into the bloodstream to assist in meeting the demand of stressors.

The endocrine pathway hormones increase body metabolism for greater energy, both during stress and during recovery from stress. Fat and protein substances are processed to form glucose, the energy provider. The body also retains extra sodium (salt) resulting in increased water retention. This in turn increases blood volume, blood pressure, and the amount of blood to be pumped by the heart with each beat. Effects from the endocrine pathway are presented in figure 3.3.

These two pathways of the stress response have evolved to provide humans with the ability to meet the demands of living. However, as the stress response became more refined during its evolutionary development, the demands of living changed drastically. New demands, rapid change, the breakdown of traditional ways of responding to life events, and countless other complexities of contemporary society have led to an assortment of stress-related problems and new challenges for its management.

## The Problem and the Challenge of Stress

The stress response of our ancestors was a survival skill and prepared them to stalk game and protect themselves from human and animal intruders. When the stress response was elicited it was for life-threatening reasons. Physical activity usually followed the stress arousal. Excess energy was burned up and hormones broken down and disposed.

We are symbolic reactors today. Rather than confronting life-threatening stressors, life today centers around events that hold symbolic meaning. Should this symbolism be perceived to be threatening, the stress response is elicited. Today's norms do not readily allow appropriate release of the available energy. Rarely is physically attacking the source of stress acceptable; neither is fleeing from it. An upcoming test, a disagreement with a friend, the boredom of a job, or the lack of money to finance school are all potential examples of situations where both fighting and fleeing are unacceptable. Each of these stressors has some symbolic representation to the person experiencing them; none is life threatening. These stressors may not bring about a complete stress reaction, but the result is significant physiological changes within the body.

Distress, or stress gone bad, can be described as encountering too many stressors within a short period of time, thus exceeding a person's ability to cope effectively. Should distress continue over time, body organs and systems can become fatigued. This wear and tear can result in illness or dysfunction. Many modern afflictions are conditions which result from a maladjustment of human beings to their physical and social environment.[7] For this reason, the stress-related disorders presented in table 3.2 have been dubbed "diseases of adaptation." This list does not include emotional and mental problems such as depression, suicide, and human abuse, which number in the millions and have also been linked to distressed individuals.

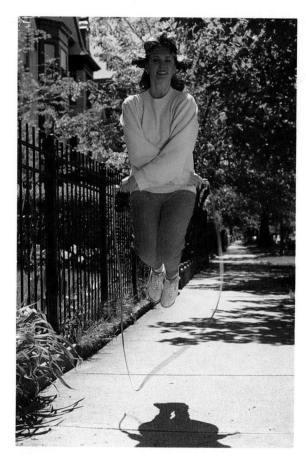

**Figure 3.4**
Physical exercise can be a positive way of managing stress.

Most diseases have multiple causes, including factors such as heredity, personality, and ability to cope. It would be inappropriate to conclude that stress is *the* cause of diseases of adaptation, or that by effectively managing stress these problems will disappear. Human beings and disease causation are far too complex to reduce to a simplistic and narrow view. (Diseases and their possible causes are discussed in more detail in chapter 15.)

**Table 3.2 Stress-Related Disorders Have Been Dubbed "Diseases of Adaptation"**

| Stress-Related Diseases | |
|---|---|
| • Coronary heart disease | • Gout |
| • Hypertension | • Diarrhea, constipation |
| • Stroke | • Allergies |
| • Diabetes | • Asthma |
| • Cancer | • Thyroid malfunction |
| • Colitis | • Headache |
| • Peptic ulcer | |

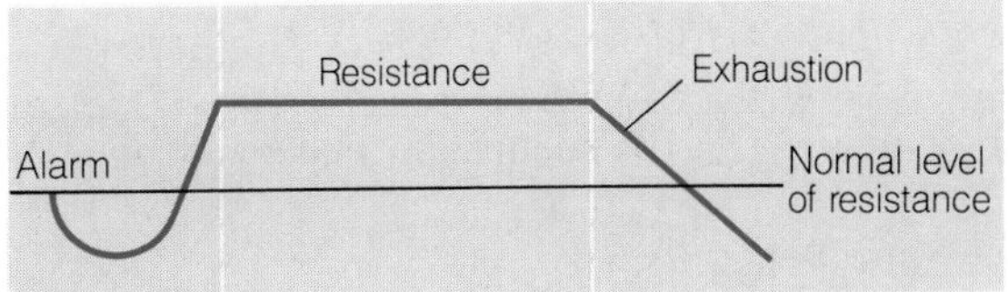


**Figure 3.5**
Stressors can cause greater susceptibility to disease and illness.
*Source:* Figure 3 (p. 39) from *Stress Without Distress*, by Hans Selye, M.D. (J. B. Lippincott Company) Copyright © 1974 by Hans Selye, M.D.

## The General Adaptation Syndrome

One theory that attempts to explain the relationship between stress and disease was advanced by Selye. As early as 1936, Selye noticed in animal experiments a predictable way of responding to stress. Later, this became known as the **General Adaptation Syndrome** or **GAS.**[8] Its three stages—(1) the alarm reaction, (2) the stage of resistance, and (3) the stage of exhaustion—describe the stress response and the adaptability of the body to stress.

When the human body experiences homeostasis, it is able to maintain a normal level of resistance to disease, and can function at an optimal level. When exposed to stressors, however, the human body reacts in the manner illustrated in figure 3.5.

**ALARM** First, during the **"alarm" stage,** the body awakens to the stressor. It is during the alarm phase that people experience the typical signs and symptoms of the stress response, such as muscle tension, a pounding heart, and butterflies in the stomach. The body gears up to deal with the stressor. During the alarm stage, general resistance to disease is decreased.

**RESISTANCE** The second stage, **resistance,** is characterized by a rebound effect aimed at resisting the stressor. During this stage, the body attempts to adapt to the stressor and return to a balanced state of functioning. Successful adaptation leads to an increased level of resistance to disease and a disappearance of the alarm reaction. All people experience the first two stages of the GAS many times. Only under extreme conditions do most people enter the third stage—exhaustion.

**EXHAUSTION** In the **stage of exhaustion** the body once again experiences the symptoms of the stress response. Exhaustion is the result of a long-continued exposure to a stressor to which the body has already adjusted. Prolonged wear and tear of stressors can cause organs to become fatigued, leading to greater susceptiblity to disease and illness. (In figure 3.5, note the line crossing below the normal level of resistance.)

Selye has stated that during the general adaptation syndrome, something gets used up. The inability to verify scientifically that something led Selye to call it **Adaptation Energy.**[9] Selye hypothesized that Adaptation Energy is finite. Each person inherits just so much Adaptation Energy at birth and, as it is depleted through life, there will be a final stage of exhaustion where death results. Prior to death, however, those organs and processes which have been called on to resist stressors and right the body become less effective and break down. When this happens, there is a shifting to other organs or systems to compensate. Eventually, entire key organs and systems fail, wrecking the whole human machinery; death occurs.

Selye and others have frequently suggested that life-style considerations are important determinants to the depletion rate of Adaptation Energy. Specifically, Selye stated, "We can squander our adaptability recklessly, 'burning the candle at both ends,' or we can learn to make this valuable resource last long, by using it wisely and sparingly, only for things that are worthwhile and cause least distress."[10] Certain life events require more utilization of Adaptation Energy than others. A brief look at life-events research may help you to understand why.

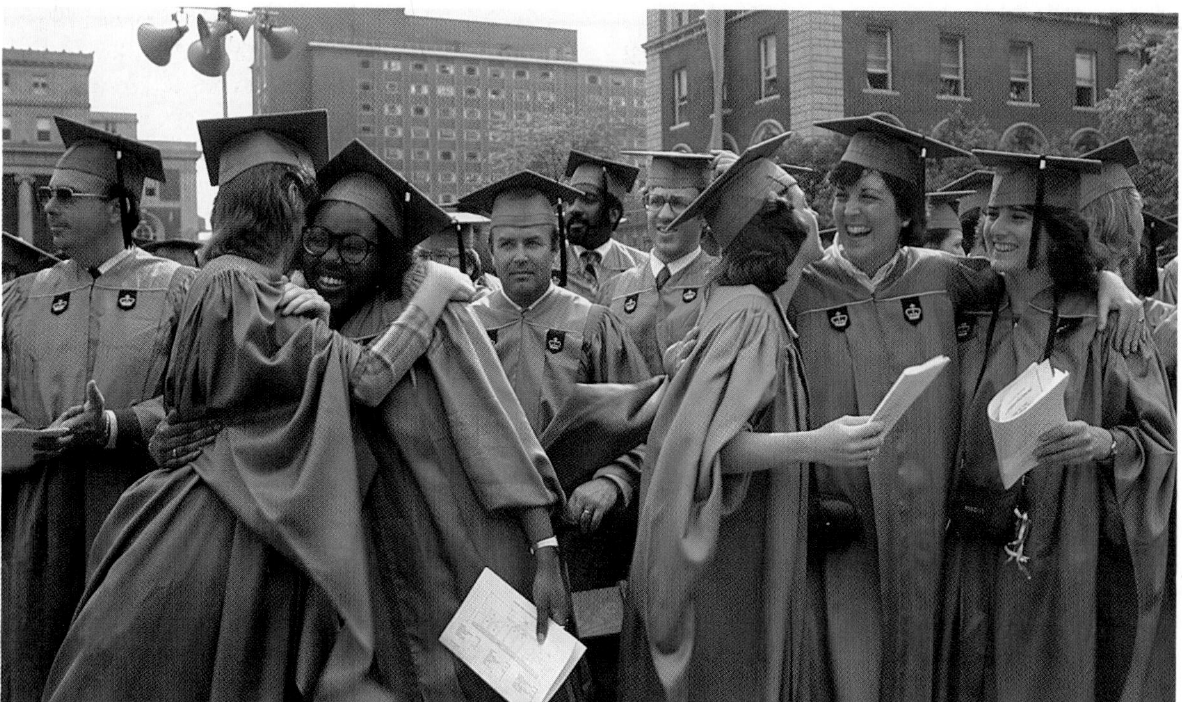

**Figure 3.6**
College graduation is the kind of marker event that can prove both exhilarating and stressful.

**CHANGE AND ADAPTATION** All change requires adjustment by the human body. Energy is used to adapt to new or novel circumstances. In contemporary society, change is inherent in the life cycle. Gail Sheehy, author of *Passages: Predictable Crises of Adult Life,* has written that throughout the life cycle there are predictable **marker events.**[11] Marker events are changes or events that are intense stressors when experienced. They are specific to developmental stages of growth, as well as to social and cultural factors which influence them. Going to school for the first time is a marker event, as are graduating from high school, marriage, divorce, singlehood, having children, beginning a new career, and retirement. Marker events, as well as other less intense life events, can be either positive or negative. Graduation, marriage, and your first child are generally viewed as positive life changes. (See figure 3.6.) Each, however, requires adaptation specific to the event as well as prior to and after the event.

It has been discovered that the number, clustering, and intensity of major life changes experienced by a person in a short time can serve as a predictor of illness, injury, or psychological problems. The original instrument used to predict this relationship was the Social Readjustment Rating Scale (SRRS) developed by Thomas Holmes and Richard Rahe.[12] The SRRS has been researched with thousands of people from all walks of life. It lists forty-three life events that require significant adaptation or coping behavior. Theoretically, the more life changes per unit of time, the greater the physiological changes and use of body energy to resist stressors. The scoring mechanism of these forty-three events makes it possible to predict with some consistency the onset of an illness, injury, or depression.

Being a college student is a marker event. Many new life changes are occurring. A version of the SRRS for college students was developed to reflect more accurately life events of college students.[13] In order to see how recent events are affecting you, see Activity for Wellness 3.1.

Before reaching conclusions about predicting illness, two important facts about major life changes must be recognized. First, people vary in their ability to handle change. Some can adjust to major change with little distress, while others do not cope as well. The scale presented here only "predicts"; it is not absolute. Some students with a very high score will remain well; others with a very low score will become ill. Second, major life changes do not and need not produce distress. The adverse effects of change can be controlled. Stimulation, challenge, and change are important ingredients for personal growth. As one health expert noted:

> It all sounds pretty grim. But there may be ways in which you can soften the blow. Change is not entirely random. You have a large amount of personal control over whether and when to marry, go to college, move or have a family. . . . So the future is not a complete blank. You can predict it to a certain degree. And to this degree, you can order your life by managing the change that is a vital part of living. You can weigh the benefits of change against its costs, pace the timing of the inevitable changes and regulate the occurrence of voluntary change to try to keep your yearly life-change score out of the danger zone.[14]

Stress can control us or we can learn to control it. Understanding more about yourself, life changes, and managing stress can equip you for stress. Stress does not have to be delegated to a painful part of life to be endured. Illness, disease, and dysfunction are only one side of the stress issue. There is a more positive side of stress; stress can also be a challenge.

Learning to control stress, not avoiding it, is the challenge. Controlling stress encourages us to view life in a positive manner regardless of our circumstances. Controlling stress is a challenge to become more sensitive to our physical selves in an artificial world. It is learning how to become more congruent, more real, and more alive. It is a challenge to make your life work better. There are no promises with this challenge. There are no guarantees that one will live longer. But those who accept the challenge to manage life's stress will tell you that it is a richer, fuller, healthier way to be alive. Developing your personal stress-management strategies and coping skills is one way to assume the challenge of managing stress.

## MANAGING STRESS

Stress management may be more appropriately referred to as **Life Management.** Life management refers to everything that you do to adapt and remain functioning as a person. It includes the simple little things that come naturally and the more complex strategies that require constant effort. To manage your life more effectively does not call for the elimination of stress. Rather, life management directs us to channel stress, thus promoting stimulation, challenge, and growth experiences. There is no single-stress management strategy that will accomplish this task. Life management is ongoing. It is learning more about who we are as human beings, why we act and react to the world around us as we do, and how to deal more effectively with life's insults and frustrations as well as its joys and pleasures. Some specific techniques are offered in this section. They are presented in light of the following principles:

1. *Awareness.* Learning to manage life and stress requires an understanding of the stress response, and appropriate management strategies to use when stress is out of control. Awareness is developed through conscious and regular assessment. It is consciously paying attention to the mental, physical, and social forces that impinge upon our lives. Awareness is learning to recognize and channel stress appropriately, thus reducing distress. You are using awareness foresight when stress is approached in this way. **Awareness foresight** is the knowledge and understanding you have about yourself that helps in making decisions. These decisons enable you to use appropriate prevention strategies prior to distress. This type of awareness is in contrast to **hindsight awareness,** an after-the-fact knowledge that stress was present but unrecognized or unmanaged. Somewhere between these two is **midsight awareness,** the realization that stress is mounting and that an increase in coping skills is required.[15]
2. *Benefiting from Distress.* Too much distress can lead to health problems, yet short-term distress forces us to turn our conscious attention to the source. We may discover a new insight, clarify a value, or modify a health habit that contributed to the distress. A wiser person emerges; personal growth has taken place. The principle is to benefit from distress by having it work for you rather than against you.
3. *A Total-Person Approach.* There is no single stress-management technique that will work for every person, or for the same person in different stress situations. The total-person

3.1 ACTIVITY FOR WELLNESS

## Scores for Life-Change Events

| Column A | | Life-Change Event | Column B | Column C |
|---|---|---|---|---|
| ______ | 1. | Entered college | 50 | ______ |
| ______ | 2. | Married | 77 | ______ |
| ______ | 3. | Trouble with your boss | 38 | ______ |
| ______ | 4. | Held a job while attending school | 43 | ______ |
| ______ | 5. | Experienced the death of a spouse | 87 | ______ |
| ______ | 6. | Major change in sleeping habits | 34 | ______ |
| ______ | 7. | Experienced the death of a close family member | 77 | ______ |
| ______ | 8. | Major change in eating habits | 30 | ______ |
| ______ | 9. | Change in or choice of major field of study | 41 | ______ |
| ______ | 10. | Revision of personal habits | 45 | ______ |
| ______ | 11. | Experienced the death of a close friend | 68 | ______ |
| ______ | 12. | Found guilty of minor violations of the law | 22 | ______ |
| ______ | 13. | Had an outstanding personal achievement | 40 | ______ |
| ______ | 14. | Experienced pregnancy, or fathered a pregnancy | 68 | ______ |
| ______ | 15. | Major change in health or behavior of family member | 56 | ______ |
| ______ | 16. | Had sexual difficulties | 58 | ______ |
| ______ | 17. | Had trouble with in-laws | 42 | ______ |
| ______ | 18. | Major change in number of family get-togethers | 26 | ______ |
| ______ | 19. | Major change in financial state | 53 | ______ |
| ______ | 20. | Gained a new family member | 50 | ______ |
| ______ | 21. | Change in residence or living conditions | 42 | ______ |
| ______ | 22. | Major conflict or change in values | 50 | ______ |
| ______ | 23. | Major change in church activities | 36 | ______ |
| ______ | 24. | Marital reconciliation with your mate | 58 | ______ |
| ______ | 25. | Fired from work | 62 | ______ |
| ______ | 26. | Were divorced | 76 | ______ |
| ______ | 27. | Changed to a different line of work | 50 | ______ |
| ______ | 28. | Major change in number of arguments with spouse | 50 | ______ |
| ______ | 29. | Major change in responsibilities at work | 47 | ______ |

approach to stress management is one that recognizes the multidimensionality of humans. The whole person is a dynamic interplay between the physical, mental, emotional, social, and spiritual dimensions. An exercise program alone is not sufficient to manage stress; nor is relaxation training, better time management, or improved communication. Each strategy serves a specific purpose, but if done to the exclusion of other strategies, and without consideration for the whole person, may be less effective.

4. *Choosing the Appropriate Skill.* Given the magnitude of options to manage stress, how a person selects the most appropriate strategy at the right time is paramount. One approach is to match the coping technique to the situation at hand. Personal management or organizing skills are particularly effective for the times when life seems out of control, when the work

ACTIVITY FOR 3.1

## WELLNESS

| A | | Event | B | C |
|---|---|---|---|---|
| _______ | 30. | Had your spouse begin or cease work outside the home | 41 | _______ |
| _______ | 31. | Major change in working hours or conditions | 42 | _______ |
| _______ | 32. | Marital separation from mate | 74 | _______ |
| _______ | 33. | Major change in type and/or amount of recreation | 37 | _______ |
| _______ | 34. | Major change in use of drugs | 52 | _______ |
| _______ | 35. | Took on a mortgage or loan of less than $10,000 | 52 | _______ |
| _______ | 36. | Major personal injury or illness | 65 | _______ |
| _______ | 37. | Major change in use of alcohol | 46 | _______ |
| _______ | 38. | Major change in social activities | 43 | _______ |
| _______ | 39. | Major change in amount of participation in school activities | 38 | _______ |
| _______ | 40. | Major change in amount of independence and responsibility | 49 | _______ |
| _______ | 41. | Took a trip or a vacation | 33 | _______ |
| _______ | 42. | Engaged to be married | 54 | _______ |
| _______ | 43. | Changed to a new school | 50 | _______ |
| _______ | 44. | Changed dating habits | 41 | _______ |
| _______ | 45. | Trouble with school administration | 44 | _______ |
| _______ | 46. | Broke or had broken a marital engagement or steady relationship | 60 | _______ |
| _______ | 47. | Major change in self-concept or self-awareness | 57 | _______ |
| | | | Total | _______ |

To find your score on this scale, place the number of times you have experienced the event listed under Column A during the past twelve months. Multiply the number under Column B by the number in Column A and place it in Column C. Remember to count *each* time you experienced the event. Finally, total Column C. If your score totals 1435 or higher, you are in the "high" category for developing an illness. If your total is 347 or less, you fall into the "low" category. The "medium" score is 890.

Source: Reprinted with permission from Mark, M. T. et al., "The Influence of Recent Life Experiences on the Health of College Freshmen," *Journal of Psychosomatic Research,* 19. 87 (1975). © 1975 Pergamon Press Ltd.

to be done exceeds the available time, or when goals are unclear and values uncertain. Valuing, personal planning, commitment, time management, or pacing might be the skill of choice when organization is the issue.

Another approach is to match the coping technique to a person's individual strengths and preferences. Although capitalizing on strengths is often helpful, it can have its drawbacks. Donald Tubesing and Nancy Tubesing stated that:

> A person who relies almost exclusively upon organizational skills . . . will probably handle certain job pressures (numerous demands, time pressures, tight deadlines, multiple responsibilities) very effectively. That same person may have difficulty responding appropriately to job or personal situations that evoke a grief reaction. The stress and pain of loss simply does not respond very well to getting better organized. In this situation the individual may want to focus on obtaining some personal support. . . .[16]

The principle is to choose the most appropriate skill based on personal preference and the situation at hand.

5. *Gradualism.* Trying to learn and implement too many new strategies at one time may become a stressor. On the one hand, you may experience frustration from trying too hard, and on the other, too much change can result in stress. Change, growth, learning new strategies, and refining old ones all take time. Walt Schaefer has stated in *Stress, Distress, and Growth* that "Wholeness is a long-term ideal, gradualism the short-run way to get there."[17] Gradualism implies taking time. Take time to gain insights about the underlying nature of your stressors. Explore a variety of skills to manage your reaction to those stressors. Experience each personal exploration to its fullest.

# COPING AND MANAGEMENT SKILLS

The primary purpose for developing coping and management skills is to reduce either the frequency or the intensity of the stress response. Daniel Girdano and George Everly have presented a categorical scheme of strategies for controlling stress (see figure 3.7).[18]

The scheme for controlling stress encompasses Social Engineeering strategies, Personality Engineering strategies, and Relaxation Training. The categories presented here have been adapted to include the work of others. This provides a greater range of specific techniques a person may choose from in learning to control stress. Medical Treatment has been added because health-care providers are important in a comprehensive approach to managing stress.

Social Engineering, Personality Engineering, and Relaxation Training involve a great number of skills that can be learned and employed by each person prior to the development of distress symptoms. These skills can be learned through self-direction or with the assistance of a professional.

Controlling and channeling stress for wellness includes employing strategies both prior to and during the stress response. Using life-management skills and techniques to prevent too much stress or to improve well-being on a regular basis helps prevent distress. Additionally, these same skills can be used as a part of a midsight approach to stress management. A midsight approach involves intervening in the stress cycle once you become aware that you are experiencing too much stress.

Although life-management strategies are presented here in four categories, it is difficult to separate them. Skills may overlap categories, and some could just as well be presented in a different category, depending upon one's intention for using the skill. For example, Brenda wants to help reduce the intensity of the stress response after taking an exam. She recognizes an increase in tension from a stressor and sets out to do a twenty-minute progressive muscle-relaxation exercise. For this purpose it is listed in the relaxation training category. Deb, however, practices relaxation daily to maintain well-being and for better sleep onset at night; for Deb, relaxation may serve as a Social Engineering strategy. How and why a skill is used determines its category. The four categories reflect various life-management strategies.

## Social Engineering

One option in dealing with the stress response is to deal with the stressor itself. In this approach, stressors are givens; for instance, you could be experiencing too many changes, frustration, overload, or any number or types of stressors. Once you have assessed the stressor, you may seek alternatives or you may modify your position rather than expend energy in trying to change the stressor. In either case, your goal is to reduce how frequently you elicit the stress response.

A simple but effective way to reduce how frequently you elicit the stress response is to analyze your stressors on paper. As you list stressors, try to determine why these events are stressors for *you.* Next, list possible ways of alleviating each stressor. This is a brainstorming session so go for quantity in listing your ideas. Alongside each of the possibilities, identify any barriers to these new ways of responding to stressors. Finally, rank your possibilities from the most feasible to implement to the least feasible.

By using this formal approach, you are getting at the source of the problem. The stressor remains the same; you have not changed it. What you have done is to use foresight awareness, and effective

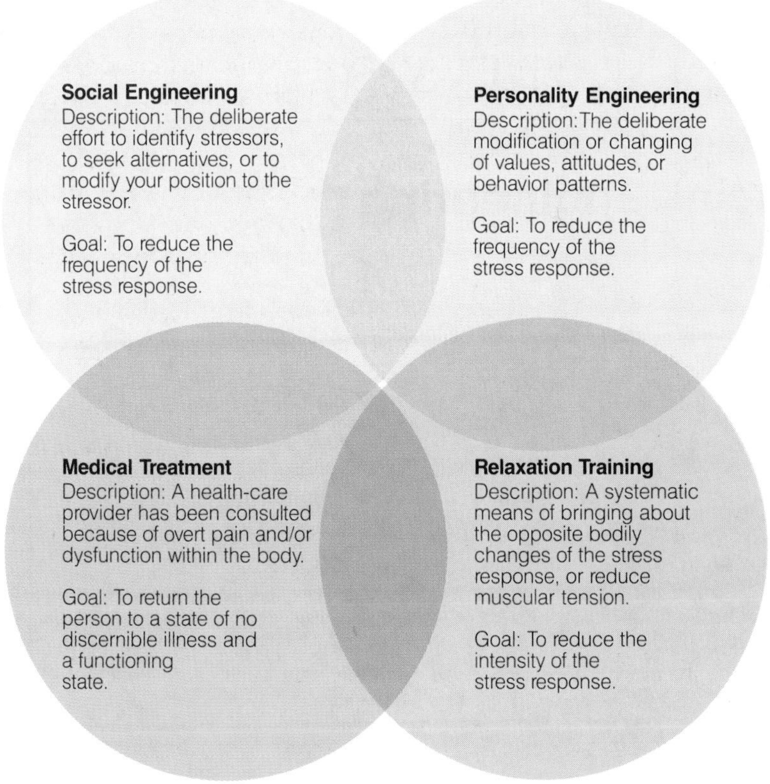

**Social Engineering**
Description: The deliberate effort to identify stressors, to seek alternatives, or to modify your position to the stressor.

Goal: To reduce the frequency of the stress response.

**Personality Engineering**
Description: The deliberate modification or changing of values, attitudes, or behavior patterns.

Goal: To reduce the frequency of the stress response.

**Medical Treatment**
Description: A health-care provider has been consulted because of overt pain and/or dysfunction within the body.

Goal: To return the person to a state of no discernible illness and a functioning state.

**Relaxation Training**
Description: A systematic means of bringing about the opposite bodily changes of the stress response, or reduce muscular tension.

Goal: To reduce the intensity of the stress response.

**Figure 3.7**
A categorical scheme of strategies for controlling stress. *Source:* From Daniel A. Girdano and George S. Everly, Jr., *Controlling Stress and Tension: A Holistic Approach.* © 1979, pp. 20–27. Adapted by permission of Prentice-Hall, Englewood Cliffs, N.J.

planning. Like most new approaches, however, it is important to do this in written form. It takes more time to write everything down, but you will quickly discover that in your analysis of stressors and in your brainstorming, there is more completeness and greater understanding of the process. Eventually, the process of alternative selection and ranking will become automatic. If what you chose does not turn out to be the best alternative for you, then you can select again from the many options you originally listed. Activity for Wellness 3.2 provides an opportunity to practice this strategy.

## Personality Engineering

Personality includes values, attitudes, and behavior patterns, all of which help to define how one perceives and reacts to stressors. **Personality Engineering strategies** help to reduce stress by deliberately modifying some aspect of one's personality that has transformed a neutral life event into a psychosocial stressor. Personality Engineering strategies also attempt to enhance one's self-concept.

**Constructive self-talk** is one technique that offers many positive stress-reduction benefits. We all talk to ourselves all the time. Much of the time our self-talk is quite negative. We say things like "Boy, was that ever a dumb thing to do!" or "I am such a weak person." This type of self-talk can be quite destructive, often keeping people in a state of stress. Self-talk, however, can also be used as a stress-control technique. People can learn to speak pleasantly to themselves, reinforcing the positive aspects of life. Statements such as "I did a good job on that," or "I will do better next time" help to enhance one's level of wellness.

Some Personality Engineering skills are directed toward offsetting distress that results from the Type-A behavior pattern. The **Type-A personality** construct was first described by two cardiologists, Meyer Friedman and Ray Rosenman.[19] They noted common behavioral characteristics in a number of their patients who had manifested cardiovascular problems. Behaviors such as a chronic sense of time urgency (always in a hurry); being time conscious, deadline oriented and impatient (hostility surfaces quickly when they are delayed); having a preoccupation with describing things in terms of numbers

3.2 ACTIVITY FOR WELLNESS 3.2

## Social Engineering

**SKILL DEVELOPMENT**

1. Identify Stressors: a conscious selection of events that cause stress.

2. Analyze underlying cause: Determine if the stressor is the result of frustration, overload, deprivation, and so on.

3. Rationally develop alternatives; seek new ways of responding to stressors.

4. List barriers to new ways of responding: determine the obstacles that may prevent implementation of alternatives.

5. Rank from most to least desirable; choose the best alternative and formulate a new plan of action.

6. Implement new plan; test the plan in your daily schedule.

7. Evaluate; examine the effectiveness of the new plan as a stress-control strategy.

8. Assess; determine the need to modify the existing plan or adopt a new approach.

**EXERCISE**

Select an academic stressor and use the above steps to change or modify your position in relation to the stressor.

| Stressor | Why | Alternatives | Barriers | Rank |
|---|---|---|---|---|
| | | | | |

(quantitative rather than qualitative in orientation); being polyphasic (attempting to do or think about more than one task at a time); and being highly competitive are major descriptors of the Type-A Personality. Persons not generally displaying these characteristics, and having seemingly less coronary disease, are referred to as Type-B individuals.

Personality Engineering strategies can be effective in offsetting some of the negative results of the Type-A person. Planning, pacing, and commitment skills are most useful for the Type-A person. The goal is not to change the personality of these individuals, but to provide skills which can help them cope more effectively with stress.

**Table 3.3 Relaxation Is Almost the Opposite of the Stress Response**

| *Stress* | *Relaxation* |
|---|---|
| Increased body metabolism | Decreased body metabolism |
| Increased heart rate | Decreased heart rate |
| Increased blood pressure | Decreased blood pressure |
| Increased breathing rate | Decreased breathing rate |
| Increased oxygen consumption | Decreased oxygen consumption |
| Increased cardiac output | Decreased cardiac output |
| Increased muscular tension | Decreased muscular tension |
| Decreased blood clotting time | Increased blood clotting time |
| Increased blood flow to the major muscle groups involved in the fight-or-flight (including the arms and legs) | |

Source: From *Learn to Relax: A 14-Day Program,* p. 19. © 1985 by John Curtis and Richard Detert. Coulee Press, LaCrosse, Wis.

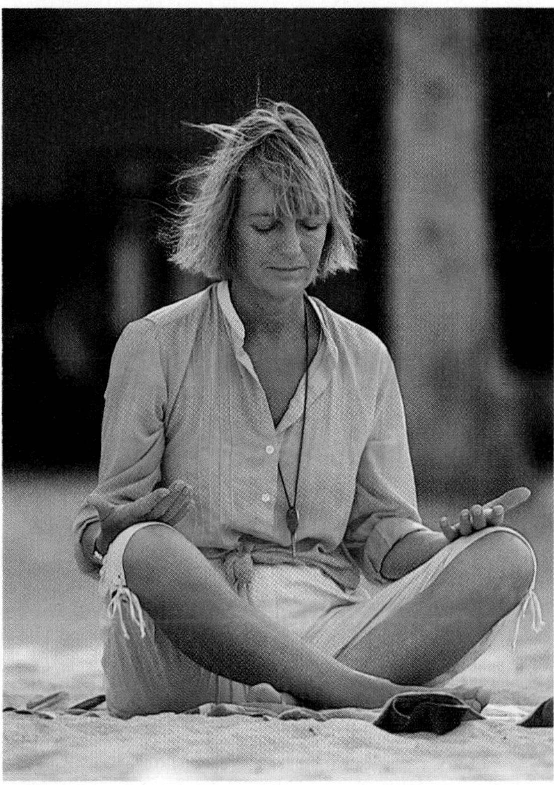

**Figure 3.8**
Relaxation skills are easily learned and, when practiced regularly, lead to important benefits.

Like Social Engineering strategies, the goal of Personality Engineering is to reduce the frequency with which the stress response is elicited. Activity for Wellness 3.3 illustrates a few Personality Engineering skills, and provides an opportunity to practice several of them.

## Relaxation Training

The third category of strategies encompasses various relaxation skills. The primary purpose of **relaxation training** is systematically to induce a physiological condition that is almost the opposite of the stress response. Table 3.3 compares the physiological response during stress and during relaxation.

There is a growing body of evidence that systematic relaxation training, when performed on a regular basis, is beneficial to health. John Curtis and Richard Detert have summarized these benefits by stating that relaxation:

1. is enjoyable;
2. can decrease symptoms of illness such as headache, nausea, rash, and diarrhea;
3. can increase levels of physical energy;
4. can increase concentration;
5. can increase the ability to handle problems and increase overall efficiency;
6. can increase social satisfaction in dealing with family, friends, and colleagues, and can increase feelings of self-confidence;
7. is helpful in the treatment of insomnia;
8. can lower blood pressure; and
9. can lower emotional arousal, which seems to explain why some individuals do not overreact to stress as much as others.[20]

Relaxation skills are easily learned (see figure 3.8). In addition, researchers have found that people who report they relax on a regular basis:

1. are more psychologically stable;
2. are more physiologically stable;
3. are less anxious;
4. feel in greater control of their lives than people who do not practice regular relaxation; and
5. achieve a faster return to a balanced state after reacting to stress.[21]

3.3 ACTIVITY FOR WELLNESS 3.3

# Personality Engineering

**SKILL DEVELOPMENT**

1. Valuing skills; developing a philosophy of life, getting in touch with a core meaning to existence.

2. Planning skills; establishing goals and choosing to pursue certain goals over others via prioritizing.

3. Commitment skills; pro-active assertiveness without feeling guilty for saying "no," without violating some one else's rights or personhood.

4. Pacing skills; determining if one is a "racehorse" or a "turtle" and developing the ability to predict how much one can handle.

5. Conversation skills; developing friendships, self-disclosing, attending to nonverbal cues, pursuing details, facilitating questions, listening with empathy.

6. Relabeling skills; viewing problems as challenges, opportunities or amusing vignettes can lead to a more positive outlook on life events, changing perceptions, attitudes, and behaviors.

7. Whisper skills; the art of positive self-talk via positive affirmations.

8. Gentleness skills; treating yourself kindly, giving yourself pats on the back, and energizing playfulness.

**EXERCISE**

Using the skills above, modify, or change an attitude, value, or behavior in regard to a large project that is due and for which you have had negative thoughts.

1. Identify a large overwhelming project that is due in several weeks ____________

____________

2. Relabel: Make a positive statement about this project several times each day using words like "challenge" or "opportunity." My statement is ____________

____________

3. Plan a steady course of action: Use the "Swiss cheese" method of identifying what needs to be accomplished by breaking it down into smaller, more manageable units according to available time or work amount.

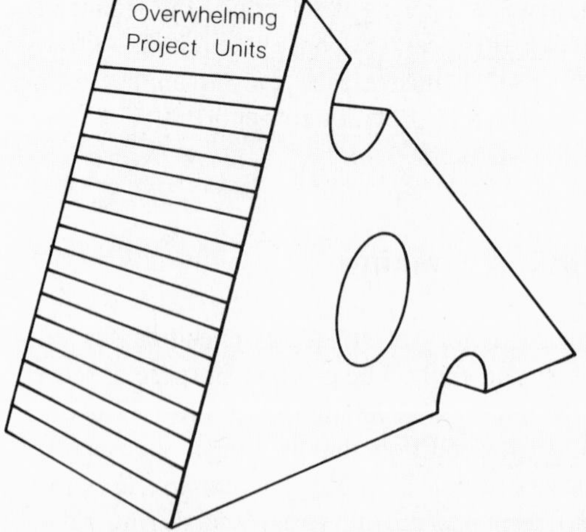


4. Begin NOW—today—on one unit.

5. Pace: maintain a steady pace by doing something every day even if it is only for fifteen minutes.

3.4 ACTIVITY FOR WELLNESS 3.4

## Relaxation Training

**SKILL DEVELOPMENT**

1. Sensory awareness skills; re-educating yourself to what is happening within your body (perceptions, functions, sensations) at a more conscious level.

2. Progressive muscle relaxation; development of "muscle sense" via alternately tensing and relaxing skeletal muscles of the forehead, face, and limbs in a progressive manner to induce physical and mental relaxation.

3. Benson's Relaxation Response; Using mental repetition of a word devoid of special meaning (such as the word "one"), a passive attitude, a relaxed posture, and a quiet environment to induce relaxation.

4. Meditation; a variety of procedures used to evoke altered states of consciousness for the purposes of peace, enlightenment, or spiritual growth.

5. Yoga; assumption of certain postures and control of breathing to increase vital capacity, flexibility, balance, and relaxation.

6. Biofeedback training; use of instruments to provide auditory or visual feedback to help yourself learn how to make changes voluntarily in body processes such as muscle tension, heart rate, and blood pressure.

7. Breathing rhythm skills; using the breathing rhythm with associative sensations to evoke desired perceptions or physiological occurrences.

8. Visualization exercises; a group of exercises that employ conscious intentional imagery, making use of self-suggestions for psychological or physiological purposes.

9. Brief relaxation exercises; awareness exercises that aid in managing muscular tension or pace without the physiological benefits of total body relaxation.

10. Mental diversion skills; activities such as hiking, gardening, reading, fishing, exercising, and the like that divert attention from stressors and help maintain physical and mental balance.

11. Massage; kneading, pummeling, and stroking of muscle groups to increase metabolism, release substances back into circulation, improve lymph drainage, and evoke mental and physical relaxation.

**EXERCISE**

Follow the guidelines for Benson's relaxation response or Bezzola's Autoanalysis relaxation exercise. Try the same exercise once each day for the next four days for a minimum of ten minutes. Do not be concerned about doing it correctly. Read the exercise description several times until you are familiar with it. Then select an environment where there is minimal interruption and begin.

There are many types of relaxation exercises that will, with regular use, lead to these benefits. Activity for Wellness 3.4 outlines a number of relaxation skills. Additionally, Activity for Wellness 3.5 provides more detailed instructions on two simple, but effective, relaxation techniques.

In addition to deep muscle relaxation exercises, there are several other skills listed in this category. Brief relaxation, massage, mental diversion, and exercise provide additional relaxing strategies. These skills do not provide deep relaxation in the same way as other relaxation procedures, but they do control mental and physical tension. Many experts, in fact, suggest that a relaxation exercise should follow twenty to thirty minutes of aerobic activity. Together, they are a powerful combination for physical, mental, and spiritual restoration.

3.5 ACTIVITY FOR WELLNESS

# Two Relaxation Techniques

**BENSON'S RELAXATION RESPONSE**

Benson's relaxation response method was developed and popularized by Herbert Benson, a cardiologist who specializes in hypertension. Dr. Benson is an associate professor of medicine at the Harvard Medical School and director of the Hypertension Section of Beth Israel Hospital in Boston. Components of Benson's method are rooted in transcendental meditation and in many major religions of the world, as well as in many secular writings. Benson has captured the basic components found in all of these writings and reduced them to a simple technique that elicits the relaxation response. His technique is not an attempt to explain meditation or prayer scientifically or to make them mechanical occurrences. Rather, it is an attempt to do what religious leaders have suggested for centuries—to use daily meditation and reflection for the benefit of mind, body, and soul.

The four components presented by Benson are:

1. A Quiet Environment: While learning to elicit the response, you need a quiet, calm environment where you can be alone for the duration of the exercise. Interruptions or background noise can, in the beginning, change your focus and prevent relaxation. A bedroom seems to be the best place in the home. At work, a private office or a conference room may be adequate. You may want to invest in a "Do Not Disturb" sign to hang on the door. (Even the bathroom can serve as your quiet place, especially if it is the only room in which you can be sure you won't be disturbed.)

2. A Mental Device: A relaxation state may be difficult to elicit because your mind is so busy with thoughts about daily activities. Repetition of a single-syllable word, in time with your exhalations, helps you to focus away from thoughts that are distracting and perhaps stressful. The word should be repeated silently or in a low, soothing tone. Some people prefer to picture a word or an object, and some gaze at an object—a flower or a stone. Traditionally, many different words, or "mantras," have been used. Because of its simplicity, follow Benson's suggestion and use the word "one."

3. A Passive Attitude: The opposite of stress and tension is relaxation. Unlike stress and tension, which can be generated within the body, relaxation cannot be forced to occur. Relaxation is a state that you can only allow to happen. Once you have learned the sequence

## Medical Treatment

In contrast to the first three categories where the individual is able to assume responsibility for the management strategies, the very nature of **medical treatment** means that some personal responsibility for controlling stress is given up. A health-care provider is frequently seen because of overt physical and mental symptoms or dysfunction. Often this results in a diagnosis and subsequent intervention efforts aimed at returning the person to a state of no discernible illness. People normally seek out a medical specialist or health-care provider as the result of midsight awareness, or after it is determined that something is wrong.

The health-care provider can prescribe medication for treating certain stress symptoms and diseases. In addition, the health-care provider has

ACTIVITY FOR 3.5
## WELLNESS

of the technique, there is no need to be concerned about whether or not relaxation is happening. The harder you work at making it happen, the less likely you are to relax. If your focus on the mental device is interrupted by sounds or people, or if your thoughts wander, passively disregard them. Just return to focusing on your exhalations and your mental device.

4. A Comfortable Position: This method can be learned in any of the basic positions. Your body needs to be comfortable and well supported, so that muscle tension is reduced as much as possible. If you find yourself drifting into sleep from a lying position, use a sitting position. Remove or loosen any tight-fitting clothes.

**BEZZOLA'S AUTOANALYSIS**

This method to relieve nervous tension was first described by Bezzola in Switzerland more than half a century ago. The body serves in the procedure as a perfect biofeedback instrument. Beata Jencks found this the most potent method for counteracting extreme nervousness. The procedure is simple.

> Sit or lie down comfortably, close the eyes, and pay attention passively to anything which goes on in the body. Put into audible words whatever happens. Do not analyze, do not intellectualize, but just pay attention and report what is sensed. Scan the body and feel more clearly what is happening in different places. For example, "Pressure in the stomach; eyes fluttering; right ear rings; throat tight; left foot itches." Omit all unnecessary words and all references to yourself such as "I" or "my." Just observe and verbalize the location and the sensations felt. Such attending brings gradually a quieting of spontaneous restlessness and a clearing of the mind.
>
> After a few minutes, sensations become fewer and a calm state, possibly sleep, follows. This simple exercise may be used as a treatment procedure by therapists, as a regular prophylactic rest period for overstressed professionals, or as an emergency tool for handling extreme nervousness. If the trainee has learned the method and is sure of his skills of relaxing with exhalations, he may combine the two.

Source: From *How to Relax: A Holistic Approach to Stress Management,* by John D. Curtis and Richard A. Detert, by permission of Mayfield Publishing Company. 

access to many of the same strategies of Social Engineering, Personality Engineering, and Relaxation Training. For example, a counselor is directly involved in facilitating individuals to examine their belief system, attitudes, or behavior patterns that may be causing distress. A patient educator might monitor a fitness program to control high blood pressure.

The promise of stress is found in the challenge of its management. There are countless strategies to develop should you decide to accept this challenge. These strategies can only be useful and growth-promoting to the degree they are utilized. Utilization or nonutilization of these management skills is often rooted in personal, social, and cultural forces. Consideration must be given to the role these forces play in enhancing or preventing individuals from employing stress-management strategies.

# PERSONAL AND SOCIAL INFLUENCES

Personal and social factors have an impact on whether stress becomes eustress or distress. Underlying all health attitudes and behaviors are a combination of cultural values, social pressures, and individual needs. The dynamic interaction of these factors can open a person to change and growth or serve as "barriers" to self-understanding and problem-solving.

Personal, social, and cultural factors are not isolated from one another. The individual develops and matures as the result of socialization experiences, which are often the result of enculturation and ethnic patterns. We learn through these life experiences how to adjust, adapt, and cope in the world. Here is a sample of factors that impact on how or whether we manage stress.

## Personal Considerations

There are many personal considerations that impact on our ability to manage stress. Several of these are discussed here.

**AN INABILITY TO PERCEIVE STRESS** Odd as it may seem, some individuals do not recognize that they are overstressed. Pressure, tension, and stress symptoms have become a "way of life." This is the way they have been, are, and will continue. Without recognition of stress, there can be little motivation for control of it.

**DEFENSE MECHANISMS** **Defense mechanisms** are our natural way to defend ourselves against stressors. For the most part they are unconscious ways of responding. They are learned and used in combination "to protect ourselves against distress . . . sometimes using fighting methods, sometimes taking flight, sometimes displacing onto others our feelings, sometimes immersing ourselves in hobbies, work, workshops, or exercise; and sometimes by getting sick."[22] Defense mechanisms can be great pressure valves and serve as a buffer to our ego and self-concept.

Defense mechanisms can also serve as barriers to managing stress effectively. When overused they can hinder the development of new and exciting ways of responding to stressful situations. They can keep people from expanding their repertoire of coping skills, thus blocking a more effective match between stressors and management strategies.

**PERSONAL PRAGMATISM** Personal pragmatism can be thought of as each person's internal standards for judging worth. Some individuals use their standard for judging the worth of stress-management efforts too quickly. Statements like "I tried it once and it didn't work" reflect a form of personal pragmatism. Learning new ways of responding to stress is different from practicing stress-management techniques until they become a part of us. When stress-management strategies are learned, *not* integrated, and then attempted during stressful situations, they can easily be evaluated as being ineffective.

Each person is the "expert" about his or her own needs; most individuals have at least a vague sense of what is needed to manage their lives better. If a person tries a strategy once and it doesn't work, it may not have been the one to use at that time regardless of the amount of time spent internalizing it. A comprehensive approach to stress management encourages personal pragmatism, experimentation, and personal freedom and choice.

## Social Influences

Social influences also affect our ability to manage stress.

**THE NEED FOR SOCIAL APPROVAL** Certain human needs are fulfilled through interaction with others. To be accepted and loved by significant others, such as family, peers, and teachers, is one of the strongest needs we have. It is one determinant of self-concept, happiness, and health status. During certain times in our lives, such as adolescence, peers have a larger influence than parents in meeting this need. During post–high-school years, individuals have given up a secure environment for one full of uncertainties; approval from others is especially important then. Pressure, real or perceived, can influence your attitudes and behaviors. Should your peers

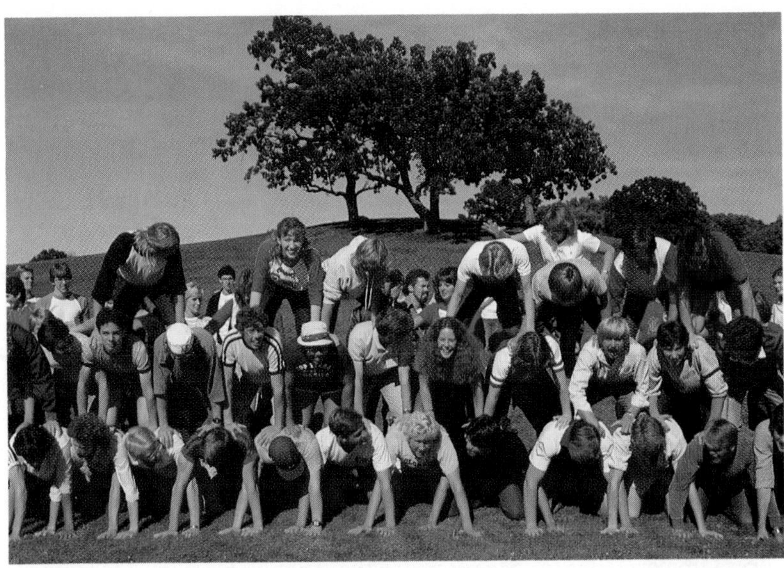

**Figure 3.9**
A strong social support network can help encourage your stress-management efforts.

view time spent at a meditation course as being a waste of time and money, you may begin to doubt its value. If the meditation also tends to conflict with your schedule of leisure activities with friends, you may discard the meditation. The need for approval from friends is a strong need and without it, stress-management efforts may be reduced.

Social approval can also be a motivator to become involved in new activities. If your friends believe in a "play" time each day to unwind from routine pressures, you gain approval by joining them. (See figure 3.9.)

**THE PACE OF AMERICAN LIFE** American society continues to be transformed at a rapid pace. In less than 100 years we moved from a predominantly agricultural society to an industrial society. The last two decades have led to another major shift—from the industrial era to the information era. In the information society, creating, processing, and distributing information "is" the job, not just a part of it. Computers are now the way to manage information. It is estimated that, within the near future, 75 percent of all jobs will include the use of computers.[23] Other major trends are currently transforming society and individual lives, including political, corporate, and population decentralization; movement from institutional help to self-help; and movement from a representative democracy to a participatory democracy. Rapid cultural changes have become the rule, not the exception. Change will continue to accelerate into the twenty-first century.[24]

Acceleration in the external environment is translated into acceleration within the internal environment. The psychological and physical arousal characteristic of the stress response is increased to accommodate rapid change. For many, the increased arousal is used to embrace change. Change is viewed as contributing to a wider range of lifestyles, increased freedom, and greater diversity. The stress response can be directed for positive adapting and purposeful functioning.

Unfortunately, the acceleration is too much for many individuals. A state of anomie develops. **Anomie** is a state characterized by confusion, disorientation, and anxiety. A person is unable to adjust adequately or to engage in adjustment strategies.

Acceleration from within also tends to increase pace. We are a people on the move; for many, good or bad days are measured by how much was accomplished. There is no time for stress management. It may be nice, but it is a low-priority item. For others, taking time to manage stress is perceived as being "lazy" or "wasting daylight hours." And for still others, taking time to manage stress signifies personal failure to keep up with others who do not appear to need recuperation. Individually, or collectively, getting caught in the mainstream of rapid pace can divert attention away from managing the pace to surviving within it.

**CAREER-ADVANCEMENT NORMS** A large portion of each day is spent at the worksite. A stimulating occupation coupled with the perceived satisfaction of pay, autonomy, peer and supervisory interaction, and security can be a rewarding and fulfilling way to spend this part of the day. Job-related stress is reduced when people are made to feel a part of the organization and have input into it.

Generally, however, the advancement norms in this country are stress producers and serve as barriers to taking action to reduce stress. Financial incentives, promotion, and retention are used as "carrots" for increased productivity. Striving for these carrots is stressful. For many it means long work days, weekends at the office, reduced personal and family time, work-related travel, and the like. The job becomes all-encompassing. Things are sacrificed in order to get the job done. Ulcers, hypertension, or headaches are used as a measure of "how hard one is working." Even when a certain measure of job success is reached, there are new stressors associated with maintaining it. Some become trapped by a desire to manage stress but an unwillingness to simplify their lives or reduce their standard of living. Our society promotes the idea that who we are as persons is closely tied to our occupation and financial status. As long as these norms are prevalent, certain barriers will exist to taking steps to reduce stress. There will always be the fear by some that to admit a need to control stress is a sign of incompetency. Theirs is the fear that one is losing "drive" or "initiative"—qualities that are highly desirable in certain occupations. If perceived in this manner, promotion, salary, reputation, or even continued employment could be at stake. Some are not willing to risk these to manage stress more effectively.

Enjoying life and its many challenges is a goal worth seeking. Channeling stress—taking the time to invest in life-management skills—is an important step toward that goal.

# SUMMARY

1. There are three important steps to managing stress for higher levels of wellness. First, assess your signs and symptoms of the stress response, the sources of stress, and appropriate stress-management techniques. Second, intervene to prevent or reduce the stress response. And third, establish a social support group that will reinforce your attempts to manage stress and experience the payoffs of wellness.

2. Stress is a state characterized by distinct physiological changes, such as an increased heart rate, increased breathing rate, increased perspiration, increased muscle tension, and a dry mouth.

3. Stressors are the stimuli that elicit the state of stress, also called the stress response.

4. Not all stressors elicit the same intensity of stress response. Some stressors may be very minor while others are quite devastating. Additionally, people perceive stressors differently—what may stimulate the stress response for you may not for a friend.

5. Selye has coined the term eustress to describe stress which is perceived as good, or leading to personal growth and fulfillment. Distress is stress which upsets our physical and psychological balance negatively, as a result of either too many stressors, or a lack of effective coping skills.

6. Physiologically, the stress response occurs through two major pathways of the body: the nervous system pathway, and the endocrine pathway. Chemical nerve transmitters and hormones activate the body to deal physically with stress.

7. In today's society there are few options for physically coping with stressors; thus we are often unable to use the stress response as it was originally intended. When fighting and running are not viable options, many people hold their stress inside and fail to cope effectively. Stress researchers believe this is one cause of the "diseases of adaptation."

8. The goal of stress management is to channel stress to promote stimulation and growth. Many skills can be learned to aid in channeling stress. Social engineering, personality engineering, relaxation, and medical care are all viable options for managing stress.

9. There are many personal considerations that directly influence one's ability to manage stress. Social norms interact with personal needs and desires and either enhance our coping skills or act as barriers to effective stress management.

### Recommended Readings

Benson, Herbert. *The Relaxation Response.* New York: Avon, 1975.

Curtis, John C., and Detert, Richard A. *How to Relax: A Holistic Approach to Stress Management.* Palo Alto, Calif.: Mayfield, 1981.

Greenberg, Jerry. *Comprehensive Stress Management.* Dubuque, Iowa: Wm. C. Brown Co., 1983.

Kriegel, Robert, and Kriegel, Marilyn Harris. *The C Zone.* Garden City, N.Y.: Anchor Press/Doubleday, 1984.

Lakein, Alan. *How to Get Control of Your Time and Your Life.* New York: Signet Books, 1973.

Selye, Hans. *Stress without Distress.* New York: Signet Books, 1974.

### References

1. John C. Curtis and Richard A. Detert, *How to Relax: A Holistic Approach to Stress Management* (Palo Alto, Calif.: Mayfield, 1981), 7–8.

2. James H. Humphrey, *A Textbook of Stress for College Students* (Springfield, Ill.: Charles C. Thomas, 1982), 6–9.

3. Hans Selye, *The Stress of Life* (New York: McGraw-Hill, 1976), 74.

4. Humphrey, *Stress,* 10.

5. Curtis and Detert, *How to Relax,* 19–20.

6. Walt Schaefer, *Stress, Distress, and Growth* (Calif.: Responsible Action, 1978), 30–31.

7. Edward Suchman, "Health Attitudes and Behavior," *Archives of Environmental Health* 20 (1970): 105–110.

8. Hans Selye, *Stress Without Distress.* (New York: Signet The New American Library, 1974), 27.

9. Selye, *Stress without Distress,* 28.

10. Selye, *Stress without Distress,* 28.

11. Gail Sheehy, *Passages: Predictable Crises of Adult Life* (New York: E. P. Dutton and Co., 1976), 20–21.

12. Thomas H. Holmes and Richard Rahe, "The Social Readjustment Rating Scale," *Journal of Psychosomatic Research* 11 (1976): 213.

13. Martin B. Mark, Thomas F. Garrity, and Frank R. Bowers, "The Influence of Recent Life Experiences on the Health of College Freshmen," *Journal of Psychosomatic Research* 19 (1975): 87–98.

14. Schaefer, *Stress, Distress, and Growth,* 147.

15. Schaefer, *Stress, Distress, and Growth,* 143–44.

16. Donald Tubesing and Nancy Tubesing, "The Treatment of Choice: Selecting Stress Skills to Suit the Individual and the Situation:" Paper presented at The First National Burnout Conference, Philadelphia, Pa., 3 November 1981.

17. Schaefer, *Stress, Distress, and Growth,* 147.

18. Daniel A. Girdano and George S. Everly, *Controlling Stress and Tension: A Holistic Approach* (Englewood Cliffs, N.J.: Prentice-Hall), 1979.

19. Meyer Friedman and Ray Rosenman, *Type A Behavior and Your Heart* (New York: Alfred A. Knopf, 1974).

20. John D. Curtis and Richard A. Detert, *Learn to Relax: A 14 Day Program.* (La Crosse, Wis.: Coulee Press, 1983), 14–15.

21. Curtis and Detert, *Learn to Relax,* 14–15.

22. Jerry Johnson, "More about Stress and Some Management Techniques," *Journal of School Health* 51.1 (January 1981): 40.

23. John Naisbitt, *Megatrends: Ten New Directions Transforming Our Lives.* (New York: Warner Books, 1982), 11–38.

24. Naisbitt, *Megatrends,* 24–38.

CHAPTER FOUR

# Nutrition: Eating for Health



Nutrition is currently a topic of great interest to many Americans. Advertisers spend large sums of money to sell us the newest culinary delights. Bookstores across the country carry hundreds of different books attempting to advise us on what and how much to eat. Community classes on healthy diets and cooking skills abound; health-food stores selling "health foods" continue to proliferate.

Nutrition may be of special interest or concern to college students. The college years are the first time many students choose or prepare their own meals. Many important nutritional questions arise for students. What are the best options for food selection in campus cafeterias? Are "fast foods" and "processed foods" nutritious options? In order to make appropriate decisions regarding personal nutritional requirements, students need a sound background in the science of nutrition.

Learning the basics of nutrition will help you decipher the many nutritional controversies prevalent today. We will also consider the impact of personal and social influences on our food choices. A tasty yet nutritious diet can add great enjoyment to life and make a considerable contribution to levels of wellness.

## THE TYPICAL AMERICAN DIET: A STATUS REPORT

American dietary patterns have changed dramatically over the past fifty years. In the early 1900s Americans consumed much greater amounts of grains, fruits, and vegetables. In fact, 56 percent of the typical American diet of the early 1900s came from carbohydrate sources such as these. At the same time, Americans at the turn of this century consumed lesser amounts of fats, salt, and refined and processed sugers. Today, the typical American diet consists of 46 percent carbohydrates, 42 percent fat, and 12 percent protein. These drastic changes in our diet have been unplanned and largely result from our affluent life-style.[1]

Many respected scientists have suggested that there are major associations between our "typical American diet" and many of the chronic and degenerative diseases prevalent today. In 1977, after much deliberation and review of expert testimony, the Senate Select Committee on Nutrition and Human Needs issued a report entitled *Dietary Goals for the United States*.[2] This major report points out that the dietary changes of the American people represent a great threat to public health, as they are linked to cardiovascular disease, cancer, hypertension, stroke, diabetes, and cirrhosis of the liver. The Senate Select Committee set as their major objective the improved health of all Americans through informed diet selection. Seven major goals were suggested by the Senate committee as a means for providing the American public with both a direction and a general magnitude for dietary change. (See table 4.1.)

These dietary goals have great potential for improving American dietary patterns. The dietary goals could intensify and expand the current nutritional consciousness of Americans. Although these goals may not be perfect, Americans in general can benefit from closely examining their dietary habits and making the recommended dietary changes. (See figure 4.1.)

**Table 4.1 U.S. Dietary Goals**

1. To avoid overweight, consume only as much energy (calories) as is expended; if overweight, decrease energy intake and increase energy expenditure.
2. Increase the consumption of complex carbohydrates and "naturally occurring" sugars from about 28 percent of energy intake to about 48 percent of energy intake.
3. Reduce the consumption of refined and processed sugars by about 45 percent to account for about 10 percent of total energy intake.
4. Reduce overall fat consumption from approximately 40 percent to about 30 percent of energy intake.
5. Reduce saturated-fat consumption to account for about 10 percent of total energy intake; and balance that with polyunsaturated and monounsaturated fats, which should account for about 10 percent of energy intake each.
6. Reduce cholesterol consumption to about 300 milligrams a day.
7. Limit the intake of sodium by reducing the intake of salt to about 5 grams a day.

Source: Select Committee on Nutrition and Human Needs, *Dietary Goals for the United States,* 2d ed. Washington, D.C.: U.S. Senate Select Committee, 1977.

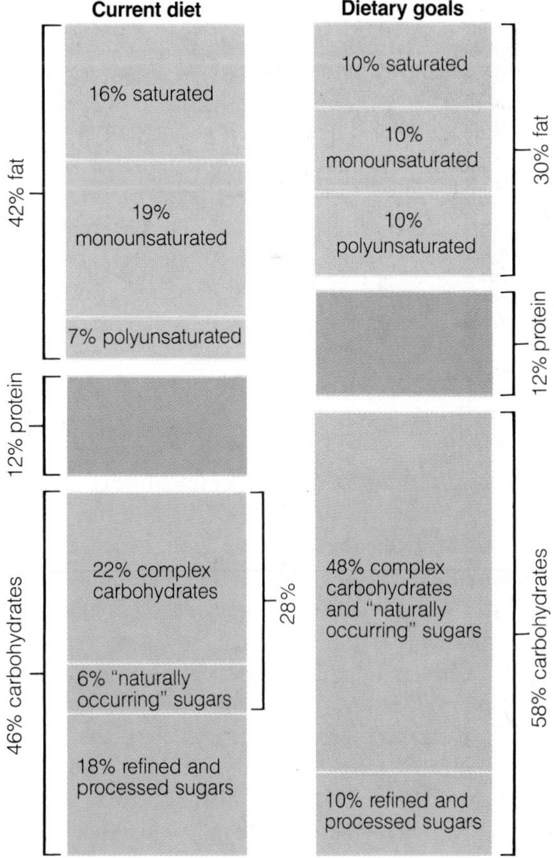


**Figure 4.1**
Percent of calories from different nutrients. *Source:* Select Committee on Nutrition and Human Needs, *Dietary Goals for the United States,* 2d ed. Washington, D.C.: U.S. Senate Select Committee, 1977.

# THE ABCs OF NUTRITION

We cannot live for long without food to fuel our bodies. Food supplies us with essential nutrients that are responsible for providing the body with energy and the materials necessary for growth and maintenance of body tissues. Of the six major nutrients, only three—carbohydrates, fats, and protein—actually contribute energy or **calories** (abbreviated kcal) to our diet. A calorie is a unit that measures the amount of energy we derive from a given food. Although they do not contribute calories, the remaining three nutrients—vitamins, minerals, and water—are important aids in utilizing the energy received from carbohydrates, fat, and protein.

In order for our bodies to function at an optimal level, we need a balanced diet that supplies us with the appropriate amounts of each of the six essential nutrient groups. The Food and Nutrition Board of the National Research Council periodically reviews the current information on nutritional needs of healthy Americans in order to set recommended amounts of the various nutrients. These recommendations are commonly known as the **RDA** or Recommended Daily Dietary Allowances. Table 4.2 presents the most recent RDA information.

## Carbohydrates

All **carbohydrates** consist of a combination of carbon, oxygen, and hydrogen atoms. Carbohydrates derive their name from the fact that their hydrogen and carbon atoms are always in the same proportion as in water—$H_2O$. Thus the name carbo (carbon) hydrate (water).

The major function of carbohydrates is to provide energy for the body. Carbohydrates are the body's preferred form of energy. Over the years, carbohydrates have been mislabeled as the "fattening nutrient." This is a fallacy of great significance. Carbohydrates provide only 4 kcal per gram, the same number of calories provided by a gram of protein and less than one-half the calories supplied by a gram of fat. In addition to their caloric value, carbohydrates can also be a rich source of vitamins, minerals, fiber, and water—all vital nutrients contributing significantly to health and levels of wellness.

Carbohydrates are typically divided into two categories: simple and complex. There are several major distinctions between these groups that merit a closer look.

### SIMPLE CARBOHYDRATES

Simple carbohydrates, often known as **simple sugars,** are the basic building blocks for carbohydrates. These simple sugars are technically known as **monosaccharides** and include glucose, fructose, and galactose. **Glucose** is the most important simple sugar in terms of optimal body functioning, as it is the major energy-supplying molecule in the body. All foodstuffs must eventually be broken down by the body to the basic glucose unit in order to be used as an energy source. Glucose is transported in the bloodstream, supplying all body tissues with energy vital for life. Appropriate blood-sugar levels are an important aspect of optimal functioning and high levels of wellness.

A second group of sugars, known as **disaccharides,** are molecules consisting of a combination of two simple sugars. Disaccharides include sucrose, maltose, and lactose.

#### Consumption of Sugar

It has been estimated that Americans eat an average of 125 pounds of sugar sweetener per person annually.[3] Of this, 76 percent is "invisible" sugars contained in processed foods and beverages which are prepared outside of the home. The next time you go to the grocery store, examine food labels for sugar—not just in baked goods, candies, and other "sweets," but in such food items as "fruit drinks," breakfast cereals, canned soups, prepared main dishes, and canned or frozen fruits. These processed foods, and many others, all contain hidden sugars. (See Activity for Wellness 4.1.)

Reading food labels will not always indicate how much sugar we are consuming. Even though food labels must list food components in decreasing proportional order, some manufacturers have found ways to confuse the consumer. Some breakfast cereal manufacturers, for instance, combine the various grains while separating the many types of sugars in their product.[4] Most manufacturers don't indicate exactly what percentage of sugar is contained in their products. This hampers the concerned consumer's attempts to estimate the sugar content of products. As a guide, *Consumer Reports* suggests looking for any word ending in "ose," such as maltose or dextrose.[5] Corn syrup, corn sugar, and corn

**Table 4.2 Recommended Daily Dietary Allowances (RDA). (Designed for the maintenance of good nutrition of practically all healthy persons in the United States.)**

| Sex-age category | Age: Years From | Age: Years To | Weight: Kilograms | Weight: Pounds | Height: Centimeters | Height: Inches | Food energy: Calories | Protein: Grams | Minerals: Calcium (Milligrams) | Minerals: Phosphorus (Milligrams) | Minerals: Iron (Milligrams) | Vitamin A (International units) | Thiamin (Milligrams) | Riboflavin (Milligrams) | Niacin (Milligrams) | Ascorbic acid (Milligrams) |
|---|---|---|---|---|---|---|---|---|---|---|---|---|---|---|---|---|
| Infants | 0 | 0.5 | 6 | 13 | 60 | 24 | kg × 115<br>lb × 52.3 | kg × 2.2<br>lb × 1.0 | 360 | 240 | 10 | 1,400 | 0.3 | 0.4 | 6 | 35 |
| | 0.5 | 1 | 9 | 20 | 71 | 28 | kg × 105<br>lb × 47.7 | kg × 2.0<br>lb × 0.9 | 540 | 360 | 15 | 2,000 | .5 | .6 | 8 | 35 |
| Children | 1 | 3 | 13 | 29 | 90 | 35 | 1,300 | 23 | 800 | 800 | 15 | 2,000 | .7 | .8 | 9 | 45 |
| | 4 | 6 | 20 | 44 | 112 | 44 | 1,700 | 30 | 800 | 800 | 10 | 2,500 | .9 | 1.0 | 11 | 45 |
| | 7 | 10 | 28 | 62 | 132 | 52 | 2,400 | 34 | 800 | 800 | 10 | 3,300 | 1.2 | 1.4 | 16 | 45 |
| Males | 11 | 14 | 45 | 99 | 157 | 62 | 2,700 | 45 | 1,200 | 1,200 | 18 | 5,000 | 1.4 | 1.6 | 18 | 50 |
| | 15 | 18 | 66 | 145 | 176 | 69 | 2,800 | 56 | 1,200 | 1,200 | 18 | 5,000 | 1.4 | 1.7 | 18 | 60 |
| | 19 | 22 | 70 | 154 | 177 | 70 | 2,900 | 56 | 800 | 800 | 10 | 5,000 | 1.5 | 1.7 | 19 | 60 |
| | 23 | 50 | 70 | 154 | 178 | 70 | 2,700 | 56 | 800 | 800 | 10 | 5,000 | 1.4 | 1.6 | 18 | 60 |
| | 51+ | | 70 | 154 | 178 | 70 | [2]2,400 | 56 | 800 | 800 | 10 | 5,000 | 1.2 | 1.4 | 16 | 60 |
| Females | 11 | 14 | 46 | 101 | 157 | 62 | 2,200 | 46 | 1,200 | 1,200 | 18 | 4,000 | 1.1 | 1.3 | 15 | 50 |
| | 15 | 18 | 55 | 120 | 163 | 64 | 2,100 | 46 | 1,200 | 1,200 | 18 | 4,000 | 1.1 | 1.3 | 14 | 60 |
| | 19 | 22 | 55 | 120 | 163 | 64 | 2,100 | 44 | 800 | 800 | 18 | 4,000 | 1.1 | 1.3 | 14 | 60 |
| | 23 | 50 | 55 | 120 | 163 | 64 | 2,000 | 44 | 800 | 800 | 18 | 4,000 | 1.0 | 1.2 | 13 | 60 |
| | 51+ | | 55 | 120 | 163 | 64 | [2]1,800 | 44 | 800 | 800 | 10 | 4,000 | 1.0 | 1.2 | 13 | 60 |
| Pregnant | | | | | | | +300 | +30 | +400 | +400 | [3]18+ | +1,000 | +.4 | +.3 | +2 | +20 |
| Lactating | | | | | | | +500 | +20 | +400 | +400 | 18 | +2,000 | +.5 | +.5 | +5 | +40 |

[1]Source: Adapted from *Recommended Dietary Allowances,* 9th ed., 1980, p. 185. Washington, D.C. 20418. National Academy of Sciences—National Research Council. Also available in libraries.

[2]After age seventy-five, energy requirement is 2,050 calories for males and 1,600 calories for females.

[3]The increased requirements cannot be met by ordinary diets; therefore, the use of supplemental iron is recommended.

**Note:** The Recommended Daily Dietary Allowances (RDA) should not be confused with the U.S. Recommended Daily Allowances (U.S. RDA). The RDA are amounts of nutrients recommended by the Food and Nutrition Board of the National Research Council and are considered adequate for maintenance of good nutrition in healthy persons in the United States. The allowances are revised from time to time in accordance with newer knowledge of nutritional needs.

The U.S. RDA are the amounts of proteins, vitamins, and minerals established by the Food and Drug Administration as standards for nutrition labeling. These allowances were derived from the RDA set by the Food and Nutrition Board. The U.S. RDA for most nutrients approximates the highest RDA of the sex-age categories in this table, excluding the allowances for pregnant and lactating females. Therefore, a diet that furnishes the U.S. RDA for a nutrient will furnish the RDA for most people and more than the RDA for many. U.S. RDA are protein, 45 grams (eggs, fish, meat, milk, poultry), 65 grams (other foods); vitamin A, 5,000 International Units; thiamin, 1.5 milligrams; riboflavin, 1.7 milligrams; niacin, 20 milligrams; ascorbic acid, 60 milligrams; calcium, 1 gram; phosphorus, 1 gram; iron, 18 milligrams. For additional information on U.S. RDA, see the "Federal Register," 38. 49 (14 March 1973): 6959–6960, and Agriculture Information Bulletin 382, "Nutritional Labeling—Tools for Its Use."

4.1 ACTIVITY FOR WELLNESS 4.1

# How Much Sugar?

Which contains a greater percentage of sugar?

1. Heinz Tomato Ketchup or Sealtest Chocolate Ice Cream?

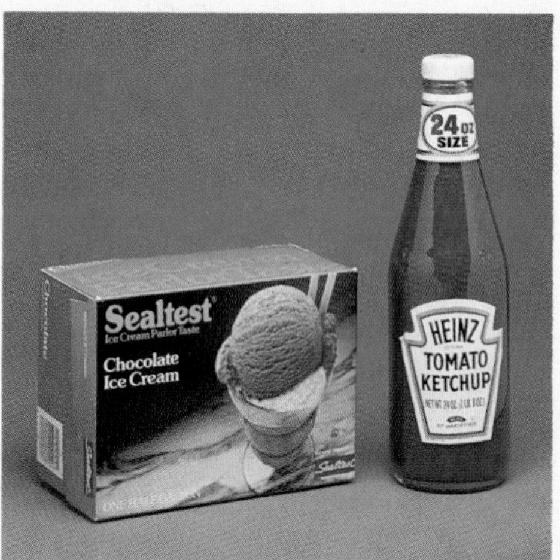


2. Wish-Bone Russian Dressing or Coca-Cola?

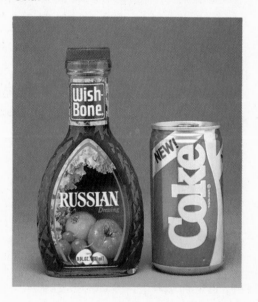


*Answers:*

1. The Heinz Tomato Ketchup is 29 percent sugar compared to 21 percent for the ice cream.
2. Wish-Bone Russian Dressing has 30 percent sugar, a proportion more than three times that of Coca-Cola (8.8 percent).
3. The Coffee-Mate, supposedly a substitute for cream, contains 65 percent sugar, compared to 51 percent for a Hershey bar.

Source: *Consumer Reports*, March 1978.

3. Coffee-Mate Non-Dairy Creamer or a bar of Hershey's Milk Chocolate?

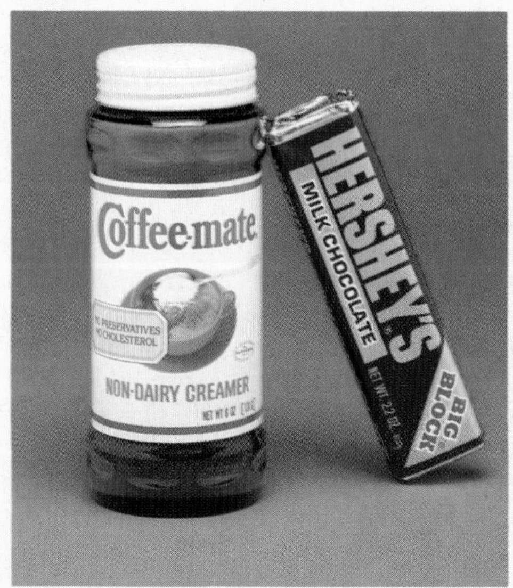

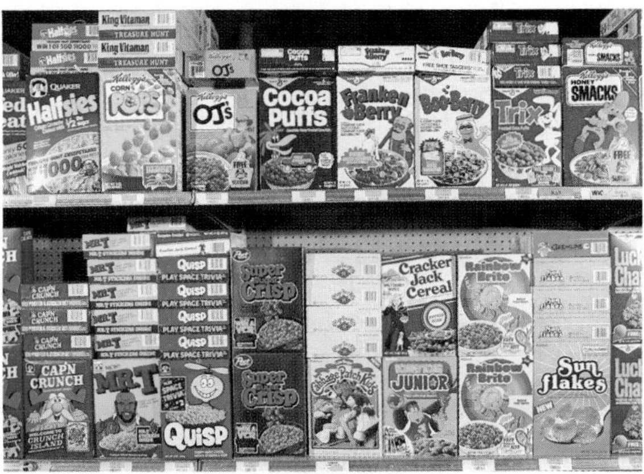


**Figure 4.2**
Breakfast cereals often contain large percentages of sugar. Start reading labels before you buy.

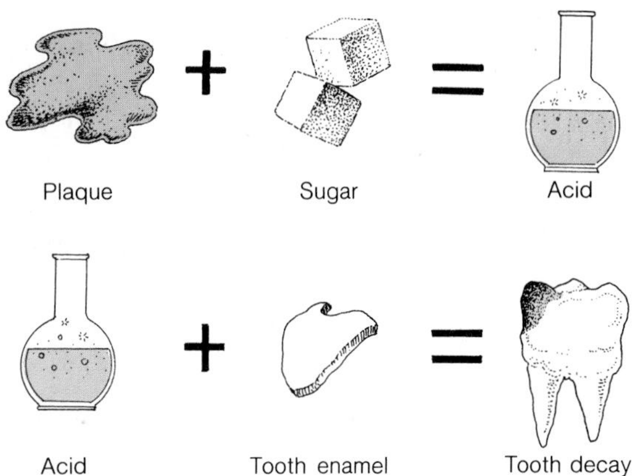


**Figure 4.3**
Tooth attack.

sweetener are other key words that indicate the addition of sugar. Some people believe that brown sugar, turbinado sugar, and honey are more "healthy" types of sugar. However, the few additional minerals they contain are so minute in quantity that they are of no practical significance in the total diet.[6] Generally, when reading labels the closer the sugars are to the top of the ingredient list, or the greater the total number of sugars listed, the more sugar that product contains.

Sugar represents between 20 and 25 percent of the calories in our diet. Just how dangerous is such a high consumption level? Nutritionist Jean Mayer believes that the evidence indicates that the typical American sugar-consumption level is highly undesirable in several ways.[7] First, sugar is a pure carbohydrate. Although it is a ready source of calories, it contains none of the other important nutrients such as vitamins, minerals, or protein. This is why sugar is often referred to as "empty calories." People who get 25 percent of their calories daily from sugar must rely on the other 75 percent of their diet to supply 100 percent of the nutrients necessary for optimal body functioning. This may be extremely difficult for the many Americans on weight-reduction (low-caloric) diets. Such individuals may be deficient in one or more of the nutrients vital for high levels of wellness.

Many books and articles have appeared in recent years linking sugar consumption with almost every noninfectious disease known today. Most medical and nutritional experts (including Mayer[8]) see little support in the research literature for these often-simplistic claims.[9] One disease, however, has been unquestionably linked to sugar consumption—tooth decay.

It has been estimated that 98 percent of American children have some tooth decay, and that by age fifty-five roughly 50 percent of Americans have no teeth.[10] **Dental caries** (tooth decay) is the most widespread degenerative disease in the Western world. Tooth decay begins with dental plaque, a sticky colorless film containing colonies of harmful bacteria that are constantly forming in your mouth. These bacteria break down food—especially sugar—changing it to an acid. The sticky plaque then holds this acid against your teeth allowing it to attack the tooth enamel. (See figure 4.3.)

Whether or not this attack will cause cavities depends on three factors: (1) the hardness of your tooth enamel; (2) the strength of the acids; and (3) the length of time the acid is on your teeth. Acids usually work on the tooth enamel for about fifteen to twenty minutes after sugary foods are eaten. If the teeth are not brushed immediately following each meal, three meals a day adds up to an hour of acid attack per day. Snacking—especially on sugary foods—increases your acid exposure.

4.2

ACTIVITY FOR
WELLNESS

## How to Brush and Floss

**BRUSHING**

For general adult usage, a straight-handled brush with soft polished nylon bristles is best. Whichever type of toothbrush is used, one should use it to brush at least twice a day, but preferably after every meal and at bedtime for maximum effect. The toothbrush is seldom used alone, most individuals use a commercial dentifrice (toothpaste, dental gel, or toothpowder) with their brush. Since all toothpastes and gels are similar, can one be better than another? Yes! How abrasive a dentifrice is and if it contains an acceptable fluoride should be the major concerns. One effective method of brushing follows:

1. Start by brushing along the gum line, moving the brush back and forth with short, gentle strokes.
2. Brush the outer and inner surface of each tooth, upper and lower.

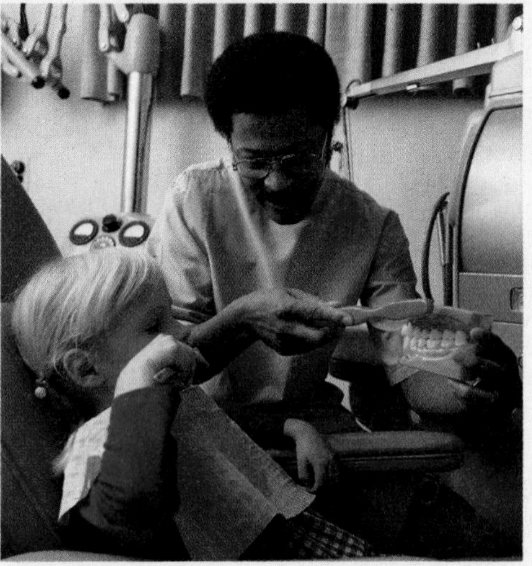

3. Brush the chewing surface of each tooth, upper and lower.
4. Brush your tongue to complete the process.

Cavities, however, do not occur overnight. It takes about three years for decay to make a hole by working its way through the enamel.[11] Changing your diet and dental-health habits may halt the decay process before a true cavity appears. Dental-health guidelines include:

1. Reduce consumption of sugars and foods high in sugar.
2. Avoid between-meal snacks of sweet or sticky foods. Replace with foods such as nuts, fresh fruits, raw vegetables, and milk.
3. Brush and floss teeth or rinse your mouth after meals and snacks—particularly after eating sweet or sticky foods.[12] (See Activity for Wellness 4.2.)
4. Use a toothpaste that contains fluoride. Studies have shown that fluoride helps in reducing cavities by reducing the tooth enamel's susceptibility to acid.[13]

**Achieving the U.S. Dietary Goals** Attempting to decrease your intake of refined and processed sugars by about 45 percent can be a challenge. The following suggestions will help you in your attempt to cut down on the sugar in your diet.

1. Limit your intake of soft drinks. This would bring many of us halfway to our goal. Substitute fruit juices or plain water for your daily beverages.
2. Processed baked goods, such as cakes, pies, cookies, and doughnuts, are estimated to be the second greatest source of sugar in the

## ACTIVITY FOR WELLNESS 4.2

### FLOSSING

A second method of disrupting the buildup of bacteria on the teeth is by using dental floss. Toothbrush bristles cannot reach plaque and small food particles caught between teeth. The following is a good technique for using floss correctly:

1. Break off a piece of floss about 18″ long.
2. Wind each end of the floss 2 or 3 times around the middle finger on each hand. If you are just beginning or have trouble manipulating the floss in the traditional way, try tying it in a loop and holding the loop between your two middle fingers. You should have about 2 inches of floss between your hands.
3. Hold the floss taut. Use your thumbs and forefingers to guide the floss gently between your teeth.
4. Keep the floss pressed against the surface of your tooth as you move it back and forth and toward the gum. Slide the floss just below the gum margin.
5. Use a straight up-and-down cleaning motion to get rid of plaque that has settled between your teeth.
6. When the floss gets soiled, move to a new section until you have finished flossing all your teeth. Make sure that you get the area behind your back molars, too.*

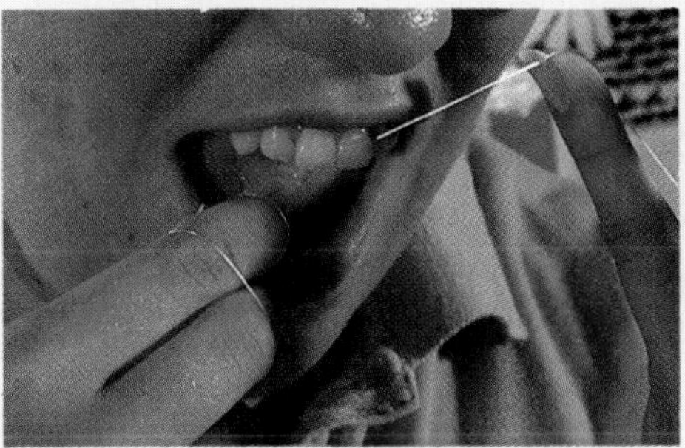

Source: Adapted from James H. Price, Nicholas Galli, and Suzanne Slenker, *Consumer Health: Contemporary Issues and Choices* (Dubuque, Iowa: Wm. C. Brown Publishers, 1985), 211–13.

*Brent Q. Hafen, *The Self Health Handbook* (Englewood Cliffs, N.J.: Prentice-Hall, 1980).

American diet.[14] Instead of eating sugary desserts, occasionally top off your meal with fresh fruit, which will satisfy your desire for something sweet while supplying valuable nutrients.

3. Many cereals are presweetened. Check the labels next time you shop and choose the unsweetened variety so that you can control the amount of sugar added.
4. If you add sugar to foods, such as coffee, tea, or cereal, gradually reduce the amount you use each time until you feel comfortable doing without it.
5. Read food labels. If some kind of sugar is listed in the top three ingredients you can be fairly certain there is a lot of sugar added to the product.
6. Begin to experiment with reducing the amount of sugar you add to foods prepared at home. Be prepared for foods that may look and taste different.

**COMPLEX CARBOHYDRATES** **Complex carbohydrates** (polysaccharides) consist of three or more simple-sugar molecules bonded together in varying patterns. The three most common types of complex carbohydrates are starch, fiber, and glycogen.

**Starch** **Starch** is a plant source of complex carbohydrate and may consist of 300 to 400 glucose molecules joined together. Common plant sources of starches include whole-grain foods, potatoes, rice,

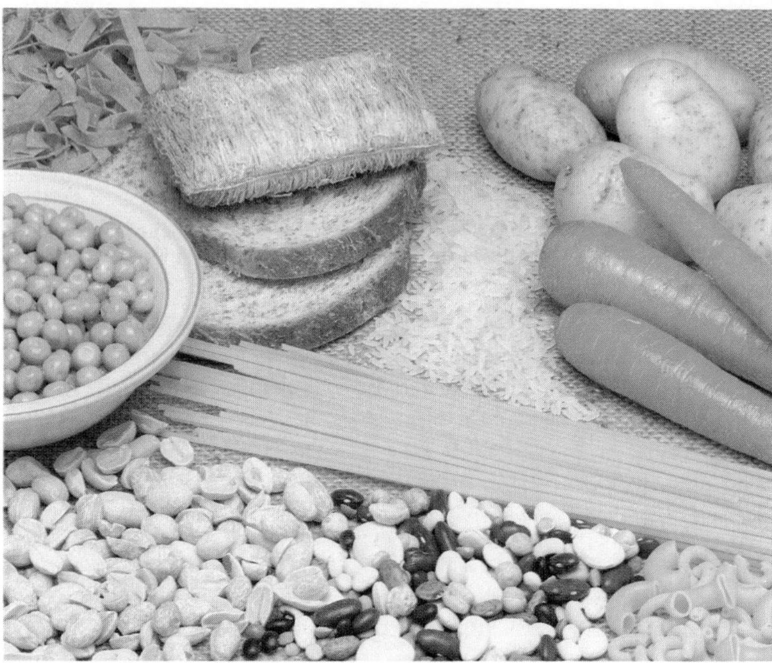

**Figure 4.4**
Starches, a plant source of complex carbohydrates, supply valuable vitamins, minerals, and protein.

beans, and vegetables. According to U.S. Dietary Goals, carbohydrates should provide the major portion of calories (energy) to our diets. Starch is the most important carbohydrate food source, supplying us with valuable vitamins, minerals, and protein in addition to calories. Wheat, corn, oats, and rice products such as bread, cereal, spaghetti, macaroni, and grits are especially good sources of nutritious starch. So are potatoes, peas, beans, nuts, and soybeans.[15] (See figure 4.4.)

**Fiber** Many of these nutritious sources of starch are also rich in fiber. **Dietary fiber** is commonly defined as the part of food that is not digested by enzymes in the small intestine, where most other foods are digested and absorbed into the bloodstream.[16] There are two major types of dietary fiber—insoluble and soluble. Both play important though somewhat different roles in our nutritional health and wellness.

**Insoluble fibers,** including cellulose, hemicellulose, and lignin, come from the cell walls of plants and are not digested by the body. Whole grains and beans are good sources of insoluble fiber, but wheat bran is by far the richest source. Insoluble fiber speeds up the movement of food through the digestive tract, absorbing water as it passes through. Insoluble fiber increases fecal bulk and contributes to regularity; it may thus play an important role in preventing constipation. Additionally, regular removal of waste from the intestines is believed to decrease the risk of developing colon cancer, ulcerative colitis, and other digestive disorders.[17] This may be due to the lowered time exposure of the intestines to toxic substances contained in the waste materials.

**Soluble fibers,** such as gums, pectins, and storage polysaccharides, are those fibers which, while remaining undigested in the small intestine, are digested and absorbed in the large intestine. Good sources of soluble fiber include oat bran, beans, and fruit, although most plant foods usually contain both soluble and insoluble fiber. Soluble fiber may play an important role in pacing the absorption of carbohydrates into the bloodstream.[18] Because these fibers tend to form gels, the nutrients in high-fiber foods are absorbed slowly over the entire length of the small intestine. This prevents dramatic swings in blood-sugar levels. Some believe soluble fiber may thus be important in controlling diabetes and hypoglycemia.[19] (See table 4.3.)

**Table 4.3 Dietary Fiber Content of Selected Foods**

| **Vegetables** | *Serving size (*½ cup cooked unless otherwise marked)* | *Total fiber (grams)* | *Soluble fiber (grams)* | *Insoluble fiber (grams)* |
|---|---|---|---|---|
| Peas | * | 5.2 | 2.0 | 3.2 |
| Parsnip | * | 4.4 | 0.4 | 4.0 |
| Potato | 1 small | 3.8 | 2.2 | 1.6 |
| Broccoli | * | 2.6 | 1.6 | 1.0 |
| Zucchini | * | 2.5 | 1.1 | 1.4 |
| Squash, summer | * | 2.3 | 1.1 | 1.2 |
| Carrot | * | 2.2 | 1.5 | 0.7 |
| Tomato | * | 2.0 | 0.6 | 1.4 |
| Brussels sprouts | * | 1.8 | 0.7 | 1.1 |
| Beans, string | * | 1.7 | 0.6 | 1.1 |
| Onion | * | 1.6 | 0.8 | 0.8 |
| Rutabaga | * | 1.6 | 0.7 | 0.9 |
| Beet | * | 1.5 | 0.6 | 0.9 |
| Kale greens | * | 1.4 | 0.6 | 0.8 |
| Turnip | * | 1.3 | 0.6 | 0.7 |
| Asparagus | * | 1.2 | 0.3 | 0.9 |
| Eggplant | * | 1.2 | 0.7 | 0.5 |
| Radishes | ½ cup raw | 1.2 | 0.3 | 0.9 |
| Cauliflower | * | 0.9 | 0.3 | 0.6 |
| Beans, sprouted | * | 0.9 | 0.3 | 0.6 |
| Cucumber | ½ cup raw | 0.8 | 0.5 | 0.3 |
| Lettuce | ½ cup raw | 0.5 | 0.2 | 0.3 |
| **Fruits** | *Serving size (raw)* | *Total fiber (grams)* | *Soluble fiber (grams)* | *Insoluble fiber (grams)* |
| Apple | 1 small | 3.9 | 2.3 | 1.6 |
| Blackberries | ½ cup | 3.7 | 0.7 | 3.0 |
| Pear | 1 small | 2.5 | 0.6 | 1.9 |
| Strawberries | ¾ cup | 2.4 | 0.9 | 1.5 |
| Plums | 2 med | 2.3 | 1.3 | 1.0 |
| Tangerine | 1 med | 1.8 | 1.4 | 0.4 |
| Apricots | 2 med | 1.3 | 0.9 | 0.4 |
| Banana | 1 small | 1.3 | 0.6 | 0.7 |
| Grapefruit | ½ | 1.3 | 0.9 | 0.4 |
| Peach | 1 med | 1.0 | 0.5 | 0.5 |
| Cherries | 10 | 0.9 | 0.3 | 0.6 |
| Pineapple | ½ cup | 0.8 | 0.2 | 0.6 |
| Grapes | 10 | 0.4 | 0.1 | 0.3 |

**Table 4.3** *Continued*

| **Breads, Cereals** | *Serving Size (*½ cup cooked unless otherwise indicated)* | *Total fiber (grams)* | *Soluble fiber (grams)* | *Insoluble fiber (grams)* |
|---|---|---|---|---|
| Bran (100 percent) cereal# | * | 10.0 | 0.3 | 9.7 |
| Popcorn | 3 cups | 2.8 | 0.8 | 2.0 |
| Rye bread# | 1 slice | 2.7 | 0.8 | 1.9 |
| Whole-grain bread# | 1 slice | 2.7 | 0.08 | 2.6 |
| Rye wafers# | 3 | 2.3 | 0.06 | 2.2 |
| Corn grits | * | 1.9 | 0.6 | 1.3 |
| Oats, whole | * | 1.6 | 0.5 | 1.1 |
| Graham crackers# | 2 | 1.4 | 0.04 | 1.4 |
| Brown rice | * | 1.3 | 0 | 1.3 |
| French bread# | 1 slice | 1.0 | 0.4 | 0.6 |
| Dinner roll# | 1 | 0.8 | 0.03 | 0.8 |
| Egg noodles | * | 0.8 | .03 | 0.8 |
| Spaghetti | * | 0.8 | .02 | 0.8 |
| White bread# | 1 slice | 0.8 | 0.03 | 0.8 |
| White rice | * | 0.5 | 0 | 0.5 |
| **Legumes** | | | | |
| Kidney beans# | * | 4.5 | 0.5 | 4.0 |
| White beans# | * | 4.2 | 0.4 | 3.8 |
| Pinto beans | * | 3.0 | 0.3 | 2.7 |
| Lima beans | * | 1.4 | 0.2 | 1.2 |
| **Nuts** | | | | |
| Almonds | 10 | 1.0 | | |
| Peanuts | 10 | 1.0 | | |
| Walnuts, black | 1 tsp. chopped | 0.6 | | |
| Pecans | 2 | 0.5 | | |

Currently, researchers use different methods to analyze dietary fiber content in foods. Until a single testing protocol is adopted, precise fiber totals will vary from laboratory to laboratory.

Meats, milk products, eggs, and fats and oils are not listed in this food-fiber survey because they are virtually devoid of fiber content.

This symbol, (#), indicates that the fiber analysis was carried out on cooked food, rather than raw food.

Source: Reprinted by permission of *Nutrition Action Healthletter*, published by the Center for Science in the Public Interest.

**Glycogen** **Glycogen,** the third major complex carbohydrate, is formed in the body by a process that binds glucose molecules. Glycogen is the principal way the body stores sugar for energy needs. Glycogen is stored mainly in the liver and voluntary skeletal muscles; it can be called on in stressful situations as a source of ready energy. During a stressful situation, the fight-or-flight response triggers the breakdown of glycogen into glucose where it is then released into the bloodstream to be used for quick energy.

**ACHIEVING THE U.S. DIETARY GOALS** Increasing your consumption of complex carbohydrates and "naturally occurring" sugars to about 48 percent of your total energy intake may present a challenge. The following suggestions will help you in your attempt to increase your intake of complex carbohydrates.

1. Include more of these foods in your meals: fruits, vegetables, breads, cereals, dry beans, and dry peas.
2. Whenever possible buy fresh fruits and vegetables, as they are likely to have greater amounts of vitamins and minerals than processed varieties. When fresh fruits and vegetables are not available, frozen produce is preferable to canned because it retains more nutrient value.[20]
3. Increase your consumption of whole-grain products, such as whole-wheat bread, whole-grain (wheat, rye, or oat) cereal, and brown rice. Refined-grain products, such as white bread, white enriched or instant rice, macaroni, egg noodles, and the like, have undergone processing that removes valuable nutrients and fiber. Some of these lost nutrients are replaced in products labeled as "enriched," but there is a danger that nutrients, both known and unknown, have been removed or altered in ways not currently understood.[21]

## Fats

**Fats,** also known as lipids, are a group of chemical compounds which, like carbohydrates, are composed of carbon, hydrogen, and oxygen atoms linked together in specific ways. Fat is the second major source of energy for the body, supplying 9 kcal for every gram of fat consumed. Because a gram of fat is a condensed source of energy, that is, it contains more than twice the amount of calories contained in one gram of protein or carbohydrate, it is a perfect way for the body to store energy. Body fat stores energy (calories) in **adipose** (fat) cells for the times you will need more energy than your diet supplies. Your adipose tissue also serves as padding to protect vital organs of the body, and helps insulate the body from extremely cold weather. Fat molecules also form the chemical core of certain hormones, and help transport and store certain vitamins. Fats are a popular food component because they add flavor and texture to our foods. Fats also contribute to a feeling of satisfaction after eating because they slow down the rate at which food is emptied from the stomach.

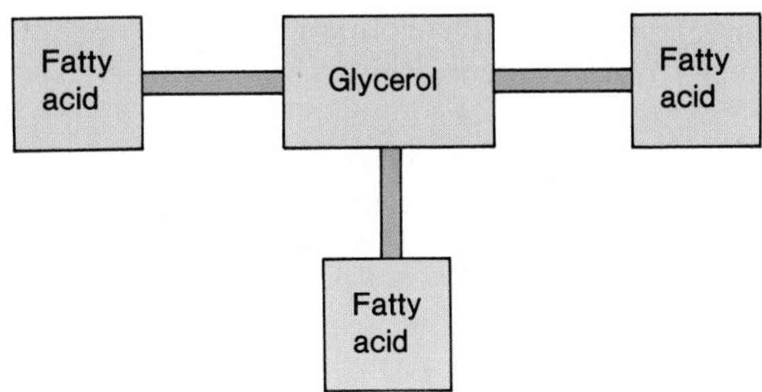


**Figure 4.5**
Structure of atriglyceride. *Source:* From Williams, Melvin H. *Nutrition for Fitness and Sport.* © 1984 Wm. C. Brown Publishers, Dubuque, Iowa. All rights reserved. Reprinted by permission.

**SATURATED AND UNSATURATED FATS** There are three major types of fat in the body: triglycerides, phospholipids, and sterols. **Triglycerides** are the major dietary source of fat; 95 percent of all fat consumed in food consists of triglycerides. Triglycerides are composed of two different clusters of atoms—glycerol and fatty acids. Each triglyceride consists of three fatty-acid molecules attached to a glycerol molecule. (See figure 4.5.)

Some triglycerides are a major source of dietary concern because of the type of fatty acid they contain. Fatty acids consist of a chain of carbon and hydrogen atoms with a few oxygen atoms on the side. If all of the carbon atoms are linked together with single bonds it allows the maximum number of hydrogen atoms to bond to the molecule. Thus, it is said to be **saturated** with hydrogen. Some fatty-acid molecules have one double bond between their carbon atoms and therefore cannot carry the maximum hydrogen atoms. This type of fatty acid is said to be **monounsaturated.** In still other fatty acids there are two or more double bonds between the carbon atoms making these fatty acids **polyunsaturated.** (See figure 4.6.)

**Saturated fats**

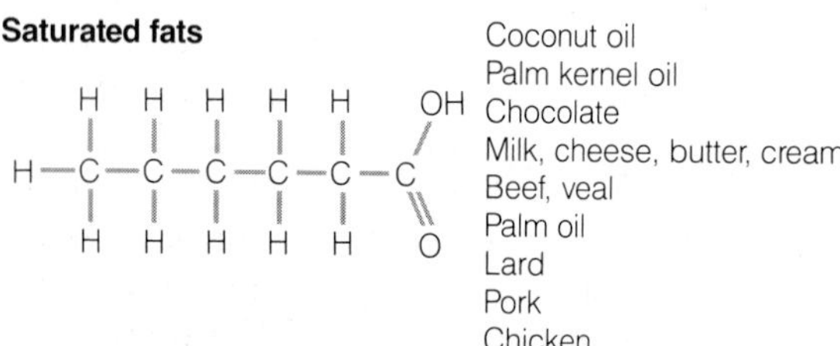


**Monounsaturated fats**

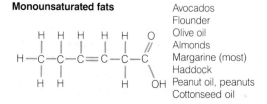

Avocados
Flounder
Olive oil
Almonds
Margarine (most)
Haddock
Peanut oil, peanuts
Cottonseed oil

**Polyunsaturated fats**

Soft margarine (most)
Sesame oil
Mayonnaise
Soybean oil
Corn oil
Sunflower oil
Safflower oil

**Figure 4.6**
Structure of saturated, monounsaturated, and polyunsaturated fats. *Source:* Reprinted by permission of *Nutrition Action Healthletter,* published by the Center for Science in the Public Interest.

Animal fats generally contain greater proportions of saturated fatty acids; plant fats usually contain monounsaturated or polyunsaturated fatty acids. Additionally, saturated fats are usually solid at room temperature while unsaturated fats tend to be liquid at room temperature. There is one major exception to these generalities. Both coconut oil and palm oil are highly saturated fats.

Once again, reading food labels to check on whether or not a product contains animal or plant sources of fat will not always tell you the complete story. Manufacturers commonly use a technique called **hydrogenation** in which they add hydrogen to polyunsaturated or monounsaturated fats. Consuming a product with hydrogenated corn oil is not the same as consuming one with plain corn oil. Even though both oils are from a plant source, the process of hydrogenation will cause the corn oil to become more saturated.

Diets high in fat, especially saturated fat, have been linked with many of the chronic and degenerative diseases prevalent today. The link appears to be strongest between saturated fat, cholesterol, and coronary-artery disease.[22] Food rich in saturated fats, such as beef, milk, cheese, coconut oil, and palm oil, have been shown to cause elevations in the blood-cholesterol levels of humans. Monounsaturated fats appear to have no influence on blood-cholesterol level; polyunsaturated fats appear to lower blood cholesterol. (See figure 4.7.)

**THE CHOLESTEROL CONTROVERSY** **Cholesterol,** the subject of great nutritional controversy, is a fatlike waxy material found in animal tissues. It is technically classified as a sterol. Cholesterol plays an important role in many body functions. It is a major constituent of cell membranes and the

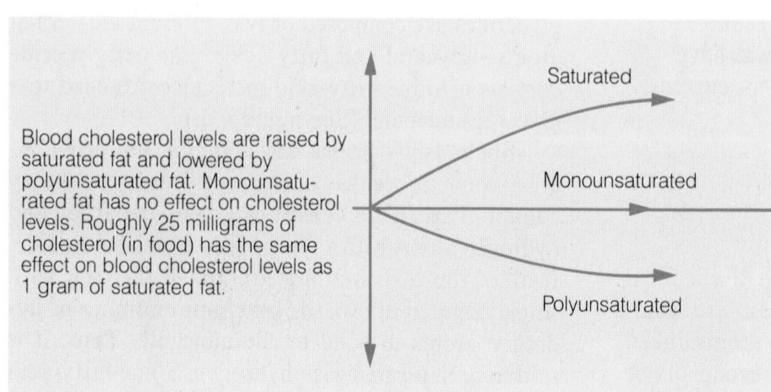

Blood cholesterol levels are raised by saturated fat and lowered by polyunsaturated fat. Monounsaturated fat has no effect on cholesterol levels. Roughly 25 milligrams of cholesterol (in food) has the same effect on blood cholesterol levels as 1 gram of saturated fat.
Saturated
Monounsaturated
Polyunsaturated


**Figure 4.7**
Effects of fats on blood cholesterol levels. *Source:* Reprinted by permission of *Nutrition Action Healthletter,* published by the Center for Science in the Public Interest.

covering that protects nerve fibers. Cholesterol also aids in the formation of vitamin D and the sex hormones androgen, estrogen, and progesterone. Cholesterol is also used by the body to produce bile acids which in turn aid in digesting fats.

The body receives cholesterol from two major sources. Cholesterol is ingested in the animal products we consume, and it is manufactured by the body itself in the liver and small intestine. (See figure 4.8.)

Cholesterol is carried in the bloodstream by special protein molecules called **lipoproteins.** The best understood in terms of their role regarding cholesterol are high-density lipoproteins (**HDL**), low-density lipoproteins (**LDL**), and very-low-density lipoproteins (**VLDL**). HDL cholesterol is sometimes referred to as the "good cholesterol," and LDL and VLDL as the "bad." LDL and VLDL carry cholesterol and other fat molecules in the bloodstream from the digestive tract to the body cells where they are needed for various body functions. If these cells receive too much fat it spills over into the bloodstream where the fat and cholesterol may tend to build up. This buildup over time may totally clog the arteries and cause heart attacks. HDL also carries cholesterol, but it carries the excess from the cells to the liver where it can be excreted by the body. Large population studies in the U.S. have shown that LDL and VLDL are associated with an increased risk of coronary-artery disease; HDL appears to protect us from this disease.[23]

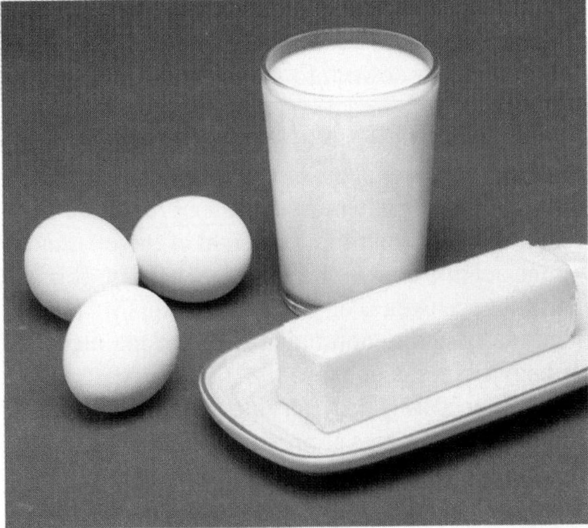

**Figure 4.8**
Cholesterol can play a beneficial role in many bodily functions—if it is consumed in moderation.

The major controversy surrounding cholesterol pertains to its relationship to coronary-artery disease. Most experts will agree that high blood-cholesterol levels are associated with a greater-than-average risk of developing coronary-artery disease.[24] Disagreement arises when some researchers and health-care providers suggest dietary changes for the American population aimed at reducing their intake of cholesterol and saturated fats. In January 1984 the first definitive study linking a reduction in blood cholesterol to a reduction in deaths from coronary-artery disease was released. In this ten-year study, experimental subjects who reduced their blood-cholesterol levels by 25 percent were found to have 50 percent less heart disease.[25] This study lends support to those experts recommending dietary changes aimed at lowering blood-cholesterol levels. There seems to be no serious risk to health or wellness from reducing fats and cholesterol in our diet and replacing them with greater amounts of complex carbohydrates and the potential benefits are great. (Heart disease and its many risk factors are discussed in greater detail in chapter 15.)

**ACHIEVING THE U.S. DIETARY GOALS** It has been recommended that Americans decrease their intake of fat to about 30 percent of their total energy (caloric) intake. They should also reduce saturated-fat consumption to account for about 10 percent of their total energy intake, while balancing it with polyunsaturated and monounsaturated fats, which should each account for about 10 percent of total energy intake. Cholesterol consumption should be limited to about 300 milligrams a day. The following suggestions should help you on your way to reducing fats and cholesterol in your diet.

1. Include more of these foods in your meals: fruits (except avocados and olives), vegetables, breads, cereals, dry beans, and dry peas.
2. Cut down on fatty meats. This includes regular ground beef, corned beef, spareribs, sausage, hot dogs, luncheon meat, and heavily marbled cuts, such as prime rib. Keep in mind that different grades of meat contain different amounts of fat. Prime beef contains more fat than Choice, and Choice more than Good.
3. Include more fish, chicken, and turkey in your diet. These foods are generally lower than many meats in fat content.

4. Leaner cuts of red meats include: flank, round, rump (beef); leg, loin (lamb); all cuts of veal.
5. Pork cuts, such as lean ham, loin, Boston butt, and picnic, are moderate in fat content and should be used only in moderation.
6. Limit nuts, peanuts, and peanut butter, which contain considerable amounts of fat.
7. Trim excess fat from meat before cooking.
8. Bake, broil, roast, stew, or barbeque foods using a rack for cooking so that fat will drain away from the food. Avoid fried foods.
9. Baste meats with wine, tomato juice, or the like, rather than using meat drippings.
10. Make stews and soups a day ahead. Chill them and scrape off the congealed fat before reheating.
11. Reduce the use of whole milk and whole-milk products, such as most cheeses and ice cream. Substitute skim or low-fat milks and their products, such as uncreamed cottage cheese, which are lower in fat content.
12. Select salad oils, cooking oils, and margarines that are high in polyunsaturated fats. Avoid hydrogenated fats.
13. Egg yolks are very high in cholesterol. Cut back your consumption of egg yolks to three per week. Try replacing breakfast eggs with high-fiber cereals.

## Protein

Like carbohydrates and fat, **protein** is composed of carbon, hydrogen, and oxygen. Protein, however, has an important distinguishing element—nitrogen. Nitrogen gives protein the important function of growth, maintenance, and regulation of body tissues and processes. All proteins are formed from varying combinations of twenty-one specific nitrogen-containing chemicals called **amino acids.**[26] These amino acids are often referred to as the building blocks of protein because they string together to form an almost-endless variety of protein molecules, much like we string together the letters of the alphabet in order to form different words.

Protein is a major component of almost every cell in the body; it helps build muscle, bone, skin, and blood. Protein is a major constituent of antibodies, an important part of our immune system, so it helps us fight infections. It also aids in the formation of hormones, such as insulin and thyroxine, which regulate our bodies' chemical processes (**metabolism**). Protein plays an important role in forming enzymes, which control the speed of various chemical reactions. Protein also carries iron, oxygen, and nutrients to all the cells of the body. Next to water, protein is the major constituent of the human body.

In addition to its many tissue-building, maintenance, repair, and regulation functions, protein can also be used by the body as a source of energy. Protein, like carbohydrates, supplies the body with 4 kcals per gram consumed. If your diet does not contain enough carbohydrates or fat to be used as energy, your body will use protein, even at the expense of building or maintaining your body tissue. On the other hand, if you consume more protein than your body needs for growth and maintenance, the extra protein is broken down to be used for calories or is converted into body fat and stored. Protein, however, is an expensive and inefficient source of calories for the body. When protein is broken down to be used for energy, not all of the protein molecule is used. The nitrogen is not needed and must therefore be excreted by the kidneys. As health writer Jane Brody wrote, "Americans excrete the most expensive urine in the world. If it were economical to collect and dry it, tons of nitrogen could be harvested from the nation's toilet bowls each day."[27]

In order to be used by the body, protein must first be broken down into amino acids. During this breakdown the human body can make many of the amino acids it needs for efficient building of body tissues. There are eight **essential amino acids,** however, which the body must consume preformed from food. Any food containing all eight of these essential amino acids is known as a **complete protein.** It is important to consume complete or high-quality protein foods daily so that optimal growth and maintenance of body tissues is enhanced.

It is relatively easy for most Americans to consume quality sources of protein daily. Meat, poultry, fish, and milk products are all good sources of complete protein. Many of these good sources of protein, however, are animal sources and thus are likely to be high in saturated fat, cholesterol, and calories.

**Table 4.4 The Percent of Fat Calories in Our Food**

**75 Percent or More**

Avocado
Bacon
Beef—Choice grade of chuck rib, sirloin, and loin untrimmed, hamburger (regular)
Coconut
Cold cuts—bologna, Braunschweiger, salami
Coleslaw
Cream—heavy, light, half-and-half, sour
Cream cheese
Frankfurters
Headcheese
Nuts—walnuts, peanuts, cashews, almonds, etc.
Olives
Peanut butter
Pork—sausage, spareribs, butt, loin, and ham untrimmed
Salt pork
Seeds—pumpkin, sesame, sunflower

**50 Percent to 75 Percent**

Beef—rump, corned
Cake—pound
Canadian bacon
Cheese—blue, cheddar, American, Swiss, etc.
Chicken, roasted with skin
Chocolate candy
Cream soups
Eggs
Ice cream (rich)
Lake trout
Lamb chops, rib
Oysters, fried
Perch, fried
Pork—ham, loin, and shoulder (trimmed lean cuts)
Tuna with oil
Tuna salad
Veal

**40 Percent to 50 Percent**

Beef—T-bone (lean only), hamburger (lean)
Cake—devil's food with chocolate icing
Chicken, fried
Ice cream (regular)
Mackerel
Milk, whole
Pumpkin pie
Rabbit, stewed
Salmon, canned
Sardines (drained)
Turkey pot pie
Yogurt (whole milk)

**30 Percent to 40 Percent**

Beef—flank steak, chuck pot roast (lean)
Cake—yellow, white (without icing)
Chicken, roasted without skin
Cottage cheese, creamed
Fish—flounder, haddock (fried), halibut (broiled)
Granola
Ice milk
Milk, 2 percent
Pizza
Seafood—scallops and shrimp (breaded and fried)
Soups—bean with pork
Tuna in oil (drained)
Turkey, roasted dark meat
Yogurt (low fat)

**20 Percent to 30 Percent**

Beef—sirloin (lean only)
Corn muffin
Fish—cod (broiled)
Liver
Oysters, raw
Pancakes
Shake, thick
Soups—chicken noodle, tomato, vegetable
Wheat germ

**Less than 20 Percent**

Beans, peas, and lentils
Bread
Buttermilk
Cabbage, boiled
Cakes—angel food, sponge
Cereals, breakfast (except granola)
Cottage cheese, uncreamed
Fish—ocean perch (broiled)
Frozen yogurt
Fruits
Grains
Milk, skim
Seafood—scallops and shrimp (steamed or boiled)
Soups—split pea, bouillon, consommé
Tuna in water
Turkey, roasted white meat
Vegetables

Source: Reprinted from *Jane Brody's Nutrition Book,* by permission of W. W. Norton & Company, Inc. Copyright © 1981 by Jane E. Brody.

Remembering to choose leaner cuts of red meat, trim off excess fat, and cook with less fat can be of much help. Poultry, fish, and low-fat milk products also contain less fat, cholesterol, and calories without losing their protein value. (See figure 4.9.)

Many plant sources of protein are lacking in one or more of the essential amino acids. Plant foods, however, can be good sources of complete protein if two or more complementary sources are combined in one meal so that one food supplies the essential amino acids missing in the other. You have, no doubt, eaten such complementary protein pairs as peanut butter and whole-wheat bread sandwiches, macaroni and cheese, or skim milk on cereal. (See table 4.5.)

According to the dietary goals, most Americans are getting adequate amounts of high-quality protein. The major change recommended for protein can be accomplished by eliminating some of our fatty sources of protein (animal products) and replacing them with complex-carbohydrate sources. However, we must be careful to remember to eat complementary sources of plant protein.

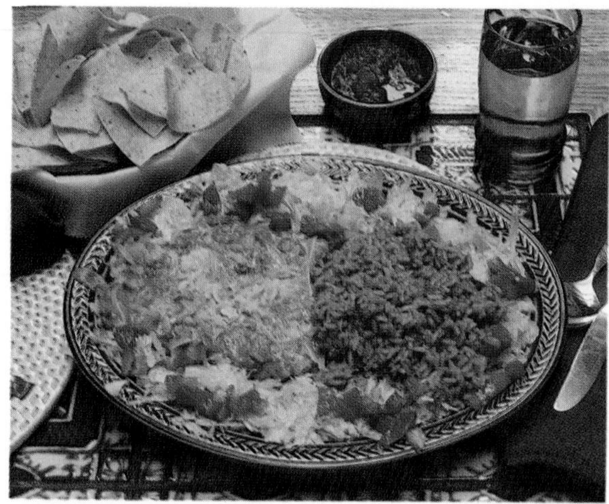

**Figure 4.9**
Mexican dinners typically feature beans and rice, two complex carbohydrates that together form a complete protein.

**Table 4.5 How to Mix and Match Protein Pairs**

To make protein-rich combinations, you can:

*Number 1—Match vegetable proteins:*
mix foods from two or more groups in column A such as: peanut butter (a legume) and whole-wheat bread (a grain).

*Number 2—Match vegetable and low-fat animal proteins:*
mix foods from any group(s) in column A with small amounts from any group(s) in column B such as: rice (a grain) and chicken (a lowfat meat).

| A | B |
|---|---|
| *Vegetable Proteins ("Incompletes")* | *Low-fat Animal Proteins ("Completes")* |
| Legumes: | Low-fat dairy products: |
| dry beans and peas—kidney, navy, lima, pinto, black, or soy beans | nonfat dry milk |
| black-eyed or split peas | skim milk |
| soy bean curd (tofu) | low-fat cottage cheese |
| soy flour | egg whites (where most of the egg protein lies) |
| peanuts and peanut butter (use wisely, has medium fat level) | Low-fat meats: |
| Grains: | poultry |
| whole grains—barley, oats, rice, rye, wheat (bulgur, cracked wheat) | fish |
| corn | lean cuts of red meat |
| pasta—noodles, spaghetti, macaroni, lasagna | |
| Nuts and seeds: | |
| almonds, cashews, pecans, and walnuts, sunflower seeds, pumpkin seeds, sesame seeds | |

*Remember:* To make the most of vegetable protein pairs, eat them at the *same* meal.

Source: *Eaters Almanac*, National Heart, Lung, and Blood Institute, National Institutes of Health, Bethesda, Md.

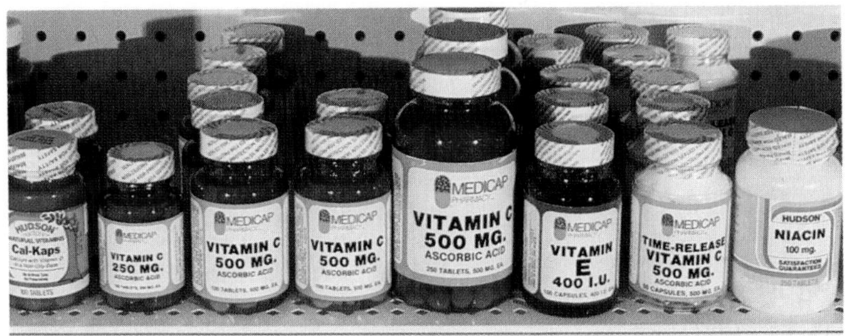


**Figure 4.10**
More is rarely better when it comes to vitamins and minerals.

## Vitamins

The body has a special need for small amounts of certain chemicals to help perform many complex chemical reactions. These chemicals are commonly referred to as **vitamins.** A substance is defined as a vitamin if it plays a vital role in human metabolism and a deficiency disease results when inadequate amounts are consumed.

Vitamins are commonly grouped into two categories: fat soluble and water soluble. **Fat-soluble vitamins** (A, D, E, and K) are transported and stored by the body's fat cells. Because the body stores these vitamins they can build up in the system and become toxic if great quantities (megadoses) are consumed. The **water-soluble vitamins** (eight B vitamins and vitamin C) are not stored by the body and therefore need to be consumed in adequate proportions in the diet daily. Tables 4.6 and 4.7 describe these vitamins, including their food sources, functions, and symptoms caused by deficiency and megadose.

Vitamin consumption is one area of health and wellness where quackery abounds. Some of the more prominent myths include:

*Myth 1. In order to maintain a healthy lifestyle, everyone should take a vitamin-pill supplement daily.* Everyone *should* have an adequate intake of vitamins to maintain good health, but, eating a varied diet is the preferred way to achieve this goal. If a vitamin supplement is used, find a supplement that supplies no more than 100 percent of the RDA for any vitamin included.

*Myth 2. If certain amounts of the various vitamins are good, more is better.* Under normal conditions the RDA will supply appropriate amounts of vitamins for living a healthy life. Excess amounts of the water-soluble vitamins are flushed out of the body daily. Therefore, consuming them in excess often leads to expensive urine rather than better health. The fat-soluble vitamins are stored and excesses often lead to toxic or harmful levels. Consumption of megadoses of fat- and water-soluble vitamins can be risky. (See tables 4.6 and 4.7.) Sometimes, a physician will recommend a vitamin supplement that contains amounts of certain vitamins which exceed the RDA. When vitamins are prescribed by a physican they should be viewed as a drug which is necessary to treat a certain medical condition. (See figure 4.10.)

*Myth 3. Natural vitamins are better than synthetic vitamins.* Natural and synthetic vitamins are chemically identical and are used exactly the same way by the human body. The major distinction between natural and synthetic vitamins is their price tag—not their health benefits.

## Minerals

**Minerals** are inorganic substances vital to many body functions. Minerals are commonly divided into two groups: macrominerals and trace minerals. **Macrominerals** are needed in large amounts (but not megadoses) by the body. Some of the known macrominerals include calcium, phosphorus, magnesium, potassium, sulfur, sodium, and chloride. **Trace minerals** serve an equally important role in body functioning but are needed in much smaller amounts. Minerals needed by the body in trace amounts include iron, zinc, manganese, copper, iodine, and cobalt. Table 4.8 presents a more detailed look at these important minerals including their common food sources, functions, and symptoms of deficiency.

Several minerals have recently been singled out by researchers and consumers alike because of their effects on health and wellness. One of the most prominent mineral controversies today surrounds the overconsumption of sodium in the typical American diet.

**Table 4.6 Fat-Soluble Vitamins**

| Vitamin | Why Needed | Important Sources | Deficiency Symptoms | Risks of Megadose |
|---|---|---|---|---|
| A | * Helps keep eyes healthy and able to see in dim light<br>* Helps keep skin healthy and smooth<br>* Helps keep lining of mouth, nose, throat, and digestive tract healthy and resistant to infection<br>* Aids normal bone growth and tooth formation through proper utilization of calcium and phosphorus | Liver, butter, fortified margarine, whole milk, vitamin-A fortified milk, deep yellow and dark leafy green vegetables, cantaloupe, apricots, other deep yellow fruits, cheese | Night blindness; impaired growth of bones and tooth enamel, eye secretions cease, infection of mucous membranes. Deficiency seldom seen in the U.S. | Headache, diarrhea, nausea, anorexia, dry skin, liver damage, blurred vision, extreme fatigue, abnormal bone growth. |
| D | * Helps promote normal growth<br>* Helps body use calcium and phosphorus for the building and maintenance of strong bones and teeth | Fish-liver oils, vitamin-D fortified milk, liver, egg yolk, salmon, tuna; sunlight produces vitamin D from a form of cholesterol in the skin | Rickets; a softening of the bones leading to bow legs and other bone abnormalities. | Early stage: weakness, fatigue, headache, nausea, vomiting, diarrhea.<br>Later stage: kidney impairment, deposits of calcium salts in the kidney, osteoporosis of the bones, calcium deposits in soft body tissue. |
| E | * Helps prevent red-blood-cell destruction<br>* Helps prevent damage to cells from oxidation | Vegetables, vegetable oils, wheat germ | Anemia due to increased red-blood-cell destruction | Little or no known toxicity in humans. |
| K | * Helps with blood clotting | Green leafy vegetables, liver, vegetable oil, tomatoes, potatoes produced by intestinal bacteria. | Severe bleeding, poor blood clotting | Few cases of toxicity are reported because it is not available in over-the-counter supplements and remedies. |

**Table 4.7 Water-Soluble Vitamins**

| Vitamin | Why Needed | Important Sources | Deficiency Symptoms | Risks of Megadose |
|---|---|---|---|---|
| C (ascorbic acid) | * Helps bind body cells together through the production of connective tissue<br>* Aids normal bone and tooth formation, maintenance, and repair<br>* Aids in healing wounds<br>* Helps the body utilize iron<br>* Helps resist infection | Citrus fruits and juices, tomatoes, green peppers, strawberries, cantaloupe, watermelon, cabbage, potatoes, broccoli, Brussels sprouts | Scurvy—degeneration of bones, teeth and gums, anemia, rough skin, wounds that don't heal | Diarrhea, bladder stones, possible $B_{12}$ deficiency; if large doses are taken during pregnancy the infant may develop scurvy after birth. |

**Table 4.7** *Continued*

| Vitamin | Why Needed | Important Sources | Deficiency Symptoms | Risks of Megadose |
|---|---|---|---|---|
| $B_1$ (Thiamine) | * Helps the body change carbohydrate foods into energy<br>* Promotes normal appetite and digestion<br>* Helps to maintain a healthy nervous system | Pork, liver, dry beans and peas, whole-grain and enriched breads and cereals, nuts | Beriberi—muscular weakness, mental confusion, cardiac abnormalities | Few cases of toxicity reported. Some people are hypersensitive to large doses resulting in cardiac abnormalities. |
| $B_2$ (Riboflavin) | * Helps release energy from carbohydrates, fat, and protein<br>* Helps keep skin healthy | Milk, liver, eggs, green leafy vegetables, lean meats, dried beans and peas, enriched breads, cereals, and pasta | Skin sores around the nose and lips, cracking of the corners of the mouth, eyes sensitive to light | None known |
| $B_3$ (Niacin) | * Helps release energy from carbohydrate, fat, and protein<br>* Helps maintain all body tissues | Tuna, poultry, lean meat, fish, liver, peanuts, peas, whole-grain or fortified breads, cereals, and pasta | Pellagra—diarrhea, mental disorders, skin rash, irritability. | Skin rash, heartburn, nausea, vomiting, diarrhea, ulcer activation, low blood pressure, fast heart rate, high blood sugar, abnormal liver function, jaundice |
| $B_6$ (pyridoxine) | * Helps the body to use protein to build body tissue<br>* Helps the body to use carbohydrate and fat for energy | Whole grains, meat, liver, fish, wheat germ, bananas, spinach, green leafy vegetables | Skin disorders, mental depression, weakness, irritability | Dependency on high doses leading to deficiency symptoms when returned to normal doses |
| $B_{12}$ (Cyanocobalamin) | * Helps the body form red blood cells<br>*Aids in normal function of all body cells | Lean meat, liver, eggs, milk, cheese (animal products) | Pernicious anemia, nervous system malfunctions, soreness and weakness in arms and legs | None known |
| Folacin (Folic Acid) | * Aids in the formation of hemoglobin in the red blood cells<br>* Necessary for the production of genetic material | Liver, green vegetables, dried beans and peas, nuts | Anemia, diarrhea, smooth red tongue | None identified in humans to date. Has produced enlarged cells in the kidneys of laboratory animals. |
| Pantothenic Acid | * Helps release energy from carbohydrate, fat, and protein<br>* Helps form hormones | Liver, whole-grain cereal and bread, green vegetables, eggs, nuts | Nausea, headache, muscle cramps, low blood sugar | Increased need for thiamin |
| Biotin | * Helps release energy from carbohydrates<br>* Helps the body synthesize fatty acids | Liver, kidney, egg yolks, green beans | None known under normal conditions | None known |

**Table 4.8 Major Minerals and Trace Elements**

| Mineral | Distribution | Functions | Sources |
|---|---|---|---|
| Calcium (Ca) | Mostly in the inorganic salts of bones and teeth | Structure of bones and teeth, essential for nerve-impulse conduction, muscle-fiber contraction, and blood coagulation, increases permeability of cell membranes, activates certain enzymes | Milk, milk products, leafy green vegetables |
| Phosphorus (P) | Mostly in the inorganic salts of bones and teeth | Structure of bones and teeth, component in nearly all metabolic reactions, constituent of nucleic acids, many proteins, some enzymes, and some vitamins, occurs in cell membrane, ATP, and phosphates of body fluids | Meats, poultry, fish, cheese, nuts, whole-grain cereals, milk, legumes |
| Potassium (K) | Widely distributed, tends to be concentrated inside cells | Helps maintain intracellular osmotic pressure and regulate pH, promotes metabolism, needed for nerve-impulse conduction and muscle-fiber contraction | Avocados, dried apricots, meats, nuts, potatoes, bananas |
| Sulfur (S) | Widely distributed | Essential part of various amino acids, thiamine, insulin, biotin, and mucopolysaccharides | Meats, milk, eggs, legumes |
| Sodium (Na) | Widely distributed, large proportion occurs in extracellular fluids and bonded to inorganic salts of bone | Helps maintain osmotic pressure of extracellular fluids and regulate water balance, needed for conduction of nerve impulses and contraction of muscle fibers, aids in regulation of pH and in transport of substances across cell membranes | Table salt, cured ham, sauerkraut, cheese, graham crackers |
| Chlorine (Cl) | Closely associated with sodium, most highly concentrated in cerebrospinal fluid and gastric juice | Helps maintain osmotic pressure of extracellular fluids, regulate pH, and maintain electrolyte balance, essential in formation of hydrochloric acid, aids transport of carbon dioxide by red blood cells | Same as for sodium |

Source: John W. Hole, *Human Anatomy and Physiology*, 3d ed. 

**SODIUM CONSUMPTION** In appropriate amounts, **sodium** plays several vital roles in body functioning. Sodium is known to help regulate blood and other body fluids, to aid in nerve-impulse transmission and heart action, and even to facilitate the metabolism of carbohydrate and protein. As important as sodium is, however, your body needs very little. The basic human requirement for sodium is only 200 milligrams daily, or about 1/10 of a teaspoon of salt. Even those who lose sodium from sweating great amounts need only a maximum of 2,000 milligrams of sodium or about one teaspoon of salt daily.

Sodium is most often consumed in our diet in the form of salt (**sodium chloride**): roughly 40 percent of table salt is sodium. Americans consume somewhere between 6 and 24 grams of salt daily, with an average of 10 to 15 grams (or an equivalent of 3 to 5 grams of sodium).[28] This level of consumption is fifteen to twenty times the amount of sodium needed by the body daily. In addition to our salt intake, we also consume many additives in processed foods which contain sodium. Monosodium glutamate, sodium bicarbonate (baking soda), baking powder, disodium phosphate, sodium alginate, sodium benzoate, sodium hydroxide, sodium

| Mineral | Distribution | Functions | Sources |
|---|---|---|---|
| Magnesium (Mg) | Abundant in bones | Needed in metabolic reactions that occur in mitrochondria and are associated with the production of ATP, plays role in conversion of ATP to ADP | Milk, dairy products, legumes, nuts, leafy green vegetables |

| Trace Element | Distribution | Functions | Sources |
|---|---|---|---|
| Iron (Fe) | Primarily in blood stored in liver, spleen, and bone marrow | Part of hemoglobin molecule, catalyzes formation of vitamin A, incorporated into a number of enzymes | Liver, lean meats, dried apricots, raisins, enriched whole-grain cereals, legumes, molasses |
| Manganese (Mn) | Most concentrated in liver, kidneys, and pancreas | Occurs in enzymes needed for synthesis of fatty acids and cholesterol, formation or urea, and normal functioning of the nervous system | Nuts, legumes, whole-grain cereals, leafy green vegetables, fruits |
| Copper (Cu) | Most highly concentrated in liver, heart, and brain | Essential for synthesis of hemoglobin, development of bone, production of melanin, and formation of myelin | Liver, oysters, crabmeat, nuts, whole-grain cereals, legumes |
| Iodine (I) | Concentrated in thyroid gland | Essential component for synthesis of thyroid hormones | Food content varies with soil content in different geographic regions, iodized table salt |
| Cobalt (Co) | Widely distributed | Component of cyanocobalamin, needed for synthesis of several enzymes | Liver, lean meats, poultry, fish, milk |
| Zinc (Zn) | Most concentrated in liver, kidneys, and brain | Constituent of several enzymes involved in digestion, respiration, bone metabolism, liver metabolism, necessary for normal wound healing and maintaining integrity of the skin | Seafoods, meats, cereals, legumes, nuts, vegetables |

propionate, sodium sulfite, and sodium saccharin are just a few sodium additives you may be consuming on a regular basis.

Excess sodium in the diet is one of several risk factors associated with high blood pressure (**hypertension**).[29] High blood pressure is of great concern because of its causative link to stroke, coronary-artery disease, congestive heart failure and kidney failure.[30] Although researchers are not completely sure of the mechanism behind the sodium-hypertension connection, many believe that certain individuals are sensitive to sodium and will develop high blood pressure when excess sodium is consumed. It has been hypothesized that some people are very sensitive to sodium and may develop high blood pressure from even small amounts of salt in the diet; others who are less sensitive will react only to salt in great excess. Some individuals may be sodium-resistant, maintaining normal blood pressure no matter how much salt they ingest.[31]

This sodium-sensitivity theory is largely responsible for the great controversy surrounding the dietary goal for salt. The U.S. dietary goals recommend that all Americans limit their intake of sodium by reducing their intake of salt (sodium chloride) to about 5,000 milligrams (5 grams) of salt

**Table 4.9 How Much Salt Did You Eat Today?**

**Processed Foods**

| *Item* | *Amount* | *Salt (mgs.)* | *Item* | *Amount* | *Salt (mgs.)* |
|---|---|---|---|---|---|
| Apple pie (McDonald's) | 1 | 1,035 | French fries (McDonald's) | 1 serving | 282 |
| Bacon, cooked (Oscar Mayer) | 2 slices | 1,725 | Frozen Turkey 3-Course Dinner (Swanson) | 1 | 4,338 |
| Beans, baked red kidney (B & M) | 1 cup | 2,025 | Green beans (Del Monte) | 1 cup | 2,312 |
| Bologna (Oscar Mayer) | 2 slices | 1,125 | Hamburger, Quarter Pounder (McDonald's) | 1 | 1,778 |
| Bread, white (Wonder) | 2 slices | 742 | Mustard (Heinz) | 1 tbsp. | 532 |
| Bread, whole wheat (Pepperidge Farm) | 2 slices | 535 | Pancakes (Hungry Jack Complete) | 3 (4″) | 2,875 |
| Butter | 1 tbsp. | 115 | Peanut butter (Jif) | 2 tbsp. | 445 |
| Cheese, natural cheddar (Kraft) | 2 oz. | 950 | Pickle, dill | 1 large | 4,820 |
| Cheese, American (Kraft) | 2 oz. | 2,225 | Pizza, frozen (Celeste) | 2 oz. | 820 |
| Cheeseburger, Quarter Pounder (McDonald's) | 1 | 3,022 | Potato chips (Wonder) | 10 | 775 |
| Chocolate shake (McDonald's) | 1 | 822 | Pudding, instant chocolate (Jell-O) | ½ cup (prepared) | 1,215 |
| Cookies, sugar (Pillsbury) | 3 | 525 | Salad dressing, Italian (Wish-Bone) | 1 tbsp. | 905 |
| Cornflakes (General Mills) | 1 cup | 762 | Soup, chicken noodle (Campbell's) | 10 oz. (prepared) | 2,625 |
| Crackers, Wheat Thins (Nabisco) | 16 (1 oz.) | 925 | Soy sauce | 1 tbsp. | 3,300 |
| Cinnamon rolls (Pillsbury) | 1 | 1,575 | Tomato catsup (Heinz) | 1 tbsp. | 456 |
| Egg McMuffin (McDonald's) | 1 | 2,285 | Tuna, in oil (Del Monte) | 3 oz. | 1,075 |
| Frankfurter, beef (Oscar Mayer) | 1 | 1,062 | Twinkies (Hostess) | 1 | 602 |

**Unprocessed Foods**

| *Item* | *Amount* | *Salt (mgs.)* | *Item* | *Amount* | *Salt (mgs.)* |
|---|---|---|---|---|---|
| Apple | 1 | 5 | Green beans | 1 cup | 12 |
| Banana | 1 | 2 | Orange juice | 1 cup | 5 |
| Beans, red kidney | 1 cup | 15 | Potato, baked | 1 | 15 |
| Beef, ground | 3 oz. | 142 | Turkey, light meat | 3 oz. | 175 |

Salt content approximate.

Source: Reprinted with permission from *Mother Jones* magazine, July 1978.

daily. Some people argue that since only a certain percentage of the population is sodium-sensitive, it doesn't make sense to recommend that all Americans cut down on sodium and salt. However, right now we have no way to identify who is sensitive to salt and who is not. Many researchers and consumers have therefore decided to control their salt and sodium intake.

There are many enjoyable and tasty ways to cut down on the amount of sodium and salt in our diet. Many people discover that foods have a much richer variety of tastes without large amounts of salt. Controlling sodium intake will involve using your creativity in experimenting with new foods and condiments as well as cutting back on certain salty foods. The following suggestions should help you on your way to a low-sodium life-style.

1. Increase your consumption of fresh or frozen fruit, fruit juices, and vegetables. Most of these foods will contain 35 milligrams or less of sodium. Frozen vegetables that contain a sauce may have a higher sodium content (140 to 460 milligrams).
2. Most grains are naturally low in sodium. Pasta and regular hot cereals cooked without salt usually contain 5 milligrams or less of sodium; white or whole-grain bread typically contain 110 to 150 milligrams.
3. Fresh meats, poultry, and fin fish usually range from 15 to 25 milligrams of sodium per ounce.
4. Be creative in your cooking. A wide variety of alternatives will contribute to a tasty yet nutritious meal. You might try lemon or lime juice, wines, onions, garlic, ground pepper, horseradish, and herbs.
5. Experiment with tasting the natural flavor of foods. Cut down on the salt used in cooking and remove the salt shaker from the table.
6. Look for salt-free beverages. Club soda and soda water, as well as diet soft drinks containing saccharin (sodium saccharin), all contain sodium.
7. Cut down on foods prepared in brine, such as pickles, olives, and sauerkraut.
8. Use less salty or smoked meat, such as bologna, corned or chipped beef, frankfurters, ham, luncheon meats, salt pork, and sausage.
9. Eat sparingly such salty or smoked fish as anchovies, caviar, salted and dried cod, herring, sardines, and smoked salmon.
10. Limit snack items such as potato chips, pretzels, salted popcorn, salted nuts, and salted crackers. Replace them with snacks like fresh fruit, raw vegetables, unsalted nuts, and unsalted unbuttered popcorn.
11. Avoid bouillon cubes, seasoned salts (including sea salt), soy sauce, Worcestershire sauce, and barbeque sauce. (See table 4.10.)

**CALCIUM CONSUMPTION** Another mineral that has received widespread attention in recent years is calcium. The body's most abundant mineral, **calcium** plays major roles in building strong bones and teeth, in regulating blood clotting, in the transmission of nerve impulses, in heart-muscle contraction, and in regulating the flow of fluids in and out of body cells.

The calcium RDA for adult men and women has been set at 800 milligrams daily. Most adults, however, take in much less. The average American woman consumes only about 500 miiligrams of calcium daily, while the average American male consumes about 750 milligrams.[32] Calcium deficiencies have been linked with several major diseases, the most notable to date being osteoporosis. **Osteoporosis** consists of a thinning of the bone materials which leads to an actual loss of bone mass. This causes bones to become brittle and prone to breakage. It is estimated that 15 million Americans have some degree of osteoporosis.[33] Women especially seem susceptible to this disease. Osteoporosis is not just a disease of the elderly. Women as young as age twenty-five are beginning to be diagnosed with signs of significant bone loss.

It was long believed that our need for calcium decreases as we age. It now seems likely that our need actually increases rather than decreases. Childhood is a time for major bone growth, but adults continue to develop bone mass until about age thirty-five.[34] Peak adult bone mass, or the largest amount of bone the body ever contains, appears to play a vital role in the process of osteoporosis. It is very important that adults consume adequate amounts of calcium during their bone-growth years.

**Table 4.10 How to Season Your Food without Salt**

| | |
|---|---|
| **Meat, Fish, and Poultry** | |
| Beef | Bay leaf, dry-mustard powder, green pepper, marjoram, fresh mushrooms, nutmeg, onion, pepper, sage, thyme. |
| Chicken | Green pepper, lemon juice, marjoram, fresh mushrooms, paprika, parsley, poultry seasoning, sage, thyme. |
| Fish | Bay leaf, curry powder, dry-mustard powder, green pepper, lemon juice, marjoram, fresh mushrooms, paprika. |
| Lamb | Curry powder, garlic, mint, mint jelly, pineapple, rosemary. |
| Pork | Apple, applesauce, garlic, onion, sage. |
| Veal | Apricot, bay leaf, curry powder, ginger, marjoram, oregano. |
| **Vegetables** | |
| Asparagus | Garlic, lemon juice, onion, vinegar. |
| Corn | Green pepper, pimiento, fresh tomato. |
| Cucumbers | Chives, dill, garlic, vinegar. |
| Green beans | Dill, lemon juice, marjoram, nutmeg, pimiento. |
| Greens | Onion, pepper, vinegar. |
| Peas | Green pepper, mint, fresh mushrooms, onion, parsley. |
| Potatoes | Green pepper, mace, onion, paprika, parsley. |
| Rice | Chives, green pepper, onion, pimiento, saffron. |
| Squash | Brown sugar, cinnamon, ginger, mace, nutmeg, onion. |
| Tomatoes | Basil, marjoram, onion, oregano. |
| **Soups** | |
| Bean | Pinch of dry-mustard powder. |
| Milk Chowders | Peppercorns. |
| Pea | Bay leaf and parsley. |
| Vegetable | Vinegar, dash of sugar. |

Source: Reproduced with permission from *Cooking without Your Salt Shaker*. © American Heart Association.

Calcium can be increased in the diet by consuming more dairy products, fish, dark leafy greens, broccoli, tofu, and legumes. Dietary supplements of calcium are not recommended as they may throw off the balance of other minerals and nutrients. Some have also been shown to contain lead, mercury, cadmium, and other toxic metals.[35]

Calcium absorption is affected by many factors. Excess protein consumption increases the amount of calcium that is excreted from the body rather than being absorbed.[36] Doubling your protein intake can increase your calcium losses by as much as 50 percent. Preliminary studies suggest that a high intake of phosphates may also increase calcium excretion. Two prime sources of phosphates in the American diet are cola drinks and meat. Substituting cola for milk is a practice of many young adults and may be an important contributing factor to the development of osteoporosis.[37]

## Water

Water is an essential nutrient. Humans can live approximately two weeks without food, but under optimal conditions can live only ten days without water. Even short-term losses of water can be life threatening due to dehydration. Approximately two-thirds of your body weight is water (65 to 70 percent water in males, and 55 to 65 percent water in females). The total amount of water in your body is directly related to the amount of lean tissue in your body, rather than to your total body weight. This is because fat tissue contains less water than lean tissue. Females typically have a greater percentage of body fat related to their secondary-sex characteristics, so they have a lesser amount of water than males.

Water is found in three major body compartments—inside your cells, outside your cells, and in your bloodstream. From these compartments, water performs a variety of functions. Water bathes all of our body cells, helping to transport oxygen and various nutrients to the cells and waste products out of the body. Water also plays an important role in regulating our body temperature by removing heat from the body during the evaporation of sweat.

Water is regulated in the body by a center in the brain that controls our thirst response. When the body needs more water we become thirsty. When there is too much water in the body the brain sends out signals to the kidney to get rid of more water in the urine.

We get water from many dietary sources. In addition to tap water, many foods are plentiful sources of water. Apples, lettuce, watermelon, green beans, broccoli, and white potatoes are only a few examples of foods that are more than 80 percent water. Milk, fruit juices, and other beverages are additional sources of water.

## NUTRITIONAL NEEDS OF SPECIAL POPULATIONS

The basic nutritional guidelines we have discussed so far apply to normal, healthy American adults. Certain groupings of Americans, such as vegetarians, athletes, women taking oral contraceptives, and the elderly, have special needs that may differ from or exceed the general guidelines.

### Vegetarians

**Vegetarians** choose to consume the majority of their calories from plant foods. Only about 1 percent of Americans are currently vegetarians, but vegetarianism appears to be becoming a more popular life-style, especially among young adults.[38]

A vegetarian diet can provide an enjoyable and nutritious diet. Although research continues, there appear to be several health benefits associated with vegetarian diets.[39] Vegetarians who select the *vegan* life-style (no animal food sources or dairy products) have been shown to have lower weights, less constipation, higher HDL cholesterol levels, and lower LDL cholesterol levels. Other groups of vegetarians have exhibited lower blood-pressure levels, low blood cholesterol, lower death rates from certain cancers, and lower rates of coronary-artery disease.

Although there appear to be major benefits from a vegetarian life-style, there are also several important dietary risks. Those of greatest concern relate to energy, protein, vitamin D, and vitamin B-12. Sufficient energy and vitamin D intake are rarely problems for adult vegetarians, but children fed a vegetarian diet may not receive adequate amounts of calories or vitamin D. Receiving enough high-quality protein (complete proteins) is a problem for all vegetarians, but especially *vegans* (those who avoid both animal food sources and dairy products).

Following the complementary protein guidelines suggested earlier in this chapter can help all vegetarians to meet their protein needs. Vitamin B-12 deficiencies are rare in most types of vegetarian diets. Vegans, however, have a special risk of these deficiencies because of their avoidance of all animal food sources and dairy products. As vitamin B-12 cannot be obtained from plant sources, it is recommended that all vegans select fortified B-12 products such as soy milk, brewer's yeast or cereal, or take a B-12 supplement equivalent to the RDA.

If you want to eat a vegetarian diet it is helpful to keep the following recommendations in mind:

1. Eat a wide variety of foods. This will help to insure that you are getting adequate amounts of the essential nutrients.
2. Pay attention to matching your plant protein sources so that you eat complementary pairs in the same meal. This will help you to take in enough complete proteins which are essential to building and maintaining your body.
3. If dairy products are a major part of your vegetarian diet, try to select low-fat dairy products such as 2 percent or skim milk and low-fat cheeses.

### Athletes

Optimal nutrition is of great importance to athletes in helping to obtain peak performance in their chosen sport or activity. Most of the nutritional requirements, however, are easily met by eating a large variety of foods in the proportions suggested by the U.S. Dietary Goals. Athletes and their coaches are often misinformed regarding nutrition and are therefore prone to health fads and quackery which, at the least, provide no additional benefits and may in fact be harmful.[40]

**Table 4.11 New American Eating Guide**

| Anytime | In Moderation | Now and Then |
|---|---|---|
| *Fruits and Vegetables (four or more servings per day)* | | |
| All fruits and vegetables except those at right | Avocado[3] | Coconut[4] |
| Applesauce (unsweetened) | Cole slaw[3] | Pickles[6] |
| Unsweetened fruit juices | Cranberry sauce[5] | |
| Unsalted vegetable juices | Dried fruit | |
| Potatoes, white or sweet | French fries[1 or 2] | |
| | Fried eggplant[2] | |
| | Fruits canned in syrup[5] | |
| | Gazpacho[2,(6)] | |
| | Glazed carrots[5,(6)] | |
| | Guacamole[3] | |
| | Potatoes au gratin[1,(6)] | |
| | Salted vegetable juices[6] | |
| | Sweetened fruit juices[5] | |
| | Vegetables canned with salt[6] | |
| *Beans, Grains, and Nuts (four or more servings per day)* | | |
| Bread and rolls (whole grain) | Cornbread[8] | Croissant[4,8] |
| Bulgur | Flour tortilla[8] | Doughnut[3 or 4,5,8] |
| Dried beans and peas | Granola cereals[1 or 2] | Presweetened cereals[5,8] |
| Lentils | Hominy grits[8] | Sticky buns[1 or 2,5,8] |
| Oatmeal | Macaroni and cheese[1,(6),8] | Stuffing (with butter)[4,(6),8] |
| Pasta, whole-wheat | Matzoh[8] | |
| Rice, brown | Nuts[3] | |
| Sprouts | Pasta, refined[8] | |
| Whole-grain hot and cold cereals | Peanut butter[3] | |
| Whole-wheat matzoh | Pizza[6,8] | |
| | Refined, unsweetened cereals[8] | |
| | Refried beans[1 or 2] | |
| | Seeds[3] | |
| | Soybeans[2] | |
| | Tofu[2] | |
| | Waffles or pancakes with syrup[5,(6),8] | |
| | White bread and rolls[8] | |
| | White rice[8] | |

Source: Reprinted from *New American Eating Guide,* which is available from the Center for Science in the Public Interest, 1501 16th St., N.W., Washington, D.C. 20036, for $3.95. Copyright 1980.

[1]Moderate fat, saturated. [2]Moderate fat, unsaturated. [3]High fat, unsaturated. [4]High fat, saturated. [5]High in added sugar. [6]High in salt or sodium. [(6)]May be high in salt or sodium. [7]High in cholesterol. [8]Refined grains.

Every athlete needs to take in enough calories to meet the extra energy demands of training and competition. Caloric requirements will vary from person to person depending on age, sex, body size, and level of activity. It is not uncommon for athletes to consume between 3,000 and 6,000 calories a day. Athletes should select their diet carefully so that about 55 percent of the calories are from complex carbohydrates, 30 percent from fats, and 10 to 15 percent from protein. If such a diet is consumed regularly, vitamin and mineral supplementation is unnecessary. Many athletes believe that supplementation enhances performance, but this is not supported by research.[41]

Some athletes, especially those participating in endurance activities such as distance running and distance swimming, participate in a nutritional regimen known as carbohydrate loading. **Carbohydrate loading** consists of depleting body stores of carbohydrate (glycogen) by exercise, followed by several days of dietary carbohydrate restriction, and then by several days of high dietary carbohydrate intake. This regimen has been shown to double the glycogen stores in the liver and large skeletal muscles of some athletes, thereby enhancing their levels of endurance.[42] Long-term effects of repeated carbohydrate loading are not known at this time, and many nutritionists and exercise physiologists therefore caution against its use. More recent evidence has

| Anytime | In Moderation | Now and Then |
|---|---|---|
| *Milk Products (three to four servings per day for children, two for adults)* | | |
| Buttermilk (from skim milk) | Cocoa with skim milk[5] | Cheesecake[4,5] |
| Low-fat cottage cheese | Cottage cheese, regular[1] | Cheese fondue[4,(6)] |
| Low-fat milk (1 percent) | Frozen yogurt[5] | Cheese soufflé[4,(6),7] |
| Low-fat yogurt | Ice milk[5] | Eggnog[1,5,7] |
| Nonfat dry milk | Low-fat milk (2 percent)[1] | Hard cheeses: blue, brick, Camembert, cheddar, Muenster, Swiss[4,(6)] |
| Skim-milk cheeses | Low-fat yogurt, sweetened[5] | Ice cream[4,5] |
| Skim milk | Mozzarella, part-skim[1,(6)] | Processed cheeses[4,6] |
| Skim-milk and banana shake | | Whole milk[4] |
| | | Whole-milk yogurt[4] |
| *Poultry, Fish, Meat, and Eggs (two servings per day; vegetarians should eat added servings from other groups)* | | |
| Cod | Fried fish[1 or 2] | Fried chicken, commercial[4] |
| Flounder | Herring[3,6] | Cheese omelet[4,7] |
| Gefilte fish[(6)] | Mackerel, canned[2,(6)] | Whole egg or yolk (limit to three a week)[3,7] |
| Haddock | Salmon, canned[2,(6)] | Bacon[4,(6)] |
| Halibut | Sardines[2,(6)] | Beef liver, fried[1,7] |
| Perch | Shrimp[7] | Bologna[4,6] |
| Pollock | Tuna, oil-packed[2,(6)] | Corned beef[4,6] |
| Rockfish | Chicken liver[7] | Ground beef[4] |
| Shellfish, except shrimp | Fried chicken in vegetable oil (homemade)[3] | Ham, trimmed[1,6] |
| Sole | Chicken or turkey, boiled, baked, or roasted (with skin)[2] | Hot dogs[4,6] |
| Tuna, water-packed[(6)] | Flank steak[1] | Liverwurst[4,6] |
| Egg whites | Leg or loin of lamb[1] | Pig's feet[4] |
| Chicken or turkey, boiled, baked, or roasted (no skin) | Pork shoulder or loin, lean[1] | Salami[4,6] |
| | Round steak or ground round[1] | Sausage[4,6] |
| | Rump roast[1] | Spareribs[4] |
| | Sirloin steak, lean[1] | Red meats, untrimmed[4] |
| | Veal[1] | |

indicated that increased glycogen stores can be attained by simply resting several days before competition and consuming a high-carbohydrate diet.[43]

A common nutritional myth endorsed by many athletes involves the belief that a substantial amount of protein is needed in order to build muscle mass, meet energy needs, and increase athletic performance. Weight lifters are especially vulnerable to protein myths. While it is true that athletes need more energy than their sedentary peers, the most efficient source of energy is complex carbohydrates and fats. Additionally, there is no sound evidence that a high protein intake builds more muscle or increases performance.[44]

Fluid replacement is a very important component of optimal athletic performance. During prolonged exercise it is possible for the athlete to lose as much as six to eight pounds of body weight due to sweating.[45] It is recommended that athletes consume proper amounts of fluids, prior to, during, and after athletic competition. Water is the best fluid-replacement choice prior to and during the event. Experts recommend drinking between ten and twenty ounces of water before the event, and five to eight ounces every ten to fifteen minutes during the event. Afterwards, orange juice, apple juice, lemonade, and Gatorade are good fluid choices.[46] Sodium and chloride losses from sweating are easily replaced by normal food intake after the competition. Salt tablets are not recommended as they can cause nausea and vomiting and lead to greater dehydration of fluid within the cells. (See figure 4.11.)

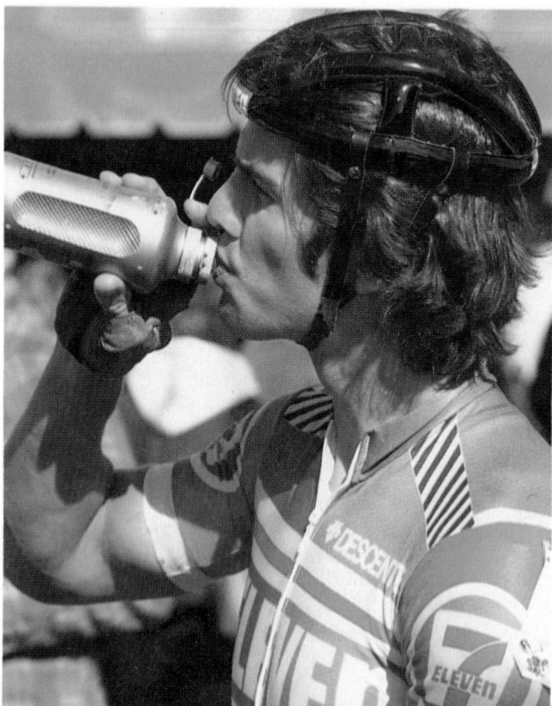


**Figure 4.11**
Athletes need to consume proper amounts of fluid before, during, and after their event.

### Women Taking Oral Contraceptives

Various studies have indicated that women taking birth-control pills may need more of certain vitamins because their bodies may metabolize them differently. Specifically, women taking birth-control pills may need to increase their intake of B-complex vitamins (especially B-6 and folic acid) and vitamin C.[47] Eating more foods rich in these vitamins is the preferred way to meet these vitamin needs. A multivitamin supplement can also be taken daily; however, it must contain folic acid and should not contain any nutrient in amounts over the RDA.

### The Elderly

Every day more people enter old age than leave it. Currently 11 percent of the U.S. population is estimated to be over the age of sixty-five.[48] As more Americans are living longer, researchers have become interested in nutritional aspects of the aging process. Careful research into nutritional requirements for the elderly, however, is still in its infancy. This leaves much room for speculation about what constitutes the best diet for our aging population.

Researchers do, however, seem to be in agreement on several aspects of nutrition and aging.[49]

1. The basic principles of good nutrition remain the same for older as for younger people. Modifying our diets toward the dietary goals is recommended for Americans of all ages.
2. Obesity may be a serious problem for older people who remain on their own. This relates directly to the decreasing energy needs of older people due to a slowing down of their metabolism. The older we get, the fewer daily calories we require to remain at optimal weight. Monitoring caloric intake and increasing activity levels are important to counteract a decreasing metabolism as we age.
3. Certain groups of elderly people may consume diets deficient in certain nutrients. Elderly widowers are one vulnerable group. A man whose wife has always prepared his meals may start to eat a diet of junk food and processed food when he is alone. Such a diet is usually deficient in one or more vitamins and minerals, and contains an excess of fat and sugar.
4. There appears to be an increasing need for calcium as we age in order to combat osteoporosis. Older women in particular need to increase their calcium intake. Currently, it is estimated that 1.5 grams of calcium each day would meet the increased needs of aging.[50] This is roughly equivalent to four glasses of milk daily. Some experts recommend that low-fat dairy products be stressed as sources for calcium.

## PERSONAL AND SOCIAL INFLUENCES

When it comes to eating, most of us are influenced by many factors other than our knowledge of the nutrients essential for optimal health. Cost, convenience, personal tastes and preferences, and habit are just a few of the many factors that interact and contribute to our food choices and ultimately to our level of wellness. (See "Natural Foods: Are You Willing to Pay More?")

4.1 EXHIBIT 4.1

# "Natural" Foods: Are You Willing to Pay More?

**HEALTH FOOD: WHY NOBODY REALLY KNOWS WHAT THAT MEANS**

Do the terms "natural," "organic," and "health food" confuse you? They should. Since the federal government has not chosen to come up with "legal" definitions, you're on your own in deciding what they mean.

The term "organic" usually refers to foods grown without the addition of agricultural chemicals and pesticides. But just because the label says "organic," there are no guarantees that this is actually true. An often-cited 1972 study revealed that many foods labeled as "organic" actually contained very small amounts of pesticide residues, just as conventional foods can. And since this type of farming process is so costly, the products are expensive, while they may be of lesser quality.

"Natural" usually means that the products are minimally processed and contain no artificial ingredients, and consumers seem to be willing to pay more for foods with this label. Consequently, "natural" has become a popular advertising term appearing on products which, upon closer inspection, hardly qualify. Products labeled "natural" can still contain additives such as locust bean, coloring, and flavor enhancers. Only a careful reading of the label will tell you for sure how "natural" a product is. The term "health food" is a misnomer because it implies that these foods are somehow better than conventional foods and have "health-giving properties." The truth is, health foods aren't necessarily better, or more nutritious, than other foods; rather, they are usually more expensive. And don't assume that health foods are lower in calories, either. Consider granola: A ¼ cupful has 125 calories. Many brands of granola are chock-full of sugar and fat (often in the form of palm or coconut oil—both saturated). And "health-food" and "natural" candy bars can be just as fattening and sugar-laden as the real thing. In addition, the sugar content is not always apparent to the consumer because the label lists corn syrup, molasses, honey, fructose, or some other form of sugar. There are even "health foods" that are being palmed off on the public as "miracle" foods. The following are some examples:

***Bee Pollens***

Promoted as an excellent source of protein and anti-aging substances, bee pollens are not only virtually worthless to humans, but potentially dangerous. The major component of pollens is carbohydrate, together with a small amount of protein. The FDA Consumer points out that even if bee pollens were a good protein source (which they aren't), there are far less expensive sources, including filet mignon! No scientific evidence exists that bee pollens have any effect on aging, either. Pollens can be especially hazardous for persons with allergies, asthma, or hay fever, and may even induce anaphylactic shock in hypersensitive persons.

***RNA Tablets***

Another waste of money is RNA tablets, which are fraudulently promoted as anti-aging. Although RNA (ribonucleic acid) is a part of the reproductive apparatus of all cells and is a specific blueprint for reproduction, when taken in tablet form it is digested by intestinal enzymes and does not enter our cells intact. In fact, if the yeast and sardine RNA being sold nationally actually worked in our bodies, it would make baby sardines and yeasts!

***Spirulina***

This blue-green alga is promoted as a nutritional supplement and appetite suppressant, despite the fact that no scientific evidence exists to substantiate these claims. It does contain some protein, vitamins, and minerals, but at an exorbitant price compared to the same amount of nutrients from conventional foods. An investigation by the California Council Against Health Fraud estimated that West Coast spirulina purchasers paid ten dollars to twenty-three dollars for the equivalent amount of protein that can be obtained from just seventy cents' worth of peanuts.

***Herbal Teas***

Many people turn to herbal teas to avoid the caffeine in regular teas and coffee. Ironically, caffeine is probably less harmful than many of the pharmacologically active substances herbal teas can contain. For example, according to *The Honest*

4.1. *continued* EXHIBIT 4.1

*Herbal,* chamomile tea, from the ragweed family, can cause anaphylactic-shock reaction in certain people. Teas containing buckthorn bark and senna leaves, flowers, and bark can cause severe diarrhea.

**WHO TO COMPLAIN TO**

Three federal agencies—the U.S. Food and Drug Administration (FDA), the Federal Trade Commission (FTC), and the U.S. Postal Inspection Service—along with a private nonprofit organization, the Better Business Bureau, are working to help protect the public against health quackery. Currently, the Council of Better Business Bureaus (BBB) and the FDA are involved in a joint campaign aimed at decreasing the number of fraudulent advertisements appearing in daily and weekly publications. The gist of the program is to alert appropriate individuals in the publishing business on how to recognize spurious ads, and inform them that BBB and FDA are available to check out questionable ads. In general, report complaints to the FDA. However, report suspected mail fraud to the U.S. Postal Inspection Service, and any questionable advertising claims to the FTC. You can also contact the Council of Better Business Bureaus, or the Better Business Bureau in the area where the company is located. Here are the addresses:

- The Food and Drug Administration, Office of Consumer Affairs, HFE-88, 5600 Fishers Lane, Rockville, MD 20857. You can also contact your district office under Health and Human Services in the telephone directory.
- The Federal Trade Commission, Office of the Secretary, 6th Street and Pennsylvania Avenue, N.W., Washington, D.C. 20580.
- Chief Inspector, U.S. Postal Inspection Service, 475 L'Enfant Plaza West, S.W., Washington, D.C. 20260-2112.
- The Council of Better Business Bureaus, 1515 Wilson Boulevard, Suite 300, Arlington, VA 22209. Or contact your local Better Business Bureau.

Source: Adaptation from *Nutritional Quackery* by Leslie Weiner. Copyright © 1985 by Scholastic, Inc. Reprinted by permission.

## DISCUSSION QUESTIONS

1. Have you ever purchased foods labeled "natural," "organic," or "health food" because you thought they were better for you? Did you have any other motivations?

2. Investigate the cost of "health foods" in your community. Do some comparison shopping, checking the price of "health foods" against similar products that do not make such claims.

3. Read the labels of some "health foods." How many types of sugar and fat do they contain?

4. What do you think are some solutions to the problem of the "health food scam"? What can the consumer do? What can the government do?

## Cost

Everyone is concerned with today's high cost of food; we all want to get the best nutrition for the least amount of money. Fortunately, this is not as difficult as it may sound. Foods that are high in cholesterol, fat, and sugar are not the best buys in terms of money or health. Generally, a diet closer to the dietary goals will tend to lower food costs. Fresh fruits and vegetables in season are usually good buys, especially if you get them at a local farmers' market where you can bypass many of the costs of processing and transportation. (See figure 4.12.) Other complex carbohydrates, such as whole-grain cereals, breads, and pasta, are also cheaper and healthier food options. With a little planning on your part it is generally easy to prepare enjoyable and inexpensive foods that make a major contribution to optimal well-being. (See Activity for Wellness 4.3.)

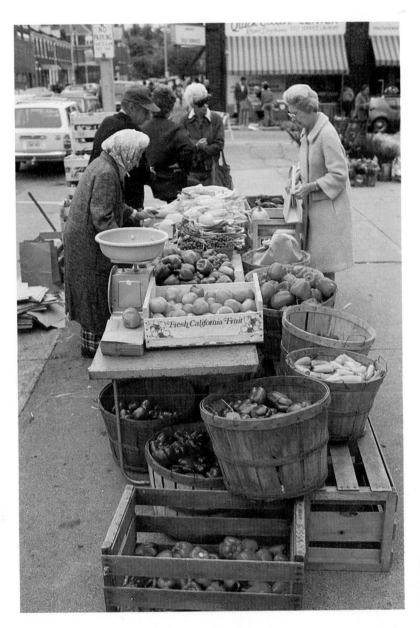


**Figure 4.12**
It is possible to buy high-quality produce at inexpensive prices from the growers themselves.

## Convenience

The college years are a busy time for most people. In addition to the many hours of study, social activities abound. Students seldom have elaborate cooking facilities. All of these factors contribute to the appeal of convenient and attractive fast foods. In the United States, food eaten away from the home accounts for about one out of every three food dollars, with over nineteen billion dollars being spent yearly at fast-food restaurants alone.[51]

Many consumers are beginning to wonder about the nutritional value of their fast-food diets. In response to consumer demand, many fast-food chains have contracted to have their foods analysed, and are beginning to make this analysis public.[52] Results indicate that most fast foods are high in calories, sodium, and fat. Additionally, they appear to have a moderate amount of carbohydrate; however, it is not clear how much is sugar and how much is starch. Most fast foods are low in fiber and vitamins, but supply adequate amounts of protein, iron, and calcium. More research needs to be done in the area of trace minerals.

4.3 ACTIVITY FOR WELLNESS 4.3

# Nine Ways to Boost Your Buying Power

1. Look for these lean meats lower in fats, calories, and price:
- "lean" versus choice and prime grades
- round and chuck versus sirloin, porterhouse, and rib roast
- lean pork and ham versus spareribs and bacon

2. Remove the excess fat from regular ground beef by breaking up, cooking, and draining the meat. Lean and extra-lean ground beef cost more than regular ground beef. After breaking up, cooking, and draining, the fat content in regular, lean, and extra-lean ground beef is about the same. So considering the meat that's left, ounce for ounce, well-drained regular ground beef (broken up) can be a cheaper, low-fat buy. But whatever type of ground beef you choose, remember to drain off the extra fat after cooking.

3. Combine vegetable proteins to help stretch your protein dollar. Many vegetable protein combinations, like rice and beans, can be combined to give you protein just as good as that in meat, but with less-saturated fats and no cholesterol. Vegetable proteins can also be paired with low-fat dairy products or small amounts of lean meats, poultry, or fish to help stretch your protein dollar.

4. Stretch your meat dollar with vegetables and starchy foods. For a tasty, more economical meat dish, try adding tomatoes, macaroni, and chili seasoning to ground beef. The Chinese stir-fry cooking style also helps cut down on fat.

5. Change gradually to low-fat dairy products. When you're buying whole milk now, try one step over to 2 percent fat milk. It has almost half as much fat, and it's hard to taste the difference. As you work your way down to skim milk, you will be saving dollars, too. You can use nonfat milk in your cooking right away and you won't notice the difference in taste.

6. Instead of butter, try a margarine that has twice as much polyunsaturated as saturated fats. Either the label or the manufacturer can give you the amount of polyunsaturated and saturated fats in a margarine. Besides costing less than butter, a margarine with at least twice as much polyunsaturated as saturated fat can help lower your blood cholesterol. However, don't forget that butter and margarine have the same amount of calories (100 calories per tablespoon), so use them sparingly.

7. Prepare more foods yourself, instead of buying more expensive convenience foods. By buying more basic foods yourself, you can use your favorite ingredients such as spices and seasonings to suit your family's tastes. You can control the amount of meat and fat in your dishes as well. Convenience foods can be high in fats and calories. They usually cost more as well. Some convenience foods are also very salty or high in sugar.

8. Choose fresh fruits and vegetables in season when there's more variety, lower prices, and better quality. Fresh fruits and vegetables have a lot more to offer: they're low in saturated fats and calories, with no cholesterol, and high in vitamins and minerals. They also give you a variety of colors and texture and are easy to prepare.

9. Use unit-pricing labels to compare similar products. Unit-pricing labels show the cost of the product per unit—such as the cost per pound or quart. If your store has unit pricing labels, use them to compare the costs of different varieties, brands, or sizes of a particular product. For example, pound for pound, a lean cut of meat like round is cheaper than sirloin or porterhouse. Lean meats and poultry can also give you the same high quality of protein without the extra fat and calories. So they are a double savings!

Source: *Eaters Almanac,* National Heart, Lung, and Blood Institute, National Institutes of Health, Bethesda, Md.

The calorie content of a fast-food meal is generally between 900 and 1,800 calories. This equals 33 to 66 percent of the total daily recommended calories for young men and 45 to 90 percent of the total daily recommended calories for young women.[53] It is not uncommon for 50 percent of these calories to be from fat. Fast-food meals could thus help to contribute to the problem of obesity for many people.

Be sure to moderate the number of fast-food meals you consume. However, it is possible to enjoy the convenience of fast foods and still maintain a good diet. In order to accomplish this you must take stock of other foods eaten on the same day. Be certain to include dairy products for additional calcium and fresh fruits and vegetables for vitamins A and C. These vegetables, in addition to whole-grain products, will also help you get needed sources of fiber. If you plan to eat more meat that day, select poultry or fish in order to cut down on total calories from fat. Many fast-food restaurants now provide salad bars that will allow you to include fresh vegetables with your other selections. Take advantage of salad bars, but watch the amount and type of salad dressing you add.

Personal and social food preferences can act to enhance our nutritional needs or serve as major barriers. An understanding of the basic nutrients and their functions is a sound foundation on which to build a diet that emphasizes the good preferences and minimizes the barriers. Eating for health can be an adventure you don't want to miss.

## SUMMARY

1. Today's "typical American diet" is too high in fats, refined and processed sugar, salt, cholesterol, and calories. Many researchers believe that this typical diet is strongly associated with many of the chronic and degenerative diseases so common in the U.S.

2. The 1977 U.S. Senate Select Subcommittee on Nutrition and Human Needs has issued seven dietary goals for Americans. These goals suggest that we eat more like our grandparents did. Specifically, we should consume a greater percentage of our calories as complex carbohydrates, such as fresh fruits and vegetables and whole-grain products.

3. Three of the six major nutrients—carbohydrates, fats, and protein—supply us with calories or energy. The other three nutrients—vitamins, minerals, and water—assist in utilizing this energy.

4. Carbohydrates are the body's preferred form of energy, and supply us with 4 calories per gram—less than one-half the calories supplied by a gram of fat. Complex carbohydrates are a rich source of important vitamins, minerals, and water.

5. Foods high in processed and refined sugars, such as table sugar, are often labeled "empty calories"; they contain few of the important nutrients such as vitamins, minerals, and protein. These foods add only calories to our diet and increase the risk of developing dental cavities.

6. Fats supply us with 9 calories per gram and thus are a condensed source of energy and a perfect energy-storage vehicle for the body.

7. A diet high in saturated fats has been strongly linked to coronary-artery disease.

8. Scientists have distinguished several types of cholesterol. HDL cholesterol may be protective against coronary-heart disease, while LDL cholesterol seems to increase the risk of this disease.

9. The major function of protein is for growth, maintenance, and repair of body tissues. Protein can also be used as a source of energy if sufficient carbohydrates and fats are lacking in the diet.

10. Protein is composed of amino acids, eight of which must be taken into the body in food at the same time daily. These are known as the essential amino acids, and are vital to tissue growth. Foods that contain all eight essential amino acids are called complete proteins.

11. Vitamins are either water soluble or fat soluble. The water-soluble vitamins (B-complex and C) are not stored by the body and must be consumed daily. Fat-soluble vitamins (A, D, E, K) are stored and can be toxic in large doses. The best source of vitamins is a well-balanced diet.

12. Minerals are inorganic substances which, in correct amounts, are vital to bodily functions. Excess or deficiency levels of minerals are considered to be health risks. For instance, excess

sodium consumption is considered a major risk factor for high blood pressure and stroke, while calcium deficiencies are believed to be a risk factor for osteoporosis.

13. Certain groupings of Americans, such as athletes, vegetarians, women taking oral contraceptives, and the elderly, have special nutritional needs. An awareness of these needs and several minor diet changes will help these groups achieve their quest for wellness.

14. Many variables, such as cost, habit, convenience, and taste, contribute to our choice of foods. Being aware of these factors and using them to your advantage will help you achieve higher levels of wellness.

## Recommended Readings

Brody, Jane. *Jane Brody's Nutrition Book.* New York: Bantam Books, 1981.

Deutsch, Ronald. *The New Nuts among the Berries.* Palo Alto, Calif.: Bull Publishing Co., 1977.

Katch, Frank, and McArdle, William. *Nutrition, Weight Control and Exercise,* 2nd ed. Philadelphia: Lea & Febiger, 1983.

Herbert, Victor. *Nutrition Cultism.* Philadelphia: George Stickley Co., 1980.

Herbert, Victor, and Barret, Stephen. *Vitamins and "Health" Foods: The Great American Hustle.* Philadelphia: George Stickley Co., 1981.

## References

1. Select Committee on Nutrition and Human Needs. *Dietary Goals for the United States,* 2d ed. (Washington, D.C.: U.S. Government Printing Office, December 1977).

2. Select Committee, *Dietary Goals.*

3. Jean Mayer, "The Bitter Truth about Sugar," *New York Times Magazine* (20 June 1976), 26, 31, 34.

4. Mayer, "Bitter Truth."

5. "Too Much Sugar?", *Consumer Reports* (March 1978): 136–42.

6. Jean Mayer, *A Diet for Living* (New York: Pocket Books, 1977).

7. Mayer, "Bitter Truth."

8. Mayer, "Bitter Truth."

9. *Consumer Reports,* "Too Much Sugar?"

10. Mayer, "Bitter Truth."

11. Frank De Fazio, "Cavity, Heal Thyself," *American Health* 3.1 (1984): 18.

12. U.S. Department of Agriculture, *Food,* Home and Garden Bulletin 228 (Washington, D.C.: U.S. Government Printing Office, 1979).

13. Aubrey Sheiham, "Changing Trends in Dental Caries," *International Journal of Epidemiology,* 13, 2 (1984): 142–47.

14. Select Committee, *Dietary Goals.*

15. G. Edward Damon, "A Primer on Four Nutrients: Proteins, Carbohydrates, Fats and Fiber," *FDA Consumer* 9.1 (February 1975): 5–13.

16. Bonnie Liebman, "Facts about Fiber," *Nutrition Action* 9.2 (March 1982): 16–17.

17. Liebman, "Facts about Fiber," 16–17; Constance Kies, "Edible Fiber: Practical Problems," *Contemporary Nutrition* 7.2 (1982); Damon, "A Primer on Four Nutrients," 5–13.

18. Liebman, "Facts about Fiber," 16–17.

19. Liebman, "Facts about Fiber," 16–17.

20. Select Committee, *Dietary Goals.*

21. Select Committee, *Dietary Goals.*

22. Marie A. Bernard, "Nutrition and Preventive Health," *Medical Times* 3.9 (1983): 113–17; Select Committee, *Dietary Goals.*

23. Ellen Ruppel Shell, "The Guinea Pig Town," *Science 82* 3. 10 (1982): 58–63.

24. William Kannel, "Recent Findings from the Framingham Study—1," *Medical Times* 106. 4 (1978): 23–27; Henry A. Solomon, "Risk Factors and CHD," *Living with Angina* 2 1 (1981):1–4, 9–11; Bernard, "Nutrition," 113–17; Select Committee, *Dietary Goals.*

25. John Langone, "Heart Attack and Cholesterol," *Discover* 5.3 (1984): 21–23.

26. John W. Hole, Jr., *Human Anatomy and Physiology.* (Dubuque, Iowa: Wm. C. Brown Publishers, 1984), 532.

27. Jane Brody, *Jane Brody's Nutrition Book* (New York: Bantam Books, 1981).

28. Michael Jacobson, "The Deadly White Powder," *Mother Jones* 3.6 (July 1978): 12–20.

29. Bonnie Liebman, "The Sodium-Hypertension Connection," *Nutrition Action* 9.10 (December 1982): 5–11; Lot B. Page, "On Making Sense of Salt and Your Blood Pressure," *Executive Health* 18.11 (1982).

30. Page, "Salt and Your Blood Pressure."

31. Liebman, "Sodium-Hypertension," 5–11.

32. Steve Findlay and Bonnie Liebman, "Brittle Bones," *Nutrition Action* 9.5 (June 1982):12–13; L. H. "Coming: Jump in Calcium RDA," *American Health* 3.1 (1984): 29–30.

33. Findlay and Liebman, "Brittle Bones," 12–13.

34. Findlay and Liebman, "Brittle Bones," 12–13.

35. L. H., "Jump in Calcium," 29–30.

36. Randi Blaun, "Preventing Osteoporosis: Calcium's the Key," *Medical Month* 2.1 (1984): 43–44.

37. Blaun, "Preventing Osteoporosis," 43–44.

38. Johanna Dwyer, "Vegetarianism," *Contemporary Nutrition* 4.6 (1979).

39. Dwyer, "Vegetarianism."

40. Robert C. Serfass, "Nutrition for the Athlete: Update, 1982," *Contemporary Nutrition* 7.4 (1982).

41. Serfass, "Nutrition for the Athlete"; Clarissa Manjarrez and Richard Birrer, "Nutritional Athletic Performance," *American Family Physician* 28.5 (1983): 105–15.

42. Manjarrez and Birrer, "Nutritional Athletic Performance," 105–15.

43. Mike Moore, "Carbohydrate Loading: Eating through the Wall," *The Physician and Sports Medicine* 9.10 (1981):97–103.

44. Manjarrez and Birrer, "Nutritional Athletic Performance," 105–15.

45. Manjarrez and Birrer, "Nutritional Athletic Performance," 105–15.

46. Manjarrez and Birrer, "Nutritional Athletic Performance," 105–15.

47. "Dietary Answers to Common Problems," *Patient Care* (15 April 1978): 42–43, 49.

48. Hamish N. Munro, "Nutritional Requirements in the Elderly," *Hospital Practice* 17.8 (1982): 143–54.

49. Myron Winick, "Nutritional Considerations for Older Americans." *Medical Times* 110.11 (1982): 31–39; Michael Freedman and J. Paul Teusink, "Food for Later Years," *Transition* 1.10 (1983): 21–32; Mary Bess Kohrs, "New Perspectives on Nutritional Counseling for the Elderly," *Contemporary Nutrition* 8.3 (1983).

50. J. M. Lane, "Osteoporosis: The Case for Sodium Fluoride and Calcium," *The Journal of Musculoskeletal Medicine* 1.8 (1984).

51. Eleanor Young, Ellen Brennan, and Gaynell Irving, "Update: Nutritional Analysis of Fast Foods," *Public Health Currents* 21.3 (1981): 9–16.

52. Young, Brennan, and Irving, "Update," 9–16.

53. Young, Brennan, and Irving, "Update," 9–16.

CHAPTER FIVE

# Weight Control: A Lifelong Challenge



Maintaining optimal body weight (and fat) is a key component of wellness for many people. People in good physical shape feel better about themselves and this in turn affects how they interact with others. Additionally, they are energetic and enjoy the many activities awaiting them each day. For people in good physical shape, weight control is part of a general style of living that is both beneficial and enjoyable.

Weight control involves more than just sporadic "crash" dieting. At any given time, about 9.5 million people are on a "diet" of some sort. However, only 20 percent of them will be successful in maintaining their weight loss. One major reason for this high failure rate is that most dieters do not attempt to establish new eating and activity habits that become part of their wellness life-style. The average dieter goes on an estimated 2.3 diets a year, each lasting an average of sixty to ninety days.[1]

Your life-style can enhance your ability to maintain optimal body weight and composition. A sound knowledge base will help you evaluate the many weight-control options available today, as well as the social supports and barriers to maintaining optimal weight and body composition.

# OVERWEIGHT VERSUS OBESITY

Our body tissue can be divided into two major categories: **fat** (or adipose) and **lean.** The fat cells of our body are very elastic and contain varying amounts of fat deposits (stored energy). Body fat has several very important functions. As we saw in chapter 4, fat helps store and transport the fat-soluble vitamins, protects and pads vital body organs, forms the chemical core of certain hormones, and helps insulate the body from extremely cold temperatures. Only small amounts of body fat, however, are needed to perform these important functions.

Our body fat can be divided into two major categories: essential fat and storage fat. **Essential fat** is that amount of fat which is necessary for normal, healthy functioning of the human body. Essential fat is stored in major body organs and tissues such as bone, muscle, heart, lungs, liver, spleen, kidneys, intestines, and the central nervous system.[2] Typically, essential fat comprises about 3 percent of body weight for men and about 10 to 12 percent of body weight for women. Women tend to have greater amounts of essential fat in order to maintain hormonal and reproductive functions specific to females. Most of us carry around considerably more body fat than this essential level. Extra fat is called **storage fat;** it tends to accumulate around the abdomen in men and in the legs, thighs, buttocks, abdomen, breasts, upper arms, chin, and face in women.[3] Storage fat is fat that accumulates in adipose or fat cells. Some storage fat is needed as it is this type of fat that protects and pads the internal organs and insulates the body during extreme cold. Lean cells make up the remainder of our body weight and include tissues such as muscle, bone, and body fluids.

## Assessing Body Fat

All too often the concepts of **overweight** and **obesity** (overfat) are used interchangeably. A prime example of this is using a scale to determine your weight, and then comparing that weight to the standard height/weight tables in order to determine how "fat" you are. A scale, which measures body weight in pounds or kilograms, can only tell you how much you weigh. It has no mechanism to allow it to tell you how much of that weight is fat versus how much is lean. As a general rule, most people who are "overweight" according to the height/weight tables are also "overfat," but there are exceptions to this rule. Take the case of many football players or bodybuilders. They typically weigh more than recommended by the height/weight tables, yet most of this weight is muscle tissue, which actually weighs more than fat. At the other extreme, some people can be considered underweight according to such tables and still be fat—that is, they maintain too great a percentage of their body weight as fat rather than lean tissue. As you can see, using a scale and height/weight tables to measure fatness or obesity may lead some people to assume they have a fat problem when they do not and it may lead others to assume they are healthy and lean when in fact they may have a problem with excess fat.

There are several good ways to measure your **percentage of body fat.** One of the best ways is called underwater weighing; it involves submersion in a tank of water in order to measure weight in water. A person's weight in water is a function of individual body density. Muscle has a greater density than fat and therefore sinks in water; fat, which is less dense, will float. Thus, the leaner you are, the more you will weigh underwater, reflecting the density of your body weight. The density figure calculated by underwater weighing is then used in an algebraic equation to estimate your percentage of body fat.

Underwater weighing is one of the most accurate ways to determine percentage of body fat. (See figure 5.1.) However, it is also one of the most expensive. This technique is also inconvenient because it must be performed in a laboratory. Fortunately, there are several other less complicated and less expensive techniques that produce reliable measures of percentage of body fat (highly correlated with underwater weighing figures).

One such measure is the skin-fold technique. Approximately one-half of the body's fat is stored beneath the skin and is referred to as **subcutaneous fat.** The skin-fold technique measures this subcutaneous fat at various body sites. These measurements are then used to estimate percentage of body fat. Special calipers measure a fold of skin and fat

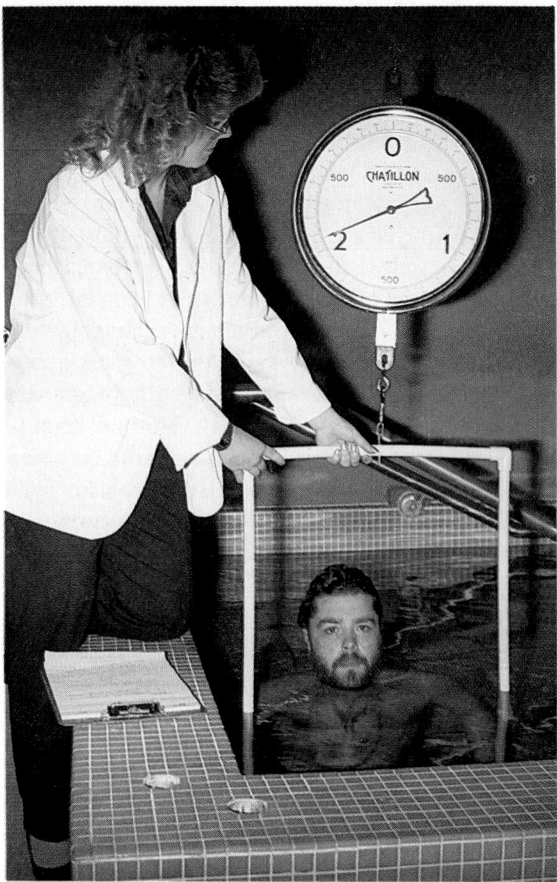


**Figure 5.1**
Underwater weighing is one of the most accurate ways to measure the percentage of body fat, although it is also expensive and time-consuming.

that is grasped firmly between the thumb and forefinger, while the skin and fat are pulled away from the underlying muscle. (See figure 5.2.) The most common sites for skin-fold measurement include the back of the right upper arm (triceps), just below the tip of the shoulder blade (scapula), just above the hipbone (suprailiac), on the abdomen an inch to the right of the navel, and on the midline of the thigh two-thirds of the distance from the kneecap to the hip.[4]

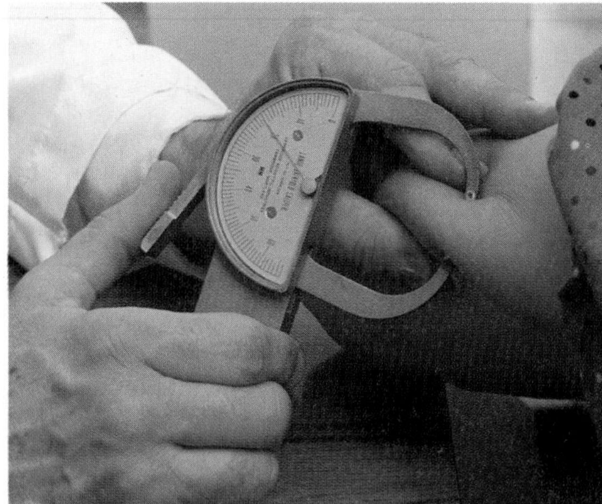

**Figure 5.2**
Measuring subcutaneous fat by the skin-fold technique is another valid way to gauge your percentage of body fat.

Many scientists have suggested standards for what percentage of our body weight should be fat. Most of these standards are based on population norms. But because many of us tend to carry excess fat, the average level of fat found in Americans may not be the goal we want to set for our wellness lifestyle. Table 5.1 presents a set of body-fat standards directed at fat levels for optimal functioning and well-being. According to these standards, women are described as fat when their percentage of body fat reaches 22 percent or higher, with obesity starting at 28 percent body fat. For men these levels are much lower; 15 to 22.9 percent body fat is described as fat and 23 percent or more is described as obese.

## Assessing Body Weight

The usual method for measuring body weight is to use a scale that determines weight in pounds or kilograms. Typically, health professionals and the general public have then turned to the Metropolitan Life Insurance Company's chart of ideal weights to interpret individual weight measures. There is growing controversy over the appropriateness of these tables for the general public. These ideal-weight charts are

**Table 5.1 Fatness Ratings of College Men and Women by Percentage of Body Fat**

| Rating | Men | Women |
|---|---|---|
| Very low fat | 5 to 7.9 | 12 to 14.9 |
| Low fat | 8 to 10.9 | 15 to 17.9 |
| Ideal fat | 11 to 14.9 | 18 to 21.9 |
| Above ideal fat | 15 to 17.9 | 22 to 24.9 |
| Overfat | 18 to 22.9 | 25 to 27.9 |
| High fat | 23+ | 28+ |

Source: Reprinted by permission from *Discovering Lifetime Fitness: Concepts of Exercise and Weight Control* by Dintiman, G. B. et al. 

based on mortality rates of people who purchase life-insurance policies. It is generally agreed that this group of people tend to be more affluent, and probably more health conscious, than the general U.S. populace.[5] Thus, these charts are not necessarily appropriate standards for all Americans. Adding to the controversy, Metropolitan Life Insurance Company recently revised their ideal-weight charts, increasing the "ideal weights." Thus, the new charts encourage many to maintain higher weights and, probably for most, higher levels of body fat. At the 1983 annual meeting of the American Heart Association, Dr. William P. Castelli, chief of the Framingham heart-disease study, stated that "recent moves toward upward revision of 'ideal' weights on standard charts are based on a misreading of mortality data and are a disservice to Americans who are 'too fat as it is'. . . . What is a good risk for the insurance companies is not necessarily a good risk for the individual who is deciding to eat more or to eat less."[6]

By using both percentage of body fat and weight measures it is possible to determine how much weight you need to lose or gain. Mary Beth, a college sophomore, weighs 145 pounds and has a percentage of body fat of 25. This tells us that 25 percent of Mary Beth's 145 pounds is fat weight. If Mary Beth wanted to attain a percentage of body fat of 19, how many pounds would she need to lose? A set of simple calculations will answer this question. First, Mary Beth needs to determine the number of pounds currently due to fat weight. This is determined by multiplying current body weight by current percentage of fat (in Mary Beth's case, 145 x .25 = 36 pounds of fat). To determine Mary Beth's current lean body weight she should subtract current pounds of fat from the current total weight. Mary Beth's lean body weight is thus 109 pounds (145 − 36 = 109 pounds of lean). By subtracting Mary Beth's desired percentage of fat (19 percent or .19) from 1.00 (1.00 − .19 = .81) it is possible to calculate an estimate of the amount she should weigh at a 19 percent body-fat level. Mary Beth's estimated target weight for 19 percent body fat is attained by dividing her current lean body weight by .81 (109/.81 = 135). Mary Beth should therefore lose about 10 pounds (145 − 135 = 10) to achieve her desired 19 percentage of body fat.

## What Causes Obesity?

In past years, many body-composition experts believed that the major cause of obesity (overfat) was an excessive intake of calories in relation to the energy requirements of the body. This explanation is commonly referred to as the caloric-balance equation. Recently, however, we have come to recognize that the balance of calories consumed and expended is only one part of the complex puzzle of obesity. There are currently several important theories that attempt to explain the causes of obesity. These include the energy-balance equation, the fat-cell theory, the set-point theory, and the insulin theory.

**THE ENERGY-BALANCE EQUATION** The **energy-balance-equation** theory tells us that a calorie is a calorie. There is no magic way to lose weight. When you take in the same number of calories that your body needs for its daily activities you will maintain your current body weight. If you happen to take in more calories daily than your body needs for its activities, you will tend to gain weight over a period of time. If you eat fewer calories than

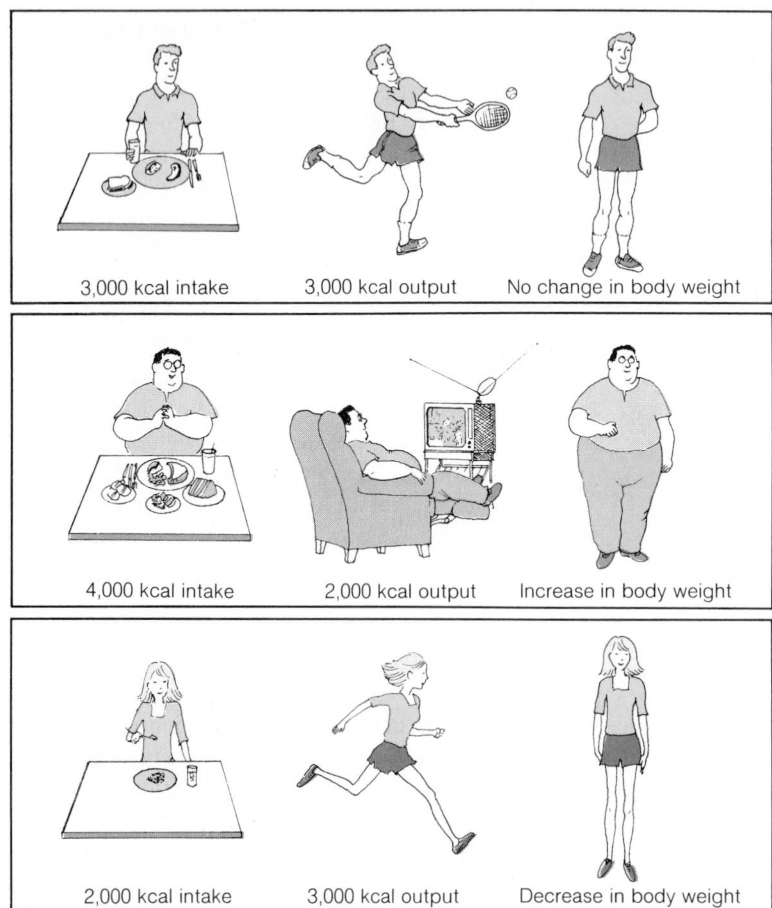
3,000 kcal intake
3,000 kcal output
No change in body weight
4,000 kcal intake
2,000 kcal output
Increase in body weight
2,000 kcal intake
3,000 kcal output
Decrease in body weight

**Figure 5.3**
The energy-balance equation.

your body needs daily for activity you will, over time, tend to lose weight. (See figure 5.3.)

One pound of body fat contains approximately 3,500 kcal. According to the energy-balance equation, each time you consume an excess of 3,500 kcal you will gain a pound of fat. Each time your body experiences a deficit of 3,500 kcal you will lose a pound of fat. It would seem obvious, based on this theory, that there are three major ways to reduce body weight. These would include decreasing caloric intake, increasing energy expenditure, or a combination of the two.

Let's look in once again on Mary Beth who, as you may remember, wants to lose 10 pounds to achieve a weight of 135 pounds and a percentage of body fat of 19. Mary Beth takes in an average of 2,175 calories daily to maintain her current weight of 145 pounds (see table 5.2). According to the energy-balance equation, Mary Beth needs a deficit of 7,000 calories weekly in order to lose 2 pounds of fat in that week. (Remember, each pound of fat contains 3,500 calories.) If Mary Beth chooses to diet only, she will need to cut her daily intake of calories to 1175. Such a drastic reduction in food may be difficult for Mary Beth. If Mary Beth decided to try weight loss by exercise alone she would lose an estimated one-half pound weekly by exercising four to five times per week. For instance, Mary Beth would burn 2,000 calories per week by adding a one-hour brisk walk, five days a week, to her schedule. If, however, Mary Beth chose to combine diet and exercise she would need to cut her calories by only 5,000 calories a week in addition to her five-day walking program. This means she could consume 1,461 calories daily—286 calories more a day than if she chose not to exercise. Mary Beth could safely lose the 10 pounds even more slowly with much less change in her life-style by decreasing her daily caloric intake by 100 calories and increasing her daily caloric expenditure by 100 calories. Specifically, Mary Beth might forgo desert or a soft drink each day and walk briskly for fifteen minutes. At this rate she would lose about 1¾ pounds per month or the 10 pounds in about six months.

**Table 5.2 Calorie Intake Calculator**

| Present Weight | Present daily intake* (Total number of calories it takes to maintain present body weight) | Daily calorie intake to lose 1 lb/wk (500 calories per day less than Present Daily Intake) | Daily calorie intake to lose 2 lbs/wk (1,000 calories per day less than Present Daily Intake) |
|---|---|---|---|
| 295 | 4,425 | 3,925 | 3,425 |
| 290 | 4,350 | 3,850 | 3,350 |
| 285 | 4,275 | 3,775 | 3,275 |
| 280 | 4,200 | 3,700 | 3,200 |
| 275 | 4,125 | 3,625 | 3,125 |
| 270 | 4,050 | 3,550 | 3,050 |
| 265 | 3,975 | 3,475 | 2,975 |
| 260 | 3,900 | 3,400 | 2,900 |
| 255 | 3,825 | 3,325 | 2,825 |
| 250 | 3,750 | 3,250 | 2,750 |
| 245 | 3,675 | 3,175 | 2,675 |
| 240 | 3,600 | 3,100 | 2,600 |
| 235 | 3,525 | 3,025 | 2,525 |
| 230 | 3,450 | 2,950 | 2,450 |
| 225 | 3,375 | 2,875 | 2,375 |
| 220 | 3,300 | 2,800 | 2,300 |
| 215 | 3,225 | 2,725 | 2,225 |
| 210 | 3,150 | 2,650 | 2,150 |
| 205 | 3,075 | 2,575 | 2,075 |
| 200 | 3,000 | 2,500 | 2,000 |
| 195 | 2,925 | 2,425 | 1,925 |
| 190 | 2,850 | 2,350 | 1,850 |
| 185 | 2,775 | 2,275 | 1,775 |
| 180 | 2,700 | 2,200 | 1,700 |
| 175 | 2,625 | 2,125 | 1,625 |
| 170 | 2,550 | 2,050 | 1,550 |
| 165 | 2,475 | 1,975 | 1,475 |
| 160 | 2,400 | 1,900 | 1,400 |
| 155 | 2,325 | 1,825 | 1,325 |
| 150 | 2,250 | 1,750 | 1,250 |
| 145 | 2,175 | 1,675 | 1,175 |
| 140 | 2,100 | 1,600 | 1,100 |
| 135 | 2,025 | 1,525 | 1,025 |
| 130 | 1,950 | 1,450 | 950 |
| 125 | 1,875 | 1,375 | 875 |

*Your weight × 15 = your daily calorie intake which maintains your present weight.
Source: From *Your Daily Portion Prescription.* © 1980 Pennwalt Corporation. Reprinted with permission, Pennwalt Pharmaceutical Division.

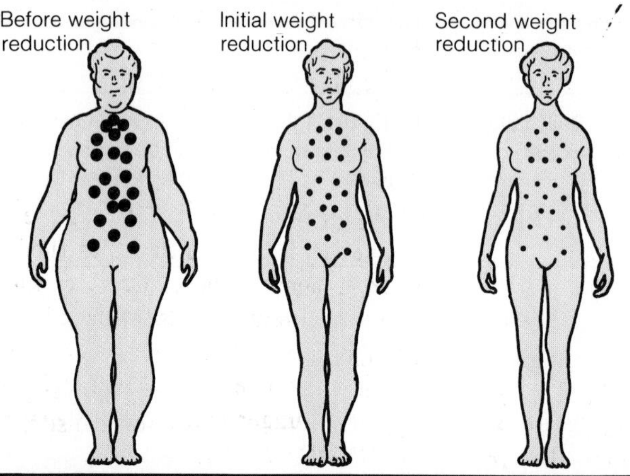


| Body weight | 328 pounds | 227 pounds | 165 pounds |
|---|---|---|---|
| Fat-cell size | 0.9 micrograms/cell | 0.6 micrograms/cell | 0.2 micrograms/cell |
| Fat-cell number | 75 billion | 75 billion | 75 billion |

**Figure 5.4**
Changes in adipose cellularity with weight reduction in obese subjects.

These calculations work out well on paper, but in recent years experts have found that there are factors other than the simple balancing of energy intake with energy output that may have dramatic influences on weight gain and loss in humans. The following theories present other pieces in the puzzle of obesity.

**THE FAT-CELL THEORY** Many experts believe that obesity is related to both the size and number of fat cells in the human body.[7] The **fat-cell** theory states that the human body increases fat storage in two ways. The first involves fat increases in already-existing fat cells; the second involves an actual increase in the number of fat cells.

Research has indicated that a major difference in the composition of fat tissue between obese and nonobese people is the number of fat cells.[8] As a general guideline, an average nonobese individual has about 25 to 30 billion fat cells, a moderately obese person about 60 to 100 billion, and a massively obese person as many as 200 billion fat cells.[9] There seem to be three critical times in our life when these fat cells are significantly increased in terms of number. These include the last three months of fetal development, the first year of life, and during the adolescent growth spurt. There is some speculation that humans can add fat cells at other times during adulthood, but long-term research is needed to address this question with any measure of certainty.[10]

Studies indicate that weight-reduction efforts can cause a reduction in the size of fat cells, but not a decrease in their number. People who gain large numbers of fat cells during childhood may be predisposed to obesity. They can reduce the amount of fat in their fat cells, but the large numbers of fat cells remain, waiting to be filled once again. This may partially explain why many people are able to lose weight (fat) but so easily gain it back. (See figure 5.4.)

**THE SET-POINT THEORY** Another interesting theory of obesity postulates that the human body maintains a **set point** for fat storage. This set point acts like a thermostat, dictating how much fat a person should carry.[11] If fat levels fall below the set point, the body will undergo certain changes designed to return the body to its set level of fat. Body metabolism will decrease causing calories to be burned at a much slower rate, thus conserving remaining fat stores and slowing down weight loss. Additionally, the brain will send out signals to increase hunger. This theory may explain the typical dieter's plateau—the point in a diet where, even with severe caloric restriction, weight loss seems to come to a standstill. Weight control by diet alone is a difficult and often-unsuccessful ordeal as it amounts to a battle against your set point.

It is believed that some people have high set points, causing them to maintain higher levels of body fat, while others seem to have low set points. Heredity may play an important role in determining variations in individual set points.[12] Practically speaking, the body weight at which you tend to stabilize when not dieting is currently the best way to estimate your personal set point.

It is not well understood exactly how the set-point mechanism works. One theory suggests that signals are given off by the body's fat cells, reflecting the amount of fat currently being stored. This signal is then thought to be interpreted by a center in the brain (possibly the hypothalamus). The brain considers input from fat cells, along with other environmental stimuli, and determines what the body's set point should be.[13] These same signals are used to maintain fat levels.

Various factors can influence set point. The taste and smell of food high in sugar and fat, as well as access to a wide variety of food, seems to increase the body's set point. Artificial sweeteners may also tend to raise set point. We have all heard people state that they can put on fat just from looking at food. According to the set-point theory this may be close to the truth. Although looking doesn't actually add calories to the diet, it may cause metabolism to slow down and hunger to increase, all in an effort to increase body fat. This tendency to increase set point would have been very important for our ancient ancestors who lived with frequent food shortages. When good foods were available their set points would rise. Thus, they would consume larger amounts of food and increase fat stores, all as a protection against times of shortage when high levels of body fat would mean survival.

Several factors are thought to decrease set point, including the drugs amphetamine and nicotine, and regular exercise. Amphetamine and nicotine, however, are *not* considered healthy ways to lower set point. The effects of these two drugs on set point last only as long as the drug is taken regularly. Both amphetamine and nicotine have numerous and well-documented harmful effects on the body with long-term use. (These drugs are discussed in detail in chapters 13 and 14.) Exercise, on the other hand, may be one of the best ways to lose fat weight. By lowering set point, exercise marshals the body to help in the attempt to lose fat, rather than fighting against itself.

**THE INSULIN THEORY** Researchers at Yale University have theorized that the kind of food you eat can have dramatic affects on both your appetite and your ability to lose weight.[14] Judith Rodin, a psychologist at Yale, believes that the explanation for this is biochemical. Specifically, insulin seems to increase hunger and food consumption, and make sweets taste better.

**Insulin** is a hormone produced by the body to help guide sugar and fat from the bloodstream into various body cells where it is then used for energy or is stored as fat. Typically, when we eat foods high in glucose our blood-sugar levels will rise. The body reacts to this by secreting more insulin. This lowers the blood-glucose level; however, it often leaves us with high blood-insulin levels for several hours. These high blood-insulin levels have been shown to make experimental subjects hungrier and more inclined toward sweet tastes.[15]

Research seems to indicate that certain foods boost insulin levels more than others. Foods high in glucose cause the greatest rise in insulin levels, while fructose produces a much slower and more moderate rise. Eating one or two large meals daily may also increase your blood-insulin levels, while eating several small meals will usually help keep insulin levels more stable. Additionally, in a group of subjects Rodin has labeled hyperresponders, insulin levels were shown to increase from merely the sight and smell of certain foods. It seems that their bodies were getting ready for the food before it ever reached their mouths. (See table 5.3.)

Being fat can contribute to a cycle of excess insulin secretion. As you gain weight, your body cells become less sensitive to insulin. Your body must then compensate by producing more insulin to accomplish the same function. It is believed that this extra insulin can increase fat tissue as well as keep you hungry. Aerobic exercise tends to have the exact opposite effect, actually increasing the body's sensitivity to insulin.

**Table 5.3 Which Foods Boost Insulin?**

In June, 1983, *American Health* published a "glycemic index" of foods, developed by Dr. David Jenkins at the University of Toronto. This list shows how quickly different foods boost blood sugar and raise your insulin. Foods with a high number act the most like glucose, leading to an insulin jump. Foods with a low index give a slow rise in blood sugar—fructose, fruits, complex carbohydrates.

| | | | |
|---|---|---|---|
| **Honey and Sugars** | | | |
| Fructose | 20 | Honey | 87 |
| Sucrose | 59 | Glucose | 100 |
| **Bread, Pasta, Corn, and Rice** | | | |
| Whole-wheat spaghetti | 42 | Brown rice | 66 |
| | | White bread | 69 |
| White spaghetti | 50 | Wheat bread | 72 |
| Sweet corn | 59 | White rice | 72 |
| **Breakfast Cereals** | | | |
| Oatmeal | 49 | Shredded Wheat | 67 |
| All-Bran | 51 | Cornflakes | 80 |
| **Fruits** | | | |
| Apples | 39 | Bananas | 62 |
| Oranges | 40 | Raisins | 64 |
| Orange juice | 46 | | |
| **Root Vegetables** | | | |
| Sweet potatoes | 48 | White potatotes | 70 |
| Yams | 51 | Carrots | 92 |
| Beets | 64 | Parsnips | 97 |
| **Dairy Products** | | | |
| Skim milk | 32 | Ice cream | 36 |
| Whole milk | 34 | Yogurt | 36 |
| **Peas and Beans** | | | |
| Soybeans | 15 | Chickpeas | 36 |
| Lentils | 29 | Lima beans | 36 |
| Kidney beans | 29 | Baked beans | 40 |
| Black-eyed peas | 33 | Frozen peas | 51 |
| **Odds and Ends** | | | |
| Peanuts | 13 | Sponge cake | 46 |
| Sausages | 28 | Potato chips | 51 |
| Fish sticks | 38 | Pastry | 59 |
| Tomato soup | 38 | Mars bar | 68 |

Source: Reprinted from *American Health: Fitness of Body*. © 1983 American Health Partners, New York.

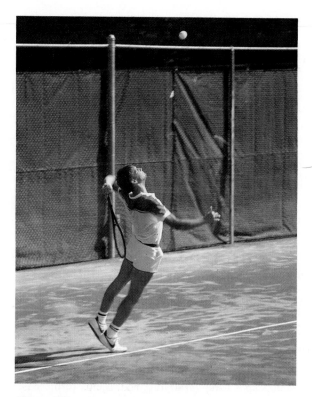

**Figure 5.5**
Ideal levels of body fat allow our bodies to function efficiently and actively.

## Why Maintain Optimal Body Composition?

Many of the enjoyable activities in life require some movement on our part. Bicycling, swimming, or playing tennis or racquetball all require some level of movement. Other daily activities, such as running to catch a bus, carrying a heavy bag of groceries, or even climbing a few flights of stairs, call on us to use our muscles in an efficient manner. Our muscles support our desire and our need to be active. Much of our body fat, on the other hand, serves only as an extra burden. The more excess fat we carry, the less efficiently our bodies can move.[16] Think about how much more difficult it is to climb three flights of stairs carrying twenty pounds of books, compared to carrying nothing as you climb. Having twenty extra pounds of fat to carry around with you daily creates a comparable work load. Maintaining an ideal level of body fat allows your body to function actively in an efficient manner, lending a valued boost to your quality of life and level of wellness. (See figure 5.5.)

5.1 EXHIBIT 5.1

## Facts about Fat

If you have a fat problem—controlled or uncontrolled—you are not alone. The more your fat increases the more problems you'll encounter in maintaining health and achieving longevity. "The longer the waistline, the shorter the lifeline" is an all-too-familiar adage. But sadly, it doesn't really sink in for many people until the insidious growth of girth creates a crisis. We're not stressing the cosmetic disabilities caused by excess fat—or the psychological problems. We are presenting the gut problem.

Shortness of breath may be a first sign of pulmonary distress and heart strain caused by obesity, which increases the heart's work load and contributes to premature death. Fat enlarges the capillary bed (tiny connective blood vessels in an area or organ of your body), which increases the amount of tissue to be nourished by the blood and through which the blood must be pumped by your heart.

In addition, the fat accumulated has to go someplace. You can see what's happening on the outside of you—now let's take a look at the inside. Fat infiltrates the liver and other organs. It's a squeeze process, an invasion. Fat compresses the heart, decreases the blood supply to the intestines, and so on. (See figures 5.6 and 5.7.) Some very fat people can't sit, because if they do, there's no space for their lungs to operate in, as the fat invades the chest. These people have to stand up or lie down all the time. They have disabled themselves. Along with all this, extra-heavy people—and even moderately overfat persons—are putting an extra burden on their backs and legs (the weight-bearing joints), which causes or increases arthritic problems.

Complications following surgery occur more frequently in fat people versus thin. Wounds don't heal as well or as fast. And again a breathing problem—overfat people can't take anesthesia as well as people with ideal fat levels.

Source: © *Medical Times*. Reprinted by permission of Romaine Pierson Publishers, Inc.

### DISCUSSION QUESTIONS

1. Obese people may be physically limited by their oversupply of fat. What are some of the activities that might be physically impossible for an obese person to take part in?
2. If being obese is such a health hazard, why don't obese people reduce their fat levels? Name several personal and social barriers to fat loss.

Research studies over the years have linked many diseases with the risk factor of "obesity."[17] There have been several common flaws in these studies, however, which have led current body-composition researchers to rethink their conclusions regarding the health risks of overweight and obesity.[18] Health professionals are beginning to distinguish between two types of obesity—moderate and morbid. **Moderate obesity** is currently defined as 20 to 40 percent overweight according to height/weight tables, while **morbid obesity** is considered anything above 50 percent over normal weight.[19] Once again, common definitions of obesity confuse the concept of weight (which includes lean and fat weight) with the concept of overfat. (See figures 5.6 and 5.7.) The percentage of body fat ratings presented earlier in this chapter suggest percentage of body fat standards for these classifications.

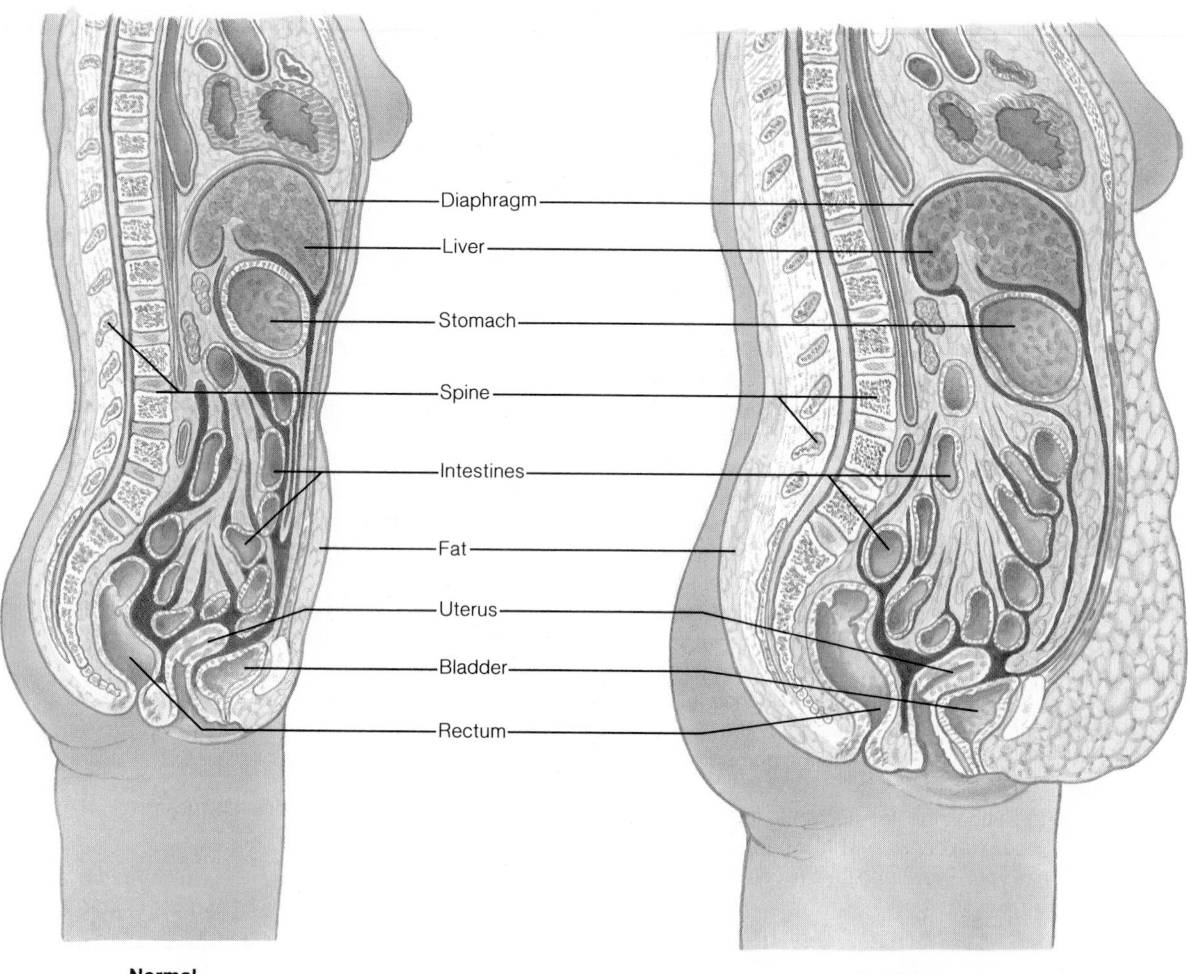


**Figure 5.6**
Normal and overfat intestinal systems. *Source:* © *Medical Times.* Reprinted by permission of Romaine Pierson Publishers, Inc.

According to the standards presented in table 5.1, the ideal fat category would give you the most efficient level of fat for an enhanced work/play capacity, leading to high-level wellness. The categories of very low fat and low fat are usually attained only by serious athletes who spend a good portion of each day in physical training. These low levels of fat are of benefit to people in situations calling for physical competition. The normal person would probably not strive for a life-style leading to these low levels of body fat. The category labeled "above ideal fat" indicates that there is a level of body fat that, while affecting quality of life in terms of work/play capacity, is probably not a health risk in and of itself. The "overfat" category corresponds with moderate obesity. Elevated blood cholesterol, hypertension, and diabetes commonly accompany this level of body fat. The percentage of body fat category "high fat" corresponds with morbid obesity. Studies have indicated that at this extreme level of body fat death and debilitating diseases such as coronary-artery disease, diabetes, and high blood pressure occur at very high rates.[20]

People who fall into the categories of "overfat" and "high fat" should make a concerted attempt to lose this excess fat. Many people with diabetes and high blood pressure benefit greatly by reducing their weight and fat levels.[21] A majority of obese hypertensives return to a normal blood-pressure range with fat loss. Obese adult-onset diabetics can often be taken off insulin medication with a loss of fat. Reductions in total blood-cholesterol levels have also been documented in obese subjects after fat loss.[22]

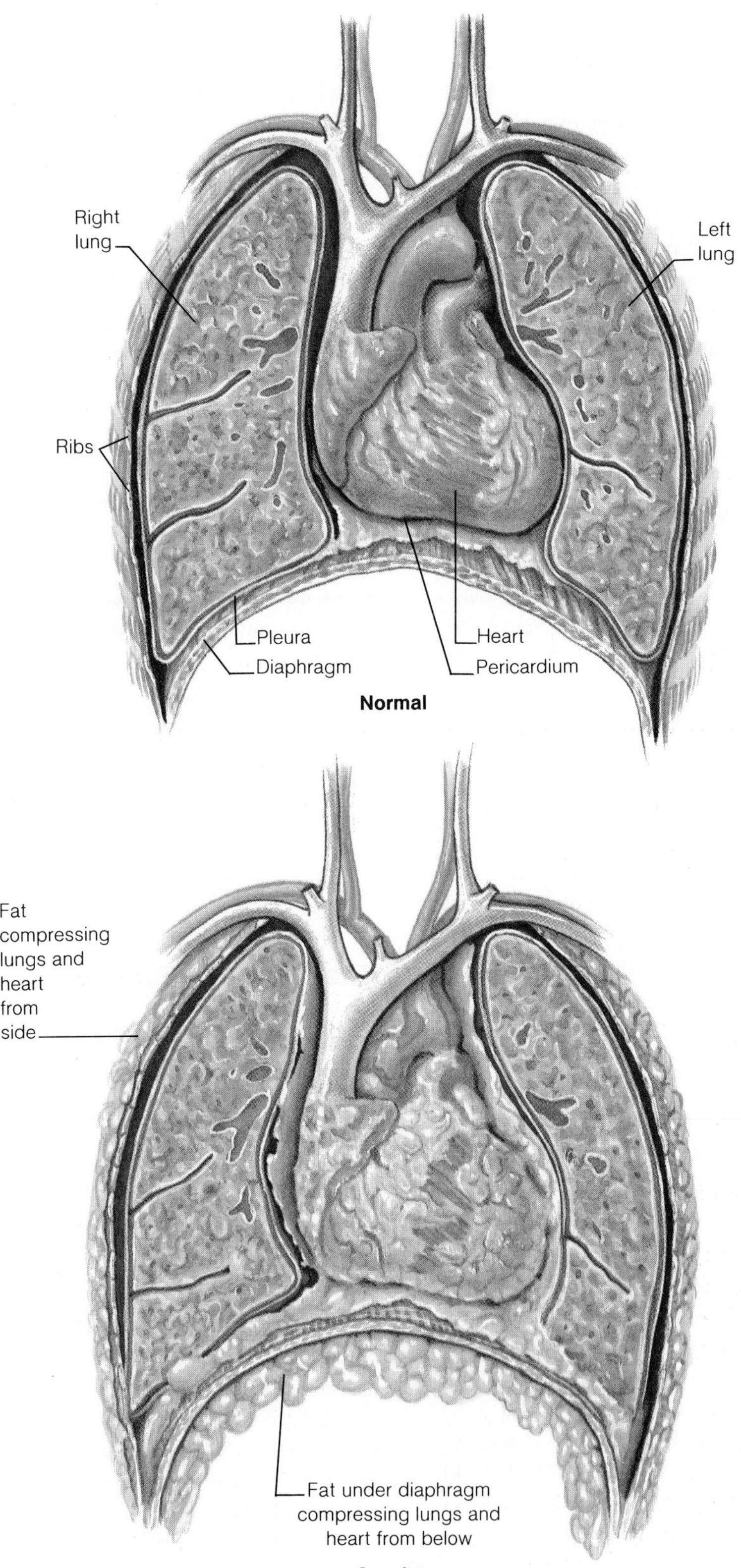


**Figure 5.7**
Normal and overfat respiratory and cardiac systems. *Source:* © *Medical Times*. Reprinted by permission of Romaine Pierson Publishers, Inc.

People in the "above ideal fat" category who have diabetes or high blood pressure will also gain such benefits from fat loss. Many people who fall in this "above ideal fat" category, however, experience no risk factors. For these people, it is doubtful if losing fat will change their disease-risk profile in any significant manner. Therefore, if they are satisfied with their personal appearance and their ability to perform activities which they consider meaningful, there is little evidence to recommend drastic revisions in life-style in order to change body composition.

## BODY COMPOSITION AND LIFE-STYLE CHANGE

When you go on a diet your body reacts in several predictable ways. We saw in chapter 4 that your body's preferred form of energy is carbohydrate. When you restrict your food intake your body will use the glycogen (a carbohydrate) stored in your muscles and liver for energy. Carbohydrates are stored with water in a 1:3 ratio (1 gram of carbohydrate for each 3 grams of water). As you use glycogen for energy you also tend to lose water. It is estimated that 70 percent of the weight lost during the first few days of a diet is due to water loss.[23] By the end of the third week of dieting, water losses are minimal. (See figure 5.8.)

As you continue on a diet, your body begins to use up its second form of preferred energy—fat. Triglycerides, which have been stored in your adipose (fat) cells, begin to be broken down into fatty acids and are secreted into the bloodstream to be taken to the liver. The liver then converts these fatty acids into glucose to be used by body cells for energy.

When you attempt fat loss solely by restricting caloric intake your body will use protein, in addition to the carbohydrates and fats, as a source of energy. This translates into a significant loss of muscle mass, as muscle cells are broken down to be used for fueling the body.

When you diet, your body interprets these signals as starvation and reacts, within twenty-four to forty-eight hours, by slowing down your metabolism as much as 15 to 30 percent.[24] This causes you to conserve energy by burning fewer calories for your daily activities, and also makes fat loss more difficult. Additionally, studies have shown that each time you diet your metabolism will decrease more rapidly, and will return to its original baseline more slowly after each diet is terminated. This is likely to translate into a progressively slower weight loss with each successive diet, as well as more rapid regaining of weight after each diet.[25]

Charlatans have found fat control to be a big moneymaker. Consumers spend over $80 million annually on weight-reduction gimmicks and fad diets.[26] Some estimates go as high as $10 billion.[27] Only 20 percent or so of those who lose weight from such diets are able to maintain their weight loss.[28] The various theories of obesity give us many plausible explanations for such failures. Too many fat cells, a low metabolism, a high set point, genetic tendencies, and a lack of exercise may all play a role. Together, however, these theories direct us to an important realization. Optimal body composition is a result of life-style changes; it does not result from isolated bouts of exercise or caloric restriction.

Research studies based on our best theories continually point to three basic approaches to fat control—aerobic exercise, a balanced low-calorie diet, and behavior-modification techniques. A healthy change in life-style, leading to optimal body composition and higher levels of wellness, would probably include an integration of all three of these approaches.

### The Need for Exercise

Some health professionals have suggested that, by 1977, Americans had reached an all-time minimal-activity level for the human species.[29] Americans have become ingenious in their inventions to avoid muscle movement.[30] Electric can openers, electric toothbrushes, electric garage-door openers, electric typewriters, and the automobile are only a few of the "time-saving" and "energy-saving" devices developed to increase our ability to be sedentary. As we "save" our energy with these devices and fill our leisure time watching others exercise, we tend to throw our energy balance out of kilter.

Inactivity has been cited by many weight-control experts as the major cause of obesity.[31] Recently, however, some experts have posed a question as to whether inactivity is a consequence of obesity rather than a cause.[32] We know that the more excess fat we carry, the less efficiently our bodies move, and the greater the number of calories we burn for a given activity. Thus, it would not be surprising to

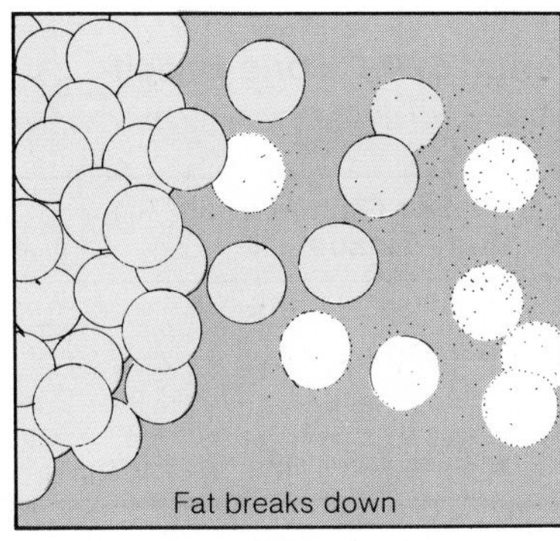

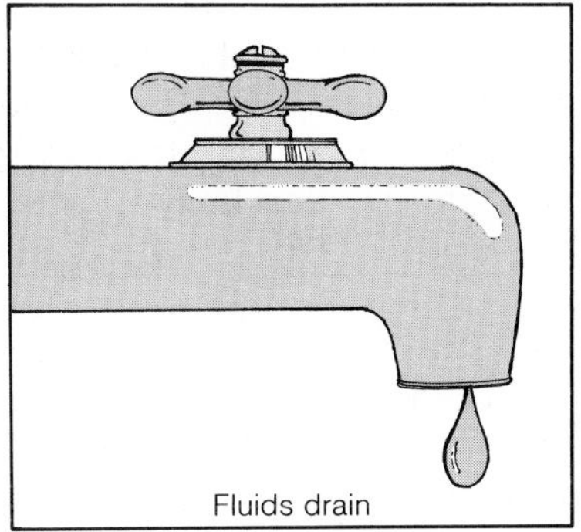

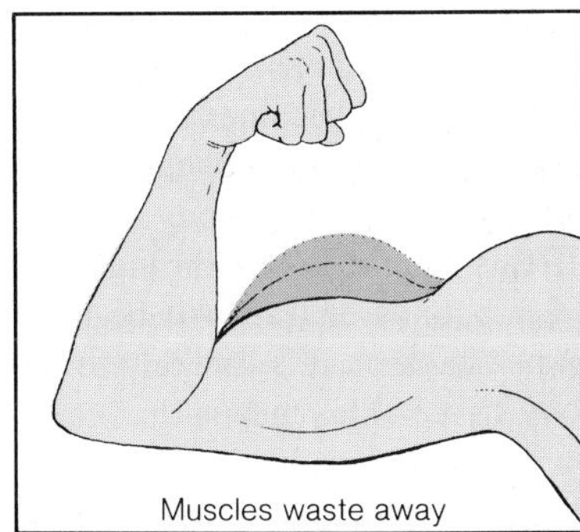

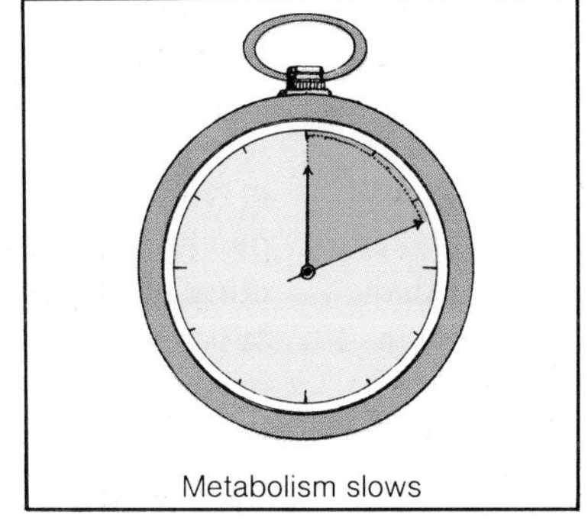


**Figure 5.8**
On a diet.

find that becoming overfat slows people down. Studies supporting this contention have shown that while obese adults are less active than their non-obese counterparts, the same is not true of obese children.[33]

Regardless of whether inactivity is a cause or a consequence of obesity, exercise is one of the primary techniques recommended by experts for losing weight and changing body composition. There are many benefits to be achieved by a regular exercise program that will aid in an attempt to lose body fat.

1. *Exercise increases metabolism.* Exercise increases the rate at which you burn calories. Extra calories are needed for any activity. Overfat people will actually burn more calories for any given activity than their leaner counterparts. It has been estimated that a 100-pound person would burn an extra 70 kcals when jogging one mile. A person weighing 200 pounds, however, would burn up an extra 140 kcal for jogging the same mile. Some people become discouraged when they realize that such a strenuous exercise as jogging a mile burns so few calories. We must remember, however, that successful fat control involves a slow change in life-style habits. People don't put on 20 pounds of excess fat overnight, nor should they expect to take it off at that rate. Most weight-control experts recommend that for a safe and healthy weight loss, a person should attempt to lose no more than 2 pounds of fat per week. Looking at fat control as a long-term improvement in life-style, the energy-expenditure benefits of exercise become more clear. For instance, a daily thirty-minute brisk walk would consume about 55,000 kcal in one year, the equivalent of almost 15 pounds.[34] Additionally, it has been shown that our bodies continue to burn an extra 30 to 50 calories per hour for six to eight hours or longer after a strenuous workout.[35] This adds at least an extra 180 to 400 calories to the total energy cost of each exercise session. This increase in metabolism is also believed by many to offset the body's natural decrease in metabolism when dieting.

2. *Exercise may lower your set point.* Proponents of the set-point theory of obesity believe that exercise may be the most healthy and natural way to lower the thermostat in the body that dictates the amount of fat your body carries.[36] A lowering of the set point is thought to cause an adjustment of food intake as well as increasing the rate at which calories are burned. A study of middle-aged men conducted at Stanford University illustrates the effect of exercise on set point. Peter Wood, a biochemist at Stanford, compared forty-eight middle-aged men involved in an aerobic-exercise program with a control group that remained sedentary over the course

**Table 5.4 Pounds of Lean and Fat Body Weight Lost on Three Different 500-Calorie Deficit Weight-Loss Programs**

| | Lost Body Weight | Lost Body Fat | Lost or Gained Lean Body Tissue |
|---|---|---|---|
| Diet group | −11.7 | −9.3 | −2.4 |
| Exercise group | −10.6 | −12.6 | +2.0 |
| Exercise-diet group | −12.0 | −13.0 | +1.0 |

Source: W. B. Zuti, "Effects of Diet and Exercise on Body Composition of Adult Women during Weight Reduction," *Physical Fitness Research Digest.* Washington, D.C.: President's Council on Physical Fitness, 5. 2 (April 1975).

of the year they were studied. The results of this study showed that the men in the exercise group who ran only a few miles a week ate less food than the sedentary controls. The exercisers' set points may have been lowered, leading to decreased food intake. The men in the exercise group who ran more than twenty-five miles each week increased their food intake in direct proportion to their increase in activity.[37] These men, however, also lost the most body fat. Activity may thus be more important than food intake for fat loss. In this experiment the men who lost the most fat were those who ate the most. It may well be that their set points were lowered by exercise, allowing them to eat more food without adding fat.

3. *Exercise decreases loss of muscle tissue during weight loss.* Studies have shown that people who diet and do not exercise lose significant amounts of lean body tissue (muscle). Aerobic exercise, however, either alone or in combination with dieting, protects against this loss of muscle. This is due, in part, to an enhanced breakdown of fat for the body's energy supply, and to the increase in the rate of protein buildup in skeletal muscles.[38] Table 5.4 presents the results of a study in which three groups of adult women were put on a weight-loss program designed to give them a 500-calorie deficit daily. One group of women was put on a diet that cut 500 calories daily from their normal food intake. Another group was prescribed an exercise program that caused them to expend an extra 500 calories daily. The third group used a combination of both diet and exercise to attain their 500-calorie deficit. As table 5.4 indicates, there was little difference in the total number of pounds lost on these three weight-control programs. Notice, however, that 2.4 pounds of the weight lost by the diet-only group consisted of muscle loss, while neither groups that included exercise in their routine lost lean body tissue. This becomes extremely important for those who engage in the phenomenon of yo-yo dieting, that is, losing 10 pounds only to quickly regain it. If this weight is lost through dieting alone, about 2½ pounds of lean will be lost. When the weight is put back on it is unlikely to be put back as lean body tissue. This means that each time someone yo-yo diets they are likely to become fatter than they were before their last diet.

4. *Exercise suppresses appetite.* Many people mistakenly believe that they should not exercise when they diet because it will increase their appetite and their food intake. Most research to date, however, points to the opposite conclusion. Studies indicate that moderate exercise has a tendency to decrease appetite.[39] This seems to be especially true for people who are very inactive to begin with, and those who tend toward obesity.

5. *Exercise changes how your body handles fat.* Obesity is associated with high levels of triglycerides, and with low levels of HDL cholesterol. Both of these factors are in turn related to coronary-heart disease.[40] Plasma triglycerides have been shown to decrease dramatically with physical training, especially in those people who have high levels to begin with. Additionally, studies conducted by Peter Wood at Stanford have provided us with evidence that exercise can increase the levels of HDL cholesterol (the good cholesterol).[41] Many weight-control experts believe that these changes in lipids (fats) may benefit the obese by lowering their risk of coronary-heart disease.

Proponents of the insulin theory believe that exercise may benefit people who are overfat by its effects on plasma-insulin levels.[42] One of the major functions of insulin is to guide blood fats into adipose cells for storage. High levels of plasma insulin seem to increase the amount of fat your body will

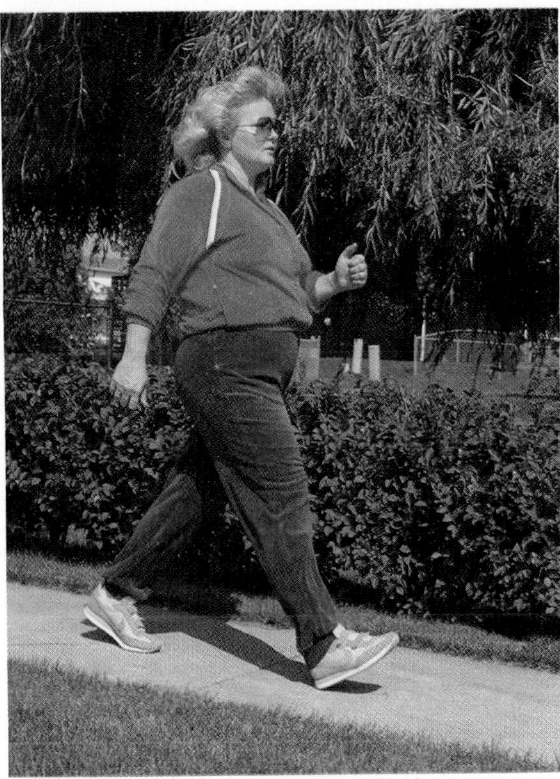

**Figure 5.9**
Walking briskly is a good way to work aerobics into your life-style and a fat-management program.

store. One of the earliest changes seen in people who undertake physical training is a decrease in their plasma-insulin levels.[43] This decrease is seen even after a single bout of exercise. Therefore, experts believe that lowered insulin is a result of the exercise itself, rather than from a secondary effect of weight loss. There is also some evidence that exercise increases the insulin sensitivity of muscle tissue.[44] This would seem to help in regulating the amount of insulin needed by the body for optimal functioning.

6. *Exercise may lower risk even without weight loss.* Several of the beneficial effects of exercise have been shown to occur even when weight loss does not accompany the exercise program. Blood lipids, such as triglycerides and high-density lipoprotein cholesterol, change favorably even without weight loss, as do plasma-insulin levels. Additionally, exercise has been shown to lower blood-pressure levels, especially in those people who had high blood pressure before beginning a regular exercise program.[45] Exercise of an aerobic nature will also increase cardiovascular functioning in general. Resting heart rate will decrease, exercise tolerance will improve, and heart rhythm abnormalities will decrease.[46] For people who fit the obese category, exercise may contribute in a significant way to a reduction in cardiovascular risk, even if weight is not lost. Even those in the "over ideal fat" range may benefit from regular exercise through an increase in their work/play capacity. Thus, people "above ideal fat" would be able to be more active with greater efficiency and less physical discomfort. (See figure 5.9.)

## AN EXERCISE PROGRAM FOR OBESITY

Our muscles depend on two different types of fuel to power them—glycogen and fatty acids. The type of activity that burns fat is commonly known as **aerobic** exercise. The word aerobic means "with air," or exercise that uses oxygen. Exercises such as sprinting or weight lifting that call for a short, intense effort, rapidly break down the glycogen through a process that does not need oxygen. This type of activity is called **anaerobic.** Glycogen, or stored sugar, is found in the large skeletal muscles and the liver and is used for short bursts of work. Your muscles can rely solely on glycogen for fuel for as long as sixty seconds. This anaerobic-energy system is not very efficient in the long run for two major reasons. First, glycogen is a bulky way to store energy. Each gram of glycogen contains only 4 kcal of energy. Second, when glycogen is used for fuel a waste product known as lactic acid will build up in the muscles. This waste must be removed from the muscles or it will injure them. Our bodies, however, have a built-in mechanism for safeguarding our muscles. There is a limited amount of time we are capable of such an all-out effort before we must stop and recover.

Aerobic exercise, on the other hand, allows us to work somewhat below our maximum level for a longer and sustained period of time. Aerobic exercises include jogging, swimming, bicycling, and brisk walking. Aerobic exercise uses the fatty acids released from the fat tissue for its fuel source. The fatty acids are combined with oxygen to give us a steady supply of needed energy. Fat is a very efficient source of fuel, containing about 9 kcal per gram.

If you want to lose fat, aerobic exercise is the type of activity to choose. For those people who are in the "overfat" and the "high fat" categories, and for those people who dislike jogging or bicycling, many fat-control experts recommend a walking program. A brisk walk can be very effective as a physical-conditioning program and fat-loss program. Whichever aerobic exercise you choose, the American College of Sports Medicine recommends that you exercise for at least twenty minutes, three days a week.[47] Some studies have indicated that people who exercised four or five times a week lost fat three times faster than those people who only exercised three times a week. For those people exercising one or two days a week, exercise was found to be completely ineffective in losing fat.[48]

In addition to a regularly scheduled exercise program, it is important for overfat people to fit more routine activities into their life-style. Routine activity might include such activities as using stairs rather than escalators and elevators, or parking the car a few blocks from your destination and walking the rest of the way.

One of the most popular misconceptions regarding exercise and fat control is the notion of "spot reducing." Strength exercises such as weight lifting and calisthenics will strengthen specific muscle groups, depending on the particular exercise performed. They do not, however, burn off fat from any particular area of the body. Remember that these activities are for the most part anaerobic and use glycogen rather than fat for their fuel source. Aerobic exercise, on the other hand, will gradually shrink existing fat cells from all sites on the body as it uses the fat for energy. Tennis players, for example, were studied by measuring fat skin folds and muscle circumference. They were found to have larger muscles in their playing arms as compared to their nonplaying arms. The levels of fat, however, did not vary between playing and nonplaying arms.

Aerobic activities should be used to reduce levels of fat on the total body. Anaerobic strength exercises can then be used in a complementary manner to tone up and strengthen specific muscle groups. Aerobic exercise and anaerobic exercise are explained in greater detail in chapter 6.

## The Role of Diet

Low-calorie diets have long been a mainstay of weight-control regimens. Decreasing your intake of food is one logical option for balancing your energy (calorie) intake and output. But is decreasing your food intake the best way to lose weight and change your body composition?

Controlling the amount of food you eat is considered by most fat-loss experts to be an important component of a sound and healthy fat-loss program. The level of caloric restriction, however, is very important, as well as the types of foods you consume. In order to meet your daily nutritional needs for protein, carbohydrates, vitamins, and minerals, most experts believe that you must consume a minimum of 1,000 to 1,200 kcal daily. Below this caloric level it becomes almost impossible for most people to meet the Recommended Dietary Allowances (RDA). Remember, too, that your body will interpret very-low-calorie diets as starvation and begin almost immediately to slow down your metabolism to counteract the decrease in food.

If the set-point theorists are correct, simply dieting may be of little help in adjusting your set point. In fact, it may begin a chain of events that will make life very unpleasant due to a continuous state of hunger and a decreased metabolism. This, in turn, may make it almost impossible to lose significant amounts of fat.

Proponents of the insulin theory believe that controlling those foods which cause sudden increases in blood-glucose levels may be an important adjunct to a fat-loss diet, as this will help maintain steady levels of both blood glucose and insulin. This may then help to control excess hunger and excess fat storage.

**A BALANCED DIET FOR FAT/WEIGHT CONTROL** A diet that seems to combine the best components of the major theories of obesity is commonly known as the **exchange diet.** Physicians, nutritionists, and health educators often recommend the exchange diet for people who are diabetics, who are overfat, or who just want to improve their health.[49] The exchange diet consists of lists of food groups that are used for menu planning at various caloric levels. The food groups found in the exchange diet consist of Milk, Vegetable, Fruit, Bread, Meat, and Fat Exchanges. Foods in any one group can be substituted or "exchanged" with other foods in the same group. Foods listed within each exchange group contain approximately the same number of calories, and the same amount of carbohydrate, protein, and fat. Following the exchange diet assures you that, even at a low-caloric level, you are eating a balanced diet that will contribute to your general level of well-being. (See Activity for Wellness 5.1.)

5.1 ACTIVITY FOR WELLNESS 5.1

# The Exchange Diet

**YOUR DAILY PORTION PRESCRIPTION**

Locate your Daily Calorie Allowance level on the chart below and read across to obtain your Daily Portion Prescription for each of the six main food groups. Insert the number for each group in the blocks provided in the next section.

| *Daily Calorie Allowance* | *Group 1. Milk Group (portions)* | *Group 2. Vegetable Group (portions from 2B)* | *Group 3. Fruit Group (portions)* | *Group 4. Bread Group (portions)* | *Group 5. Meat Group (portions)* | *Group 6. Fat Group (portions)* |
|---|---|---|---|---|---|---|
| 2,100 | 2½ | 2 | 6 | 7½ | 8 | 6 |
| 2,000 | 2½ | 2 | 5 | 7½ | 8 | 5 |
| 1,900 | 2½ | 2 | 5 | 7 | 7 | 5 |
| 1,800 | 2½ | 2 | 4 | 6 | 7 | 5 |
| 1,700 | 2½ | 1 | 4 | 6 | 6 | 5 |
| 1,600 | 2 | 1 | 4 | 6 | 6 | 5 |
| 1,500 | 2 | 1 | 4 | 5 | 6 | 4 |
| 1,400 | 2 | 1 | 3 | 5 | 6 | 3 |
| 1,300 | 2 | 1 | 4 | 4 | 5 | 3 |
| 1,200 | 2 | 1 | 4 | 4 | 5 | 1 |
| 1,100 | 2 | 1 | 4 | 3 | 5 | 0 |
| 1,000 | 2 | 1 | 3 | 2 | 5 | 0 |
| 900 | 1½ | 1 | 3 | 2 | 5 | 0 |
| 800 | 1½ | 1 | 2 | 1 | 5 | 0 |

**YOUR GUIDE TO PROTECTIVE EATING**

This dietary guide is a flexible one that divides foods into six main groups. All the portions for the foods listed in a group have the same energy (calorie) value and the same Protein, Carbohydrate and Fat value, as indicated under each main heading.

***Group 1. Milk*** ☐

***Each portion = 170 calories***

***(12 grams Carbohydrate, 8 grams Protein, 10 grams Fat)***

| ***Milk*** | ***Portion*** |
|---|---|
| Whole | 1 cup |
| Skim* | 1 cup |

5.1 *continued*

## ACTIVITY FOR WELLNESS

| ***Milk*** | ***Portion*** |
|---|---|
| Evaporated | ½ cup |
| Powdered, whole | ¼ cup |
| Powdered, skim (nonfat dried milk*) | ¼ cup |
| Buttermilk | |
| From whole milk | 1 cup |
| From skim milk* | 1 cup |

*Add 2 Fat portions to your meal for each cup you use of skim milk or buttermilk made from skim milk.

### *Group 2. Vegetables* ☐

A. These vegetables may be used as desired in ordinary amounts. Carbohydrates and calories are negligible.

| | |
|---|---|
| Asparagus | Rhubarb |
| Broccoli | Sauerkraut |
| Brussels sprouts | Squash, summer |
| Cabbage | String beans, young |
| Cauliflower | Tomatoes |
| Celery | "GREENS" |
| Chicory | Beet |
| Cucumbers | Chard |
| Eggplant | Collard |
| Escarole | Dandelion |
| Lettuce | Kale |
| Mushrooms | Mustard |
| Okra | Spinach |
| Pepper | Turnip |
| Radishes | |

B. Vegetables: 1 serving equals ½ cup equals 100 grams (about 3 ounces)

Each Portion = 36 Calories (7 grams Carbohydrate, 2 grams Protein)

| | |
|---|---|
| Beets | Pumpkin |
| Carrots | Rutabaga |
| Onions | Squash, winter |
| Peas, green | Turnips |

### *Group 3. Fruit* ☐

***Each portion = 40 calories (10 grams Carbohydrate)***

| ***Fruit*** | ***Portion*** |
|---|---|
| Apple (2″ diam.) | 1 small |
| Applesauce | ½ cup |
| Apricots, fresh | 2 medium |
| Apricots, dried | 4 halves |
| Banana | ½ small |
| Berries: Straw., Rasp., Black. | 1 cup |
| Blueberries | ⅔ cup |
| Cantaloupe (6″ diam.) | ¼ |
| Cherries | 10 large |
| Dates | 2 |
| Figs, fresh | 2 large |
| Figs, dried | 1 small |
| Grapefruit | ½ small |
| Grapefruit juice | ½ cup |
| Grapes | 12 |
| Grape juice | ¼ cup |
| Honeydew melon (7″ diam.) | ⅛ |
| Mango | ½ small |
| Orange | 1 small |
| Orange juice | ½ cup |
| Papaya | ⅓ medium |
| Peach | 1 medium |
| Pear | 1 small |
| Pineapple | ½ cup |
| Pineapple juice | ⅓ cup |
| Plums | 2 medium |
| Prunes, dried | 2 medium |
| Raisins | 2 tbsp. |
| Tangerine | 1 large |
| Watermelon | 1 cup |

Remember that snacks can add many extra calories to the daily total. Budget between-meal snacks from your daily food portions.

***The following foods may be used as desired:***

| | |
|---|---|
| Coffee* | Pickles, unsweetened dill |
| Tea* | |
| Clear broth | |
| Bouillon (without fat) | Gelatin, unsweetened |
| Rennet tablets | Cranberries |
| Pickles, sour | |

*Use with milk from daily allowance and artificial sweeteners, if desired.

ACTIVITY FOR 5.1

# WELLNESS

Choose these portions according to your portion prescription size for each group. You can eat any combination of these foods anytime in the day so long as you do not go over the portion sizes.

***Group 4. Bread*** ☐
***Each portion = 68 calories (15 grams Carbohydrate, 2 grams Protein)***

| ***Bread*** | ***Portion*** |
|---|---|
| Bread | 1 slice |
| Biscuit or roll (2″ diam.) | 1 |
| Muffin (2″ diam.) | 1 |
| Corn bread (1½″ cube) | 1 |
| Flour | 2½ tbsp. |
| Cereal, cooked | ½ cup |
| Cereal, dry (flake or puffed) | ¾ cup |
| Rice or grits, cooked | ½ cup |
| Spaghetti, noodles, etc., cooked | ½ cup |
| Crackers | |
| Graham (2½″ square) | 2 |
| Oyster | 20 (½ cup) |
| Saltines (2″ square) | 5 |
| Soda (2½″ square) | 3 |
| Round, thin (1½″ diam.) | 6–8 |
| Vegetables | |
| Beans or peas, dried, cooked (lima, navy, split peas, cowpeas, etc.) | ½ cup |
| Baked beans, no pork | ¼ cup |
| Corn | ⅓ cup |
| Parsnips | ⅔ cup |
| Potatoes | |
| White (2″ diam.), baked, | 1 |
| boiled, mashed | ½ cup |
| Sweet or yams | ¼ cup |
| Sponge cake, plain (1½″ cube) | 1 |
| Ice cream (omit 2 fat portions) | ½ cup |

***Group 5. Meat*** ☐
***Each portion = 73 calories (7 grams Protein, 5 grams Fat)***

| ***Meat*** | ***Portion*** |
|---|---|
| Meat or poultry (med. fat) beef, lamb, pork, liver, chicken, etc. | 1 oz. |
| Cold cuts (4½″ × ⅛″ thick): salami, bologna, liverwurst, luncheon loaf, minced ham | 1 slice |
| Frankfurter (8–9 per pound) | 1 |
| Fish | |
| Cod, haddock, mackerel, trout, etc. | 1 oz. |
| Salmon, tuna, crab, lobster | ¼ cup |
| Oysters, shrimp, clams | 5 small |
| Sardines | 3 medium |
| Cheese | |
| Cheddar, American | 1 oz. |
| Cottage | ¼ cup |
| Egg | 1 |
| Peanut Butter | 2 tsp. |

***Group 6. Fat*** ☐
***Each portion = 45 calories (5 grams Fat)***

| ***Fat*** | ***Portion*** |
|---|---|
| Butter or margarine | 1 tsp. |
| Bacon, crisp | 1 slice |
| Cream, light | 2 tbsp. |
| Cream, heavy | 1 tbsp. |
| Cream cheese | 1 tbsp. |
| French dressing | 1 tbsp. |
| Mayonnaise | 1 tsp. |
| Oil or cooking fat | 1 tsp. |
| Nuts | 6 small |
| Olives | 5 small |
| Avocado (4″ diam.) | ⅛ |

***The following seasonings may be used as desired:***

| | |
|---|---|
| Chopped parsley | Mint |
| Garlic | Nutmeg |
| Celery | Cinnamon |
| Pepper and other spices | Vinegar |
| | Mustard |
| Lemon | Onion |

Source: *Are You Really Serious About Losing Weight?* © 1980 Pennwalt, Corporation. Reprinted with permission, Pennwalt Pharmaceutical Division.

**Food Diary**
Day of the week

| Time | Food type and quantity | Feeling while eating | Activity while eating | Minutes spent eating | Degree of hunger | Location of eating |
|---|---|---|---|---|---|---|
| 6:00–11:00 A.M. | | | | | | |
| 11:00–4:00 P.M. | | | | | | |
| 4:00–9:00 P.M. | | | | | | |
| 9:00 P.M.–6:00 A.M. | | | | | | |

**Figure 5.10**
A detailed food diary is essential to successful weight control.

Remember that the best combination for fat loss is aerobic exercise and a balanced, reasonably low-calorie diet. This combination promotes the greatest amount of fat loss without losing muscle tissue at the same time.

## Modifying Eating and Exercise Behaviors

Often we need help in learning new behavior patterns, such as beginning an exercise program or changing our eating habits. Psychologists have had some measure of success in helping people lose fat with a technique called **behavior modification.**[50] Behavior modification includes four distinct phases: (1) describing the behavior to be modified; (2) replacing the established behaviors with more desirable behaviors; (3) developing techniques to control behaviors; and (4) using positive reinforcements or rewards for successful behavior changes.[51]

**MODIFYING EATING BEHAVIORS** The first step in modifying eating behaviors is to determine the behaviors to be modified. This is usually accomplished by keeping a detailed food diary which describes the type and quantity of food you consume, the time of day you consume it, how you feel while eating, any activites you are involved with while eating, how long you spend eating, where you eat, and how hungry you were before eating. This food diary should be kept for a minimum of three days, and may be used for several weeks in order to get an adequate picture of your dietary habits. (See figure 5.10.) Usually when people analyze their food diaries, they find that they have very predictable behavior patterns regarding food. Possibly you might notice that you eat every time you turn on the television, or that you always eat when certain people are with you. Some people find that their food consumption is tied to an emotional state such as feeling angry, sad, bored, or lonely. Others may typically binge on sweets after an argument with their boyfriend or girlfriend. In behavior-modification terms, these moods, activities, or even certain people, are considered to be **cues** to eating.

Once your cues to eating have been documented, they can be replaced with more acceptable and healthy behavior patterns. For instance, if you find that you always eat ice cream after an argument with your boyfriend or girlfriend, you could choose to go for a brisk walk after an argument instead. If you find that you usually eat a candy bar in the morning on your drive to campus, try and sing along with the radio instead. The possibilities of acceptable alternatives are endless and are bound only by your creativity.[52] Your goal is to establish new behaviors for the environmental cues you receive. It is also helpful to establish some techniques you can use to control the act of eating. (See Activity for Wellness 5.2.)

Finally, it is important to reward yourself for short-term goals you have successfully accomplished. Your rewards should be things other than food that you would not have given yourself if you hadn't completed the short-term goal you set. Buying some new clothes, going to a movie, or taking a trip are all good options for rewards. Keeping charts and

5.2 ACTIVITY FOR WELLNESS 5.2

## Techniques to Control the Act of Eating

There are many useful techniques to gain control over eating habits once undesirable environmental cues have been identified. How many of the following techniques do you use? Check the items you have tried.

[ ] 1. Make the act of eating food a ritual; limit eating to one place in the house and no matter what foods you eat, follow a set routine. Use a place mat, set the table with silverware, and use the same dishes at each meal. Do this for main meals as well as for snacks. One dieter who continually snacked between meals curbed this habit by dressing up in a tuxedo and eating by candlelight for each meal and snack. He soon stopped snacking between meals.

[ ] 2. Use smaller dishes; the impetus to finish the meal may not be the food per se, but the desire to view an empty plate or glass.

[ ] 3. Eat slowly. Fight the urge to eat quickly by taking more time at meals. You can do this by cutting food into smaller pieces and chewing each piece ten to fifteen times before swallowing. Another technique is to place the knife, spoon, or fork back on the table after each two or three bites and allow for a one- or two-minute rest pause between mouthfuls.

Source: From Katch, F. I. and McArdle, W. D., *Nutrition, Weight Control, and Exercise.* Lea & Febiger, Philadelphia, 1983.

records of your fat loss and behavior change is also a motivating and reinforcing technique that is helpful for many people.

**MODIFYING EXERCISE BEHAVIORS** The process for modifying your exercise behaviors parallels that of modifying eating behaviors. The first step is to identify what behaviors need to be modified. This is done by keeping a diary of your activities for a period of time ranging from several days to several weeks. An analysis of your diary will indicate how active you really are and where you could make realistic changes in your exercise routines.

Adding exercise and activity to your life-style doesn't have to be thought of solely in terms of a regularly scheduled "exercise session." Although this is extremely helpful, it is also useful to consider more routine ways in which you could fit more activity into your daily life. (See Activity for Wellness 5.3.)

Rewarding and reinforcing yourself for successfully adding more activity to your life is very important. Many people make their exercise session a social occasion by exercising with a group of friends. You could also try running in fun runs, keeping charts to record your progress, or plotting the miles you cover through walking, running, bicycling, or swimming, on a map route leading to some faraway destination. Again, the possibilities are endless—being creative in your reward system is part of the fun!

5.3 ACTIVITY FOR WELLNESS 5.3

# Substituting Alternate Exercise Behaviors

There are many ways to increase energy expenditure within the time allotted to daily routines. The important considerations are to determine when and how to make changes. How many of these substitutes would you be willing and able to try? Make a check next to those items.

[ ] 1. When driving to work, park a half mile away and walk the remaining distance. Brisk walking to and from the car each day, five days a week, will burn up the caloric equivalent of about seven pounds of fat in one year.

[ ] 2. When taking public transportation, get off eight or ten stops early and walk the remaining distance.

[ ] 3. When traveling relatively short distances, walk instead of taking a cab or bus.

[ ] 4. Don't go to a restaurant for lunch; participate in some form of physical activity, such as walking, which you can continue for thirty to forty-five minutes.

[ ] 5. Wake up a half hour early and take a brisk walk, bicycle, or swim before breakfast.

[ ] 6. Replace the cocktail hour with twenty minutes of exercise.

[ ] 7. Replace coffee breaks with exercise breaks.

[ ] 8. Walk up and down several flights of stairs after each hour of work.

[ ] 9. Sweep the sidewalks in front of your house or apartment. We know of one world-renowned seventy-four-year-old scientist who sweeps around a four-square-block park in San Francisco, two-and-one-half hours a day, five to six days a week!

[ ] 10. When going on a family outing, allow time for exercise: (a) Get out of the car before reaching your destination; let your family drive the rest of the way while you walk. (b) Instead of eating at halftime or intermission at sports events, walk around the stadium or arena. Climb up and down stairs instead of using elevators or escalators.

[ ] 11. Replace the hired help and undertake some of these tasks yourself:
- [ ] a. Gardening
- [ ] b. Mowing the lawn
- [ ] c. Painting
- [ ] d. Washing and waxing the car
- [ ] e. Walking the dog

[ ] 12. During television commercials, run in place, jump rope or jog up and down stairs.

[ ] 13. Replace power tools and appliances with manually operated devices:
- [ ] a. Lawn-care equipment
- [ ] b. Automatic household appliances such as vacuum cleaners, eggbeaters, ice-cream makers, juicers
- [ ] c. Saws
- [ ] d. Drills
- [ ] e. Snow shovelers
- [ ] f. Garage doors

[ ] 14. Play golf without a golf cart or caddy.

[ ] 15. Walk or jog up and down the beach in addition to sunbathing.

Source: From Katch, F. I. and McArdle, W. D. *Nutrition, Weight Control, and Exercise.* Lea & Febiger, Philadelphia, 1983.

# PERSONAL AND SOCIAL INFLUENCES

Our society supports many notions and activities that may serve as barriers to attaining an optimal level of body fat. Many of these barriers involve support and reinforcement for life-style factors that oppose wellness. Others involve the widespread availability of fad diets and "weight-control" quackery. To succeed in reaching your goals regarding body composition, it is helpful to have some insight into these possible barriers.

## Life-style Barriers

Our culture and social-support systems often reward us for living a sedentary life-style. New technological innovations at work and in the home "save" us energy. What do we do with this saved energy? Too many of us choose to store it by sitting in front of the television and watching other people exercise. Additionally, some nutrition experts now believe that prime-time television shows are sending implicit messages to viewers that overeating and indulging in junk food and alcohol are harmless. One study conducted at the University of Pennsylvania found that during a typical week's prime-time programming, eating, drinking, or talking about food occurs an average of nine times per hour.[53] A similar study completed at Rutgers University noted that, of the references to food, 34 percent were to alcohol, soda pop, or other beverages (excluding milk); 28 percent were to cakes, pies, cookies, chips, gum, candy, and ice cream; 12 percent were to meat, fish, and poultry; and only 13 percent were to fruits, vegetables, and grain and dairy products combined.[54] These researchers point out that more houses in the U.S. have television sets than have plumbing, and that these television sets are turned on for an average of 6.3 hours each day. Television viewing could indeed be fattening, due to its reinforcement of a sedentary life-style and overconsumption of a variety of nonnutritious foods.

Many of us carry with us and practice mistaken notions about "diet foods." The salad bar is one notorious example. How many times have you selected to eat only the salad bar for lunch or dinner, telling yourself the reason for this was because you were on a diet? As figure 5.11 so graphically illustrates, the typical American salad could have as many calories, and possibly even more, than the typical luncheon entree. Hidden fats and refined sugar have even infiltrated the salad bar.

No one food in and of itself is "fattening." The overall selection of a reasonable amount of nutritious food and a physically active life-style seem to correlate best with optimal body composition and high levels of wellness.

## Fad Diets and Diet Quackery

Pick up any current issue of a popular magazine, or even the Sunday newspaper, and you are likely to find dozens of advertisements for weight-loss products. Estimates indicate that consumers may spend as much as $10 billion a year for diets, gadgets, pills, and potions promising to take off those ugly pounds *fast*.[55]

Advertisements for fad diets have several common characteristics:[56]

1. *The promise of a quick fix.* Many diets will promise a magical loss of weight (but not fat) within a matter of hours or days. Beware the advertisement that promises weight losses of over two to four pounds per week. The weight lost on these "quick" diets will most often be water weight. Remember that carbohydrate retains three times its weight in water. When you consume less than 60 grams of carbohydrate your body will start to lose water. This water weight is quickly replaced as soon as you return to your regular diet or consume fluids.
2. *A strong sexual overlay.* Most of the models in weight-loss advertisements are beautiful, curvaceous women or handsome, muscular men. The only "fat" people are those in the "before" photographs. These ads often blatantly suggest that love is available only to thin, beautiful people.
3. *No pain, no strain.* Many fad diets promise pounds off fast with no exercise, and no restrictions on food intake. By using their magic lotion, belt, pills, and the like, you can help your body "melt away unwanted fat."

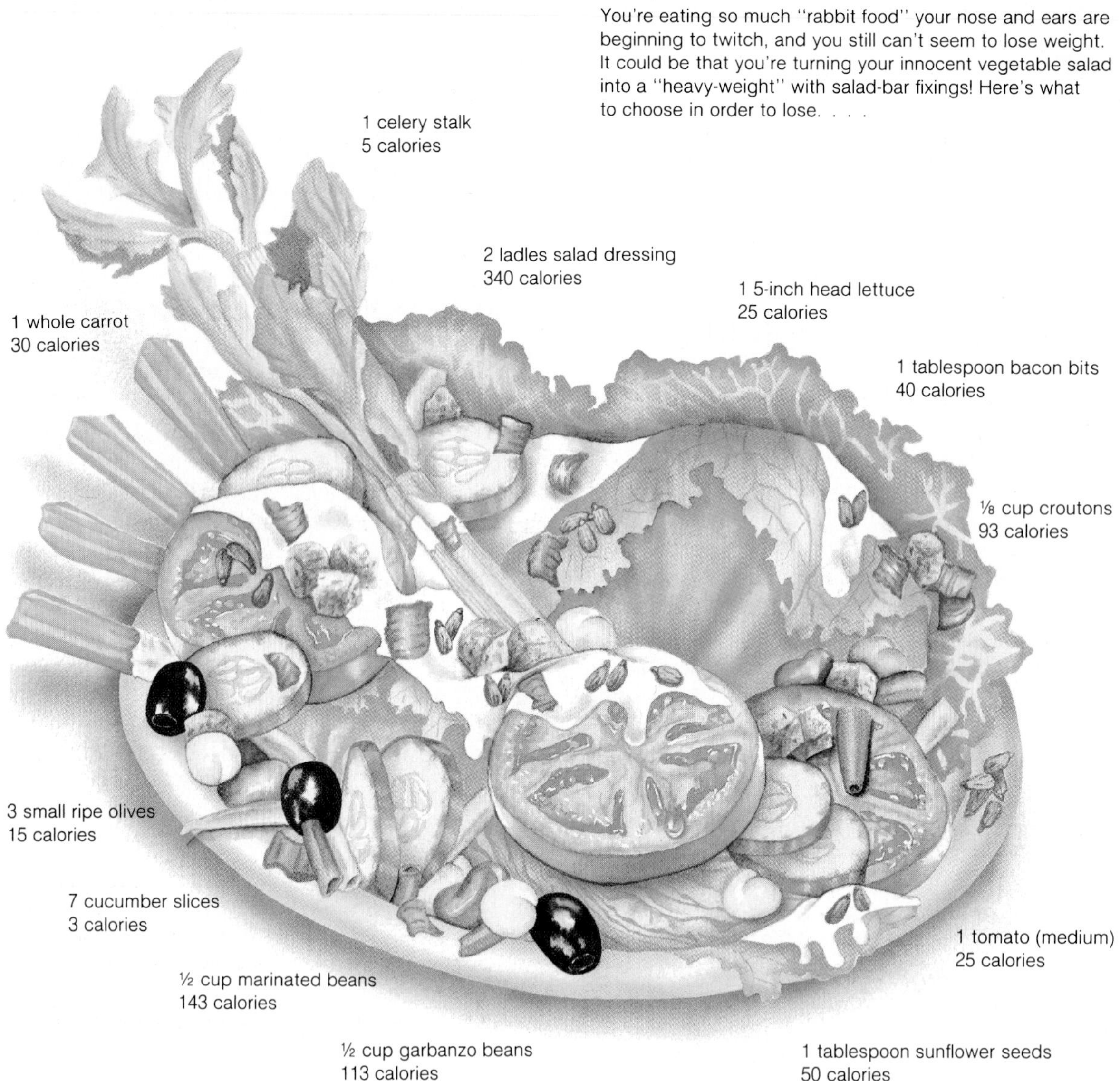


**Figure 5.11**
The 884-calorie salad.

4. *Testimonials.* Most fad diets rely on testimonials from "the person on the street" who has tried this great diet. Often the weight losses reported are incredible—sixty pounds or more. Some of these testimonials have been attained by paid solicitation.
5. *The Imprimatur of Experts.* Fad-diet advertisements are almost all based on the research or beliefs of "scientists," "doctors," and "medical experts" from "medical schools" or "medical laboratories" across America. Few of these experts or institutions are ever identified by name.
6. *Figments and Fragments of Science.* Many diets use medical jargon to persuade the consumer. For example, one diet promises a "hypocaloric effect" (medical jargon for calorie restriction) and states that on their diet the food will be metabolized and oxidized in as little as two to three hours after eating (this is the normal physiological time frame).

Fad diets appear with a frequency so great that it is almost impossible to keep up with them. Table 5.5 presents some of the more popular current fad diets. When attempting to analyze any new diet that may become popular, there are several major questions you should use to test its effectiveness and safety.[57]

1. Is the diet nutritionally well balanced, including an adequate number of calories?
2. Is the person or organization promoting the diet well respected and knowledgeable about nutrition and fat loss?
3. Does the diet represent and follow the recommendations of the best fat-loss authorities?
4. Does the diet allow for individual preferences, practices, and taste?
5. Could you live on this diet for the rest of your life?

If your answers to these questions are affirmative it is likely that the diet is sound and will help you on your journey to optimal body composition.

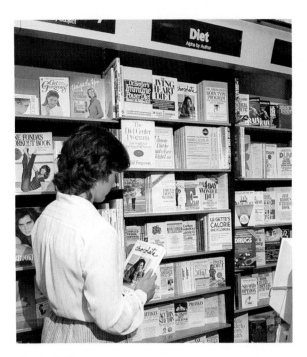


**Figure 5.12**
Many diet books promote ineffective and sometimes dangerous fad diets.

Table 5.5 **Popular Current Fad Diets**

| Name of Diet | Category | Kcal | Technique Employed | Comments |
|---|---|---|---|---|
| The Beverly Hills Diet | — | not specified | This plan is based on eating foods in the "correct" order and offsetting high-calorie binges with "corrective" feasts of fruit.<br>Fruit is the main component of the six-week weight-loss phase of the diet. | This diet contains no source of complete protein until the nineteenth day of the diet.<br>Weight loss is mainly through dehydration associated with diarrhea.<br>Potential hazards: severe diarrhea leading to shock; potassium deficiency, heart arrhythmias, and hair loss. |
| Liquid protein diets | High protein | 300 to 500 kcal/day | Consumption of only liquefied protein substances. | Many of the liquefied protein mixtures are made from low-quality (incomplete) protein sources.<br>More than forty sudden deaths have been reported as associated with this type of diet.<br>Other complications include: low potassium, a dramatic drop in blood pressure experienced upon standing, fainting, irregular heart rhythm, muscular weakness, cramps, dry skin, and hair loss. |

**Table 5.5** *Continued*

| Name of Diet | Category | Kcal | Technique Employed | Comments |
|---|---|---|---|---|
| The Cambridge Diet | Low calorie | 330 kcal/day | A mixture consisting of 33 grams of protein and 44 grams of carbohydrate is the sole source of nutrition for periods of up to four consecutive weeks. | Provides too little protein leading to a loss of lean body mass over a period of weeks.<br>Other complications include: weakness, dizziness, dehydration, a dramatic drop in blood pressure experienced upon standing up, and cardiac irregularities.<br>As of 1982, the F.D.A. had reports of 138 illnesses (including 6 deaths). |
| The Complete Scarsdale Medical Diet | High protein/low carbohydrate | Averages 750 kcal/day | A rigid fourteen-day high-protein, very low-carbohydrate diet.<br>$<$ 35 percent carbohydrate, 30–35 percent protein, and $>$ 35 percent fat. | Much of the weight loss is water weight.<br>This diet is a poor source of thiamine, niacin, calcium, iron, and magnesium. |
| The Doctor's Quick Weight-Loss Diet (Stillman's) | High protein/low carbohydrate | 1,500 to 1,800 kcal/day | A very low-carbohydrate diet.<br>Recommends drinking eight or more glasses of water daily | High in saturated fats and cholesterol.<br>Intake of calcium, iron, and vitamins C and A is inadequate.<br>Dizziness, fatigue, headache, and nausea have been reported. |
| Dr. Atkin's Diet Revolution | High fat/low carbohydrate | 1,500 to 1,600 kcal/day | This diet consists of 20 to 40 grams of carbohydrates, unlimited fats, large amounts of meat and eggs for protein, and omits breads and cereals.<br>60–70 percent fat, 23–27 percent protein, and $<$ 10 percent carbohydrate. | High in saturated fats.<br>Likely to be low in iron, magnesium, and vitamin $B_6$. May also be low in vitamins A and D, and calcium if cheese and butter are not used.<br>Fatigue and low blood pressure have been reported. |
| The Pritikin Diet | High carbohydrate (complex) | 650 to 1000 kcal/day | Very low in fat (10 percent), 10 percent protein, and 80 percent carbohydrates.<br>Stresses consumption of vegetables. Sugars, salt, cholesterol and processed foods are severely restricted.<br>An exercise plan accompanies this diet. | Extremely high in fiber.<br>Low amounts of complete protein sources.<br>Probably a poor source of calcium, iron, and vitamin $B_{12}$. |

Sources: (1) "Cambridge diet 'experimental,' FDA reports," *American Medical News,* 21 January 1983. (2) "The Beverly Hills Diet: Experts Call Its Science Slim, Its Claims Puffery," *Medical World News* 22. 5 18 (1981): 6–7. (3) E. B. Feldman and T. T. Kuske, "Health Hazards of Popular Reducing Diets," *Consultant* 22. 5 (1982): 46–51. (4) Richard B. Friedman, Phillip Kindy, and Judith A. Reinke, "What to Tell Patients about Weight-Loss Methods," *Postgraduate Medicine* 72.4 (1982): 73–80. (5) Bonnie Liebman, "Diet Plan Update," *Nutrition Action* 9.9 (1982): 15. (6) Richard S. Rivlin, "Obesity: Dispelling Some Hormonal and Nutritional Myths," *Consultant* 21. 6 (1981): 125–28. (7) Thomas A. Wadden, Albert J. Stunkard, Kelly D. Brownell, and Theodore B. Van Italie, "The Cambridge Diet: More Mayhem?", *Journal of the American Medical Association* 250.20 (1983): 2833–34.

5.2 EXHIBIT 5.2

# How to Write Your Own Diet Book

A *New York Times* editorial during the summer of 1981 marked the decline in American literary taste: The most popular books on the paper's best-seller list were guides to losing weight and volumes of cat cartoons. At present, cat books have gained the greater share of the market, but more diet manuals are surely waiting in the wings. Because no diet works for long, millions of people are caught in the lose-gain trap. And writing a diet book with a new angle, however strange, can be the surest way to a publishing fortune.

What counts in this kind of work is the formula, and diet books follow a pattern as rigidly as Gothic romances or spy stories. We plowed through as many diet books as we could stand (at twenty or so, we hit our limit) in an effort to divine their guiding principles. From this arduous labor we devised a ten-point plan for writing a successful diet book—a set of instructions that, needless to say, we hope fewer and fewer writers will follow.

1. *Tell 'em who you are.* It helps to be a physician—like Drs. Atkins and Stillman, and the late Dr. Tarnower—or an osteopath like Robert Linn, the liquid-protein man. But laymen, too, can cut themselves into the deal. Consider *The Amazing Diet Secret of a Desperate Housewife* and *The Hollywood Emergency Diet.* (The actor who wrote the latter, the advertisement boasts, "is not a scientist or a doctor. He's not even a college graduate.") Nathan Pritikin, who has made a fortune on his diet-and-exercise plan, began as an inventor in Chicago. And Judy Mazel, author of *The Beverly Hills Diet,* explains herself thus: "I do not purport to be a medical doctor. . . . If medical experts had conclusively proven the causes of fat, we'd all be thin. I have simply pulled together scattered facts and synthesized them. . . ."

2. *Pick a catchy title.* This is essential. In 1958, Richard Mackarness published a high-fat, low-carbohydrate diet with the bland title *Eat Fat and Grow Slim.* It went nowhere. Just three years later, Herman Taller, M.D., published a similar diet plan called *Calories Don't Count.* It stayed on the best-seller lists for the better part of a year. Drama is everything. Robert Linn's liquid-protein plan sold well over a million paperback copies as *The Last Chance Diet*—even though the title became funereally apt when deaths were attributed to liquid-protein diets.

3. *Get 'em into the tent.* Dieting is a drag. To be motivated, your readers need both a carrot and a stick. Tell them that they'd better listen to you if they don't want to die young. Sound the familiar warning that extra weight leads to heart disease, cancer, lumbago, diabetes, gout, and arthritis, and throw in one or two diseases they've never heard of. Then turn around and play the sympathetic friend. Promise to help them with a plan—based on newly discovered scientific principles—that makes it easy to lose weight and will improve their sex lives simultaneously.

4. *Present . . . The Master Plan.* This takes ingenuity. As a general rule of thumb, the diet should be as unnatural and unbalanced as possible: There is, by now, no other way to make it seem special. A tried-and-true method is to tell people to eat only certain food groups and exclude others. The most serviceable villains are carbohydrates—bread, sugar, even fruits and vegetables. A bolder approach is to base a diet on a single food. Eggs and grapefruit are now hallowed by tradition; one recent count turned up no fewer than fifty-one diets based on these two staples. People get sick of eggs and grapefruit, and will certainly lose weight if that's all they eat; but they may also become sick of your diet altogether. Your readers may also suspect that you think they're simpleminded.

Judy Mazel has cleverly surmounted these obstacles in *The Beverly Hills Diet.* Her rigid six-week plan is based largely on single-food days, but the food-of-the-day *varies* in a programmed way. Watermelon, grapes, pineapples, and other fruits predominate. Such a diet, of course, can lead to diarrhea, which Mazel applauds. "If you have loose bowel movements, hooray! Keep in mind that pounds leave your body two main ways—bowel movements and urination. The more time you spend on the toilet, the better. On watermelon days especially, you can expect to urinate a lot. That's the idea."

## 5.2 *continued* EXHIBIT 5.2

5. *Break out the textbooks.* However unbalanced your diet is, you shouldn't be hard put to find some scientific-sounding rationale for it. Old diet books are a good place to look, also any book on folk medicine. Low-carbohydrate diets have been recycled, with the same justification, for a century. If you can't find a ready-made reason for your gimmick, look through some articles on nutrition and metabolism, take a few quotes out of context, and make something up. Inspiration comes from unlikely places: Mazel found hers in a book on enzymes that she picked up in a health-food store, where she went to buy cashew nuts. Don't be shy about theorizing. Remember that human nutrition is still very poorly understood.

6. *Pad, pad, pad.* You don't really have much to tell your readers, so fill up the book with recipes, anecdotes, homilies, and reprints of government nutrition tables (which aren't copyrighted). One famous author broke up his diet book into twenty-five short chapters, each with its own title page. Like fiber, this adds bulk.

7. *Foretell the future.* Your readers know that weight lost is quickly regained. Tell them that you know this too, and have designed your diet to help them change their eating habits permanently—even if the plan is so bizarre that only a monomaniac could stick to it for more than a week.

8. *Contemplate exercise.* But ignore it as much as possible; don't make yourself a bore by pushing sweat.

9. *Blame the victim.* Most of your readers will get nothing whatever from your book. Absolve yourself of any responsibility. Follow Robert Linn's example. In *The Last Chance Diet,* he claims that "the program cannot fail. Only you can fail." End of discussion.

10. *Cover yourself.* Somewhere, in large type or small, advise the reader to consult her or his physician before going on your diet.

Source: From *The Dieter's Dilemma: Eating Less and Weighing More,* by William Bennett and Jack Gurin. Copyright © 1982 William Bennett and Jack Gurin. Reprinted by permission of Basic Books, Inc.

## DISCUSSION QUESTIONS

1. How many diet books do you own?

2. Take a look at a couple of diet books (in a public library or bookstore if you don't own any). Can you find most of the ten points listed by Bennett and Gurin in these diet books?

3. Why do you think people continue to fall prey to diet books and gimmicks?

Optimal body composition and related levels of wellness are a result of your life-style choices. Isolated diets or sporadic exercise routines are unlikely to have much positive impact. Developing a life-style of sound dietary practices and activity can be approached as an adventure. Seek out new activities and new and nutritious foods. Your life-style is your choice.

## SUMMARY

1. Body weight is composed of fat cells and lean cells. The fat cells are elastic and store fat deposits. The lean cells make up all other body cells, such as bone, blood, muscle, and organs.

2. Fat can be divided into two categories: essential and storage fat. Essential fat is necessary for normal body functioning. Some storage fat is necessary to pad vital organs and insulate the body. The rest of storage fat is used to store energy or calories.

3. Scales and height/weight tables are *not* good ways to measure body fat, as they have no mechanism to differentiate fat weight from lean body weight. The skin-fold technique and underwater weighing are better methods for fat measurement as they are able to estimate percentage of body fat.

4. There are several good theories that attempt to explain the cause of obesity. The energy-balance-equation theory, the fat-cell theory, the set-point theory, and the insulin theory all add important pieces to the puzzle of obesity causation.

5. Maintaining optimal levels of body fat helps to facilitate optimal and efficient body function. This lends a valuable boost to your wellness life-style.

6. Body-composition experts suggest that people who are moderately to morbidly overweight are at risk for hypertension, diabetes, elevated blood cholesterol, and coronary-artery disease. These people would benefit from a disease-prevention program aimed at reducing percentage of body fat.

7. Dieting, by itself, causes water and protein loss, as well as fat loss. Additionally, body metabolism slows down by as much as 15 to 30 percent.

8. The optimal way to lose body fat is to combine aerobic exercise with a well-balanced, low-calorie diet.

9. Exercise increases metabolism, lowers the set point, decreases muscle loss, suppresses appetite, and changes how your body handles fat. All of these contribute to safe and effective fat loss.

10. Aerobic exercise uses fatty acids for its energy source and is thus the best type of fat-loss exercise.

11. Behavior-modification techniques can help people learn new food and exercise habits. Three steps are involved with behavior modification: assessing eating and exercise cues, modifying diet and exercise habits, and reinforcing positive changes.

12. There are many barriers to attaining and maintaining optimal body composition. Factors that support sedentary life-styles and overindulgence in food are primary barriers. The abundance of fad diets and "weight-control" quackery are additional barriers.

13. Optimal body composition involves life-style changes that can add to life's adventure. Begin to explore new activities and taste new foods. Try to view your fat-control efforts as adding a new, positive direction to your life.

## Recommended Readings

Bailey, Covert. *Fit or Fat.* Boston: Houghton Mifflin, 1978.

Bennett, William, and Gurin, Joel. *The Dieter's Dilemma.* New York: Basic Books, 1982.

Berland, T. *Consumer Reports, Rating the Diets.* New York: Signet Books, 1984. (Updated yearly.)

Katch, Frank, and McArdle, William. *Nutrition, Weight Control and Exercise,* 2nd ed. Philadelphia: Lea & Febiger, 1983.

Williams, M. H. *Nutrition for Fitness and Sport.* Dubuque, Iowa: Wm. C. Brown Co. Publishers, 1983.

## References

1. Maria Simonson and Joan Rattner Heilman, *The Complete University Medical Diet* (New York: Rawson Associates, 1983).

2. Frank I. Katch and William D. McArdle, *Nutrition, Weight Control, and Exercise,* 2nd ed. (Philadelphia: Lea & Febiger, 1983), 103.

3. Maria Simonson, "Obesity as a Health Factor," *The Female Patient* (September 1978); William E. Straw, "Managing Obesity," *Family Practice Recertification* 1. 5 (1979): 21–27.

4. Katch and McArdle, *Nutrition,* 124.

5. International Medical News Service, "Raising of 'Ideal' Weights Held a Disservice," *Family Practice News* 13. 2 (1983): 2, 85.

6. International Medical News Service, "Raising of 'Ideal' Weights," 2, 85.

7. Michael Weintraub, "A New Look at Obesity," *Drug Therapy* (August 1981): 141–47; Katch and McArdle, *Nutrition,* 134–35; Pauline S. Powers, "Evaluating and Treating Patients for Obesity," *Physician and Patient* 1. 2 (1982): 7–14.

8. Katch and McArdle, *Nutrition,* 136.

9. Katch and McArdle, *Nutrition,* 138–39.

10. Powers, "Evaluating Obesity," 1982; Katch and McArdle, *Nutrition.*

11. William Bennett and Joel Gurin, *The Dieter's Dilemma* (New York: Basic Books, 1982).

12. W. Bennett and J. Gurin, *Dieter's Dilemma.*

13. W. Bennett and J. Gurin, "Book Bonus: How the Body Outwits the Dieter," *American Health* 1. 2 (1982): 44–51.

14. J. Rodin, "Taming the Hunger Hormone: Is Insulin the Key to Weight Control?", *American Health* 3. 1 (1984): 43–47.

15. Rodin, "Taming Hunger Hormone," 43–47.

16. Melvin H. Williams, *Nutrition for Fitness and Sport* (Dubuque, Iowa: Wm. C. Brown Co. Publishers, 1983).

17. Norman M. Kaplan, "The Bottom Line About Fat," *The Saturday Evening Post* 255. 3 (April 1983): 18–23, 100.

18. Kaplan, "Bottom Line," 18–23, 100; Thomas R. Knapp, "A Methodological Critique of the 'Ideal Weight' Concept," *Journal of the American Medical Association* 250. 4 (1983): 506–10; Faith T. Fitzgerald, "Weight Reduction: Science vs. Scam," *National Forum LXIV.* 1 (1984): 31–33.

19. Kaplan, "Bottom Line," 18–23, 100.

20. Kaplan, "Bottom Line," 18–23, 100.

21. Kaplan, "Bottom Line," 18–23, 100.

22. Kelly D. Brownell and Thomas A. Wadden, "Treating the Overweight Patient," *Medical Times* 111. 6 (1983): 117–21.

23. Williams, *Nutrition.*

24. Kelly D. Brownell and Albert J. Stunkard, "Physical Activity in the Development and Control of Obesity," in Albert J. Stunkard, *Obesity* (Philadelphia: W. B. Saunders Co., 1980).

25. Brownell and Stunkard, "Physical Activity."

26. Simonson, "Obesity."

27. Daniel Q. Haney, "Girth Control," *Greensboro News and Record* (4 December, 1983).

28. Simonson, "Obesity."

29. Bennett and Gurin, "Body."

30. Grant W. Gwinup, "Aerobic Program for Obesity," *The Female Patient* 8.34/8–34/9, (1983).

31. Jean Mayer, *A Diet for Living* (New York: Simon & Schuster, Pocket Books, 1977); Frank Konishi, *Exercise Equivalents of Foods: A Practical Guide for the Overweight.* (Carbondale, Ill.: Southern Illinois Univ. Press, 1973); Bennett and Gurin, "Body."

32. Brownell and Stunkard, "Physical Activity."

33. P. Wilkinson, J. Parklin, G. Pearloom, H. Strong, and P. Sykes, "Energy Intake and Physical Activity in Obese Children," *British Medical Journal* 1.756, (1977).

34. William E. Straw, "The Dilemma of Obesity: Current Concepts of Causes and Management," *Postgraduate Medicine* 72.1 (1982): 121–26.

35. George B. Dintiman, Stephen E. Stone, Jude C. Pennington, and Robert G. Davis, *Discovering Lifetime Fitness* (St. Paul, Minn.: West Publishing Co., 1984); Bennett and Gurin, "Body."

36. Bennett and Gurin, "Body."

37. Bennett and Gurin, "Body."

38. William Zuti, "Effects of Diet and Exercise on Body Composition of Adult Women during Weight Reduction," doctoral dissertation, Kent State University, 1972, as reported in *Physical Fitness Research Digest* 5.2. Washington, D.C., *President's Council on Physical Fitness,* Series 5, No. 2 (April 1975).

39. Brownell and Stunkard, "Physical Activity."

40. Brownell and Stunkard, "Physical Activity."

41. P. D. Wood, W. Haskell, H. Klein, et al. "The Distribution of Plasma Lipoproteins in Middle-Aged Male Runners," *Metabolism* 25 (1976): 1249–57; P. D. Wood, H. Klein, S. Lewis, et al., "Plasma Lipoprotein Concentrations in Middle-Aged Male Runners," *Circulation* 50 (suppl.) (1974): 115.

42. Rodin, "Taming Hunger Hormone," 43–47.

43. P. Bjorntrop, K. de Jounge, L. Sjostrom, et al. "Physical Training in Human Obesity II: Effects on Plasma Insulin in Glucose-Intolerant Subjects without Marked Hyperinsulinemia," *Scandinavian Journal of Clinical Laboratory Investigations* 32 (1973): 41–45.

44. P. Bjorntrop, L. Sjostrom, and L. Sullivan, "The Role of Physical Exercise in the Management of Obesity," in Munro, J. F., ed., *The Treatment of Obesity.* (Lancaster, England: MTP Press, 1979).

45. Brownell and Stunkard, "Physical Activity."

46. Brownell and Stunkard, "Physical Activity."

47. "American College of Sports Medicine Position Statement: The Recommended Quantity and Quality of Exercise for Developing and Maintaining Fitness in Healthy Adults," *Medicine and Science in Sports* 10. 3 (1978): vii–x.

48. Leonard Epstein and Rena Wing, "Aerobic Exercise and Weight," *Addictive Behaviors* 5 (1980): 371–88.

49. American Diabetes Association, *Exchange Lists for Meal Planning* (New York: American Diabetes Association, 1976).

50. Gloria R. Leon, "The Behavior Modification Approach to Weight Reduction," *Contemporary Nutrition* 4. 8 (1979).

51. Katch and McArdle, *Nutrition,* 176.

52. Katch and McArdle, *Nutrition,* 178.

53. Susan Holden, "Why Television Is Fattening," *Nutrition Action* 9. 2 (1982): 9.

54. Holden, "Television Is Fattening."

55. Fitzgerald, "Weight Reduction."

56. Fitzgerald, "Weight Reduction."

57. Theodore Berland, *Rating the Diets* (New York: Signet Books, 1983).

CHAPTER SIX

# Fitness Potentials: Discovering Your Play



One of the most visible wellness trends in America today is a growing interest in physical fitness. At least 50 percent of adult Americans are estimated to participate in some form of exercise on a regular basis.[1] Some of the more popular fitness activities include jogging, walking, bicycling, swimming, aerobic dance, weight lifting, racquetball, and tennis. Health spas and fitness centers are springing up in most communities to cater to this thriving interest in fitness. Newsstands, too, mirror public interest with a variety of new fitness journals.

While the interest in fitness remains high, it does not necessarily translate into beneficial and safe exercise programs for the American public. Unfortunately, there are many charlatans only too eager to capitalize on our lack of knowledge and high interest regarding the process of becoming more physically fit. This chapter will introduce you to the concept of fitness and its various dimensions. Additionally, it will help you learn how to set up safe, beneficial, and enjoyable fitness activities. Becoming more active will enhance your quest for a wellness lifestyle.

## FINDING YOUR PLAY

According to Dr. George Sheehan, cardiologist and author of numerous exercise articles and books, the key to enhancing your level of wellness through activity is to find your play.[2] We should ask ourselves "What activities bring joy and creativity into our lives?" and "What activities do we consider to be fun?"

Play is an attitude that can transform any activity into a joyful, rewarding experience. As children, we looked forward to the moment we were set loose for recess or the end of the school day. We couldn't wait to get outside to run, play tag, climb in trees or on monkey bars, ride bikes, roller skate, or jump rope. We called this play! What has happened in our transition to adulthood that turned so many of these activities into work? Why do so many of us now finish a day at school or the office and rush home, only to turn on the television set and watch others play for us? What have we done with our play?

One of the best motivations for physical activity is enjoyment. As you contemplate ways to become physically fit, keep in mind that you are looking for "play" as much as for a "workout." Experiment with many different activities until you find those that truly enhance your life and well-being. (See Exhibit 6.1.)

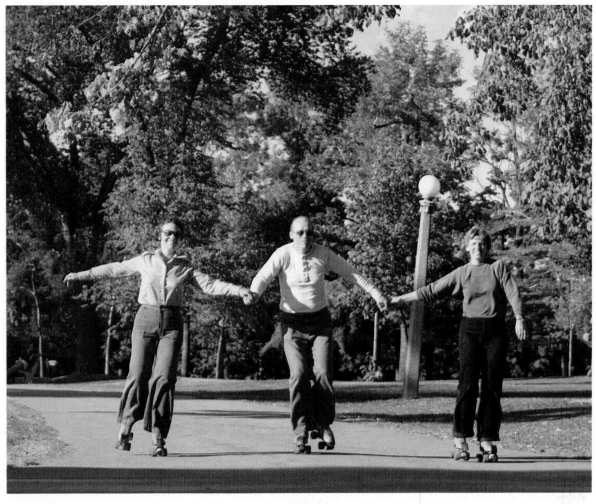

**Figure 6.1**
It is important for both adults and children to find playful physical activity.

6.1 EXHIBIT

## If the Spirit Is Willing, the Flesh Will Follow

On a recent radio show I discussed exercise with a woman who did not exercise. "The spirit is willing," she told me, "but the flesh is weak."

I had, of course, heard that excuse many times before. But for the first time, it occurred to me that the opposite was true.

The flesh is willing. It is the spirit that is weak. Our bodies are capable of the most astounding feats, but the horizons of our spirits do not reach beyond the television, the stereo, and the car.

The flesh is not only willing, it is wanting and waiting to be put into action. The flesh is filled with everything the spirit lacks: grit, pluck, nerve, and determination. We come from a breed that crossed continents on foot and trekked from pole to pole. And even now we see teachers running marathons, stockbrokers in Outward Bound, retired executives climbing Everest.

Our flesh asks for more challenges and seeks new frontiers. What is missing is not physical energy. Physical energy is there for the using. The fuel is there. It is waiting to be ignited. We need something to light the fire, something to get us into action.

This can be seen from the moment we wake up. We lie abed waiting the third, and last, and now frantic call. The alarm clock, the radio, and the family have taken turns trying to get us up. Still we lie immobile until the last possible minute.

Survey this scene and tell me that the spirit is willing but the flesh is weak. How many calories does it take to get out of bed? Whose bodies are so exhausted that they can't get their feet on the floor?

I can plead that I'm in a semicoma, not yet ready for coordinated action, but the same inertia happens again and again throughout the day. The body is ready and willing and able, but the spirit is becalmed. Where there is no emotion, there is no motion, either.

What is missing is the spiritual energy, what the Greeks called "enthusiasm." There are, of course, many other desirable qualities missing as well, but enthusiasm is the key.

It is from lack of enthusiasm that the failures of the spirit multiply during the day. We must, as the word implies, be filled with and possessed and inspired by a divine power or spirit.

When we are enthusiastic, we take on the qualities that go with it. We develop a determination to equal the endurance of our muscles, a fortitude to match the courage of our hearts, and

# BENEFITS OF PHYSICAL ACTIVITY

Many people are physically active because of the benefits they experience as a result of choosing this life-style. Benefits of physical activity thus serve as incentives and motivators. What are the benefits of regular, vigorous physical activity?

## Psychological Benefits

Vigorous activity can lead to improvements in perception of body image, a more positive self-concept, and decreases in levels of both anxiety and depression.[3] All of these changes have been linked to the state that habitual exercisers refer to as "the feeling-better sensation."[4]

Many people use exercise as one of their primary stress-coping skills. The physiological mechanisms associated with the stress-handling benefits

## EXHIBIT 6.1

a passion to join with the animal strengths of our bodies.

To succeed at anything, you need passion. You have to be a bit of a fanatic. If you want to move anyone to act, you must first be moved yourself. To instigate, said Emerson, you must first be instigated. I am aware of this every time I lecture. For an hour before the talk, I can be seen walking alone, muttering to myself, gradually building myself to a fever pitch.

But the spirit has more to offer than just this excitement. It gives us motivation and incentive when the excitement is missing. This spirit is what gets us through when everything else fails. In his paper on "Factors in Human Endurance," Oxford professor Ralph Johnson states that a man's ability to survive depends on the qualities of his personality.

This thought is particularly striking in the accounts of explorers and mountain climbers, people stretched to their limits and beyond. The explorer Captain Scott, writing of one of his men, said, "Browers came through the best. Never was there such a sturdy, active, undefeated man." Of Scott himself one of his companions wrote, "Scott was the strongest combination of a strong man in a strong body that I have ever known. And this because he was weak. He conquered his weaker self and became the strong leader we went to follow and came to love."

So behind the enthusiasm, behind the inspiration, behind the passion, there must be the will. What finally and irrevocably separates us from the rest of the world is our will.

We can choose. We can decide. We can will to do it our way. And when we do, nothing can prevail against us.

Source: From George Sheehan, M.D., "If the Spirit is Willing, the Flesh Will Follow," in *The Physician and Sports Medicine* 7.3 (March 1979): 39. Reprinted by permission of The Physician and Sports Medicine, a McGraw-Hill publication.

## DISCUSSION QUESTIONS

1. Do you agree with Dr. Sheehan's statement, "the flesh is willing. It is the spirit that is weak"?

2. What could (or does) motivate you to exercise? Try to list at least three motivators.

3. What activities do you consider to be play? How does this label of "play" affect your willingness to participate?

of physical activity are not well understood at this time. In studies at the University of Southern California, Herbert deVries has observed that muscle tension (a widely used measure of stress) decreases after physical activity.[5] Additionally, it has been suggested that moderate physical activity is incompatible with maintaining skeletal-muscular tension, and thus apparently leads to a relaxation response.

Many runners have reported experiencing positive psychological states during long-distance runs which they have labeled "exercise highs." Some researchers have proposed that an increase of a substance known as beta-endorphin, a morphinelike chemical produced by the body, may be responsible for this elevated mood.[6] More research is needed to aid in our understanding of this phenomenon, as well as other psychological benefits of physical activity. (See Exhibit 6.2.)

6.2 EXHIBIT 6.2

## Take a Walk, Not a Mars Bar

The best pick-me-up is not long distance, as phone ads and marathon runners say. Nor is it munching a candy bar. The shortest route to feeling better may be a ten-minute walk outdoors.

In a series of experiments, in the lab and on the campus of California State University in Long Beach, Dr. Robert Thayer has been studying the effects of brisk walking on energy and tension levels. First he asked volunteers for written diaries on their levels of energy and tension. They described how they felt at ten-minute intervals starting an hour before and continuing an hour past a ten-minute treadmill walk. For half an hour after the walk, they reported more energy.

In a second experiment, he asked subjects to roll dice at an appointed time each day, and then, depending on the number, either walk around the block or eat a candy bar. The outdoor walk boosted energy for up to two hours and lowered tension. The candy bar, on the other hand, boosted energy only briefly and, after thirty minutes, tension levels went way up.

In a third experiment, Thayer found that the energy boost from walking is probably the best temporary remedy for depression. Unfortunately, many of the depressed subjects who enthusiastically began the study could not complete it. They couldn't bring themselves to walk, says Thayer, because they felt too little energy.

Dr. Herbert deVries, a USC physiologist, has measured corresponding decreases in neuromuscular tension after light exercise. According to deVries, rhythmic exercises like walking, jogging and cycling for five to thirty minutes at 30 percent to 60 percent of maximum capacity give the best "tranquilizer effect." Neither that amount of time nor that intensity will build your heart, but it may bring some peace of mind.

Source: Reprinted from *American Health: Fitness of Body.* © 1983 American Health Partners, New York.

### DISCUSSION QUESTIONS

1. Have you ever noticed that about thirty minutes after eating simple sugars, such as a candy bar, your tension level goes up?

2. Do you currently use mild, rhythmic exercise, such as walking or jogging, as a coping mechanism for tension or stress? If so, how do you feel after you exercise?

3. If you do not currently take advantage of mild, rhythmic exercise for stress reduction, how could you fit ten minutes of walking into your daily lifestyle? Are you willing to do this?

## Cardiovascular Benefits

Physically active individuals may experience a cardiovascular conditioning or **training effect.** Regular vigorous activity helps to strengthen the heart muscle. The walls of the heart become thicker and stronger, allowing it to pump more blood per beat than an untrained heart. This, in turn, helps the heart to work more efficiently, both during exercise and at rest. One measure of the heart's efficiency is the resting heart rate. Normal resting heart rates for adults vary between sixty and eighty beats per minute. It is not uncommon to see resting heart rates of forty-five to fifty-five beats per minute in individuals who regularly participate in vigorous activity. This indicates that the heart is able to pump enough blood to meet the body's needs by doing less work. Another sign of the heart's efficiency is the heart-rate level during and immediately following physical activity. During an exercise session, the trained

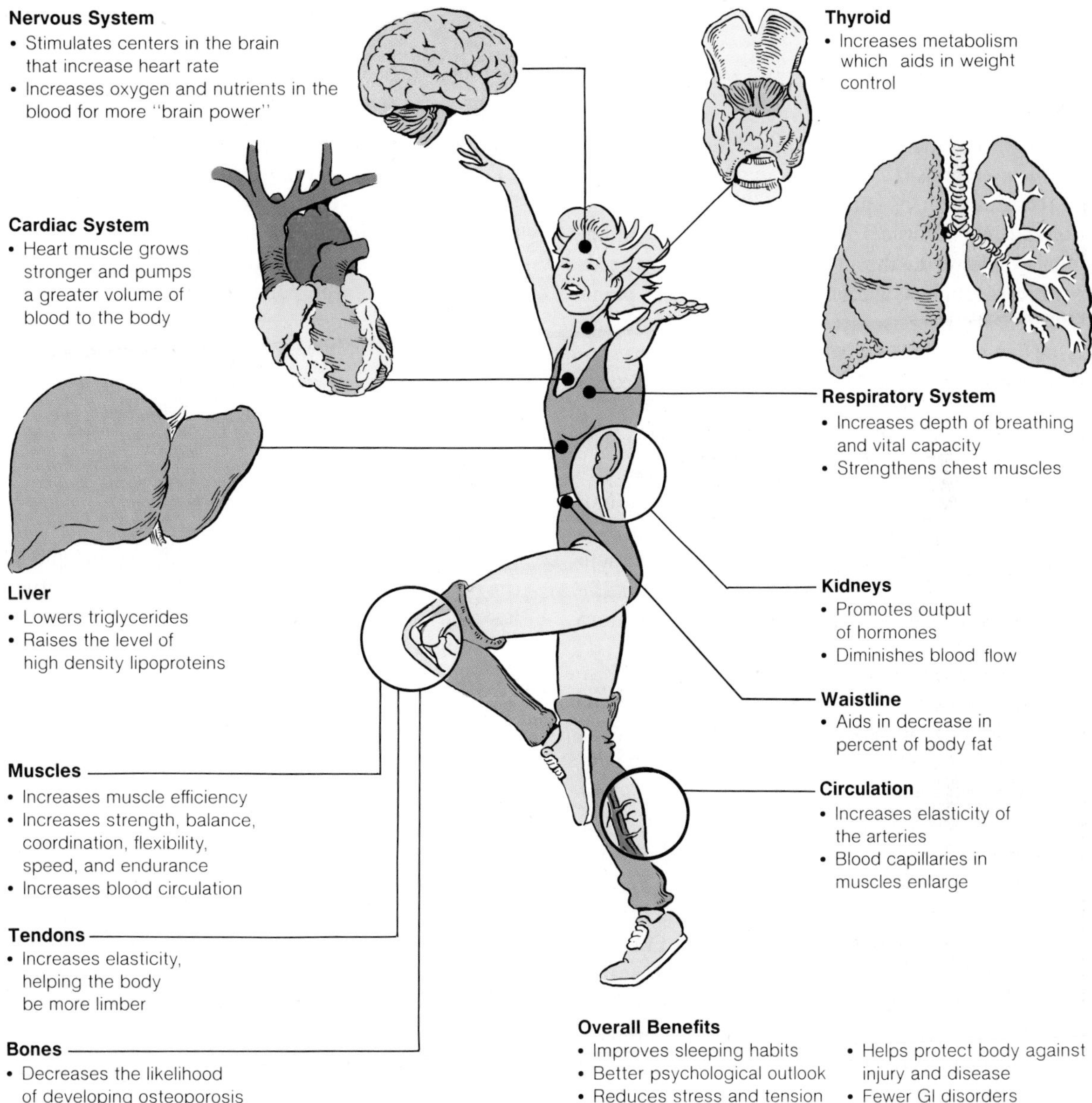
Nervous System
• Stimulates centers in the brain that increase heart rate
• Increases oxygen and nutrients in the blood for more "brain power"
Thyroid
• Increases metabolism which aids in weight control
Cardiac System
• Heart muscle grows stronger and pumps a greater volume of blood to the body
Respiratory System
• Increases depth of breathing and vital capacity
• Strengthens chest muscles
Liver
• Lowers triglycerides
• Raises the level of high density lipoproteins
Kidneys
• Promotes output of hormones
• Diminishes blood flow
Waistline
• Aids in decrease in percent of body fat
Muscles
• Increases muscle efficiency
• Increases strength, balance, coordination, flexibility, speed, and endurance
• Increases blood circulation
Circulation
• Increases elasticity of the arteries
• Blood capillaries in muscles enlarge
Tendons
• Increases elasticity, helping the body be more limber
Bones
• Decreases the likelihood of developing osteoporosis
• Improves joint motion
Overall Benefits
• Improves sleeping habits
• Better psychological outlook
• Reduces stress and tension
• Increases energy
• Helps protect body against injury and disease
• Fewer GI disorders
• Promotes better posture

**Figure 6.2**
Some benefits of exercise.
*Source:* © *Medical Times.* Reprinted by permission of Romaine Pierson Publishers, Inc.

heart will be able to pump more blood per beat than the untrained heart; therefore, the trained heart rate response will be lower for any given exercise intensity. After the activity, the trained heart will return more quickly to a normal heart rate—it recovers faster.

Cardiovascular training also leads to improvements in an individual's ability to utilize oxygen during physical activity. Increases in both the amount of blood pumped per minute and changes in the body's ability to extract and utilize oxygen carried in the bloodstream lead to an increased consumption of oxygen. Meanwhile, the lungs are also increasing their capacity to bring more oxygen into the system to be carried in the bloodstream of the exerciser. These changes translate into the ability to perform an activity more strenuously or for a longer period of time than could a person whose cardiovascular system is untrained.

## Contributions to Effective Weight Control

Exercise contributes to the maintenance of ideal body composition in many ways. Exercise can increase metabolism, resulting in the burning of greater numbers of calories during and after vigorous activity. Physical activity may also have an influence on lowering the amount of fat our body needs to store through its action on the body's set point. Additionally, exercise decreases the loss of muscle tissue during weight-loss attempts, and helps to suppress appetite (especially for those of us who are inactive or obese). Physical activity also changes the way our bodies handle fat. Insulin, which is responsible for guiding fat into body cells for storage, decreases in the bloodstream after just one bout of exercise. Muscle tissue also becomes more sensitive to the insulin. All these changes are thought to help regulate the amount of insulin circulating in the bloodstream. We discussed these benefits in more detail in chapter 5.

## Disease Prevention

Vigorous physical activity is believed to reduce the risk of several chronic disease conditions. One such disease is **osteoporosis,** a chronic disease consisting of a thinning of bone materials, such as calcium, leading to an actual loss of bone mass. Women seem to be especially susceptible to this problem. Exercise programs have been studied as a possible preventive measure. The exact mechanism for the protective effects of vigorous activity are still unknown; however, it has been suggested that vigorous activity, in combination with adequate amounts of dietary calcium, either increase the mineral content and size of bones in the limbs used for the activity,[7] or decrease the loss of calcium from bones during the aging process.[8] Osteoporosis is discussed in greater detail in chapter 20.

Heart disease is another chronic condition for which exercise has been suggested as a preventive measure. One of the major risk factors for coronary-artery disease is a high blood-cholesterol level. We discussed the relationship between diet, cholesterol, and heart disease in chapter 4. High LDL cholesterol levels have been linked with an increased risk of coronary heart disease; HDL cholesterol may actually protect us from this disease. Vigorous physical activity has been associated with lower levels of LDL cholesterol and higher levels of HDL cholesterol.[9] Vigorous exercise has also been shown to exert a beneficial influence by slowing down blood clotting.[10] These factors in combination are likely responsible for a large portion of the cardiovascular preventive benefits of vigorous exercise. Coronary-heart disease and its many risk factors are discussed in greater detail in chapter 15.

# WHAT IS FITNESS?

Fitness means different things to different people. Is the person who plays baseball every Saturday afternoon physically fit? What about the avid golfer or the weight lifter? Exactly what do we mean when we talk about physical fitness? (See figure 6.3.)

Exercise specialists commonly describe **physical fitness** as "a state which characterizes the degree to which a person is able to function efficiently."[11] The American College of Sports Medicine has delineated three major classifications of activities that contribute to fitness: (1) cardiorespiratory endurance; (2) flexibility, coordination, and relaxation; and (3) muscular strength and endurance. **Cardiorespiratory endurance** refers to the body's ability to sustain strenuous activities for long periods of time. Cardiorespiratory endurance relies on the ability of the circulatory and respiratory systems to supply the necessary oxygen for this sustained activity. **Muscular strength** is described as the maximum amount of force that can be exerted by a muscle in a single effort. **Muscular endurance** is defined as the ability of specific muscles to sustain effort over a long period of time. The final component of fitness—**flexibility**—refers to the ability of a specific joint to move through its entire range of motion. Each of these types of fitness activities make unique and important contributions to our level of physical fitness. Some activities make their major contribution to one aspect of fitness, while others give a broader range of benefits. Table 6.1 presents a list of sports and their contribution to the major components of fitness.

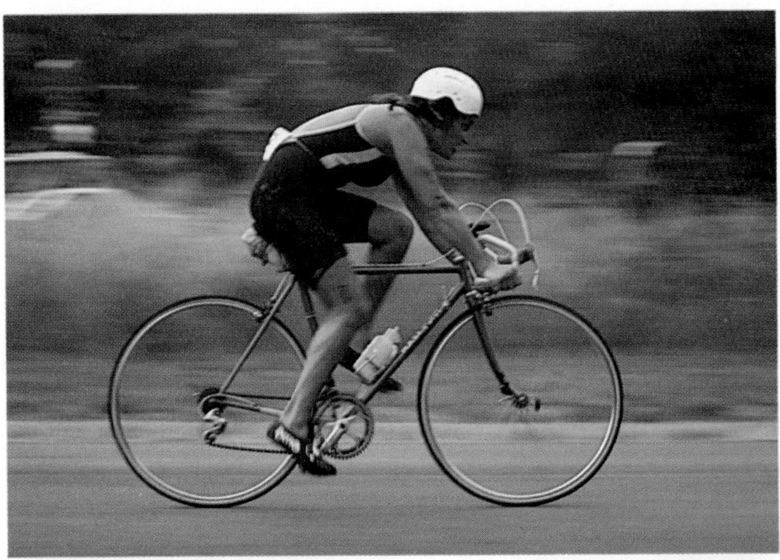

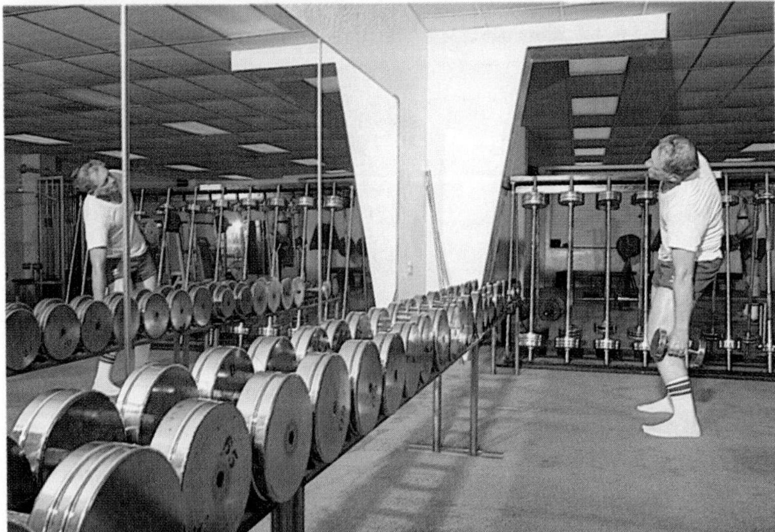

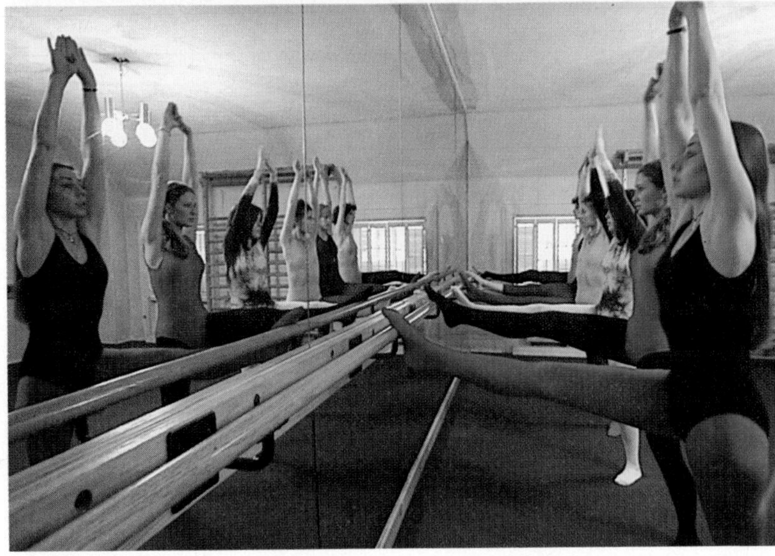

**Figure 6.3**
What is fitness?

**Table 6.1 What Some Sports Do for You**

| Activity | Heart | Muscle Endurance | Muscle Power | Coordination | Balance | Flexibility |
|---|---|---|---|---|---|---|
| Aerobic dancing | * | * | * | * | * | * |
| Archery | | | * | | | |
| Badminton | * | * | | * | | |
| Bicycling | * | * | * | | * | |
| Bowling | | | | * | | |
| Canoeing (bow) | * | * | | | * | |
| Canoeing (stern) | * | * | * | * | * | |
| Fly fishing | * | * | * | | | |
| Golf (walking) | * | * | | * | | |
| Golf (with cart) | | | | * | | |
| Handball | * | * | * | * | * | * |
| Hiking | * | * | * | | * | |
| Horseback riding | | | * | | * | |
| Jogging | * | * | | | * | |
| Long brisk walk | * | * | | | | |
| Mountain climbing | * | * | * | * | * | |
| Rowing | * | * | * | * | | |
| Short walk | * | | | | | |
| Softball | | * | | * | | |
| Square dancing | * | * | | * | * | |
| Surf-casting | | * | * | * | * | |
| Swimming | * | * | * | * | | * |
| Table tennis | * | | | * | | |
| Tennis | * | * | * | * | * | * |
| Upland game hunting | * | * | | | * | |
| Walk run walk | * | * | | | * | |

(Asterisk indicates beneficial effect)

Source: From *The Shape of Things to Come: Fitness Facts for Women.* Courtesy California Raisin Advisory Board.

## Principles of Fitness

There are four principles of fitness that apply to cardiovascular endurance, as well as to the flexibility and muscular strength/endurance activities. The four principles are: overload, specificity, individual differences, and reversibility.

**OVERLOAD** The first principle of fitness is **overload.** The whole concept of fitness is based on physiological adaptations that our bodies make in response to certain activities. In order for these adaptations to occur an individual must exercise the body at a level of activity greater than that to which it is accustomed. We can carry out the principle of overload in three ways: (1) we can increase the number of days that we exercise (frequency); (2) we can increase how strenuously we exercise for a given time period (intensity); or (3) we can increase the length of time that we exercise at a given intensity.

For an illustration of the concept of overload, let's examine the fitness program of Gary, a college sophomore. Gary has developed a fitness program for himself that consists of swimming at a local pool three days a week, for thirty minutes each session. Gary has followed this routine for about six months and has just noticed that his fitness potential is not improving as it had been in the beginning of the program. Gary could continue to improve his fitness level by implementing the principle of overload. He could, for instance, swim four days a week rather than three. Or, if three days were all Gary could fit into his schedule this semester, he could choose instead to swim faster (and thus farther) during his thirty-minute sessions. If, for some reason, Gary did not want to alter his pace, he could swim at his normal speed and distance but for forty minutes each time. All of these would place Gary in a state of overload and gradually increase his level of fitness.

**SPECIFICITY** Another important principle of fitness is called the principle of **specificity.** Physiological adaptations to activity are specific to the type of activity and overload. Let's look again at Gary's fitness program. Gary swims as his major fitness activity; after six months he has developed a good level of physical fitness. Many of the fitness adaptations his body has made, however, are specific to swimming. This became very obvious to Gary when he decided he would go on a twenty-five-mile bicycle trip with several of his friends. He found that he had great difficulty keeping up with the pace set by his friends. Additionally, he had some very sore muscles when the trip was over. As the principle of specificity points out, many of the muscles needed for bicycling had not been trained by Gary's swimming program.

**INDIVIDUAL DIFFERENCES** The third principle of fitness is the principle of **individual differences**. This principle tells us that individuals attain the many fitness benefits at varying rates. One of the biggest determinants of fitness gains is an individual's relative level of fitness at the start of a program. People who begin with low levels of fitness often see more dramatic improvements early in their fitness programs. The principle of individual differences is one of the major reasons that exercise specialists like to give individualized fitness prescriptions. These prescriptions will be discussed later in this chapter.

**REVERSIBILITY** The fourth principle of fitness is that of **reversibility.** This principle is best summed up by the maxim "use it or lose it." Once you have trained your body and started to receive the benefits of regular exercise, you must continue to keep physically active or you will begin to lose those benefits. David Costill, Director of the Human Performance Laboratory at Ball State University, has studied the effects of "detraining" and found that if a person is unable to exercise for just one week the aerobic energy of their specifically trained large muscles may decline by as much as 50 percent of their trained level.[12] The capacity of the heart to pump blood during strenuous activity also begins to decline. Generally, it is safe to say that there is no major loss of cardiovascular exercise benefits for the first five to seven days of missed physical activity.

Keeping these four general principles in mind, let's investigate cardiovascular fitness, the component many experts believe to be the most important fitness key to wellness.

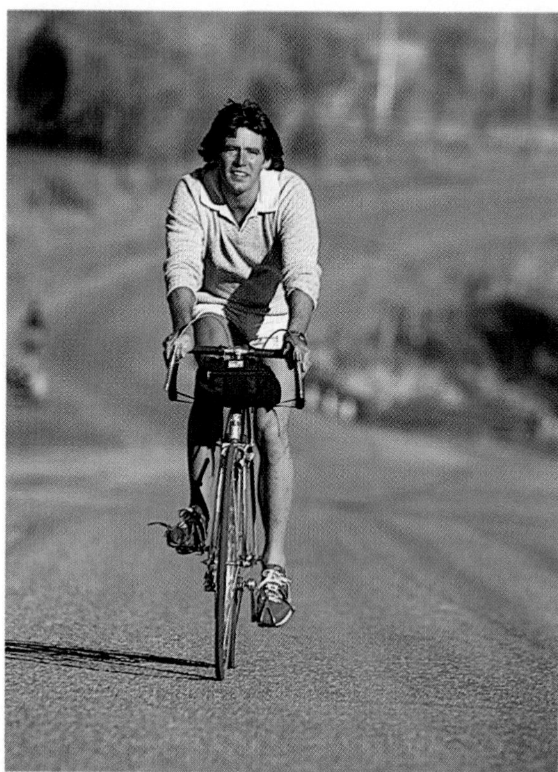

**Figure 6.4**
Bicycling is a good form of aerobic activity.

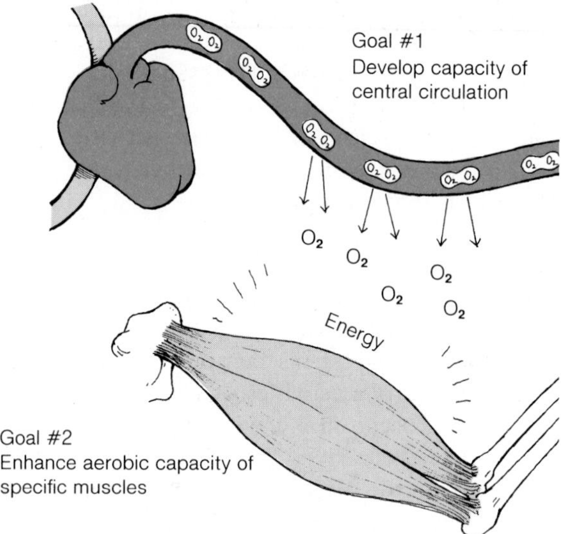


**Figure 6.5**
The two major goals of aerobic conditioning. *Source:* From McArdle, W. D., Katch, F. I., and Katch, V. L., *Exercise Physiology—Energy, Nutrition and Human Performance.* Lea & Febiger, Philadelphia, 1981. Reprinted by permission.

# CARDIORESPIRATORY ENDURANCE

Cardiorespiratory-endurance activities, more commonly known as **aerobic exercises,** are activities that cause a sustained increase in heart rate and use the large muscles of the body continuously for an extended period of time. (See figure 6.4.) Many experts believe that cardiovascular endurance is the most important component of physical fitness.

## Aerobic Exercises

Aerobic exercises have two major goals.[13] The first goal is to improve the general circulatory system (heart and lungs) so that greater amounts of blood and oxygen can be circulated throughout the body. The second goal is to improve the ability of specific muscles to consume greater amounts of oxygen. (See figure 6.5.) The particular muscles used for a given activity will be those targeted for aerobic improvements. If you are a runner, for instance, the muscles of your legs will increase their ability to use more oxygen, while your lungs increase the oxygen to the bloodstream and your heart adapts to pump greater amounts of blood each minute.

The key to aerobic exercise is oxygen (the word aerobic literally means "with oxygen"). As we saw in chapter 5, aerobic activities rely on oxygen in order to use fatty acids as their prime source of energy. The duration of exercise is one of the major determinants of the source of energy used. Continuous activity lasting longer than four minutes is considered to be aerobic. This means that, for exercise lasting longer than four minutes, the body is able to bring in enough oxygen to meet all, or almost all, of the energy demand during the actual activity.[14] Running, stationary cycling, jumping rope, and cross-country skiing are some of the better aerobic activities.

## Anaerobic Exercises

**Anaerobic exercise,** on the other hand, is exercise that does not rely on oxygen. Anaerobic exercises use glycogen stored in the liver and skeletal muscles for its energy source. Glycogen can be broken down into glucose without the presence of oxygen. Glycogen stores, however, are rapidly depleted. This

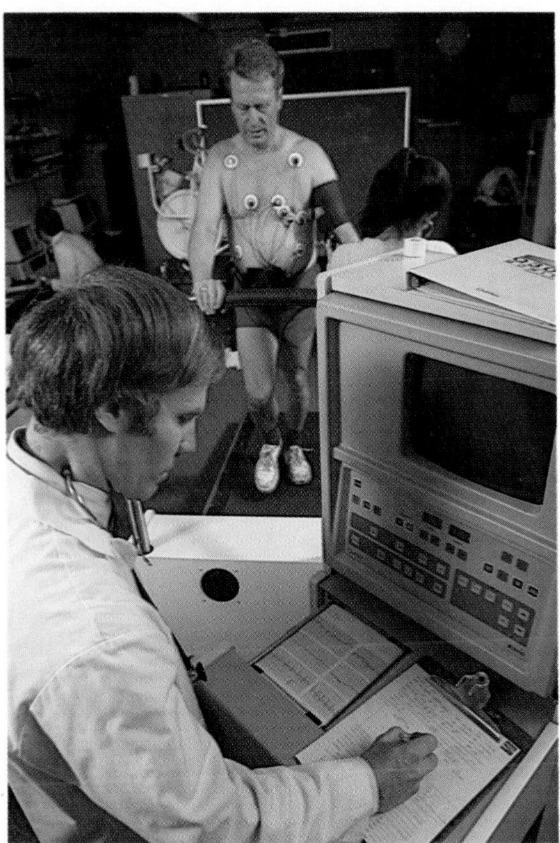

**Figure 6.6**
Stress testing is one of the more accurate ways to measure aerobic fitness.

means that after a very short time of maximal effort (ten to ninety seconds) an individual must stop in order to take in enough oxygen to be able to use the more plentiful fatty acids as an energy source. Anaerobic activities are described as those requiring an intense, maximum burst of energy.[15] Activities such as the 100-yard dash or the tennis serve would be considered anaerobic. During these activities, which require intense, short bursts of energy, waste products build up in the muscles and an oxygen debt occurs. By slowing down, or stopping, the body is able to take in needed oxygen and remove waste products from the muscles.

## Designing an Aerobics Program

Before you begin an individualized aerobic activity program you will need to assess your present level of cardiovascular fitness.

**AEROBICS FITNESS TESTING** Currently, the most accurate way to test cardiovascular fitness is to take what is known as a **stress test.** This test involves running on a treadmill or riding a stationary bicycle while trained medical and fitness personnel monitor your heart-rate and blood-pressure response to strenuous exercise. (See figure 6.6.) Although it is a fairly accurate measure of aerobic fitness, stress testing is unavailable to many Americans and, when available, is very costly.

Dr. Kenneth Cooper, a well-known aerobics researcher, has developed several fitness tests that are more easily completed by the average person and are highly correlated with results obtained from stress testing. One of these tests is the **Twelve-Minute Walking/Running.** To complete this fitness test you would run, walk, or a combination thereof, for a period of twelve minutes, keeping track of how far you are able to go during that time. Your aerobic fitness level is then calculated according to your age, sex, and the distance you covered in twelve minutes. In order to receive a "good" aerobic fitness level, a male under twenty years of age would need to run 1.57 to 1.72 miles in twelve minutes; a female under twenty years of age would need to run 1.3 to 1.43 miles. (See Activity for Wellness 6.1.)

Once you have determined your current level of aerobic fitness you are ready to design your aerobics program. In designing your program, you must keep in mind three major components. These components are easily remembered as the F.I.T. Guidelines: **Frequency, Intensity,** and **Time.**[16]

**F.I.T.: FREQUENCY** The first F.I.T. Guideline is frequency. The American College of Sports Medicine suggests that, in order to receive optimal benefits, you should exercise three to five times each week.[17] If you choose to exercise only three days each week you will find that exercising every other day will lead to the greatest benefits and to a decreased risk of muscle injury. Additionally, there should not be more than two days of rest between each exercise session or benefits will begin to be lost.

Some people enjoy aerobics so much that they participate six or seven days each week. Exercising this frequently may increase the likelihood of muscle, bone, and joint injury.[18] If you decide to participate six or seven days a week you can lower the risk of injury by slowing your pace every other day, or by

6.1 ACTIVITY FOR WELLNESS 6.1

## Twelve-Minute Walking/Running Test (Distances (miles) covered in twelve minutes)

| Fitness Category | | Age (years) 13–19 | 20–29 | 30–39 | 40–49 | 50–59 | 60+ |
|---|---|---|---|---|---|---|---|
| I. Very Poor | (men) | <1.30* | <1.22 | <1.18 | <1.14 | <1.03 | < .87 |
| | (women) | <1.0 | < .96 | < .94 | < .88 | < .84 | < .78 |
| II. Poor | (men) | 1.30–1.37 | 1.22–1.31 | 1.18–1.30 | 1.14–1.24 | 1.03–1.16 | .87–1.02 |
| | (women) | 1.00–1.18 | .96–1.11 | .95–1.05 | .88– .98 | .84– .93 | .78– .86 |
| III. Fair | (men) | 1.38–1.56 | 1.32–1.49 | 1.31–1.45 | 1.25–1.39 | 1.17–1.30 | 1.03–1.20 |
| | (women) | 1.19–1.29 | 1.12–1.22 | 1.06–1.18 | .99–1.11 | .94–1.05 | .87– .98 |
| IV. Good | (men) | 1.57–1.72 | 1.50–1.64 | 1.46–1.56 | 1.40–1.53 | 1.31–1.44 | 1.21–1.32 |
| | (women) | 1.30–1.43 | 1.23–1.34 | 1.19–1.29 | 1.12–1.24 | 1.06–1.18 | .99–1.09 |
| V. Excellent | (men) | 1.73–1.86 | 1.65–1.76 | 1.57–1.69 | 1.54–1.65 | 1.45–1.58 | 1.33–1.55 |
| | (women) | 1.44–1.51 | 1.35–1.45 | 1.30–1.39 | 1.25–1.34 | 1.19–1.30 | 1.10–1.18 |
| VI. Superior | (men) | >1.87 | >1.77 | >1.70 | >1.66 | >1.59 | >1.56 |
| | (women) | >1.52 | >1.46 | >1.40 | >1.35 | >1.31 | >1.19 |

*< Means "less than"; > means "more than."

This simple exercise will help you assess your current level of aerobic fitness. Time yourself for twelve minutes. During that twelve minutes run or walk as far and as fast as you can. You should try and pace yourself so that you are at your maximum effort output at the end of the twelve minutes (i.e., you just can't go any further). Keep track of how far you go and then locate your distance, sex, and age on the chart above. Circle your fitness category.

Source: From *The Aerobics Program for Total Well-Being* by Kenneth H. Cooper, M.D., M.P.H. Copyright © 1982 by Kenneth H. Cooper. Reprinted by permission of the publisher, M. Evans & Co., Inc., New York, N.Y. 10017.

alternating daily the muscle groups you use by changing the type of aerobic activity. Karen, for instance, is an avid jogger; her day isn't complete without at least a short run. Karen runs five miles every other day on a scenic trail through the park near her apartment. The other days, however, she runs at a slightly slower pace and limits herself to two miles. Bob runs with Karen on her five-mile runs, but chooses to swim on the alternate days. In this way Bob can train his upper-body muscles with swimming, while jogging increases the aerobic capacity of his lower-body muscles.

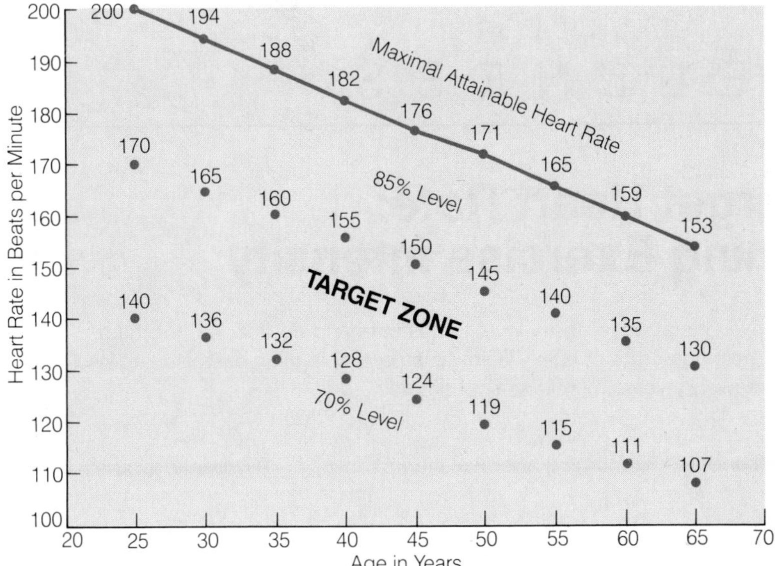


Figure 6.7
Maximal attainable heart rate and target zone. *Source:* From Zohman, Lenore, M.D., *Beyond Diet: Exercise Your Way to Fitness and Heart Health.* © 1974 CPC International, Inc. Englewood Cliffs, N.J. Reprinted by permission.

**F.I.T.: INTENSITY** The second F.I.T. Guideline is intensity. An important key to accruing aerobic benefits is the "pace" you maintain during the activity you choose. If the intensity is too low you will receive little or no aerobic benefits, but if the intensity is too great it may be too stressful for the heart. One general guideline that you can use to gauge the intensity of your aerobic activity is the *talk test.* You should exercise at a pace that allows you to talk to a fellow exerciser in a slightly halting, but not gasping, manner.[19] If huffing and puffing stop you from conversing with someone you should slow down.

A more scientific method of monitoring your intensity is to calculate your **target heart rate.** The target heart rate is the range you should aim for when exercising, and will vary from person to person. This is one part of the exercise prescription where the principle of individual differences is clearly seen.

The target-heart-rate range depends on the individual's **maximal heart rate,** or the highest heart rate reached during an all-out aerobic effort. The best way to measure maximal heart rate is to take a stress test and measure the heart rate immediately at the end of the test, but there are other ways to estimate your maximal heart rate. Generally, we know that the maximal heart rate decreases as we age. By subtracting your age from 220 you can get a rough estimate of your maximal heart rate. The target-heart-rate range is then calculated by taking a percentage of the estimated maximal heart rate. For beginners the percentages range between 70 percent and 80 percent of maximal heart rate, while more advanced participants may have a target range between 75 percent and 85 percent. (See figure 6.7.) Age and fitness level are generally reflected by the heart rate; Matti Karvonen has developed a method of determining the ideal target-heart-rate range that takes these variables into account. Activity for Wellness 6.2 illustrates this method of determining the target-heart-rate range.

In order to use your target-heart-rate prescription you will need to know how to take your heart rate or pulse. (See figure 6.8.) When you stop exercising you must quickly locate your pulse. Your heart rate will drop rapidly once you stop exercising. One place to take an exercise heart rate is over the blood vessels on your neck (the carotid arteries), which are located directly to the left or right of your Adams apple. Another good place to take an exercise heart rate is over the artery on the inside of your wrist just below the base of your thumb (the radial artery). Lightly place your index and middle finger over one of these arteries. As soon as you find your pulse, count the beats for ten seconds starting with zero as the first count. Multiply your ten-second count by six to determine if you are in your target range. If your heart rate is too high, you need to slow down. If it is too low, you will need to increase your pace in order to receive the optimal aerobic benefits.

6.2 ACTIVITY FOR WELLNESS 6.2

## Target Heart Rate: Determining Exercise Intensity

It is important for individuals to exercise at an intensity level that is safe and appropriate for them. Intensity is measured by taking one's heart rate or pulse. Below is an example of an exercise target-heart-rate prescription for Gary, a twenty-year-old college sophomore.

1. *Resting heart rate (RHR)*
   Count your pulse for sixty seconds in the morning after waking up. __70__ beats/minute
2. *Maximum heart rate (MHR)*
   220 − your age = MHR (estimated) __200__ beats/minute
3. *Adjusted heart rate*
   MHR − RHR = Adjusted heart rate
   __200__ − __70__ = __130__
4. *Work rate*
   Adjusted heart rate × Percent of MHR (60 percent, 70 percent, 80 percent, etc.) = Work rate
   __130__ × __.70__ = __91__
5. *Target heart rate (THR)*
   Work rate + RHR = THR
   __91__ + __70__ = __161__
6. *Exercise heart rate*
   Count your pulse for ten seconds IMMEDIATELY after excercising and multiply by six.

Source: From Mullen, Kathleen D. and Gerald D. Costello, *Health Awareness Through Self-Discovery: A Workbook.* © 1981 Burgess Publishing Co., Minneapolis, Minn. Adapted by permission.

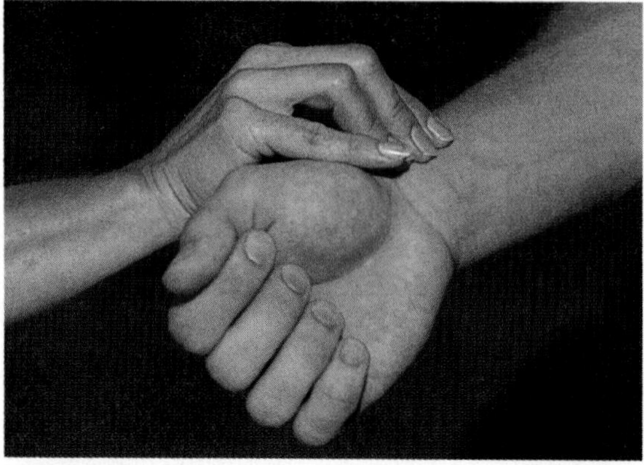

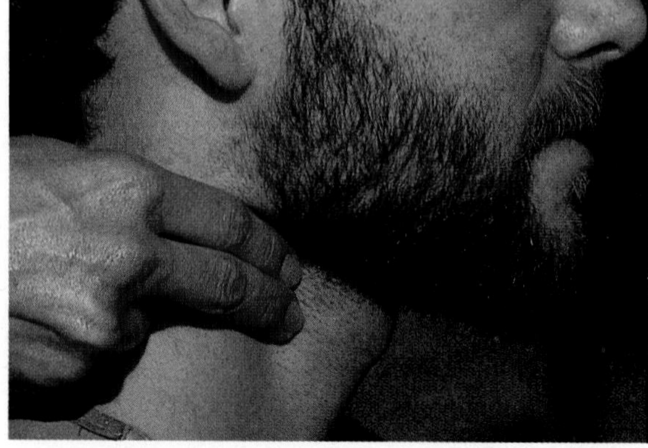

**Figure 6.8**
Learning how to take your exercise heart rate will help you to monitor your exercise intensity.

**Table 6.2 Cardiovascular-Fitness Benefits of Various Exercises**

| A<br>Do Condition Heart and Lungs | B<br>Can Condition Heart and Lungs | C<br>Do Not Condition Heart and Lungs |
|---|---|---|
| Cross-country skiing | Bicycling | Baseball |
| Hiking (uphill) | Downhill skiing | Bowling |
| Ice hockey | Basketball | Football |
| Jogging | Calisthenics | Golf (by cart) |
| Jumping rope | Field hockey | Softball |
| Rowing | Handball | Volleyball |
| Running in place | Racquetball | Weight lifting |
| Stationary bicycling | Soccer | |
| | Squash | |
| | Swimming | |
| | Tennis (singles) | |
| | Walking | |

Source: *Exercise and Your Heart,* no. 81–1677 (May 1981):34–35. National Heart, Lung, and Blood Institute, National Institutes of Health, Bethesda, Md.

A prime determinant of the amount of cardiovascular benefit that an activity will contribute to your fitness level is its ability to raise your heart rate into the target zone for a continuous period of time. Some exercises, such as running, jumping rope, and stationary cycling, easily maintain the heart rate in the target zone for continuous lengths of time. This qualifies them as the best aerobic activities, or those which give the most cardiovascular benefits for the least amount of time investment. Other activities are more "stop and go" and therefore do not maintain the heart rate in the training range the entire time. Tennis is a good example of a moderately aerobic activity. During tennis volleys there is a level of intensity that will raise your heart rate to its training zone. Between volleys, however, there are many pauses that allow your heart rate to drop below the training zone. In general, to get optimal cardiovascular benefits from moderately aerobic activities such as singles tennis, basketball, and racquetball, you should plan on spending twice the amount of time each session that you would for a more vigorous aerobic activity. Table 6.2 presents various types of activities and how they contribute to your cardiovascular-fitness level.

**F.I.T.: TIME** The third F.I.T. Guideline considers the amount of time you need to devote to each exercise session. The American College of Sports Medicine has determined that for vigorous aerobic activities (column A of table 6.2) you will receive optimal aerobic benefits if you exercise in your target-heart-rate zone for twenty to thirty minutes. For the more moderate aerobic exercises you will need to devote a little more time because of their "stop-and-go" nature. You should aim for a range of forty to sixty minutes each time for moderate aerobic exercises such as those listed in column B of table 6.2.

**PUTTING IT ALL TOGETHER** Now that you have determined your exercise prescription (frequency, intensity, and time) you are ready to begin your program. Before you start each exercise session it is very important to **warm up.** A general warm-up before exercise will gradually increase the amount of blood your heart pumps each minute, the blood flow to active muscles, and your internal body temperature. This gradual increase is thought to aid in preventing injuries. Good activities for the beginning of a warm-up include brisk walking, or for those with a good fitness level, a slow jog. Once you have gradually increased circulation to the active muscles, you should engage in some limited stretching activities. (See Activity for Wellness 6.3.) Stretching activities will also contribute to your total fitness by improving your flexibility. When stretching, it is important to remember the following points:[20]

1. Maintain your normal breathing throughout the stretch. Do not hold your breath while exercising. Try to exhale during the stretch.

6.3 ACTIVITY FOR WELLNESS

## Stretch

### BACK AND HAMSTRING STRETCH

1. Lying on your back, pull one leg toward your chest (figure A) and hold for thirty counts. (Keep the other leg as straight as you can. If possible, try to keep the back of your head on the mat rug; if you can't, that's OK.)
2. Lower your leg and repeat with the other leg.

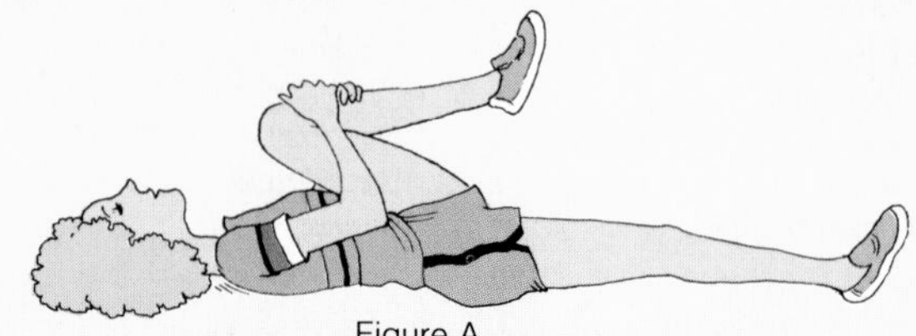
Figure A

### BACK AND HAMSTRING STRETCH

1. Sit as shown (figure B).
2. Slowly bend forward (from the hips) toward the foot of your outstretched leg until you feel a slight stretch (figure C). Hold stretch for a count of twenty. (Do not bounce!)

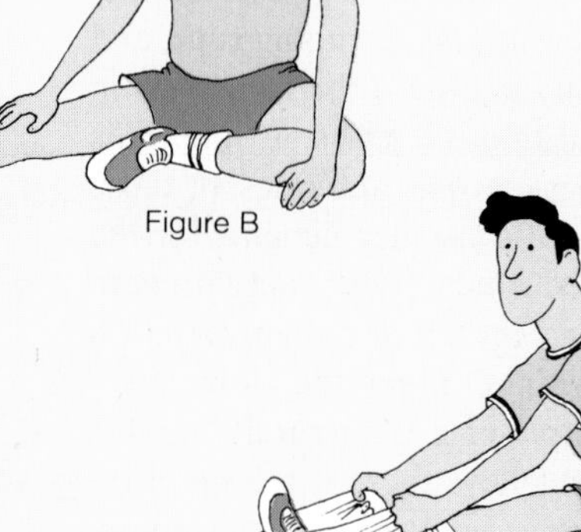
Figure B

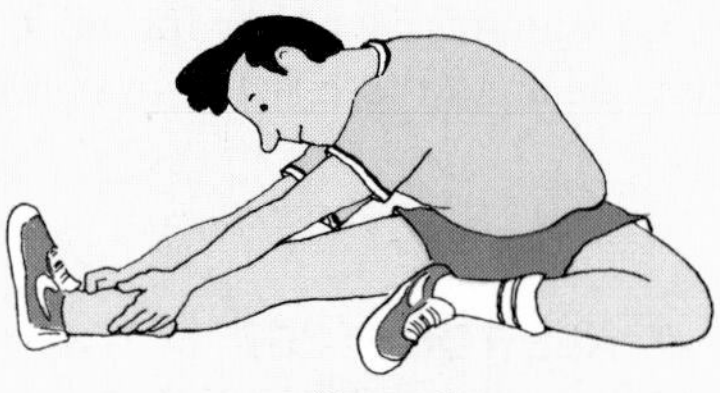
Figure C

3. Now stretch a little more and hold stretch for twenty more counts; use a towel to help you stretch if you cannot reach your feet easily (figure D). Repeat with other leg.

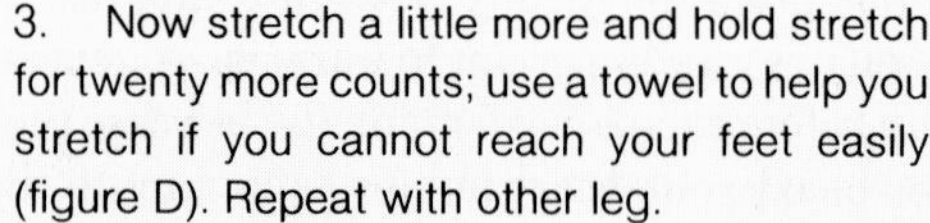
Figure D

2. Do not use bouncy or jerky movements while stretching. Perform each stretching exercise slowly, briefly holding the stretch in a comfortable position.
3. Go through your entire range of motion, to the best of your ability, without straining.
4. Concentrate on doing each stretch correctly, not quickly.
5. Listen to your body. Don't overdo it. If you stretch regularly, you will begin to feel more limber each day.

Just as it is important to warm up properly before you exercise, it is equally important to **cool down** after you exercise. The activities that make up a good cool-down are the same as those described for the

ACTIVITY FOR
WELLNESS 6.3

**QUADRICEPS AND KNEE STRETCH**

1. Hold the top of one foot with the *opposite* hand (figure E) and gently pull your foot toward your buttocks. Hold for a count of thirty. Repeat with other leg.

**CALF AND ACHILLES TENDON STRETCH**

1. Stand about three feet away from a wall or other solid support and lean on it with your forearms (rest your head on your hands). Bend one leg and place it in front of you; place the other leg straight behind you (figure F).
2. Slowly move your hips forward while keeping your lower back flat. The heel of your outstretched leg should be on the ground, and the toes should be pointed forward, or slightly turned in.
3. Hold a *comfortable* stretch for thirty counts. (Do not bounce!) Repeat with other leg.
4. By bending your outstretched back leg at the knee *slightly,* and lowering your hips, you can also gently stretch your Achilles tendon (back of your ankle). (Remember to keep your lower back flat, your heels on the ground, and your toes pointed forward.)

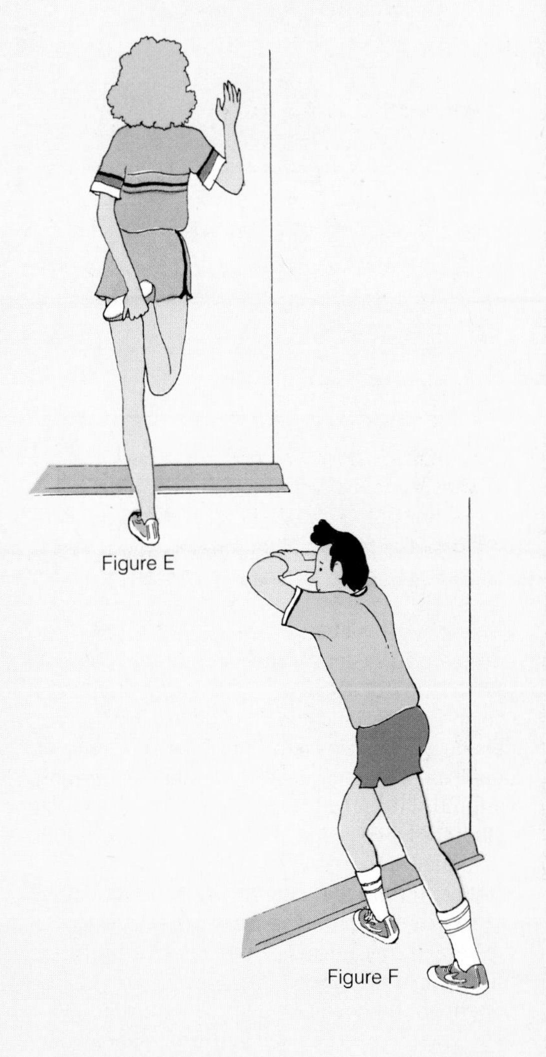
Figure E

Figure F

Source: *The HOPE Newsletter,* published by the Bob Hope Heart Research Institute, Seattle, Wash. Reprinted with permission.

warm-up. Generally, you should keep moving once you finish your aerobic activity. Walk slowly to keep the blood circulating and prevent it from pooling in the legs. This may also help remove waste products that have accumulated in the muscles during the exercise. It is important to let your heart rate drop gradually from the training zone toward a resting rate. The best time to do stretching activities is probably during the cool-down from aerobic exercise. At this time your muscles will be warmed up and will be less likely to be injured. Figure 6.9 illustrates how the whole pattern of aerobic exercise fits together. It shows the progression from warm-up, to a period of twenty to thirty minutes of aerobic activity in your target-heart-rate range, and finally to cool-down and recovery.

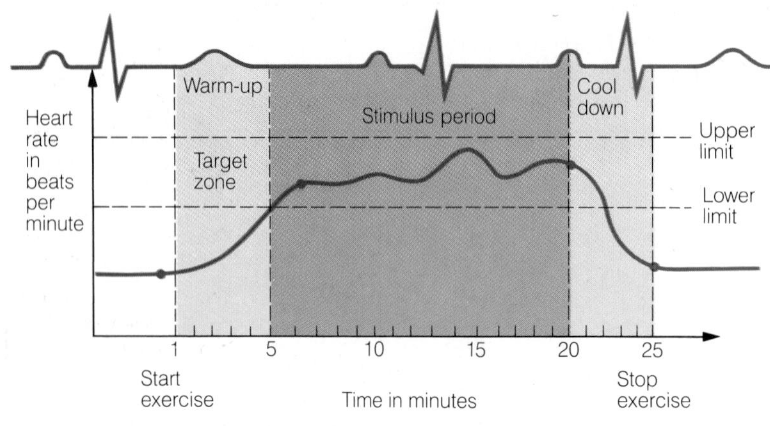


**Figure 6.9**
A typical exercise session. *Source:* Unknown.

6.3 EXHIBIT

# Progressive Resistance Exercise

Progressive Resistance Exercise (P.R.E.) is a general exercise system which incorporates three different forms of exercise. This system has been shown to be effective in rehabilitation, increasing athletic performance, and changing physical appearance. The three forms are: **weight training, weight lifting,** and **body building.** All are similar in that they involve the use of resistance (weights) in gradually progressive amounts. However, each is different from the other in terms of outcome of the exercise system. The primary gains for any of the P.R.E. forms are that of **muscular strength** and **muscular endurance.** The specific gain will be dependent on how the variables associated with this type of exercise system are manipulated. These variables include:

- **Resistance** (load)—This is the amount of weight that is being used with a specific exercise.
- **Repetitions** (reps)—The number of times an exercise movement is repeated.
- **Sets**—The number of times an exercise of specified reps will be performed.
- **Repetitions maximum**—The number of reps a maximum amount (load) of weight can be performed.

Equipment is necessary in P.R.E. and may take many forms. Barbells, weight plates, dumbbells, and the Universal Machine are some such equipment.

Increases in strength of muscle will only occur if the principle of **overload** is used. This is done by lifting gradually increasing resistance during each exercise session thus forcing adaptation and muscular **hypertrophy.**

By increasing the number of repetitions while keeping resistance constant the gain will be primarily that of muscular endurance.

As a general rule in P.R.E., increases in resistance will create increased strength, while increases in repetitions will create increased muscular endurance.

P.R.E. contributes little if anything to cardiorespiratory fitness primarily due to the fact that the actual work phase of exercise is quite short, lasting only a few seconds. Consequently, it does not qualify as an exercise which induces the aerobic training effect.

**Weight training** is that part of P.R.E. which involves the use of resistance exercises in the development of strength and/or muscular endurance as an aid in general body conditioning,

# STARTING YOUR PERSONAL EXERCISE PROGRAM

One of the most important things to remember as you start your aerobic-exercise program is to *start slow.* Proceeding gradually to your fitness goals will help make your activities more enjoyable and make you less prone to injury. The American College of Sports Medicine has delineated three stages of progress for aerobic exercise.[21] The three stages are the initial-conditioning stage, the improvement-conditioning stage, and the maintenance stage.

## Initial-Conditioning Stage

The **Initial-Conditioning Stage** consists of low-level aerobic exercises, some mild stretching, and light calisthenics. The beginning exerciser with a low level of fitness should begin with twelve minutes for each exercise session and gradually increase toward the goal of twenty minutes. For many beginners this phase may last four to six weeks. Monitor your heart-rate response to exercise to determine when to progress to the next stage. As the heart becomes trained it becomes stronger and thus pumps fewer times each minute in order to do the same amount of exercise. As you become more fit, you will need to increase your pace and the amount of time you spend each session in order to stay in your target-heart-rate zone.

### EXHIBIT 6.3

improvement of sport skills, and changes in body contour (physical appearance).

**Weight lifting** involves a competitive approach to P.R.E. where the primary goal is maximum lift capacity in selected exercises or lifts. Weight lifting is an Olympic sport as well as being an international competitive event in non-Olympic years.

**Bodybuilding** is also a form of P.R.E., which has as its goal the creation of maximum muscular hypertrophy and body symmetry. The individuals who enjoy this approach have competitions which lead to such titles as Mr. America, Mr. Universe, and Mr. World. It is not unusual for individuals pursuing this goal to have incredible degrees of muscle hypertrophy.

Until rather recently P.R.E. had been considered the domain of "men only." Fortunately, this taboo has been broken and women have become familiar with the offerings that "weight training" holds. Contrary to popular opinion the idea of "muscle-boundness" does not occur with this system of training. Women do not have to fear the tremendous degrees of hypertrophy which make them look "too masculine." The reason is that the hormone testosterone will control the degree of hypertrophy and this hormone is present in much higher levels in men than in women. However, there are cases where some women athletes have maximized their inherited tendencies with weight training to produce considerable muscularity.

Source: J. D. LePanto and F. C. Jenkins, *Exercise: For the Health of It,* 3d ed. Copyright © by Kendall/Hunt Publishing Company. Reprinted by permission.

### DISCUSSION QUESTIONS

1. Why isn't progressive resistance exercise (P.R.E.) considered an aerobic activity?

2. If you wanted to increase your muscular endurance, would you need to include many reps, or only a few reps with heavy weights?

3. Why do you think more women are becoming interested in weight training and bodybuilding?

6.4 ACTIVITY FOR WELLNESS 6.4

## Should I Consult a Doctor Before I Start Exercising?

Most people do not need to see a doctor before they start since a gradual, sensible exercise program will have minimal health risks. However, there are some people who should seek medical advice.

To find out if you should consult a doctor before you start, use the following checklist. Mark those items that apply to you:

- ☐ Your doctor said you have heart trouble, a heart murmur, or you have had a heart attack.
- ☐ You frequently have pains or pressure—in the left or midchest area, left neck, shoulder, or arm—during or right after you exercise.
- ☐ You often feel faint or have spells of severe dizziness.
- ☐ You experience extreme breathlessness after mild exertion.
- ☐ Your doctor said your blood pressure was too high and is not under control. Or you don't know whether or not your blood pressure is normal.
- ☐ Your doctor said you have bone or joint problems such as arthritis.
- ☐ You are over age sixty and not accustomed to vigorous exercise.
- ☐ You have a family history of premature coronary-artery disease.
- ☐ You have a medical condition not mentioned here which might need special attention in an exercise program (for example, insulin-dependent diabetes).

Source: *Exercise and Your Heart,* no. 81–1677 (May 1981):34–35. National Heart, Lung, and Blood Institute, National Institutes of Health, Bethesda, Md.

## Improvement-Conditioning Stage

The second stage of progression is called the **Improvement-Conditioning Stage.** During this stage you will advance more rapidly. You should be able to increase the duration of your exercise session every two to three weeks, eventually reaching your goal of thirty minutes. Additionally, during this stage your target heart rate will be raised to 75 to 85 percent of your estimated maximal heart rate. This is the stage where many of the cardiovascular benefits we discussed earlier in this chapter will be experienced.

## Maintenance Stage

The final stage of conditioning is the **Maintenance Stage.** This stage typically begins about six months into a regular aerobic-fitness program. Many people reach a point in their aerobics program where they are completely satisfied with the level of cardiovascular fitness they have attained. At this point they are interested in maintaining the benefits of their program rather than continuing to improve. This is accomplished by maintaining the program they have established during the improvement-conditioning stage. For most people this will consist of twenty to thirty minutes of aerobic exercise at the target-heart-rate range, for three to five days each week.

**Table 6.3 Choosing Aerobic Exercises**

**Choose an Aerobic Exercise that Fits!**

The following chart is a general guide that can help you choose an aerobic exercise (or a combination of exercises) that fits your needs, interests, and life-style.

| | Aerobic dance | Aerobicize | Basketball | Bicycling (indoors) | Bicycling (outdoors) | Cross-country skiing | Handball, racquetball | Jogging | Jumping rope | Mini-trampoline | Rowing (indoor) | Skating (ice or roller) | Soccer | Swimming indoor laps | Tennis singles | Walking |
|---|---|---|---|---|---|---|---|---|---|---|---|---|---|---|---|---|
| If you're out of shape | • | | | • | • | | | | | • | • | • | | • | | • |
| If you're in *great* shape | • | • | • | • | • | • | • | • | • | | • | • | • | • | • | |
| If you want to be alone | | | | • | • | | | • | • | • | • | • | | • | | • |
| If you like company | • | • | • | | • | • | • | • | | | | • | • | | • | • |
| If you hate to sweat | | | | | | | | | | | | | | • | | |
| If you love the indoors | • | • | • | • | | | • | | • | • | • | • | | • | | |
| If you love the outdoors | | | | | • | • | | • | | | | • | • | | • | • |
| If you have joint problems | | | | • | | | | | | • | | | | • | | • |
| If you don't have much time | | | | • | | | | • | • | • | • | | | | | |
| If you're *easily* bored | • | • | • | | • | • | • | | | | | • | • | | • | |
| If you're competitive | | | • | | • | | • | • | | | | • | • | • | • | |
| If you can't spend much | | | • | | | | | | • | | | | • | | | • |
| If you want to be flexible | | | • | | | • | • | | | | | • | | • | • | |
| If shorts are too revealing | | | | • | • | • | | | | • | • | | | | | • |

Source: *The HOPE Newsletter,* published by the Bob Hope Heart Research Institute, Seattle, Wash. Reprinted with permission.

In selecting an aerobic exercise it is important to consider your needs, interests, and life-style. (See table 6.3.) If you like social gatherings you might enjoy joining an aerobic-dance class where you would meet other people who share your interest in exercise. If you are really out of shape you might want to consider beginning with a walking program, at least for the initial progression stage. If you have a very competitive nature you might enjoy a game such as racquetball. Remember, however, that if you select a moderately aerobic game such as racquetball or tennis you will need to invest a greater amount of time in order to achieve optimal aerobic benefits. It also helps to select a partner whose skill and fitness level are similar to your own, as the amount of time you will spend in your target range will probably be increased. One study showed that in racquetball games where opponents were equally skilled and fit the typical match lasted fifty minutes rather than the average thirty-four minutes between opponents of varying abilities and fitness levels.[22]

6.5 ACTIVITY FOR WELLNESS 6.5

## Effective Ways to Avoid Injuries

The most powerful medicine for injuries is prevention. Here are some effective ways to avoid injuries:

1. Build up your level of activity *gradually* over the weeks to come.
   - Try not to set your goals too high—otherwise you will be tempted to push yourself too far too quickly.
   - For activities such as jogging, walking briskly, and jumping rope, limber up gently and slowly before and after exercising.
   - For other activities, build up slowly to your target zone, and cool down slowly afterwards.
2. Listen to your body for early warning pains.
   - Exercising too much can cause injuries to joints, feet, ankles, and legs. So don't make the mistake of exercising beyond early warning pains in these areas or more serious injuries may result. Fortunately, minor muscle and joint injuries can be readily treated by rest and aspirin.
3. Be aware of possible signs of heart problems such as:
   - Pain or pressure in the left or midchest area, left neck, shoulder, or arm during or just after exercising. (Vigorous exercise may cause a side stitch while exercising—a pain below your bottom ribs—which is not the result of a heart problem.)
   - Sudden dizziness, cold sweat, pallor, or fainting.

Ignoring these signals and continuing to exercise may lead to serious heart problems. Should any of these signs occur, stop exercising and call your doctor.

Source: *Exercise and Your Heart,* no. 81-1677 (May 1981):34-35. National Heart, Lung, and Blood Institute, National Institutes of Health, Bethesda, Md.

## PERSONAL AND SOCIAL INFLUENCES ON ACTIVITY

One of the largest barriers to an active life-style is our own attitudes. The list of excuses for our inactivity is almost endless. We don't have the time, or exercise is boring, or we don't have the right equipment and clothes. What excuses do you use?

Time is a valued commodity for most of us. When it comes to physical activity we just can't seem to "find" the time. To overcome this hurdle, you need to realize that you will never "find" the time. You must learn to "make" the time. (See figure 6.10.) Fortunately that won't be as difficult as it sounds. One way to make the time is to cut down on the number of hours you watch television. The typical American family spends an estimated four to six hours of each day watching television.[23] By carefully selecting the programs you watch on television you should be able to free up at least thirty minutes a day, three days a week, that you could use for experimenting with aerobic activity. The time of day you select to participate in your physical activity will also present potential barriers and benefits. Table 6.4 presents some of these advantages and disadvantages.

Many of us have developed the notion that exercise is boring. If you find yourself saying these words you need to look behind this vague generality and identify exactly what it is about your fitness activity that leads you to feel this way.[24] Is it possible that you have structured your exercise sessions so

## Table 6.4 Squeezing Exercise into a Too-Tight Schedule

You might as well give up trying to *find* the time to exercise. For most of us, time to exercise can't be *found;* it has to be *made.*

The good news is that getting regular exercise doesn't have to be a big deal and doesn't have to take much time. Studies have shown that getting (and staying) in shape need not take more than thirty minutes, three times a week (every other day).

So when's the best time to exercise? That depends on you and your life-style. The important thing is not *when* you exercise, but *whether*. . . .

| Exercise Time | Possible Disadvantages | Possible Advantages |
|---|---|---|
| Morning (before breakfast) | • Sometimes hard to get out of the sack. | • Clears the fog so you can begin your day refreshed and alert.<br>• You have to take a shower anyway.<br>• Outside exercisers can enjoy the peace and quiet of their sleepy neighborhood.<br>• Done in the morning, it's "out of the way." |
| Noon (before lunch) | • This is not possible if you have a short lunch period, or if showers are not available at work or school. | • Enables you to work off morning tensions.<br>• Can help curb lunch appetite.<br>• Refreshes you to meet afternoon demands. |
| Early evening (before dinner) | • Easy to postpone exercise due to coming home from work late, feeling "too tired," etc. | • Clears day's tensions.<br>• Helps you avoid "just home from the office" bingeing/snacking.<br>• Can help curb dinner appetite.<br>• Refreshes you for evening activities. |
| Late evening (before bed) | • Easy to postpone exercise due to eating late, wanting to watch a good TV program, telling yourself you'll get up early the next morning to do it, etc.<br>• Necessary to wait an hour or so after a heavy meal. | • Can help you relax and clear your mind of the day's problems so you can sleep more soundly. |

Source: *The HOPE Newsletter,* published by the Bob Hope Heart Research Institute, Seattle, Wash. Reprinted with permission.

rigidly that there is no room for creativity, spontaneity, and play? If you find yourself doing the same exercise, on the same day, at the same time, year in and year out, maybe you need to vary your routine. Try a new aerobic activity now and then, or ask a friend to share your fitness activities and make it a social occasion. You could even combine the two and join a friend or associate who is already involved in a different kind of activity. Let people show you the ropes of their favorite exercise. Remember, variety is the spice of life. (See figure 6.11.)

The best way to assure yourself of leading an active physical life-style is to choose aerobic activities you enjoy. If jogging is not for you, try swimming, bicycling, aerobic dance, or any of the other many activities that offer aerobic benefits. Investigate your chosen activity. (See table 6.5.) Seek out a support group to participate with. And most of all, have fun.

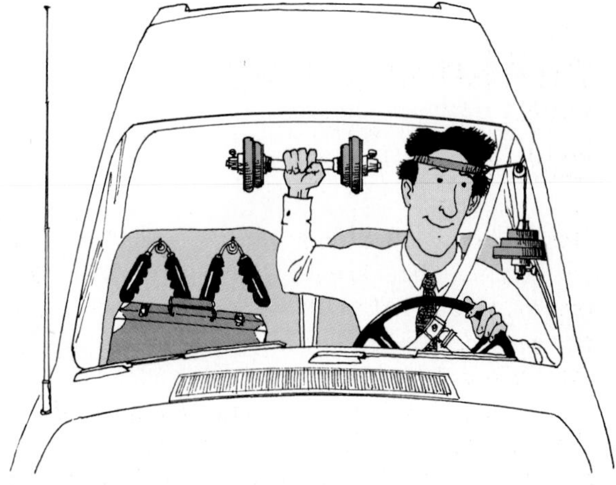

**Figure 6.10**
You don't find the time, you make the time to exercise.

## Table 6.5 Aerobic Exercise

**Where to Go for More Information:**

*Bicycling*

Bikecentennial—The Bicycle Travel Association
P.O. Box 8308
Missoula, MT 59807
(406) 721-1776
A publications list is available from Bikecentennial. They will answer questions on all aspects of bike touring.

*Hiking/Backpacking*

Sierra Club
530 Bush Street
San Francisco, CA 94108
(415) 981-8634
The national office will answer inquiries on hiking, camping, backpacking, canoeing, and other outdoor activities.

*Racquetball*

American Amateur Racquetball Association
815 North Weber Street
Colorado Springs, CO 80903
(303) 635-5396
The AARA will respond to requests for information on racquetball.

*Running/Jogging*

American Running and Fitness Association
2420 K Street NW
Washington, DC 20037
(202) 965-3430
The ARFA serves as a clearinghouse of information on running and jogging. Their Runner's Referral Service can match you with a runner of similar ability in your area.

*Swimming*

International Amateur Swimming Federation
200 Financial Center
Des Moines, IA 50309
(515) 224-1116
The IASF will respond to mail and telephone requests for information on swimming.

*Walking*

Walking Association
4113 Lee Highway
Arlington, VA 22207
(703) 527-5374
This association will respond to inquiries on walking.

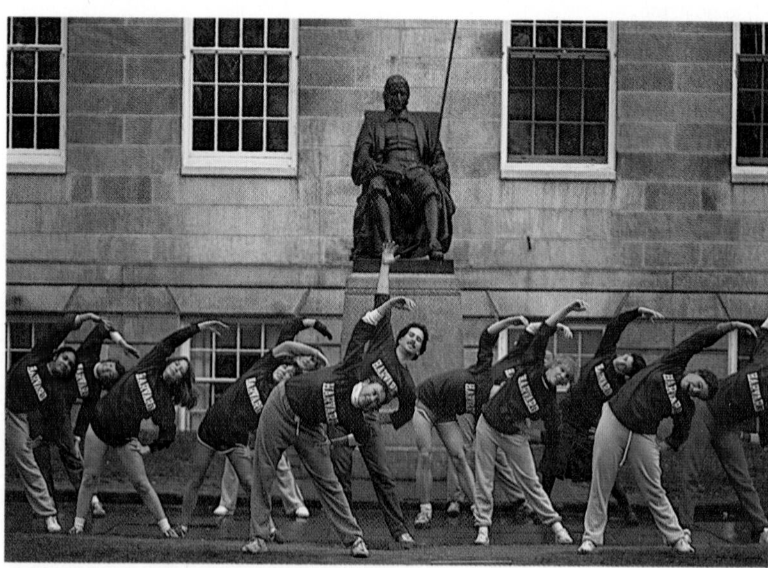

**Figure 6.11**
Sharing fitness activities can help make exercise a social occasion.

# SUMMARY

1. The key to leading a physically active wellness life-style is to find aerobic activities that you consider play.

2. There are many benefits of physical activity, including psychological, cardiovascular, weight control, and disease-prevention benefits.

3. Fitness can be described as the ability to function efficiently. The American College of Sports Medicine has delineated three major components of fitness: cardiorespiratory endurance; flexibility, coordination, and relaxation; and muscular strength and endurance.

4. There are four generally accepted principles of fitness: overload, specificity, individual differences, and reversibility.

5. Aerobic exercise causes a sustained increase in heart rate and uses the large muscles of the body for an extended period of time. Long-distance running, bicyling, and swimming are considered good aerobic activities.

6. Aerobic exercise has two major goals: to increase the total amount of blood and oxygen circulated throughout the body during exercise and to improve the ability of the large skeletal muscles to utilize the oxygen circulated.

7. Anaerobic exercise requires an intense, maximum burst of energy, and is of short duration (ten to ninety seconds). A tennis serve and a 100-yard dash are examples of anaerobic exercise.

8. There are many ways to measure physical fitness. A treadmill stress test and Cooper's Twelve-Minute Walk/Run Test are two good ways to measure aerobic-fitness levels.

9. When designing an aerobic-exercise program it is important to consider frequency, intensity, and time (F.I.T.). The American College of Sports Medicine recommends that aerobic exercise be done three to five days each week, maintaining the target heart rate for twenty to sixty minutes each session.

10. Target heart rate is the specific percentage of an individual's maximal heart rate; it is the rate which is the goal when exercising aerobically.

11. It is important to begin each exercise session with an appropriate warm-up period, and end it with a cool-down period. Warm-ups and cool-downs help to prevent exercise injuries.

12. Stretching exercises are good activities to include in the warm-up and cool-down periods. Stretching also makes an important contribution to total fitness by increasing flexibility.

13. Progressive resistance exercises (P.R.E), such as weight lifting and bodybuilding, make important contributions to muscular endurance and strength.

14. The American College of Sports Medicine suggests that aerobic-exercise programs progress gradually from very low-level activities to more strenuous activities. Three stages of conditioning are recommended: the initial-conditioning stage; the improvement-conditioning stage; and the maintenance stage.

15. People don't *find* the time to exercise. They must *make* the time. Choosing activities that are enjoyable and playful will help with "making the time," as will building a support network for play. Experiment with physical activity as one avenue to a wellness life-style.

### Recommended Readings

Allsen, P. E., Harrison, J. M., and Vance, B. *Fitness for Life: An Individualized Approach.* Dubuque, Iowa: Wm. C. Brown Publishers, 1983.

Anderson, B. *Stretching.* Bolinas, Calif.: Shelter Publications, 1980.

Cooper, K. *The Aerobics Program for Total Well-Being.* New York: M. Evans and Co., 1982.

Dintiman, G. B., Stone, S. E., Pennington, J. C., and Davis, R. G. *Discovering Lifetime Fitness.* St. Paul, Minn.: West Publishing, 1984.

Katch, F. I., and McArdle, W. D. *Nutrition, Weight Control, and Exercise*, 2nd ed. Philadelphia: Lea & Febiger, 1983.

Wescott, W. L. *Strength Fitness: Physiological Principles and Techniques.* Boston: Allyn & Bacon, 1982.

## References


1. H. T. Milhorn, "Cardiovascular Fitness," *American Family Physician* 26 (1982): 163–69.

2. George Sheehan, *Running and Being: The Total Experience* (New York: Warner Books, 1978), 71–83.

3. Richard A. Dienstbier, "The Effect of Exercise on Personality," in *Running as Therapy: An Integrated Approach,* edited by M. L. Sachs and G. W. Buffone (Lincoln, Nebr.: Univ. of Nebraska Press, 1984), 253–72.

4. William L. Haskell and Robert Superko, "Designing an Exercise Plan for Optimal Health," *Family and Community Health* 7.1 (1984): 72:88.

5. Ben Yogoda, "Relaxation," *Esquire* 101.5 (1984): 125–28.

6. Kevin McKeon, reported by Wayne Villanueva, "Exercise: 72 Million Americans Can't Be Wrong—or Can They?", *Discover* 3.8 (1982): 84–88; Haskel and Superko, "Exercise Plan."

7. Haskell and Superko, "Exercise."

8. R. Sanders Williams, "How Beneficial Is Regular Exercise?", *Journal of Cardiovascular Medicine* 7.11 (1982): 1112–20; Villanueva, "Exercise."

9. Haskell and Superko, "Exercise."

10. Haskell and Superko, "Exercise."

11. James D. Lepanto and F. Compton Jenkins, *Exercise: For the Health of It,* 3rd ed. Dubuque, Iowa: Kendall/Hunt Publishing Co., 1984.

12. David L. Costill, "Use It or Lose It," *The Runner* 7.2 (1984): 41–42, 59.

13. Frank Katch and William McArdle, *Nutrition, Weight Control and Exercise,* 2nd ed. (Philadelphia: Lea & Febiger, 1983).

14. Katch and McAardle, *Nutrition, Weight Control, and Exercise.*

15. Katch and McAardle, *Nutrition, Weight Control, and Exercise.*

16. "How Much? How Often? Minimum Guidelines for Squeezing Aerobic Exercise into a Too-Tight Schedule," *Independence Health Plan Newsletter* 4.1 (1984): 4–5.

17. American College of Sports Medicine, *Guidelines for Graded Exercise Testing and Exercise Prescription,* 2nd.ed. (Philadelphia: Lea & Febiger, 1980).

18. Bonnie G. Berger, "Running Strategies for Women and Men," in *Running as Therapy: An Integrated Approach,* edited by M. L. Sachs and G. W. Buffone (Lincoln, Nebr.: Univ. of Nebraska Press, 1984), 23–62.

19. Franklin Payne, "Exercises that Help Bodies Stay Healthy," *Consultant* 23.8 (August 1983): 188–204.

20. "Photostory: Warm-Up/Cool-Down Exercises for Joggers," *Patient Care* (30 April 1979): 168–77; "STRETCH," *Independence Health Plan Newsletter* 3.10 (1983):3.

21. American College of Sports Medicine, *Guidelines.*

22. "Racquetball Players," *Independence Health Plan Newsletter* 2.3 (1982).

23. "How Do You Spell Exercise? B-O-R-I-N-G," *Independence Health Plan Newsletter* 2. 4 (1982).

24. "How Do You Spell Exercise?"

# UNIT TWO

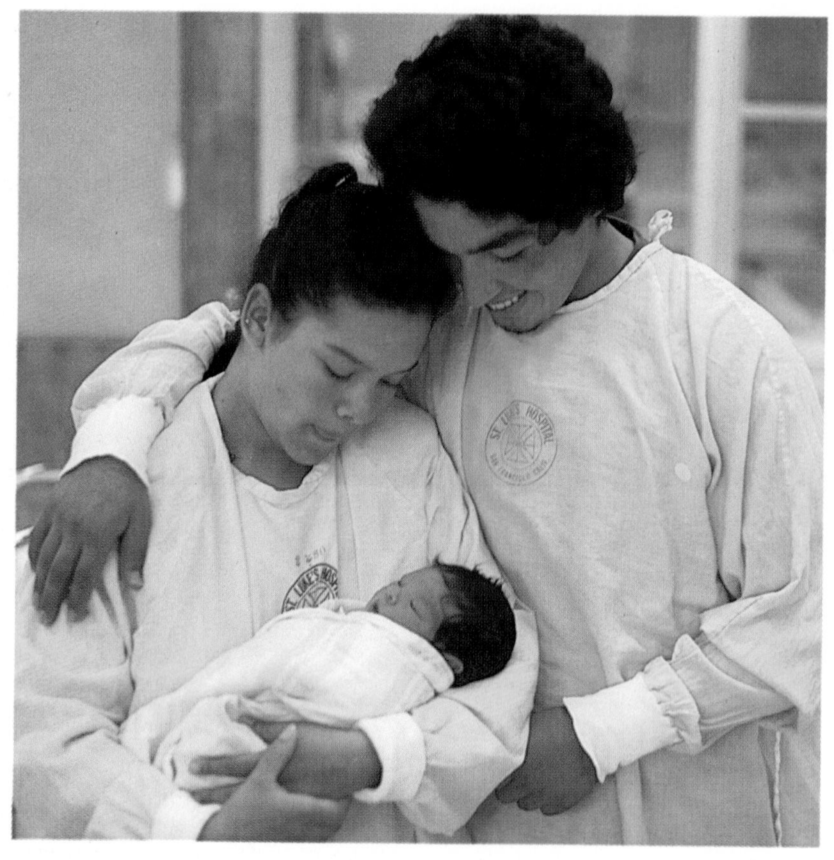

# Personal Intimacy and Well-Being

Unit 1 concentrated on your wellness level as an individual. Intimate relationships with other people are also an essential part of wellness. In unit 2 we will consider personal relationships from a wellness perspective. We will see how sexuality, birth control, pregnancy, and parenting can affect wellness. Chapters 7 through 10 will give you the information you need to make decisions regarding personal intimacy and well-being, helping you to maximize your wellness potential.

In chapter 7, you will learn about sexual behavior and life-style choices, as well as the factors that influence those choices. Sexuality is a basic component of high-level wellness, so decisions about sexual life-style options can have a profound effect on your wellness.

A better understanding of the reproductive and sexual response systems can also help you make decisions about your sexual lifestyle. Chapter 8 discusses the structure and function of the primary male and female reproductive organs. The human sexual response system is described, as well as common sexual dysfunctions.

Birth control makes possible many of the sexuality life-style options available today. Chapter 9 presents the major forms of birth control, how they work, and their advantages and disadvantages. Your decision to use a particular birth control method, or none at all, will strongly affect your level of wellness.

Another important decision affecting your life style is whether or not to have children, and if you do, how to parent them. Not all people can become natural parents, however. Chapter 10 will discuss both fertility and infertility, as well as provide information about pregnancy and childbirth. In addition, you will be asked to seriously consider what it means to be a parent.

CHAPTER SEVEN

# Human Sexuality: Sexual Behavior and Life-Style Choices



Are men born males? Are women born females? What factors influence the way people see themselves and their sex roles? What factors influence sexual behavior and life-style choices?

This chapter will explore the many factors that influence human sexual behavior. It will also describe some common sexual life-style options. The chapter will give you a better understanding of several important sexual issues and topics. With this enhanced understanding, we hope you will be better prepared to appreciate your sexuality as a basic component of high-level wellness.

# PERSONAL AND SOCIAL INFLUENCES ON SEXUALITY

Societies often perceive nonconforming behaviors and ideas as threats. Sexual behaviors and sexual attitudes are certainly no exception to this practice. There are often customs and laws in place to maintain the status quo. These subtle but pervasive forces sometimes get in the way of facts and objectivity.

When examining sexual behavior it is important that you distinguish between what is a fact and what is a belief. Sometimes the line between fact and belief is clear, but often this distinction is not easily recognized. Understanding more about sexuality requires separating correct information from misinformation.

## Sexuality Research

It is a difficult task to describe the sexual behavioral profile of a particular society. Paper-and-pencil questionnaires, telephone surveys, mail surveys, and personal interviews make up the majority of data-collection techniques used in sexuality research. These techniques are prone to error.

Some people do not respond to sexuality surveys, so the results of many studies reflect only the sexual attitudes and behaviors of those people who did respond. It is quite possible that people who respond to sexuality surveys are different from nonresponders, especially regarding sexual behavior. Because of this nonresponse factor, it is difficult for researchers to construct a sample of people who are representative of all Americans, or even smaller groups such as southerners or Washingtonians.

Another problem with sexuality research involves time. Sexuality studies tend to represent people's attitudes and behaviors for a certain time frame. Ten years, ten months, or even ten days later, people's attitudes may have changed.

Certain groups of people, such as the very rich, the very poor, and the young, are generally inaccessible to researchers. Additionally, social institutions often erect barriers to sexuality research. For instance, public schools have traditionally discouraged research examining the sexual behaviors of students.

Another major limitation of sexuality research involves the need to rely on the memories of subjects. People who respond to surveys may be unable to recall the details of their sexual behavior, especially five, ten, or twenty years after the fact. Others may feel that their answers are too personal to share with strangers. So even though our libraries are overflowing with "sex research," our knowledge of sexual behavior, like many other types of human behavior, is incomplete.

# DEFINING HUMAN SEXUALITY

Much has been written about human sexuality, but there is not one widely accepted definition. Although we know much about human sexuality, its true nature and meaning is elusive. Theories that attempt to explain human sexuality fall into three general categories: genetic, intrinsic, and social.

## Genetic Theories of Sexuality

**Genetic theories** suggest that sexuality is determined by a person's genetic gender. There are chromosomal variations, but virtually everyone is either a genetic male or a genetic female. Genetic blueprints, established at the moment of fertilization, will cause the fetus to develop either male or female internal and external reproductive organs. These blueprints will also dictate the emergence of either male or female secondary-sex and reproductive characteristics.

Maccoby and Jacklin suggest four gender differences that have been well established in the literature: (1) males are more proficient than females in visual-spacial abilities and (2) in mathematical abilities;[1] (3) females have a greater verbal ability than males; and (4) males are more aggressive than females.

One possible explanation for these gender differences is found in a recent area of research called brain dimorphism.[2] Brain dimorphism suggests that the male and female brains are structurally and functionally different. Thus, emotional and intellectual differences between males and females may not be caused by social learning, but by physiological brain differences dictated by genetic gender. Certain male and female traits may turn out to be genetically predetermined at birth.

The genetic gender of a person is the only part of sexuality that is not influenced by society. However, genetic science has recently played a more active role in manipulating sex chromosomes and reproductive hormones.

## Intrinsic Theories of Sexuality

**Intrinsic theories of sexuality** suggest that sexual behavior is a result of inner sexual drive. These theories focus on some inner force, controlled by the brain, which affects sexual behavior. For example, in 1931 Warden demonstrated that male rats were willing to cross an electrified grid in order to copulate.[3] In fact, the longer the male rats were denied a mate, the more times they would cross the grid to copulate.

Freud named the human sex drive the "libido." He believed that most human behavior was motivated by this powerful drive. Freud suggested that the libido was one of the two major forces influencing human behavior, the other drive being "Thanatos" or the death instinct.

Another intrinsic theory suggests that there is a pleasure center in the brain and humans crave its activation through sexual stimulation. Researchers have taken Warden's experiment one step further by electrically stimulating the area of the lower brain responsible for pleasure sensations. Animals have been observed to reject behaviors such as eating and copulating in favor of having their pleasure centers electrically stimulated.

Intrinsic theories of sexuality are often criticized because the findings from animal research may not be applicable to humans. It is also difficult to study the subconscious mind and theoretical abstractions such as the "libido."

## Social Theories of Sexuality

**Social theories** attempt to explain human sexual behavior as a product of social expectations and imitation. Such theories place great importance on social rewards and punishments as molders of peoples' sexuality.

Social-learning theory suggests that society directs a child's development of either male or female characteristics. The reinforcement of stereotypic gender roles is pervasive and can be found in educational, courting, marital, and occupational settings. Each culture has its own idea of how males and females should behave. That is why masculine behavior in one culture may be feminine behavior in another. For example, Greek males hold hands while dancing and this is well within the Greek masculine stereotype. (See figure 7.1.) However, U.S. males have been socialized generally not to hold hands or dance together, and this is within the U.S. masculine stereotype.

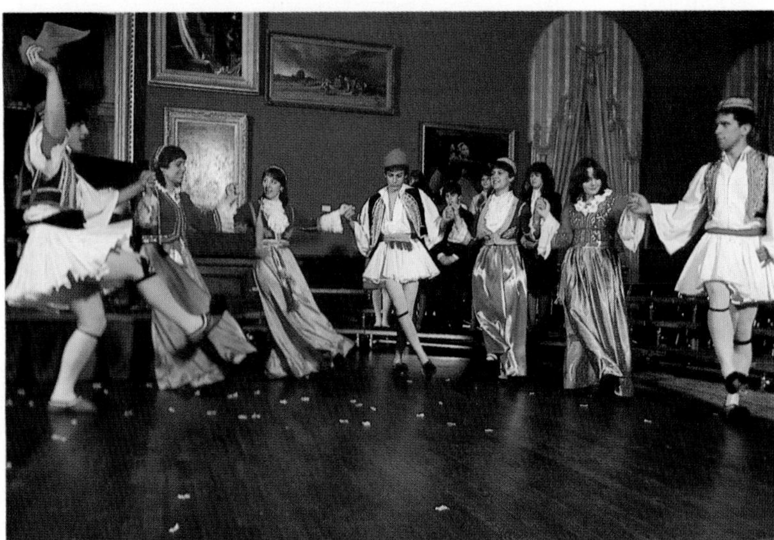

**Figure 7.1**
Each society defines its own stereotypic gender behavior. The Greek males regularly hold hands when dancing.

In the U.S., infant boys may be treated more roughly than infant girls. Boys are more likely to be physically punished, whereas girls are more likely to be verbally scolded. Males are generally expected to be more aggressive, athletic, ambitious, and unemotional than girls. Females are generally expected to be more affectionate, tender, maternal, and outwardly emotional than boys. When young children take on behaviors associated with the opposite sex-role stereotype they may be called a "sissy" or a "tomboy." When adults stray from their gender-role stereotype it is not unusual for them to be classified as "queer" or "gay." These labels are ways of notifying people that their behaviors are outside expected gender roles. The social-learning theory suggests that cultures, through example and social reinforcement, encourage people to think and act within gender-role stereotypes.

Some researchers believe that sexuality is determined by a combination of genetic gender and culture.[4] Although biology may dictate sex, it is culture that determines how males and females should think and behave sexually. Such views embrace the notion that you are a product of "nature" (your genes) and "nurture" (your environment).

**Human sexuality,** then, is a mixture of things. "Sexuality refers not only to reproduction and the pursuit of sexual pleasure but also to our need for love and personal fulfillment. . . . Sexuality includes our awareness of and reaction to our own maleness or femaleness and that of everyone with whom we interact."[5]

## SEX ROLES AND SOCIETY

Each society has historically devised a variety of gender-role guidelines for males and females. Despite the many variations between societies, within each society there is a minimum of duplication between gender roles. In addition, gender roles within a society are often compatible, even though they may be quite specialized. In a given society, the male may be the provider and the female the preparer. The male may be the model of strength and the female the model of compassion, and so on.

Over the centuries such specialized roles developed from social idiosyncracies and from the belief that males and females were biologically and intellectually different, and therefore best suited for different life tasks and roles. Before, as now, people tended to live their lives according to a set of gender-role guidelines.

Only recently have arguments been made for the case that males and females are human beings first and neither gender has a monopoly on a given emotion, ability, or intellectual vocation. Furthermore, stereotypic gender roles have been perceived to stifle human development and serve only to limit the range of emotional and personal options in life.

Are females better suited for domestic responsibilities and rearing children? Are males better suited for careers outside the home? Some people believe the ideal gender identity is neither male nor female, but rather an androgynous one. An **androgynous person** is not limited to a menu of either male or female behaviors or thoughts. Androgynous people utilize a wide range of available emotional and life-style options. (See figure 7.2.)

This recent challenge to gender-role stereotypes has caused many people to reexamine their sex roles, but the promotion of androgynous roles is not without

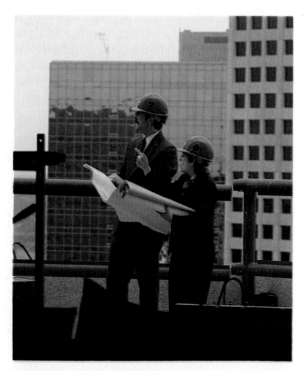

**Figure 7.2**
The distinction between "woman's work" and a "man's job" has blurred in recent years.

critics. People who support traditional gender-role stereotypes argue that males and females are physiogenically and intellectually different.

As the debate continues, the acting out of specific male and female roles will be pleasing to some and antagonistic to others. Social pressures will exist to convert housewives to corporate managers, or firemen to domestic engineers. There will also be social pressure to maintain the status quo.

In our society, there are always certain individuals and organizations trying to influence others to adopt particular sets of gender-role behaviors. Because gender-role behaviors are not necessarily right or wrong, each of us can create our own individual sexual identity. The choices among androgyny, traditional masculinity, traditional femininity, or a combination of these gender roles are available to each person. (See Activity for Wellness 7.1.)

7.1 ACTIVITY FOR WELLNESS 7.1

## Defining Male and Female Activities

How much of your masculinity and femininity do you understand and accept? To help you to determine the answer to this question, list below the "typical" male and female chores and activities that you routinely perform:

| ***Male Chores and Activities*** | ***Female Chores and Activities*** |
|---|---|
| 1. | 1. |
| 2. | 2. |
| 3. | 3. |
| 4. | 4. |
| 5. | 5. |
| 6. | 6. |
| 7. | 7. |
| 8. | 8. |
| 9. | 9. |
| 10. | 10. |

Would you want to do away with one of these lists? Why?

Are there any actions on either list that you would be embarrassed to perform in front of others? Why or why not?

Are there any chores or activities on your lists that should be performed by males only? Females only? Why?

What do you do that you would be embarrassed to do in front of males? Females? Why?

The answers to these questions will help you decide whether or not you are comfortable with both the masculinity and femininity in your personality. You should be aware of how you express both your maleness and your femaleness (i.e., your humanness) and be comfortable with that expression.

Source: From Greenberg, Jerrold et al., *Sexuality: Insights and Issues.* 

# LOVE

Two terms that are often associated with human sexuality are love and sex. Although often related, they can be very different kinds of human experience. A couple giving pleasure to each other through sex play is one way of expressing love. A father taking his daughter to the movie theater and watching her delight in the day's outing is another way to express love.

Societies place many codes and values on sexual activity. One common belief is that people must be in love before they engage in sexual intercourse. Another belief is that orgasm should occur only during sexual intercourse. These kinds of mores have linked love, sexual intercourse, and orgasm into a seemingly single-dimensional human event. Whether or not they should be linked is a matter of personal beliefs. However, the understanding that love, sexual intercourse, and orgasm are three separate human experiences allows them to be examined as unique parts of the human life experience.

Terms such as family love, puppy love, and erotic love have been used to describe the various types of human love. Often the definitions describe love in terms of what is going on in the relationship. For example, "puppy love" is used to define two young people who have found an interest in each other. Puppy love is usually defined as a relationship without sexual intercourse, and carried on at an immature level.

Rather than search for a collection of behaviors that represent true love, it might be better to define love in terms of a commitment. A common thread in love is that people who are in love often make a commitment to their lover. Through love relationships people realize their own self-worth and fulfill personal needs.

We will discuss two types of love—altruistic love and anterotic love.

## Altruistic Love

**Altruistic love** is the unselfish concern for the welfare of another person. Altruistic lovers want to satisfy the needs of the people they love, requiring nothing in return for their love. Altruistic lovers may heal someone's wounds, pay someone's bills, or work to meet another person's needs. In return, altruistic lovers do not expect or desire gratitude, recognition, or even repayment for their gifts of love from the person they love.

People such as humanitarians, Good Samaritans, or adoptive parents may qualify as altruistic lovers. The motives behind someone entering an altruistic love relationship are many. It is possible that altruistic lovers are meeting their own needs by being in such a love relationship. They may believe that by meeting other people's needs, they will be rewarded by God, or improve their self-worth, or repay past improprieties or past good fortune. Whatever the driving force, altruistic lovers expect nothing in return for their love from the person they love.

## Anterotic Love

The second type of love relationship is called **anterotic love,** named after the Greek god Anteros (an′ - te-ros).[6] Anteros punished people who did not reciprocate love. Most humans expect something in return for their love. "I'll love you if you cook and clean for me." "I'll have sexual intercourse with you if you promise to marry me." "I'll marry you if you promise to love me forever." These expectations become the conditions of the anterotic love relationship.

Probably the most common expectation of an anterotic lover is to be loved back, which seems reasonable. Often the anterotic lover expects to be loved in the way he or she defines being loved. A person may require a phone call each day from a working spouse, or a lustful sexual partner each evening after dinner. The anterotic lover may expect a faithful, supportive lover.

Lovers usually have different expectations for each other, which can make the anterotic love relationship a tenuous one. Anterotic lovers need to consider that their partner is probably not capable of meeting all of their expectations or may be unwilling to do so. Their partner might not be as thoughtful, or as witty, or as domestic as they would like. Anterotic lovers might want their lovers never to change, or to change radically. They may imply, or use statements such as, "If you really love me you'll . . . take out the trash, move to California, or have children!" Inevitably there will be times the anterotic lover will feel shortchanged.

Anterotic lovers are constantly in a process of giving and receiving. It may be that one lover is giving much more than the other. This is not automatically a poor love relationship. Some people may be "givers" while others are "receivers." On the surface, parental love usually involves considerably more giving on the part of the parents than the child. Nevertheless, each lover takes from the love relationship something they value or desire. It may be a feeling or a touch. It may be that the greatest joy some people seek is simply to be able to give their love to someone. Whatever it is, there is no true way of determining which lover receives the greatest benefit from a love relationship.

There is one additional consideration in all beginning anterotic love relationships, and that is timing. Falling in love does not usually occur simultaneously between two people. Anterotic lovers may become frustrated because their love is not reciprocated. Anterotic lovers often invest their love in the hope that it will be returned sometime in the near future. So the mother begins to love her newborn, and the suitor displays his affections for his newfound love.

Timing is often the critical factor in anterotic love. During different stages of people's lives they may be more receptive or less receptive to making a love commitment. Some potential lovers do not want to get involved when the school session is drawing to a close. They realize that they will soon be separated by time and distance. Some lovers may be very receptive to a commitment when they have just landed a high-paying job, or graduated, or moved to a town where they have few friends or family. Some lovers who have recently been rejected by another lover may also be very receptive to a love commitment. Timing can both promote and prevent love relationships.

## Love Relationships

Humans seemingly have always given advice to each other about love relationships. There are scores of theories and thousands of suggestions. If two people want to fall in love they will find a way. However, there are at least three essential elements of mature love relationships: accordance, communication, and time.[7]

**ACCORDANCE** A love relationship involves **accordance**—the harmony of minds and wills. Two people agree on individual and mutual goals. They realize that any decision affecting one of them affects the other. In turn, each partner becomes responsible to the other for his or her decisions.

**COMMUNICATION** A second component of love relationships is communication. Lovers communicate by word, by action, and by reaction. Lovers constantly express their concern, satisfaction, dissatisfaction, or disinterest. Lovers often develop private languages which may include primordial noises, baby talk, door slamming, fragrances, body movements, and other inventive techniques. Lovers can thus communicate back and forth, sometimes in a form that is only understood by them.

In love relationships it is essential that lovers communicate important feelings and thoughts. In order to accomplish this, lovers need to have a fairly clear and up-to-date notion of what is important to each of them. If one person does not communicate his or her needs to the other, it is possible that those needs will not be met. Sometimes people have their partners guess at what they require. Such people run the risk that their partners might not guess correctly, or might not even be aware that they were supposed to guess!

The key to communication is interpretation and response. At times a partner may be quite direct in making a request, and interpretation becomes simple—for example, "You're late!" Your lover is upset with the fact you were late and you can respond to that need. Sometimes, however, a partner is quite indirect and interpretation is difficult. Consider this statement: "You have never asked me once if I needed some help with the chores around the house!" This statement can be interpreted at face value, or it may be that the person is sending up a "help signal." Maybe this person had a bad day, or someone was hateful toward them, or today they are dissatisfied with themselves.

Before giving a response to a statement, it is important to be fairly certain of the correct interpretation. If a husband drops the sugar bowl and the wife says, "I'm leaving you," clearly the sugar bowl had little to do with the problem. One way to respond to this help signal is by asking an open-ended

7.1 EXHIBIT

## Gut-Level Communication

When we speak of revealing our "true selves" (self-disclosure), we need to understand that our true nature is not a fixed or static reality but a dynamic process in a constant state of change. We are what we think, feel, judge, value, honor, esteem, love, hate, desire, hope for, believe in, and are committed to. When we see our friends today, we must not assume that they are exactly the same people we knew yesterday. Now they have experienced more of life—more love, pain, pleasure, and hurt—and now they are different. And, of course, we are different today ourselves.

We communicate with each other at many levels of self-disclosure. The least intimate form of communication is "cliché communication" in which we reveal nothing of our inner feelings. "How are you?" "Just fine, thank you." "Sure is warm today." "Sure is." From this level of noncommunication, we gradually proceed through levels of revelation culminating in the open expression of deepest, innermost feelings, which John Powell calls "gut-level communication." In his classic *Why Am I Afraid to Tell You Who I Am?* (1969), Powell lays down five "rules" for gut-level communication:

1. Gut-level communication never implies a judgment of the other. We can reveal our emotional reactions to the other's actions: "I feel really (hurt, angry, good, nervous, etc.) when you (whatever action it is)." Here we reveal our response to that specific action, but we do not judge the whole person on the basis of that action. We do not force the other into defending his or her whole being, but we do allow for discussion and possible modification of a specific behavior pattern.

2. Emotions are not moral—they are neither good nor bad. They are simply factual—they exist. Most of us have emotions to which we do not want to admit. We may feel ashamed of our fears or guilty about our anger or sexual desires. Before we can freely communicate our feelings, we need to accept that everyone experiences all of these same emotions and that they are neither good nor bad and that feeling them does not make us either good or bad persons.

3. Emotions need to be integrated with the intellect and the will. This means that while we must experience, recognize, and accept our emotions fully, we must not always act on those emotions. To do so is to allow our emotions to control our lives. Thus, while we want to feel free to admit our fears, we need not be paralyzed by them. While we can freely admit our anger, we cannot feel free to punch out the person whose actions cause us to feel angry.

4. In gut-level communication, emotions are reported. For one thing, when we do not speak out our emotions, we act them out in temper tantrums, acts of violence, or our own psychosomatic health

question, such as: "You are upset because. . . ?" Let your partner help you in understanding his or her needs. Together you can identify the need, and then both of you can respond to that need.

This process, like any other communication technique, will work best when the partners are not demonstrating anger toward each other. Although it is possible to interpret what is said during a display of anger, often it is hard to reason with each other at that moment. Patience and the willingness to absorb your lover's anger without retaliation is a loving response to your lover's help signal. When tempers have cooled, lovers can then discover what needs are not being met.

Once you have interpreted your lover's need, then you can respond. The response might be straightforward or it may involve compromise. As two people agree on a response, they form another bond in their love accordance.

In love relationships lovers also communicate support for each other. There are many ways lovers can communicate their support and reaffirm that their love is alive.

## EXHIBIT 7.1

problems. But also, when we base our relationships on anything less than openness and honesty, they fail to stand the test of time. They soon crumble, leaving neither partner fulfilled by the experience.

5. With rare exceptions, emotions are best communicated at the time they are being experienced. It is much easier and feels much "safer" to report an emotion after it has become history. It is almost like talking about another person. And, in a sense, that was another person. As we have said, we each are a different person every day. But the emotions that are most meaningful with respect to our current relationships are those that we are feeling right now—and that is when they are most profitably communicated. (One exception to this rule is when the person to whom you would communicate your feelings is currently so disturbed with him- or herself that your report would be distorted by that person's emotional state. Another is when your interaction with that person is so transient (for example, a discourteous clerk) that it is hardly worth your time to tell him or her your emotional reaction.)

Honest disclosure of feelings has at least two major benefits. The more obvious reward is the type of intimate relationships it allows. But it also results in a more clearly defined sense of self-identity for each of the people in the relationship. For only by disclosing ourselves to others can we really know who we are. As we said earlier, we are what we think, feel, value, etc. And only through communicating these things to others can we really understand ourselves.

Source: Kenneth L. Jones, Louis W. Shainberg, and Curtis O. Byer, *Dimensions of Human Sexuality.* 

## DISCUSSION QUESTIONS

1. Do you use gut-level communication techniques in your love relationships?

2. Do you agree with the statement "only through communicating . . . to others can we really understand ourselves"?

**TIME** A third element of love relationships is time. Lovers spend time together in many ways. First, they spend time in direct interaction. Such interaction may include talking to each other, planning a vacation, playing various board games, and giving emotional and physical pleasure to each other. These moments bring their intellect, emotions, and bodies together for sharing and experiencing. Second, lovers spend time together as companions, watching television, attending social events, or living together. Lovers also spend time together by thinking about each other. Their thoughts range from passion to companionship. New lovers may spend a good deal of their waking and sleeping hours thinking about their partners. Separated lovers may find solace in their memories of moments together and in their anticipation of being together again.

Each love relationship has varying amounts of accordance, communication, and time. Love relationships develop from people first spending time together, then communicating, and finally reaching an accordance. Love relationships often dissolve, however, when people are not in accordance, do not communicate, and finally do not spend time together.

These three elements of a love relationship are only parts of love. Love is more than its elements; it will forever remain more than its description.

# SEXUAL BEHAVIORS

People may participate in sexual behaviors by themselves or with other persons. The menu of sexual behavior includes activities such as kissing and touching, masturbation, manual and oral-genital stimulation, and sexual intercourse.

## Kissing and Touching

Sexual stimulation can be communicated through all sensory receptors in the body. Two common avenues for communicating sexual stimulation are kissing and touching. These behaviors, however, are not always intended as sexual behaviors. Many people use a kiss or a touch to communicate love and emotional commitments which do not involve sex. A mother kissing her child, or one friend hugging and kissing another friend after a long absence are examples of nonsexual intentions.

Sexual activity with another person often begins with kissing and touching. Many parts of the human body are receptive to stimulation from both kissing and touch. Areas of the body that are especially receptive to sexual stimulation are known as **erogenous zones,** and commonly include the mouth, ears, inner surfaces of the thighs, the breasts, and the genitals. (See figure 7.3.)

## Masturbation

Usually a person's sexual experience begins with self-discovery of his or her own body and the pleasures of being sexually aroused. Self-stimulation of the body for the purposes of sexual pleasure is defined as **masturbation.**

Most Americans begin masturbating in their teen years. By the age of fifteen approximately 75 percent of U.S. males have masturbated at least once and by their early twenties more than 90 percent of males have masturbated. By the age of fifteen approximately 33 percent of U.S. females have masturbated at least once. By age sixteen about 50 percent and by their early twenties 75 percent of U.S. females have masturbated.[8]

A considerable proportion of males and females continue to masturbate throughout their lifetimes. Many continue to masturbate and also maintain active sexual relationships with their spouses or partners. Some couples include partner or mutual masturbation as a part of their sex play.

Over the years the American culture, like other cultures, has attempted to discourage people from masturbating. Scores of myths and tales have been invented to terrify and discourage the would-be masturbator. There is no evidence to indicate that masturbation causes any physical harm to the body, especially the brain. Some aggressive masturbating

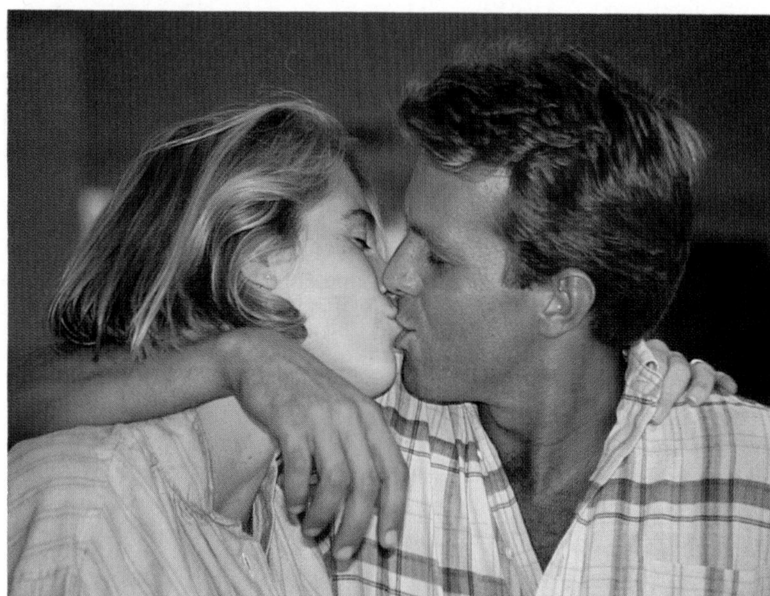

**Figure 7.3**
Kissing is one way of stimulating and communicating sexual arousal.

techniques may leave the genitals temporarily tender or inflamed, but masturbation does not cause blindness, deafness, cancer, epilepsy, mental illness, acne, sterility, or hairy palms.

## Oral-Genital Stimulation

A sexual behavior which is becoming more popular among heterosexual American couples is oral-genital stimulation. **Heterosexual cunnilingus** is the term used to describe the male orally stimulating the female genitals. **Heterosexual fellatio** is the term used to describe the female orally stimulating the male genitals. Cunnilingus and fellatio are also popular sexual behaviors among homosexual couples.

Estimates range widely on the percentage of American heterosexual couples and marrieds who have participated in oral-genital stimulation. Hass reported that 35 percent of the sixteen-year-olds he surveyed had experienced fellatio and cunnilingus.[9] A general estimate is that approximately 90 percent of Americans by age thirty-five have performed or received oral-genital stimulation at least once in their lifetimes.

## Sexual Intercourse

Societies have always been interested in human sexual behavior. This interest is reflected in the mores, laws, and rituals governing sexual intercourse. **Sexual intercourse** is technically defined as insertion of the penis into the vagina. The traditional view of sexual intercourse was that it should be used only by married couples to procreate (produce children). By the middle of the twentieth century this view was softened to accept sexual intercourse for pleasure, but only among married couples.

What do we know about contemporary sexual behavior in the U.S.? Today the majority of people experience sexual intercourse for the first time outside of marriage. Zelnik and Kantner reported that 69 percent of the fifteen-to-nineteen-year-old never-married females and 77 percent of the same-age never-married males they studied were nonvirgins.[10] Studies done in the last forty years indicate that the group most responsible for the recent proportional increase in never-married nonvirginity was young females.[11] By the end of this decade it is possible that the percentage of never-married nonvirgin females will equal that of never-married nonvirgin males.[12]

Several researchers dispute the notion that never-married sexually active people are having indiscriminant sexual intercourse. They contend that never-married couples engaging in sexual intercourse are more likely to be emotionally involved with their partners than just casual friends or strangers.[13] However, Zelnik and Kantner reported that 14 percent of the eighteen-to nineteen-year-old nonvirgin females they studied had eleven or more sexual partners and 86 percent had one to five sexual partners.[14]

Americans seem to believe that sexual intercourse can be shared by people who are emotionally involved with each other but not necessarily married, that sexual intercourse is for procreation but is also an acceptable activity for pleasure. This is not to say that all Americans collectively accept these beliefs. There are individuals and organizations that hold to more traditional views of sexual intercourse.

### EXTRAMARITAL SEXUAL INTERCOURSE

Research indicates that the proportion of spouses who participate in sexual intercourse with partners other than their spouses has not dramatically changed in the past few decades. Approximately half of married men and one quarter of married females have experienced extramarital sexual intercourse. The group showing the greatest proportional increase is females under the age of twenty-five.[15] Some researchers suggest that the female rate of extramarital sexual intercourse will equal the male rate of 50 percent by the end of this decade.[16] (See Activity for Wellness 7.2.)

7.2

ACTIVITY FOR WELLNESS

## It's Up to You: Decisions about Sex

(The following is based on an excellent brochure prepared by the Los Angeles Planned Parenthood—World Population organization. While the brochure is intended for teenagers, much of it applies to adults as well.)

How do you know when you're ready for sex? Many people will tell you what to do, and this can be very confusing. As a teenager, you are physically capable of having and enjoying sex. But there's more involved than physical needs, including your feelings, your relationship, and your view of yourself. Sex is used by people for many purposes. Although most people desire the pleasure of sex, it is often used for other reasons, many of which lead to pain. Sex can be one of life's most pleasurable experiences, or it can be equally as devastating. Because sex can be such a strong force, deciding when you are ready for sex is not a decision to be made in a moment of passion. It is a decision that you alone can make. Because remember—in the end, it's up to *you.*

Answering the following questions should help you in making decisions about your sexual activity.

**YOU**

1. Have you thought about your sexuality?
2. Are you prepared to make sure an effective form of contraception is used?
3. If you don't use contraception, are you prepared to cope with a pregnancy?
4. There are many types of sexuality; which will you choose?
5. How will you handle it if your sexual experience is unpleasant?
6. Sexually transmitted diseases are a definite risk. Can you deal with that?
7. If the sexual life-style you choose is not legal (for example, prostitution), are you willing to deal with the consequences?
8. Do you use sex to shock people?
9. How will you feel the next day?

**YOUR RELATIONSHIP**

1. Is there mutual consent to have sex?
2. Is sex being used as a weapon or bribe?
3. Do you or your partner feel like a sex *object* or feel exploited?

# LIFE-STYLE OPTIONS AND SEXUALITY

In general, Americans are marrying later in life than years ago and more females proportionately are nonvirgins at the time of their first marriage. There is also a greater proportion of people who remarry. More unmarried people today are living together than years ago. Additionally, more people spend a greater number of years single or in single households. More married couples are postponing having children or deciding to remain childless.

## Factors Affecting Sexual Life-Styles

Many developments have contributed to the changes in American sexual life-styles. Some of the more prominent factors include prolonged adolescence, increased life span, fertility technology, leisure time, and occupational opportunities for women.

**PROLONGED ADOLESCENCE** Four hundred years ago people married in their early teens, about the time they reached puberty. Seventy years ago Americans married in their late teens, just a few

## ACTIVITY FOR WELLNESS 7.2

4. Is sex a last resort to hold the relationship together?
5. What kind of commitment are you willing to make to one another?
6. Can you have a good relationship without sex?
7. Do you feel comfortable talking about sex with one another?
8. Will sex enhance your relationship?

**YOUR PARENTS**

1. How will your parents react?
2. Have you ever discussed sex with your parents? Or their values about sex?
3. Will you have to lie to your parents? Can you cope with that?
4. Are you using sex as a way to hurt your parents?
5. How have your parents' attitudes toward sex influenced you?

**YOUR FRIENDS**

1. Do you feel pressured to have sex?
2. Would you be considered "out of it" if you didn't have sex?
3. Do you need to be sexually active to be popular?
4. Are you tempted to have sex when and if you get high or drunk?
5. Does it really matter what your friends think?

**BACK TO YOU**

Many of these questions can be answered only by you. To answer them, it is helpful to understand your personal values, needs, and desires, as well as the consequences of your actions. If any of these questions are difficult to answer, perhaps you need more time to think before you make a decision or take an action. These questions should help you in making the best decision for yourself, because, basically, *it's up to you.*

Source: Courtesy of Planned Parenthood, Los Angeles, California.

years after they reached puberty. Today Americans marry in their early twenties, about one decade after they reach puberty. There is now a ten-year time lag from when most young people seek out sexual relationships to when they get married.

Prolonged adolescence has been necessitated by society's ever-increasing need to have trained and educated workers. More and more young people today wait to complete college before starting a career and marriage. Although society has extended the youth's occupational training period, it is not able to postpone the youth's desire for human intimacy and sexual relationships.

Prolonged adolescence encourages young people to enter into sexual relationships of convenience which do not hinder or jeopardize their future education or career goals. This pattern of mate selection encourages relationships in which the participants place personal goals before relationship needs. The pressure to marry when "you are ready," or when the "timing is right" is brought to bear by both friends and family.

**INCREASED LIFE SPAN** Increased lifespan has also influenced Americans' sexual relationships. During colonial times the average American life span was about thirty-five years. If you married and had children at age sixteen you would probably not live to see your grandchildren or your twenty-fifth anniversary. Today if you marry at age eighteen it could be a sixty-year commitment! This has caused some people to question the wisdom of marriage without the option of divorce. On the other hand, it has caused others who oppose divorce to be even more committed to the view that marriage and family are the foundation of society and bind it together. (See figure 7.4.)

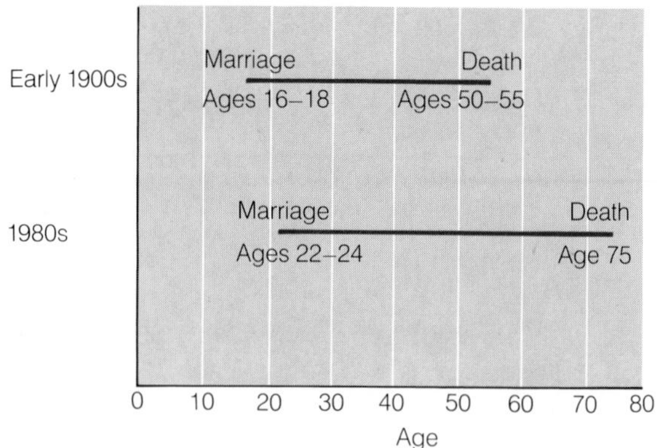


**Figure 7.4**
Graph of age at marriage and death, 1900 versus now. *Source:* From Jones, Kenneth L., Louis W. Shainberg, and Curtis O. Byer, *Dimensions of Human Sexuality.* 

**FERTILITY TECHNOLOGY** A third factor challenging sexual relationships is fertility technology. Today people have the option to postpone procreation or to procreate artificially (artificial insemination, surrogate mothers, sperm banks). Unwanted pregnancies can be prevented and people can choose to be sexually active and not procreate before they believe they are socially ready. This makes sexual intimacy during prolonged adolescence less a threat to an individual's future marital and career goals. Young people can continue to pursue their educational, occupational, and sexual goals without having a pregnancy jeopardize their plans. The number of females having their first child between the ages of thirty and thirty-four increased 82 percent from 1972 to 1981. The number of females having their first child between the ages of thirty-five and thirty-nine increased 33 percent in the same time period.

Single people can become parents. Married couples can remain childless. Remarried people can remain childless or decide to procreate and start a second family. Fertility technology has added several new options to the American sexual life-style.

**LEISURE TIME** A fourth factor influencing sexual life-styles is leisure time. As the number of average working hours decreases Americans gain more free time. This increased leisure time grants people additional opportunities to locate sexual partners. In turn, Americans have more time to invest in one or more ongoing sexual relationships. Leisure time has contributed to the number of relationships and social options open to single and married people.

**OCCUPATIONAL OPPORTUNITIES FOR WOMEN** The fifth factor affecting sexual relationships is improved occupational opportunities for women. New opportunities provide women with the independence and freedom to maintain their single life-styles indefinitely. Occupational opportunities give married and single females the economic independence to move from one relationship to another. Occupational opportunity also increases mate selection opportunities. The more people someone is able to meet, the greater the chance for a relationship to develop. Working acquaintances and friendships have the possibility of developing into loving relationships for married as well as single people.

## Single Life-Style

Everyone is single at some point during their lifetime. However, the traditional goal was to get married. Today there is a greater proportion of men and women remaining single for longer periods of time. There are more never-married single males than single females up to the age of fifty-five. However, the number of never-married single females has increased significantly over the last decade.

Traditionally, being single after the expected age of marriage was a social stigma, but this stigma is losing its control over people. An increasing proportion of people believe that their career has a higher priority than marriage in their lives.[17] These people may postpone marriage or remain single throughout their lifetime.

Singles expend considerable resources and energy locating partners. For the never-married high-school or college student there are usually ample opportunities to meet eligible partners with similar interests and backgrounds. Employed singles, on the other hand, have limited opportunities to meet eligible partners with similar interests and backgrounds and may face the task of placing themselves in social situations which will improve their chances of locating a partner. Employed singles may rely more on family and friends to meet potential partners. (See Exhibit 7.2.)

**COHABITATION** **Cohabitation** describes a living arrangement in which two people who are not married to each other share both bed and board. Cohabiting couples in essence act as married couples without being legally married. Although the term cohabitation is generally applied to heterosexual couples, homosexual couples also participate in this living arrangement. However, there is little data on cohabiting homosexuals.

Estimates vary but it is believed that about 15 percent of college students are cohabiting at any one time, and about 25 to 33 percent of all college students have cohabited.[18] It is also estimated that 2 percent of American households are formed by people cohabiting.[19] Glick and Norton reported that 40 percent of the cohabiting couples they studied eventually married.[20] There is no clear indication of whether or not cohabiting with a future spouse improves the chances for marital success.[21]

Not all cohabiting couples view their living together as a prelude to marriage.[22] Many couples cohabit in order to experience the heightened emotional and personal sharing generated by living together.

## Marriage

Marriage is the personal commitment of two people to share forever their feelings, thoughts, failings, and triumphs. The marriage bond is a legal bond and is often practiced as a spiritual bond. The marriage ceremony is the formal act of two people announcing to the state, and possibly their God, that they have joined their lives forever.

In the traditional view, marriage creates a foundation for the family that serves as the workshop for human emotional, spiritual, physical, intellectual, and social development. The husband and wife form a human bond of purpose, which unites them to their ancestors. Each spouse becomes responsible for the other and for any children they might bear. Man and woman become one, each responsive to the other's needs and dedicated to their chosen union.

Americans today overwhelmingly seek out this traditional form of marriage. (See figure 7.5.) Proportionately more people are getting married today than at any other time in American history, making marriage the most popular life-style in the U.S.[23] Americans tend to marry partners who are similar to themselves in terms of economic, racial, and religious backgrounds.[24] Additionally, Americans tend to marry spouses who have lived or are living close to their homes. First-time marrieds tend to marry

7.2 EXHIBIT 7.2

# Advertising for Partners

Share my farm, view of the mountains, wood-splitting, animal chores, and bed. Twenty-eight-year-old Taurus female seeks equal partnership with gentle, hard-working male. Your animals welcome.

Intelligent, peace-loving, reasonably good-looking male, thirty-three, with secure income seeks honest female companion for exploration of life's joys. No drugs, smoking, or religious fads, please.

Gay white female, warm and loving, looking for affectionate, feminine gay female for potential relationship, ages twenty-five to thirty-five.

Extraordinary lady, early thirties, highly intelligent, very attractive, discriminating tastes, incurably romantic, seeks scintillating Jewish professional. No man who likes polyester suits or discos, has dependents, or wears toupee need apply.

Gay white male, thirty-two, six feet, 190, strong build, wants small, cuddly, young gay lover.

Film producer, mature male, harassed but successful, seeks quiet, intelligent, slender, athletic young woman for fun and whatever.

Very shy male artist, age twenty-seven, seeks to meet warm female for companionship.

Exuberantly sensual thirty-five-year-old female with open marriage seeks enthusiastic daytime partners. Prefer masculine types with good build. Any race.

Gay father, thirty-two, with two preschool children, seeks to share home, parenthood, and companionship with compatible gay father. I'm considerate, quiet, athletic, into cross-country skiing, hiking, nature photography, and classical music.

Professional black female, twenty-seven, tall and aristocratic, desires to meet educated, expressive, proud black male.

Personal ads fill pages of certain newspapers and often spell out the desired exchange in great detail. Do people write them for kicks? Does anyone answer? Carole Goldberg (1979) ran an informal survey of people who have taken out personal ads in the *New Haven Advocate*. One finding: Ads placed by females draw far more responses than ads placed by males. Goldberg encountered one man who had done a little research on his own. He placed an ad seeking a female companion for himself, as well as a phony one by "an attractive female wishing to meet men." His ad got one reply. The fake female ad drew 100 responses.

What kind of people answer the ads? According to one male, the women who responded to his ad were "nice, . . . high-class, quality people" except for one who was "a little crazy." Women who place these ads seem pleased with their experiences, too. One woman had met her spouse through a personal ad, and so had her brother met his.

What kind of people place personal ads? Goldberg found that motives vary from loneliness to lust to playfulness. Those placing ads seem willing to take the initiative in looking for partners. But they want to maintain some kind of buffer between themselves and utter strangers. Placing an ad gives them a chance to be selective without risking their self-esteem, as they would if they were trying to meet people by going to bars, discos, or "new age" workshops. As one gay male pointed out, it's a relatively safe way to explore the unknown, "a romantic, almost quaint, old-fashioned way to meet. . . . If you get a lot of letters it's like having your own harem. You get to pick and choose by your own criteria" (Goldberg 1979, p. 42).

Source: From *Sexual Choices: An Introduction to Human Sexuality* 2d ed., by Nass, G. D., R. W. Libby, and M. P. Fisher. Copyright 1984, 1981 by Wadsworth, Inc. Reprinted by permission of Wadsworth Health Sciences Division, Monterey, Calif. 93940.

## DISCUSSION QUESTIONS

1. Have you ever considered submitting or answering an ad in the personals?

2. Do you think personal ads are an appropriate way to meet people?

3. Why do you think personal ads are becoming so popular?

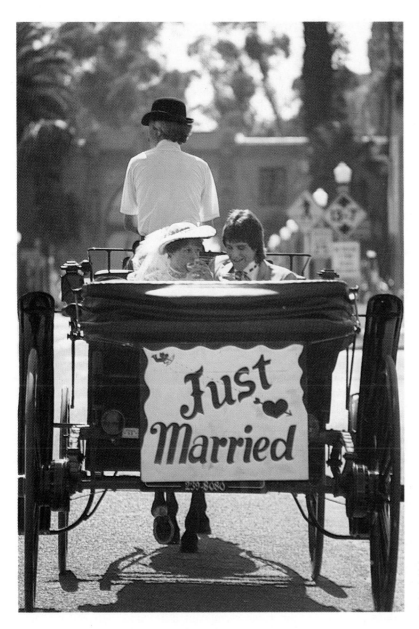


**Figure 7.5**
Proportionately more people are getting married today than at any other time in U.S. history.

spouses close to their own age. The average marital age of American males is twenty-four and of females twenty-two. Approximately 22 percent of all marriages involve at least one spouse who was previously married.

There are two basic mores of marriage. The first is that the husband's and wife's sexual activity is limited to each other. The second is that the husband and wife are personally and socially responsible for each other and their children. The spouses are the family providers, protectors, teachers, and counselors.

Why are so many people attracted to marriage as a life-style? Marriage offers people the chance to experience intense human compassion and support for a lifetime. Married people can build their relationship over time until love and friendship become one. They can be molders and givers of life and love. They can share their compassion with children. Additionally, marriage offers economic benefits and support, as well as providing a heritage of ancestors and the possibility of heirs.

## Divorce

In the last thirty years the American divorce rate has doubled. For every two couples who married in 1980 there was one couple who divorced. Based on this divorce rate some people may conclude that the institution of marriage is failing. Approximately 80 percent of divorced people, however, remarry.[25] In one study, 75 percent of remarried people were found to be happy in their new marriages.[26] It is reasonable to assume that Americans are more likely divorcing their spouses than divorcing marriage. The average age at which American men are divorced is twenty-nine; the average woman is twenty-eight.

Divorced people are faced with the task of reassembling their lives and life-styles. They must deal not only with the legal matters of divorce but also with the emotional and social aspects. In some cases divorced persons must sever ties with family, friends, and neighbors. They will probably seek out another mate, and this will require that they reenter the dating arena. Divorced people may learn that the dating rules have changed considerably in the years they were married.[27] They may also learn new dating rules that apply to divorced people. In most cases divorced people will be anxious about their new life-style and possibly apprehensive over their ability to readjust. This increased stress could explain why some researchers see a correlation between divorce and suicide.[28]

There are researchers who believe that the trauma of divorcing a spouse is a greater burden than the trauma of becoming a widow or widower.[29] In the case of the death of a spouse there is usually no one "at fault." Death is also final; there is no chance of bringing back a dead spouse. With divorce there is a propensity to establish fault and encourage guilt; there is also the chance that the couple could remarry or maintain communication and emotional ties. Divorce carries the possibility for immediate and long-term emotional upset for all family members.

On the positive side, most divorced people do adjust and find a new sense of independence and self-worth. Sometimes the feeling of being freed from a marriage is a tremendous personal relief.

**DIVORCE AND CHILDREN** It is estimated that 50 percent of American children will soon come from divorced households.[30] There is an ongoing debate as to whether there are any ill effects of divorce on children. It has been reported that adolescent girls from divorced households had a higher prevalence of drug involvement and sexual behavior associated with psychiatric referral.[31] Presently there are studies that suggest that divorce adversely affects children[32] and studies that suggest that divorce is not necessarily harmful to children.[33] Most researchers do agree that divorce is a stressful and emotionally upsetting experience for children.

## Homosexuality

**Homosexuals** are people who prefer to engage in sexual activities with persons of their own gender. There are homosexual males and homosexual females. Homosexuality is not the norm in the majority of societies.[34] For centuries societies have attempted to discover why some people are homosexual although the vast majority are heterosexual.

One theory suggests that homosexuality is caused by genetic inheritance. Kallam, in his study of identical twins, reported that this was true.[35] However, later studies reported that there was no link between people's genes and their sexual preferences.[36]

A second theory suggests that an excess or deficiency of certain hormones causes homosexuality. Several researchers have discovered different testosterone levels in homosexual versus heterosexual males. Hormonal differences have also been reported between homosexual and heterosexual females.[37] There are additional studies, however, which report no significant differences between the hormonal levels of homosexuals and heterosexuals.[38]

A third theory suggests that homosexuals are products of families in which their same-gender parent was missing or submissive. Some speculate that there were inadequate male and female role models during the homosexual's childhood.[39] But there are other studies that dispute this theory.[40] There are also studies that suggest that homosexual parents do not necessarily raise homosexual offspring.[41]

The attempt to explain what causes homosexuality generates a lot of theories, but there is no conclusive evidence available. It may be that each theory is actually correct for a select group of homosexuals. It is also possible that none of the current theories are correct and the right theory has yet to be discovered.

The discovery that a person has homosexual preferences usually occurs during adolescence for males and a bit later for females.[42] Homosexual individuals may live as singles or couples. In one study 57 percent of female homosexuals reported between five and twenty-five homosexual partners whereas 43 percent of male homosexuals reported more than 500 partners.[43]

Common sexual behaviors for female homosexuals are manual stimulation of the genitals and cunnilingus.[44] Contrary to popular belief, female homosexuals are not particularly likely to use electric devices to reach orgasm. Fellatio is a common practice among male homosexuals. Additionally, approximately 20 percent of homosexual males have experienced anal penetration by a penis.[45] (See Exhibit 7.3.)

Most homosexuals have had heterosexual experiences including sexual intercourse. Approximately 35 percent of the homosexual females and 20 percent of the homosexual males studied by Bell and Weinberg were currently heterosexually married.[46] Davis estimates that there are 1.5 million homosexual female parents in America.[47] There are relatively few homosexual male parents in America because they are generally unable to gain custody of their children in divorce cases.[48]

Today homosexuals are more willing to make their life-style known publicly ("come out of the closet"). Homosexual communities can be found in major cities and rural areas. Like other minorities, homosexuals have organized and are working toward obtaining open approval and guaranteed rights. They are challenging those who believe that homosexuality is a sexual perversion and a socially unproductive life-style.

7.3 EXHIBIT 7.3

## Some Common Myths about Homosexuality

Each of the following common myths about homosexuality is partly correct but is partly, or even mostly, incorrect. Each is true of some homosexual individuals but is not true of some or most others.

**Myth:** *You can always tell homosexual people by the way they look and act. Gay men always dress, talk, walk, and act in an effeminate way. Men who seem feminine must be gay. Gay women always have short haircuts, deep voices, and act like men. Masculine-seeming women must be lesbians.*

**Facts:** These stereotypes may sometimes prove accurate, but they do not apply to the majority of gay people (Krajeski 1981). There are gay men and lesbian women who do fit the stereotypes in terms of mannerisms, and there are also many heterosexuals who fit these stereotypes. Appearances are often unreliable in judging a person's sexual orientation.

In some communities, some of the gay people conform to a particular manner of dress and hairstyle. Such fashions vary from place to place and constantly change in any one given place. For example, among males in San Francisco in 1981, if one had short hair, a moustache, and wore blue jeans, work boots, and a leather jacket, one was presumed to be gay and very likely was gay. However, in a Midwestern farm town in 1981, a male with the same appearance was presumed to be heterosexual.

For individuals who are insecure with their own masculinity or femininity, it may seem important to be as unlike a homosexual person as possible. To accomplish this, these insecure individuals may maintain in their minds the stereotype of the effeminate gay male or masculine lesbian and thus view themselves as more sexually adequate in contrast (Krajeski 1981). Such individuals are very disturbed and threatened when they encounter gay people who fail to fit their stereotyped concept.

7.3 *continued* EXHIBIT 7.3

**Myth:** *Homosexual people never marry. People who never marry are probably gay. People who marry and have children can be presumed to be heterosexual.*

**Facts:** Many homosexual people do marry and have children, and many people who never marry are strictly heterosexual. Hunt (1977) and Maddox (1982) estimate that about one out of every five gay men and one out of every three lesbians enter into heterosexual marriage at some time. Hunt further estimates that at least 2 to 3 percent of currently married American men are bisexual and have sex with other men at least once in a while in addition to having sex with their wives.

**Myth:** *Homosexual people are all undersexed. Or, homosexual people are all oversexed. (It's heard both ways.)*

**Facts:** Like heterosexuals, gay people represent a broad range of sexual desire. A few gay males are extremely sexually active, exceeding the sexual capacities of almost all straight men (Hunt 1977), but they are the exception rather than the rule. The sexual activity level of most gay people is not significantly different from that of most heterosexual people.

**Myth:** *The number of gay people has increased tremendously in the past few years. Gay people are constantly trying to convert straight people to homosexuality.*

**Facts:** First, the incidence of homosexuality has remained fairly constant for at least thirty years (Kinsey 1948; Marmor 1980). However, homosexual individuals are more visible now than in the past. Many have stopped keeping their sexual preferences secret and have come out in the open, one very beneficial result of the gay liberation movement. But apparently the percentage of people of primarily homosexual orientation has changed little.

As to trying to seduce straight people, a few homosexual individuals do try to seduce straights, just as a few heterosexual people enjoy trying to seduce gays. But the great majority of gay people do not. They just are not attracted to people who are not attracted to them. And since, as we have seen, sexual orientation is apparently determined quite early in life, any efforts to convert straight people to homosexuality (or vice versa) are highly unlikely to succeed.

Source: Kenneth L. Jones, Louis W. Shainberg, and Curtis O. Byer, *Dimensions of Human Sexuality.* 

## DISCUSSION QUESTIONS

1. Have you heard these myths before? Did you believe any of them?

2. Why do you think so many myths are generated regarding homosexuality?

# SUMMARY

1. Genetic theories of sexuality suggest that sexuality is determined by biologic gender. Intrinsic theories of sexuality suggest that sexuality is a result of a person's inner sexual drive. Social theories of sexuality attempt to explain human sexual behavior as a product of social norms and imitation.

2. Sexuality is a term that describes someone's perception of sex roles, love, reproduction, sexual and personal fulfillment, and interaction with others.

3. There is no set of gender-role behaviors that any science can conclusively claim as right or wrong.

4. Altruistic love is the unselfish concern for the welfare of another person.

5. Anterotic lovers expect the people they love to reciprocate.

6. Three essential elements of a mature love relationship are accordance, communication, and time.

7. Masturbation is defined as self-stimulation of the body for the purposes of sexual pleasure.

8. Cunnilingus is defined as oral stimulation of the female genitals. Fellatio is defined as oral stimulation of the male genitals.

9. The majority of Americans experience their first sexual intercourse outside of marriage. When considering how Americans behave it seems that they subscribe to the belief that sexual intercourse can be shared by two people who are emotionally involved with each other, but not necessarily married.

10. Many factors have affected American sexual life-styles in the last several decades. Five of the more important factors are prolonged adolescence, increased life span, fertility technology, increased leisure time, and increased occupational opportunities for females.

11. Today a greater proportion of Americans remain single for longer periods of time.

12. Ninety percent of Americans will marry by age thirty-five and ultimately 95 percent of all Americans will marry.

13. In the last thirty years the American divorce rate has doubled. It is estimated that 50 percent of American children will soon come from divorced households.

14. Homosexuals are people who prefer to engage in sexual activities with persons of their own gender. Like other minorities, homosexuals have organized and are working toward obtaining open approval and guaranteed rights.

### Recommended Readings

Jones, Kenneth L., Shainberg, Louis W., and Byer, Curtis O. *Dimensions of Human Sexuality.* Dubuque, Iowa: Wm. C. Brown Publishers, 1985.

Katchadourian, H. *Human Sexuality: A Comparative and Developmental Perspective.* Berkeley: Univ. of California Press, 1979. Reissued in Ira, *Family Systems in America.* 3d ed. New York: Holt, Rinehart, and Winston, 1980.

Rathus, S., and Nevid, J. *Adjustment and Growth: Challenges of Life.* New York: Holt, Rinehart, and Winston, 1983.

Zelnick, M., and Kantner, J. "Sexual Activity, Contraceptive Use, and Pregnancy among Metropolitan-Area Teenagers," *Family Planning Perceptives* 12 (1980): 230–37.

## References


1. E. Maccoby and C. Jacklin, *The Psychology of Sex Differences* (Stanford, Calif.: Stanford Univ. Press, 1974).

2. K. Dohler et al., "Pre-Postnatal Influence of Testosterone Propionate and Diethylstilbestrol on Differentiation of the Sexually Dimorphic Nucleus of the Preoptic Areas in Male and Female Rats," *Brain Research* 302 (1984): 291–95; Tom Mazur and John Money, "Prenatal Influences and Subsequent Sexuality," in *Handbook of Human Sexuality,* edited by Benjamin B. Wolman and John Money (Englewood Cliffs, N.J.: Prentice-Hall, 1980); R. Whalen, "Brain Mechanisms Controlling Sexual Behavior," in *Human Sexuality in Four Perspectives,* edited by F. Beach (Baltimore: Johns Hopkins Univ. Press, 1977).

3. C. J. Warden, *Animal Motivation: Experimental Studies on the Albino Rat* (New York: Columbia Univ. Press, 1931).

4. H. Gardner, *Developmental Psychology* (Boston: Little, Brown, 1978).

5. Kenneth L. Jones, Louis W. Shainberg, and Curtis O. Byer, *Dimensions of Human Sexuality* (Dubuque, Iowa: Wm. C. Brown Publishers, 1985).

6. Philip Belcastro, "Sexuality and Love," unpublished manuscript, 1980.

7. Belcastro, "Sexuality and Love."

8. A. Hass, *Teenage Sexuality: A Survey of Teenage Sexual Behavior* (New York: Macmillan, 1979); M. Hunt, *Sexual Behavior in the 1970's* (Chicago: Playboy Press, 1974).

9. Hass, *Teenage Sexuality.*

10. M. Zelnick and J. Kantner, "Sexual Activity, Contraceptive Use, and Pregnancy among Metropolitan-Area Teenagers," *Family Planning Perceptives* 12 (1980): 230–37.

11. R. R. Bell and J. B. Chaskes, "Premarital Sexual Experience among Coeds, 1958 and 1968," *Journal of Marriage and Family* 32 (1970): 81–84.

12. P. Belcastro and T. Nicholson, "An Explanation of Convergence between Male and Female Adolescent Sexual Behaviors," paper presented at the 111th meeting of the American Public Health Association, Dallas, 1983.

13. Hunt, *Sexual Behavior;* D. Jedicke, "Sequential Analysis of Perceived Commitment to Partners in Premarital Coitus," *Journal of Marriage and the Family* 37 (1975): 385–90.

14. M. Zelnick and J. Kantner, "Reasons for Nonuse of Contraception by Sexually Active Women Aged 15–19," *Family Planning Perspectives* 11 (1979): 289–96.

15. Hass, *Teenage Sexuality.*

16. Lynn Atwater, "Getting Involved," *Alternate Lifestyles* 2 (1979): 33–68.

17. I. H. Frieze et al., *Women and Sex Roles: A Social Psychological Perspective* (New York: Norton, 1978).

18. D. W. Bower and V. A. Christopherson, "University Students' Cohabitation: A Regional Comparison of Selected Attitudes and Behavior," *Journal of Marriage and the Family* 39 (1977): 447–53; Paul R. Newcomb, "Cohabitation in America: An Assessment of Consequences," *Journal of Marriage and the Family* 41 (1979): 597–602.

19. I. L. Reiss, *Family Systems in America,* 3d ed. (New York: Holt, Rinehart and Winston, 1980).

20. P. Glick and A. H. Norton, "Marrying, Divorcing and Living Together in the U.S. Today," *Population Bulletin* 32 (1978): 3–38.

21. Newcomb, "Cohabitation"; J. Jacques and K. Chason, "Cohabitation: Its Impact on Marital Success," *Family Coordinator* 28 (1979): 35–39; M. Newcomb and P. Bentler, "Assessment of Personality and Demographic Aspects of Cohabitation and Marital Success," *Journal of Personality Development* 4 (1980): 11–24.

22. E. Macklin, "Review of Research on Nonmarital Cohabitation in the United States," *Exploring Intimate Life Styles,* New York, Spring 1978.

23. A. Pietropinto and J. Simenauer, *Beyond the Male Myth* (New York: New York Times Books, 1977).

24. G. Leslie and E. Leslie, *Marriage in a Changing World* (New York: John Wiley & Sons, 1977).

25. Glick and Norton, "Marrying, Divorcing."

26. B. Murstein, *Love, Sex and Marriage through the Ages* (New York: Springer, 1974).

27. Morton Hunt and Bernice Hunt, *The Divorce Experience* (New York: McGraw-Hill, 1977).

28. S. Stack, "The Effects of Marital Dissolution on Suicide," *Journal of Marriage and the Family* 42 (1980): 83–92.

29. S. A. Rathus and J. S. Nevid, *Adjustment and Growth: The Challenges of Life* (New York: Holt, Rinehart and Winston, 1983).

30. Glick and Norton, "Marrying, Divorcing"; A. Plateris, "Divorces and Divorce Rates," *Vital and Health Statistics* series 21, no. 29, National Center for Health Statistics (Washington, D.C.: U.S. Government Printing Office, 1979).

31. M. Kalter and J. Remsar, "The Significance of a Child's Age at the Time of Parental Divorce," *American Journal of Orthopsychiatry* 51 (1981): 81–100.

32. T. Parrish, "The Relationship between Factors Associated with Father Loss and Individual's Level of Moral Judgement," *Adolescence* 15 (1980): 534–41.

33. S. Grossman, J. Shea, and G. Adams, "Effects of Parental Divorce during Early Childhood on Ego Development and Identity Formation of College Students," *Child Development* 7 (1978): 313–26.

34. F. Beach, *Human Sexuality in Four Perspectives* (Baltimore: Johns Hopkins Univ. Press, 1977).

35. M. Diamond and A. Karlen, *Sexual Decisions* (Boston: Little, Brown, 1980).

36. Diamond and Karlen, *Sexual Decisions;* B. Zuger, "Monozygotic Twins Discardant for Homosexuality: Report of a Pair and Significance of the Phenomenon," *Comprehensive Psychiatry* 17 (1978): 661–69.

37. J. Money, "Human Hermaphroditism," in F. Beach, ed., *Human Sexuality in Four Perspectives* (Baltimore: Johns Hopkins Univ. Press, 1977); J. Money and M. Schwartz, "Dating, Romantic and Nonromantic Friendships, and Sexuality in 17 Early Treated Adrenogenital Females, Aged 16–25," in P. A. Lee et al., eds., *Congenital Adrenal Hyperplasia* (Baltimore: University Park Press, 1977).

38. H. Meyer-Bahlburg, "Sex Hormones and Male Homosexuality in Comparative Perspective," *Archives of Sexual Behavior* 6 (1977): 197–325; G. Tourney, "Hormones and Homosexuality," in J. Marmor, ed., *Homosexual Behavior* (New York: Basic Books, 1980).

39. A. Bandura, *Principles of Behavior Modification* (New York: Holt, Rinehart, and Winston, 1969); M. T. Saghir and E. Robins, *Male and Female Homosexuality* (Baltimore: Williams & Wilkins, 1973).

40. J. Marmor, ed., *Homosexual Behavior* (New York: Basic Books, 1980); W. H. Masters and V. E. Johnson, *Homosexuality in Perspective* (Boston: Little, Brown, 1979).

41. B. Hoeffer, "Children's Acquisition of Sex-Role Behavior in Lesbian-Mother Families," *American Journal of Orthopsychiatry* 51 (1981): 536–44; M. Kirkpatrick, C. Smith, and R. Roy, "Lesbian Mothers and Their Children: A Comparative Survey," *American Journal of Orthopsychiatry* 51 (1981): 545–51.

42. R. R. Troiden and E. Goode, "Variables Related to the Acquisition of a Gay Identity," *Journal of Homosexuality* 5.4 (1980): 383–92.

43. A. P. Bell and M. S. Weinberg, *Homosexualities: A Study of Diversity among Men and Women* (New York: Simon & Schuster, 1978).

44. P. Califia, "Lesbian Sexuality," *Journal of Homosexuality* 4.3 (1979): 255–66.

45. Bell and Weinberg, *Homosexualities.*

46. Bell and Weinberg, *Homosexualities.*

47. R. Davies, "Representing the Lesbian Mother," *Family Advocate* 1 (1979): 21–24.

48. R. Green, "Should Homosexuals Adopt Children?" in J. P. Brady and H. K. Brodie, eds., *Controversy in Psychiatry* (Philadelphia: Saunders, 1978).

CHAPTER EIGHT

# Sexuality: The Human Reproductive System and Sexual Response



The goal of this chapter is to describe how the human reproductive and sexual response systems function. A better understanding of the reproductive and sexual response systems can increase your ability to maintain wellness. This chapter will focus on what is known about human reproduction. It will also address male and female sexual response—their similarities and differences.

This chapter will give you a background for future decisions regarding your sexuality and its relationship to high levels of wellness. There are and always will be many new philosophies regarding sexuality, as well as social and medical options that will directly affect your sexuality and sexual life-style. Each year these new developments become increasingly more sophisticated. Understanding the human reproductive system will enable you to make decisions regarding sexuality that are appropriate for you, your mate, and your family.

## PERSONAL AND SOCIAL INFLUENCES

For centuries, human reproduction and sexual response were mysteries, because sexual intercourse was secret. People believed that "talking about sex" would increase the likelihood of promiscuous sexual behavior. So generations grew up learning in school about the digestive system, respiratory system, and other systems, while parents and clergy supposedly taught children about the reproductive system. Unfortunately, most parents and clergy reneged on their duty to teach children and young adults about the human reproductive and sexual response systems. Thus, for most of us, friends, television, movies, and other media became the primary "sex teachers" by default.

Ironically, much structured "sex education" has contributed its share of misinformation. School sex education courses are under constant pressure from external influences such as PTAs, churches, health departments, and political groups. In addition, many courses are taught by people not academically or emotionally prepared for sound instruction. Only rarely does a school employ a full-time teacher trained specifically in human sexuality. (See figure 8.1.)

Such factors have kept the workings of the human reproductive and sexual response systems a confidential subject. People thus tend to judge sexual functioning in terms of their own sexual experience. Although personal life experiences are valuable cognitive tools, a lifetime of experiences does not equal the experience of lifetimes. As in other areas of human knowledge, scientific research can tell us more than personal observation alone.

## THE REPRODUCTIVE SYSTEM

The human species is **dimorphic** because it has two unique reproductive forms, a male and a female. Together the male and the female form the human reproductive system. Not all living creatures are dimorphic. There are species of animals that are asexual and consequently have no male or female form. Dimorphic species have more variation and adaptability because two individual members are contributing genes to their offspring. In the case of humans, each genetic parent (male and female) contributes his or her genes to their offspring. The genes combine and form a single cell, called a **zygote.** The zygote will develop into a new adult member of the human race. The creation of a zygote is called **fertilization** and its development into a new human being is the mission of the human reproductive system.

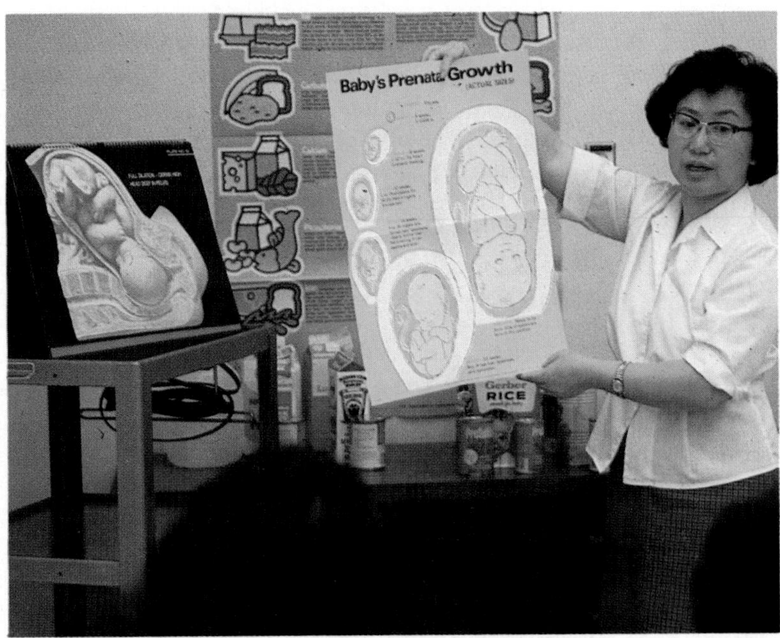


**Figure 8.1**
Full-time teachers trained in human sexuality are a rarity in most U.S. schools.

## The Primary Reproductive Organs

The primary human reproductive organs are the **testes** in males and **ovaries** in females. The testes and ovaries have several important functions. First, the sperm produced by the testes and the eggs produced by the ovaries carry genetic information. Each sperm carries either an X or Y sex chromosome. Each egg carries one X chromosome. If a zygote is formed by an X carrying sperm the offspring will be female, because the new pair of sex chromosomes will both be X chromosomes. If the zygote is formed by a Y carrying sperm the offspring will be male, because the new pair of sex chromosomes will be one X and one Y. The second function of the testes and ovaries is to produce the hormones (estrogen and testosterone) that cause **secondary sex characteristics,** the physical changes that lead to sexual maturity. And third, the testes and ovaries produce hormones that maintain the viability of the reproductive organs and associated sexual functions.

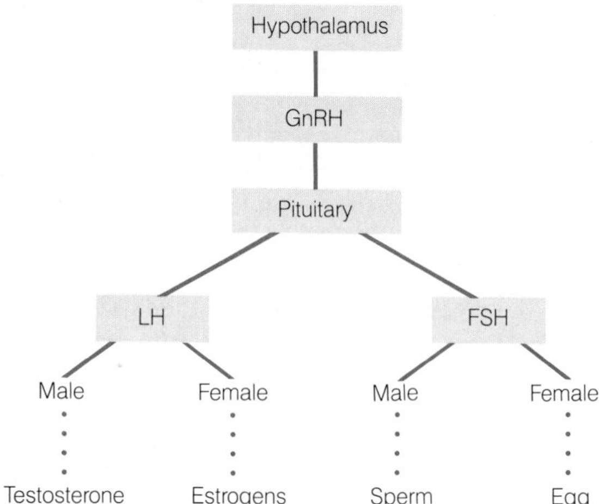


**Figure 8.2**
Hormonal control of the human reproductive system.

## Gonadotropins

The brain is responsible for the regulation of the human reproductive system. The part of the brain that monitors and regulates the reproductive system is the **hypothalamus.** (See figure 8.2.) The hypothalamus communicates its directions with **hormones,** chemicals that stimulate organs of the body into performing certain tasks. The hormone used by the hypothalamus to stimulate the testes and ovaries is called the **gonadotropin-releasing hormone,** or **GnRH.** The purpose of GnRH is to set off a chain of chemical events which will cause the testes to produce sperm and the ovaries to produce eggs, as well as producing additional hormones to maintain the reproductive organs. There are several gonadotropins, but we will focus on just two of them, luteinizing hormone and follicle-stimulating hormone.

**LUTEINIZING HORMONE** When GnRH is secreted by the hypothalamus it causes the pituitary to secrete **luteinizing hormones (LH)** into the bloodstream. In males LH stimulates the testes into producing **testosterone,** the primary male sex hormone. Although the physiological process is not completely understood, testosterone prevents atrophy (wasting away) of the male reproductive organs. Testosterone has been suggested to be partially responsible for males' socially and sexually aggressive behavior. Additionally, testosterone causes the adolescent male to develop the adult male physique, including broad shoulders, pubic hair, enlargement of the penis and scrotum, enlargement of the larynx and vocal chords, and thickening of the skin.

In females LH stimulates the ovaries to produce the primary female hormone **estrogen,** which has several functions. In preadolescent females estrogens cause the development of the breasts. Estrogens also cause the female to develop the feminine physique by adding fat deposits in the abdomen, buttocks, and hips. Estrogens are also responsible for the enlargement of reproductive organs. In postpubertal females, estrogens stimulate and maintain the female reproductive organs. Estrogens also cause eggs to mature and prepare the uterus for pregnancy.

**FOLLICLE-STIMULATING HORMONE** When GnRH is secreted by the hypothalamus it causes the pituitary to secrete the gonadotropin known as the **follicle-stimulating hormone (FSH).** In females FSH stimulates the ovaries to produce eggs. In males FSH stimulates the testes to produce sperm.

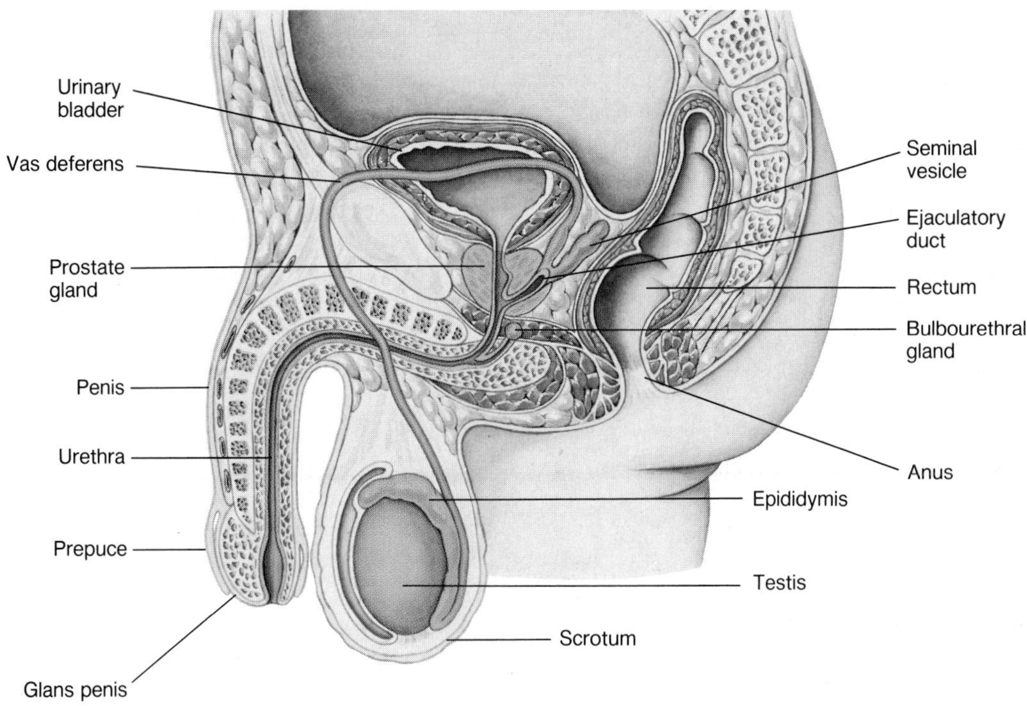


**Figure 8.3**
Male reproductive organs. *Source:* From Hole, John W., Jr., *Human Anatomy and Physiology,* 3d ed. © 1978, 1981, 1984 Wm. C. Brown Publishers, Dubuque, Iowa. All rights reserved. Reprinted by permission.

## Male Reproductive System

In order to understand the male reproductive system, you need to know about the scrotum, testes, epididymis, vas deferens, semen, seminal vesicles, prostate gland, urethra, bulbourethral glands, penis, sperm, ejaculation, sperm count, and fertilization. (See figure 8.3.)

**SCROTUM** The scrotum, a skin sac suspended in the groin area at the base of the penis, houses the two testes. The scrotum is suspended from the body in order to maintain the temperature of the testes at approximately 3.6 degrees (Fahrenheit) cooler than normal body temperature. This lower temperature is necessary for the production of sperm. Muscle fibers in the scrotum contract and relax in response to external temperature. In cold weather, the muscle fibers contract and move the scrotum and testes closer to the body for warmth, whereas in warm weather the muscles relax and move them further away from the body.

**TESTES** The testes are the primary male reproductive organs. The testes produce sperm and testosterone. One legend has it that the word testify comes from an early custom of men placing their hands over their testes when taking an oath . . . "to testify."[1]

There are two testes in the scrotum. The testes contain numerous highly coiled tubes known as the **seminiferous tubules.** It is in these seminiferous tubules that sperm are produced. In the spaces between the seminiferous tubules lie the **Leydig cells,** which produce testosterone. (See figure 8.4.)

**EPIDIDYMIS** As sperm mature, they empty from the seminiferous tubules into the **epididymis.** The literal meaning of the word epididymis is "over the testes," which accurately describes their location. The epididymis provides a fluid for storing sperm. In addition, there is evidence that some defective sperm are removed by the epididymis.[2]

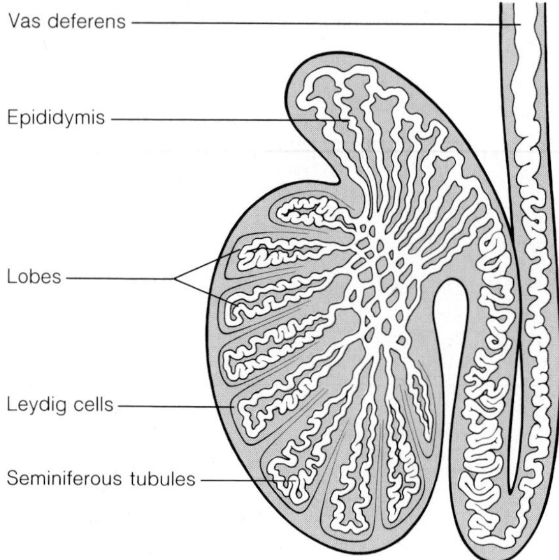


**Figure 8.4**
Cross section of scrotum.

It takes approximately seventy-four days to manufacture sperm. The male manufactures approximately 200 million sperm per day. Viable sperm remain stored in the epididymis for approximately two to four weeks. After this time they are reabsorbed by the body.

**VAS DEFERENS** Each epididymis empties into a **vas deferens.** The vas deferens are approximately eighteen inches long and are partially housed inside the scrotum. The vas deferens circle the bladder and ultimately join with the urethra. The walls of the vas deferens are lined with cilia. Contraction of the vas deferens, coupled with the action of the cilia, combine to transport sperm through the vas deferens.

**SEMEN** When exiting the body, sperm reside in a fluid called **semen.** Seminal fluid is produced by the epididymis and the accessory male reproductive organs which include the seminal vesicles, prostate gland, and bulbourethral glands.

**SEMINAL VESICLES** The **seminal vesicles** are two small glands found at the end of each vas deferens, just before the vas deferens enter the prostate gland. The seminal vesicles produce a fluid containing a simple sugar which provides nutrition for sperm. About 60 percent of the total volume of semen is made up of the fluid produced by the seminal vesicles. The seminal vesicles also secrete prostaglandins, which stimulate the sperm into undulating their tails for locomotion. Prostaglandins also stimulate the female's reproductive tract into contractions. These combined actions help to transport sperm through the female reproductive tract.

**PROSTATE GLAND** The **prostate gland** is a small walnut-shaped gland located at the base of the bladder. The ejaculatory duct and the urethra pass through the prostate gland. The prostate secretion, which makes up about 15 to 30 percent of the semen, is alkaline, opalescent in color, and possesses the characteristic seminal odor. The prostate secretions neutralize: (1) the waste products of sperm, (2) the acid found in the male urethra, and (3) the acidic environment of the female reproductive tract. Without the neutralizing action of the prostatic fluid many sperm would die, making fertilization of the egg impossible.

**URETHRA** The urethra has two functions. It is the tract that urine passes through from the bladder to the penis and the tract that semen passes through.

**BULBOURETHRAL GLANDS OR COWPER'S GLANDS** Two **bulbourethral glands** (or Cowper's glands), the shape and size of peas, are connected to the urethra as it enters the penis. These glands create an alkaline secretion that sometimes appears as a droplet prior to ejaculation. Occasionally this droplet may contain viable sperm. The exact purpose of the bulbourethral glands' secretion is not known. One popular theory is that their fluid lubricates the end of the penis.[3] Its major function, however, is more likely that of neutralizing any urine in the urethra prior to ejaculation.

8.1 EXHIBIT 8.1

## Do You Recommend My Newborn Son Be Circumcised?

No medical indication exists for routine circumcision, and the final decision should be left to the parents after they have received proper counseling and can make an informed decision,* according to the American Academy of Pediatricians (AAP). But in the minds of most Americans, circumcision of the infant boy is almost a matter of course, and the *elective* operation has become practically routine: According to various estimates, 85–90 percent of all boys born in the U.S. undergo circumcision. Recent medical literature abounds with letters and articles decrying this trend.

"I tell parents that this is not an operation I am *medically* recommending for their son," says Robert Marino, M.D., a surgeon at the University of Oklahoma Tulsa Medical College, who has written a leaflet on care of the foreskin.**

In providing counseling, Dr. Marino encourages parents to keep an open mind. He considers primarily whether the uncircumcised penis would be likely to receive adequate hygiene throughout the infant's life. Thus, he thinks circumcision is indicated for infants who are mentally retarded, who will probably be living in areas where there is little soap and water available, or who may live in an environment where inadequate hygiene is common.

Dr. Marino considers good hygiene "the viable alternative to circumcision." To help parents decide between the two, he describes in detail, with the aid of his leaflet, the steps in proper hygiene for the uncircumcised penis. He also mentions potential complications of circumcision—mainly bleeding, infection, and a predisposition to meatitis and meatal stenosis.

Dr. Marino says the role of the physician is not to advocate a course of action based on his or her opinion, but to provide parents with enough data to enable them to make informed decisions. He acknowledges that most parents he advises remain adamant in their desire for the operation. He usually accedes to their wishes, especially if they want their child circumcised for religious reasons. He advises parents who say they want their child circumcised despite limited finances that the money might be better spent elsewhere. "An automobile safety seat is much more important," he says.

"But in the final analysis," Dr. Marino says, "only the parents can decide whether the increased ease of hygiene is worth amputation of some normal anatomy of the body."

*Committee on Fetus and Newborn: Report of the Ad Hoc Task Force on Circumcision. *Pediatrics* (1975) 56: 610–11.

**For more information contact Robert Marino. M.D., University of Oklahoma Tulsa Medical College, 2808 S. Sheridan Rd., Tulsa, OK 74129.

Source: Reproduced with permission from *Patient Care* (29 February 1984). 

### DISCUSSION QUESTIONS

1. Do you believe male infants should be circumcised?

2. Were you aware that there are no medical reasons for circumcision?

**PENIS** The reproductive function of the penis is to deposit semen in the female reproductive tract. The approximate length of the adult male penis when flaccid (not stimulated) is between 2½ and 4½ inches. This increases to approximately 6 inches when erect.

The head of the penis, called the **glans,** is an especially sensitive area of the penis, containing many nerve endings. The glans is covered by loosely fitting skin called the **prepuce** or **foreskin.** It has been a common practice in the U.S. to remove the foreskin at birth or soon after. This operation is called **circumcision.** Present research indicates that there is no medical or health benefit resulting from male circumcision.[4]

Internally, there are three spongelike chambers which run the length of the penis. When the male is sexually stimulated these chambers fill with blood and the penis becomes erect.

**SPERM** The sperm cell is truly unique. The sperm has three basic parts, the head, middle piece, and the tail. Atop the head is the acrosome, a structure that contains an enzyme which breaks down the coating of cells that surround the egg, enabling a sperm to penetrate it. The middle piece, or body of the sperm, is partially responsible for generating energy. The tail is responsible for the sperm's mobility. (See figure 8.5.)

Sperm can swim about one inch an hour. However sperm, on the average, reach the fallopian tubes sixty to ninety minutes after being deposited into the female reproductive tract. The female tract is much longer than two inches, and this suggests that the sperm's journey is aided by the contractions of the female reproductive tract.

**EJACULATION** Sperm leave the body via ejaculation. **Ejaculation** is the expulsion of semen from the urethra, and is usually associated with orgasm. Ejaculation and orgasm, however, can occur independently. Semen and sperm leave the urethra in the following order: first the fluid from the bulbourethral glands is expelled, then the prostatic fluid, followed by sperm. Finally the seminal fluid is released.

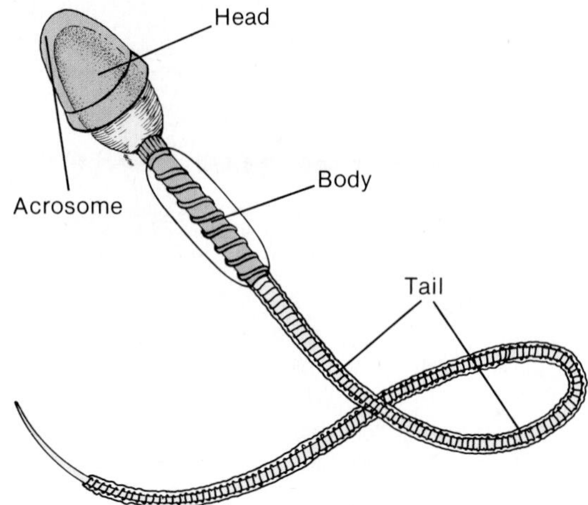


**Figure 8.5**
Sperm. A sperm is a cell highly adapted for reaching and penetrating a female egg. *Source:* From Hole, John W. Jr., *Human Anatomy and Physiology,* 3d ed. © 1978, 1981, 1984 Wm. C. Brown Publishers, Dubuque, Iowa. All rights reserved. Reprinted by permission.

**SPERM COUNT** There are several factors which can reduce the male's **sperm count,** or the number of sperm found in one ejaculation. These factors range from fever to tight underwear. Altitude (either living in elevations well above sea level or traveling frequently in airplanes) can also reduce sperm count. Stress, whether caused by the battlefield or emotional distress, can also reduce the male's sperm count. Several diseases, such as mumps, diabetes mellitus, and gonorrhea can also affect a male's sperm count.

The average ejaculation contains 3 milliliters of semen with anywhere from 10 to 100 million sperm per milliliter. There are reports of males fathering children with only 2 to 4 million sperm in their entire ejaculate. As a benchmark, however, it seems that when the male's sperm count drops below 10 million per milliliter, fertilization of the egg becomes difficult.[5]

**FERTILIZATION** When the egg is penetrated by a sperm, their genes unite and form the very first cell of a new individual called a zygote. The formation of a zygote is called **fertilization.** Only one sperm is required for fertilization. From the 300

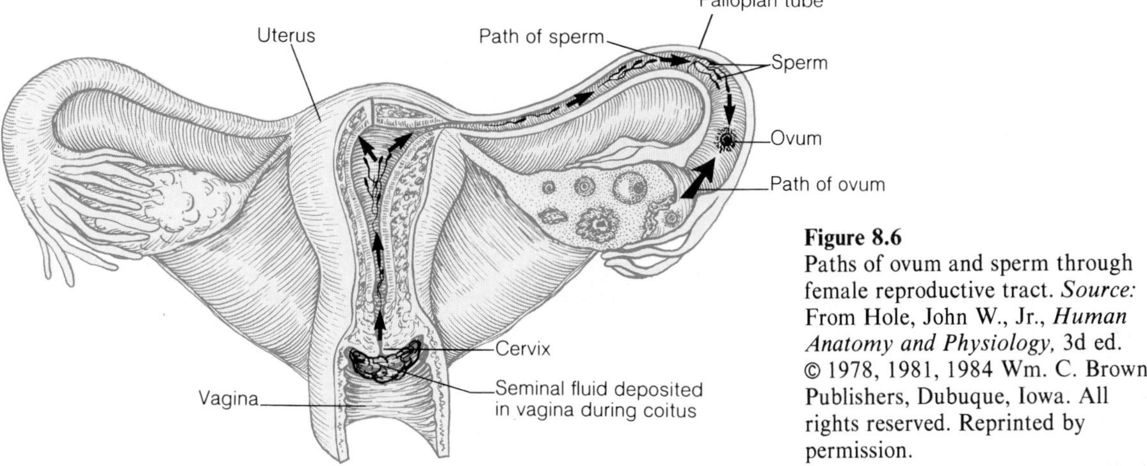


**Figure 8.6**
Paths of ovum and sperm through female reproductive tract. *Source:* From Hole, John W., Jr., *Human Anatomy and Physiology,* 3d ed. © 1978, 1981, 1984 Wm. C. Brown Publishers, Dubuque, Iowa. All rights reserved. Reprinted by permission.

million or so sperm deposited into the female reproductive tract (see figure 8.6 ), only about 300,000 will reach the female's fallopian tubes. Half of those will enter the fallopian tube without the egg, while only 2,000 sperm will actually reach the egg.

The egg is covered with a clear membrane. When a sperm penetrates this membrane it is drawn into the nucleus of the egg. This causes the secretion of polysaccharides which makes the membrane impermeable to the remaining sperm. A zygote is formed.

## Internal Female Reproductive System

After puberty the male can biologically father a child every day of his adult life. From a strictly biological viewpoint, once the male has deposited his sperm into the female's reproductive tract his reproductive role is complete. In comparison, for the female there are only a few days out of three or four weeks in which fertilization can occur. The female reproductive system is not only responsible for helping to create a zygote, it is also responsible for (1) nurturing the zygote's development during pregnancy, (2) childbirth, and (3) producing milk to nourish the newborn infant.

The female reproductive cycle has often been referred to as the menstrual cycle. The word menstruation is derived from the Latin word menses, which means month. This is a fairly accurate description of the duration of the female reproductive cycle, because it averages from twenty-five to thirty-two days.

**Menstruation** is the cyclical bleeding that signifies the beginning of the next reproductive cycle. Since menstruation is only one part, and not the central function of the female reproductive cycle, we will not refer to the female reproductive cycle as the menstrual cycle. We will focus on the primary function of the female reproductive cycle, which is procreation (the creation of a zygote), gestation (the development of a fetus), and parturition (childbirth). (See figure 8.7.)

**OVARIES** The ovaries are the primary female reproductive organs and have two main functions: to produce eggs and to produce estrogen and progesterone. Females have two ovaries which weigh about 6 grams each and measure a little over an inch across.

The female is born with all the potential eggs she will use throughout her reproductive lifetime—about one million in each ovary. Each premature egg is surrounded by a thin tissue called a **follicle.** Each month several follicles begin to mature; however, only one of these follicles will eventually be released by the ovary. The other follicles stop maturing and are dissolved in the ovary. The one follicle which completely matures is known as the **Graafian follicle.**

**Ovulation** When fully matured, the Graafian follicle's wall becomes thin. Soon after this, the Graafian follicle ruptures, releasing the egg from the ovary into the fallopian tube. This event is called **ovulation.** Some women experience discomfort, pressure, or pain around the time of ovulation. This phenomena is called **mittleschmerz,** meaning middle

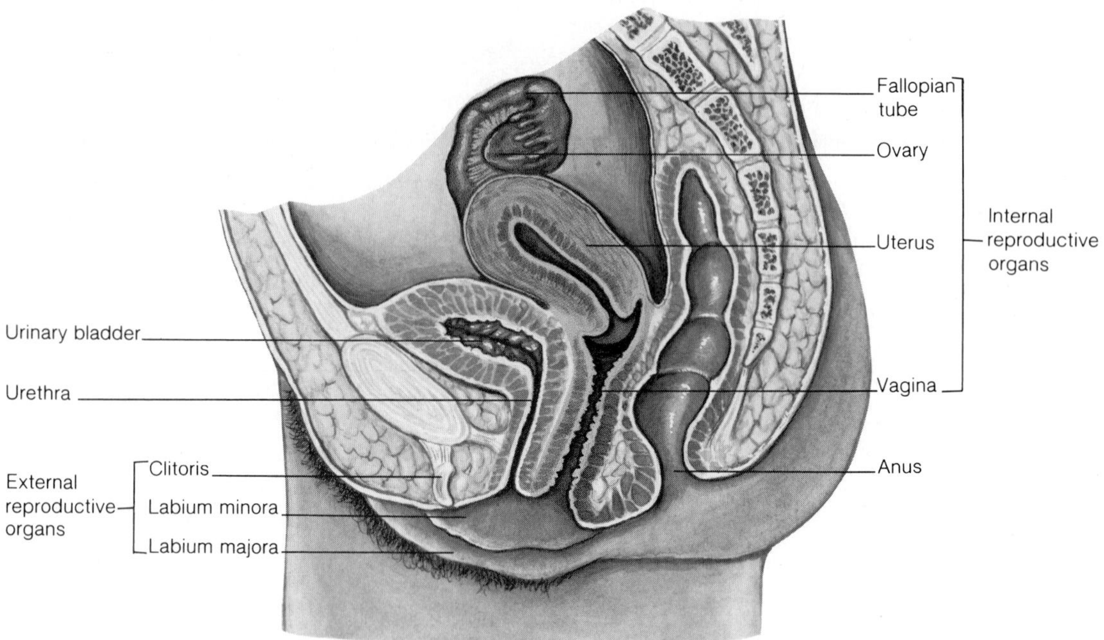


**Figure 8.7**
Side view of the organs of the female reproductive system. *Source:* From Hole, John W., Jr., *Human Anatomy and Physiology,* 3d ed. © 1978, 1981, 1984 Wm. C. Brown Publishers, Dubuque, Iowa. All rights reserved. Reprinted by permission.

pain. Mittleschmerz may occur on either side of the abdomen, depending on which ovary is ovulating. (See figure 8.8.)

Cells from the ruptured Graafian follicle that remain in the ovary are transformed by the action of LH into the **corpus luteum,** a temporary endocrine gland which secretes hormones. If fertilization occurs and a zygote is formed, the corpus luteum becomes the corpus luteum of pregnancy. The corpus luteum of pregnancy continues to secrete hormones for several months into the pregnancy. The continued secretion of hormones into the bloodstream informs the hypothalamus that the female is pregnant. If fertilization does not occur, the corpus luteum becomes the corpus luteum of menstruation. By the twenty-fourth day of the female's cycle the corpus luteum begins to degenerate. The absence of hormones in the bloodstream informs the hypothalamus that the female is not pregnant. This event results in menstruation, and a new reproductive cycle will soon follow.

**FALLOPIAN TUBES** Once the egg is released by the ovary, it enters a fallopian tube. Each **fallopian tube** is approximately four inches long and is connected at one end to the uterus. The other end of the fallopian tube consists of fingerlike projections called fimbriae that lie very close to the ovaries. Because the fimbriae are not directly connected to the ovary, there is some speculation about the process by which an egg leaves the ovary and is subsequently "picked up" by the fallopian tube.

At the time of ovulation the fallopian tubes become enlarged with blood and begin to contract, bringing the fimbria closer to the ovaries. When the egg leaves the ovary it is surrounded by a layer of cells which makes the entire mass sticky. It is possible that this "sticky mass" is picked up by the fimbria.

Through the fallopian tube contractions, and the action of its cilia, the egg is pushed to approximately the halfway point in the fallopian tube, where it remains and awaits fertilization. The egg travels at the rate of about one inch per hour. With rare exceptions, fertilization will take place in the fallopian tubes.

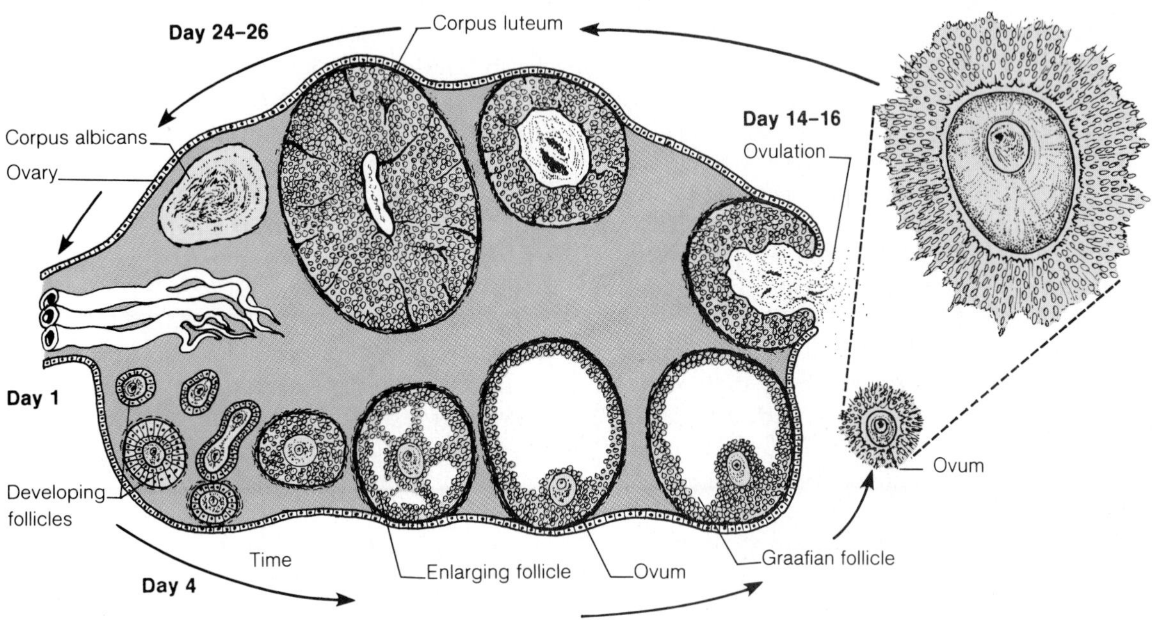


**Figure 8.8**
The ovarian cycle. At no one time are all the structures illustrated present. At the beginning of the ovarial cycle, several follicles start to develop. One of these matures into a graafian follicle, while the others regress. Near the middle of the cycle (day 14 to 16), the mature follicle releases its ovum (ovulation). The follicle then becomes a corpus luteum. If there is no fertilization, the corpus luteum starts to regress in about ten days (day 24 to 26) and ends the cycle as a scar called the corpus albicans. *Source:* From Hole, John W., Jr. *Human Anatomy and Physiology,* 3d ed. © 1978, 1981, 1984 Wm. C. Brown Publishers, Dubuque, Iowa. All rights reserved. Reprinted by permission.

The estimated time an egg can be fertilized after ovulation ranges from as short as two hours to as long as two days. There have been viable sperm found in the fallopian tubes seventy-two hours or more after being deposited in the vagina. This enhances the likelihood of fertilization. Thus it is possible for a female to have intercourse one day, ovulate the next day, and become pregnant the next day. If an egg is not fertilized it soon begins to degenerate. If an egg is fertilized it becomes a zygote and quickly begins to divide into a mass of vibrant cells as it completes its trek through the fallopian tube, on its way to the uterus.

**UTERUS** The **uterus** is a hollow, muscular, pear-shaped organ that is approximately three inches long and two inches wide in its nonpregnant state. During pregnancy the uterus will increase in size by 200 times. The opening of the uterus into the vagina is called the **cervix.** The uterus has several important functions. It is the preferred site for **implantation,** or the attachment of the zygote to the uterus, because the uterus has the necessary vascular arrangements for nurturing a fetus. The uterus also assists in transporting sperm up to the fallopian tubes and moving the fetus through the reproductive tract during childbirth. Finally, the uterus provides the necessary muscle contractions for menstruation.

The uterus has three layers, the perimetrium, myometrium, and endometrium. The **perimetrium** is the outermost layer. The **myometrium** is the muscular layer (*myo* means muscle) which is essential for birthing and menstruation. The **endometrium** is the innermost layer and is responsible for secreting fluids and nutrients for the developing fetus. The endometrium is where the fertilized egg will usually implant.

The uterus undergoes a series of changes in preparation for a zygote. In the beginning of the reproductive cycle estrogens cause the endometrium to thicken about one-eighth of an inch. This layer of tissue and fluids is necessary for the preservation and development of an embryo. Estrogens cause the mucus around the cervix to change in its consistency and become less acidic. The mucus becomes clear and elastic. This change in the cervical mucus enhances the probability of sperm penetrating the cervix and continuing on to the fallopian tube. There is also growing evidence that the cervical mucus prevents defective sperm from passing on through the fallopian tubes.[6]

If the egg is not fertilized, the corpus luteum of menstruation disintegrates causing a marked decrease of hormones in the bloodstream. About twenty-four hours after this decrease in hormonal blood levels menstruation commences. The myometrium begins to contract and the layer of blood, mucus, and membranes attached to the endometrium is sloughed off through the cervix and vagina. The menstrual phase usually takes from two to five days. During menstruation the hypothalamus will detect the reduced levels of hormones in the bloodstream and release GnRF to start the next reproductive cycle.

**VAGINA** In its unstimulated state the **vagina** is approximately three to five inches long, and connects the cervix to the external genitals. The cervix actually protrudes into the vagina. The vagina functions to transport sperm to the uterus and to transport the products of menstruation to the external genitals; it is also the passageway for childbirth. The vaginal walls have the ability to expand markedly in order to accept the penis during intercourse, or to pass the fetus during labor.

## Female Reproductive Cycle

The female reproductive cycle is plotted from the first day of menstruation to the day before the onset of the next menstruation. Average female reproductive cycles range from twenty to forty-five days. The part of the female reproductive cycle which causes the greatest time variation is the follicular phase, which is the time from menstruation up until ovulation. However, for most females, the time from ovulation to menstruation is about the same, approximately fourteen days.

The first menstruation for a female is called **menarche,** which usually occurs between the ages of eleven and fifteen for American females. The cessation of menstruation is called **menopause,** which usually occurs between the ages of forty-five and fifty for American females. During menopause the menstrual cycle becomes irregular and less frequent. In a period of usually one to two years the menstrual cycle will eventually cease.

There are scores of factors which may alter a female's reproductive cycle. These factors include the most obvious—pregnancy—to the more subtle such as diet and stress. Seemingly unrelated factors may affect the healthy functioning of the female reproductive organs. Many such factors have been suggested including tight-fitting clothing, fabric softener, brands of toilet paper, laundry detergent, bubble bath, and deodorant tampons.[7]

Discomfort, pain, unusual bleeding, foul odor, or discharge are indicators of potential health problems. Females should be aware of what is normal for them regarding their reproductive cycles. A female who is experiencing a cycle which is unusual for her should contact her physician. Together they can decide what course of action, if any, is necessary.

**DYSMENORRHEA** **Dysmenorrhea** is painful menstruation. The majority of females, at one time or another, experience dysmenorrhea. Dysmenorrhea can be caused by high levels of prostaglandins in the bloodstream which cause the uterus to contract. There are prescription medications available that inhibit natural prostaglandin secretions, thus relieving pain.

**PREMENSTRUAL SYNDROME** **Premenstrual Syndrome (PMS),** a chronic disorder which encompasses emotional, behavioral, and physical symptoms, has received a great deal of attention in recent years. Yet despite such attention, the cause and effective treatment of PMS are largely unknown. PMS symptoms (see table 8.1) usually occur a week prior to the onset of menstruation, and end at the onset of menstruation.[8]

PMS can occur at any age during the reproductive years, but seems to occur more often in women over the age of thirty.[9]

**Table 8.1 Common Symptoms of PMS**

| | |
|---|---|
| **Physical Symptoms** | |
| Abdominal bloating | Edema |
| Breast tenderness | Fatigue |
| Constipation | Headache |
| **Emotional Symptoms** | |
| Anxiety | Irritability |
| Confusion | Mood swings |
| Depression | Paranoia |
| Hostility | |
| **Behavioral Symptoms** | |
| Binge eating | Crying spells |
| Increased alcohol intake | Violence toward self or others |

Source: David B. Brecher and Richard B. Birrer, "Premenstrual Syndrome Update," *The Journal of Family Medicine* 113.4 (1985): 14 FM.

Many treatments have been suggested as potential remedies for PMS. Treatment suggestions range from life-style alterations (see table 8.2) to drugs such as mild tranquilizers and diuretics. One of the more controversial treatments is the use of progesterone. Advocates of progesterone therapy have labeled it "barely short of miraculous," but opponents call it "the laetrile of the 80's."[10] Progesterone treatment for PMS does not have FDA approval, but many physicians and clinics continue to use it for treating PMS. FDA-approved research, currently underway at Vanderbilt and Duke Universities and the National Institute of Mental Health, should shed light on the progesterone controversy in the near future. (See Exhibit 8.2.)

**Table 8.2 Common Remedies for PMS**

| **Remedy** | |
|---|---|
| Caffeine | May help or may make it worse. Caffeine is a diuretic and reduces body water content, thus helping the bloating, breast tenderness, and weight gain. But caffeine can also produce or amplify feelings of irritability and cause insomnia and headaches. Caffeine products include coffee, tea, chocolate, and many soft drinks. |
| Over-the counter medicines | Contain very common ingredients. Midol and Pamprin are most commonly used. Midol contains aspirin (prostaglandin blocker) for pain and caffeine for water retention. Pamprin contains acetaminophen (Tylenol) and pamatrom, a diuretic, for water retention. |
| Potassium | Diuretics flush potassium out of the body. Potassium is needed for healthy nerves and muscles. Potassium-rich foods (bananas, apricots, dairy products) increase potassium levels and help in reducing cramps. |
| Vitamins | Vitamins $B_6$, C, and E may help in combating menstrual cramps. Supplemental vitamin $B_6$ seems to be needed by women using oral contraceptives. |
| Minerals | A good balance of minerals is needed for normal body functioning. Thus, a mineral supplement or plant source foods, which are high in minerals, may help some women to alleviate menstrual cramps. |
| Low-sodium | Reducing sodium (table salt and other sodium-containing foods) will reduce water retention and decrease bloating and weight gains due to water retention. |
| Sleep | An adequate amount of sleep is important. Fatigue just makes pain seem worse. |
| Exercise | Perspiration removes excess water. Exercise increases blood flow to muscles increasing the amount of oxygen they obtain. This increases the muscles' ability to function without producing cramps and pain. |

Source: Kenneth L. Jones, Lewis W. Shainberg, Curtis O. Byer. *Dimensions of Human Sexuality.* 

8.2 EXHIBIT

# A Dangerous Fad Therapy for Premenstrual Syndrome?

Virtually everything concerning premenstrual syndrome is vague. The list of symptoms attributed to it—ranging from nausea to violent behavior—makes it extremely hard to diagnose. The list of theoretical causes—ranging from hormonal imbalance to immune disorders—makes it even harder to treat. But suddenly a lot of physicians say that despite all the unknowns, there's a sure path to relief: megadoses of progesterone.

In the past three years or so, more than 200 PMS clinics and education and referral services have opened across the U.S., most of them dedicated to progesterone treatment. In addition, about 3,500 private physicians are prescribing the hormone, sometimes in dosages as high as 4,000 milligrams a day. All told, possibly 100,000 American women are on the therapy.

Yet the Food and Drug Administration has refused to approve progesterone for PMS, and many gynecologists fear women taking huge doses for extended periods are risking cardiovascular problems, diabetes, and possibly even ovarian or uterine cancer. In short, we may be seeing the beginnings of yet another women's health disaster—a variation on the themes of diethylstilbestrol and high-dose oral contraceptives.

The guru of the progesterone movement is British gynecologist Katharina Dalton. She's been quietly prescribing high doses of the hormone since the late 1940s, but only in recent years has she gained widespread attention. Her 1979 book, *Once a Month,* helped, but probably what really put her on the map was the sensational murder trial that same year of a London barmaid. Dalton convinced the jury that the defendant stabbed a fellow barmaid to death because she was in the throes of PMS, and convinced the judge progesterone therapy would allow the barmaid to return to society without posing a threat. The woman's sentence: three years' probation, provided she receive daily progesterone.

Dalton and her followers believe progesterone is the key to PMS because symptoms occur only between ovulation and menstruation. It's then that the corpus luteum, the emptied egg sac, manufactures and secretes the hormone.

Only natural progesterone, not the synthetic progestogens in oral contraceptives, is considered effective. Explains ob-gyn Steven Greenberg, assistant professor at Temple University Medical School in Philadelphia and founder of Focus on PMS, a suburban clinic, "Progestogens take up the progesterone binding sites, blocking endogenous production and in effect intensifying the hormone imbalance." The synthetics also have estrogenic and androgenic effects that can worsen symptoms.

But natural progesterone, a cholesterol derivative manufactured from yams and soybeans, is broken down too quickly when taken orally; when taken by IM injection, one possible alternative, it creates too rapid a rise in blood levels. Instead, it's usually given via vaginal or rectal suppositories, which provide a steadier rate of absorption. Nevertheless, contend progesterone advocates, it's possible that because of poor overall absorption, as little as 10 percent of the prescribed dose ever reaches the bloodstream. And the rate of absorption seems to vary from one woman to another, and even from one stage of the cycle to another, possibly because of postpregnancy-related tolerance or inadequate uptake.

Dalton and her followers insist that progesterone treatment is "pure, safe, and natural." The London doctor claims that after treating thousands of patients over three decades, she has yet to encounter any serious side effects.

But critics of megadose progesterone therapy point out that it changes nearly all women's cyclical patterns, and breakthrough bleeding is common while suppositories are in use. A few women even bleed continuously, "a little or a lot, but every day since starting treatment," as one

EXHIBIT 8.2

woman reports. The menstrual flow may be dull red or brownish, usually a sign of an anovulatory cycle—becoming pregnant may be difficult—but possibly indicating abnormal endometrial development. And the flow itself may be scant.

Another worry is that women are tempted to manipulate their own dosages. By continuing to take progesterone beyond the prescribed time period, women prevent the drop in hormone level required for menstruation—leaving them "in control" and reportedly symptom-free. This raises something of a paradox: In women with PMS who are *not* taking progesterone, menstruation generally relieves symptoms. Yet some physicians suggest that progesterone treatment works precisely because it eliminates the normal menstrual cycle.

That theory may simply reflect the "backlash" phenomenon some women suffer when progesterone use abruptly stops. Forgetting a suppository in mid-treatment can precipitate a migraine, mood swings, or a bout of anxiety or depression. Many women report feeling agitated or "out of sorts" several hours after using the last suppository of the cycle. In some, symptoms begin appearing during formerly asymptomatic times.

As a result, doctors are finding some patients taking progesterone for increasing lengths of time—some every day of the month. And as months of treatment continue, steadily increasing dosages are often needed as well, to attain the same effectiveness. That pattern has led a few doctors to suspect that a tolerance develops, creating, in effect, progesterone addiction.

Such prolonged high-dose use further compounds the problem of stopping treatment, since the endometrium continues to build up as long as the hormone is taken, mimicking a continued pregnancy. When a patient does finally discontinue use, abnormally heavy bleeding may occur. The longterm effects on the endometrium itself or on the levels of other hormones are not yet known.

Even if women don't extend their treatments and take the hormone as directed, they can suffer a wide range of reactions: vaginal irritation, uterine cramping, insomnia, decreased libido, euphoria, and unpleasant leakage from the suppositories. And opponents of treatment report patient complaints of a more serious nature: vaginal swelling, itching, and infections; bloating and weight gain; feeling "incredibly pregnant"; dizziness and fainting; inability to concentrate; chest pain and palpitations; and, oddly, some of the symptoms treatment is meant to suppress—breast tenderness, hot flashes, mood swings, fatigue, increased appetite, and cravings for salty foods.

In terms of long-range residual effects, fears center on the possibility of thrombi, atherosclerosis, cardiovascular problems, diabetes, and cancer of the reproductive organs. Dalton, Norris, and other leaders in the progesterone movement contend that such effects are associated with synthetic progestogens, but will not occur with the natural hormone, which has a different chemical structure. But, "Whenever progesterone side effects appear, they seem similar to those associated with progestogens," counters psychiatrist and obstetrician-gynecologist Howard Osofsky, clinical professor at the University of Kansas Medical School, and director of the Meninger Clinic's PMS Clearinghouse.

Osofsky's view is, at least for the time being, the same as the Food and Drug Administration's. FDA has every reason to move cautiously, says the agency's Roger Eastep, a consumer safety officer, who cites past experiences with "safe" drugs: diethylstilbestrol, which caused vaginal and uterine cancer in the daughters of women who took it; estrogen replacement therapy, linked to endometrial and breast cancer; the early birth-control pills, associated with thromboemboli, strokes, heart attacks, polyps, benign tumors, and breast, cervical, and uterine cancer.

Some skeptics go several steps further, doubting whether progesterone is, in fact, therapeutic at all. The Meninger Clinic's Howard Osofsky says, "We're seeing the same results with diet, exercise, and stress management." Eastep points out that the "placebo effect is tremendous"; one doctor, who requested anonymity, asserts, "You can give PMS patients anything and 60 percent will improve." And, though it's easy to write off that

8.2 *continued* EXHIBIT

claim to the old "it's all in her head" line of thinking, even women's advocates acknowledge there's a psychological component to relief. Estimates Bonnie Oas, director of the Woman's Research and Treatment Center, a gynecology clinic in Milford, N.H., "As many as 80 percent of patients receive relief simply by professional acknowledgment that their symptoms are not imaginary."

Interestingly, despite devoting much of her career to progesterone therapy, Dalton has never performed a double-blind study to test for the placebo effect. Only two such studies have been reported, by S. L. Smith in a 1976 issue of *Clinical Obstetrics and Gynecology* and by Gwyneth Sampson in a *British Journal of Psychiatry* in 1979. In both studies, a majority of patients reported relief of symptoms regardless of whether they'd received progesterone or an inert suppository. In the Sampson study, the placebo was rated *more* effective, and was preferred because it lacked any side effects.

Nor have there been any studies comparing the results of progesterone with those of symptomatic treatment or health and life-style modifications. Maintains Osofsky, of the Meninger Clinic, "Most women don't need this kind of experimental treatment." He and others support trying more "benign" measures first—nutritional improvements, including reduction of salt and caffeine intake, avoidance of sugars and alcohol, ensuring adequate vitamin and mineral intake, and five or six small meals a day; a regular exercise program; and methods of handling stress.

Despite critics' assertions and concern, though, the effects of progesterone are, according to enthusiasts, barely short of miraculous. "My life was a nightmare," testifies one New Yorker." Right before my period I suffered terrible migraines and mood swings. I felt like Dr. Jekyll and Mr. Hyde. Now, I feel more relaxed and in control." Her reaction is typical, comments Beth Jones, training director of PMS Action, a Madison, Wis., clinic: "I'd say 96 percent of the women I see are getting good to excellent results."

Given the time, trouble, and cost of treatment, the women who stick with it must be convinced of its value. The suppositories "are a bother to use and remember," notes one. Just obtaining them is a bother, too. Without FDA approval for treatment, mass manufacture and marketing is not being done; the suppositories must be compounded on a per prescription basis, and most pharmacists are unequipped or unwilling to do it. As a result, patients tell of "traveling across the country" to find a source, and quasilegal mail-order supply houses are getting into the business. Treatment, when available, is also expensive: The suppositories range from $1 to $5 apiece, and an initial clinic visit costs from $250 to $400, a fee that's not covered by most insurance plans. Some

**TOXIC-SHOCK SYNDROME** Between January 1979 and April 1982, a total of 1,660 **toxic-shock syndrome (TSS)** cases were recorded for adult females, premenarchial females, and males. Of these reported cases 5.6 percent were fatal. TSS is an infection caused by a common staphylococcus bacterium. The signs and symptoms of TSS are fever, headaches, sore throats, diarrhea, rash, vomiting, hypertension, dizziness, and disorientation. Women account for 92 percent of TSS cases with the average age being 22.9 years.

In 1980 a commercial superabsorbent tampon was linked to TSS. TSS has also been associated with use of the contraceptive sponge. Females can markedly reduce their risk of TSS by not using tampons. Women who choose to wear tampons can decrease their TSS risk by wearing them intermittently during menstruation.[11] Women who use the contraceptive sponge should follow the directions carefully, especially the time limits for keeping the sponge in the vagina.

## EXHIBIT 8.2

clinics also charge steep fees for blood tests, even though these can *not* effectively diagnose the condition.

Critics charge the clinics don't provide adequate screening, and that progesterone is prescribed indiscriminately, before other treatments are tried and despite contraindications—histories of emboli, coronary disease, angina, hepatitis or impaired liver function, stroke, undiagnosed abnormal vaginal bleeding, cystic fibrosis, or known or suspected cancer of the breast, uterus, cervix, ovaries, or vagina.

Comments a spokesman for the American College of Obstetricians and Gynecologists, which has not taken a position on PMS therapy, "We've heard of clinics where 90 percent of the women who walk in are given progesterone." Yet, as the Meninger Clinic's Osofsky emphasizes, "Diligent medical, endocrine, and psychological assessments should be made" over a period of at least three months before progesterone should even be considered. "Under strict PMS evaluation, 90 percent of women won't qualify for this treatment."

So far, there's no reliable count of just how many women are receiving progesterone treatment—or of how many have become disillusioned with it and stopped. But, says the FDA's Roger Eastep, the entire issue "may just die out from lack of legitimate investigative findings." Adds Lee Horner, founder of PMS Research Foundation, a Las Vegas information and referral service, "Progesterone may turn out to be the laetrile of the '80s. I predict ten years from now no one will be using it."

For some women, the benefits of progesterone have already proved illusory. Says one, "After almost a year I gave it up. I didn't like what it was doing to me. Now, I'm on nutritional and attitudinal therapy for my PMS and that seems to be working much better. I guess progesterone wasn't the answer for me after all."

Source: Adapted from Witt, Reni L., "PMS: A Dangerous Fad Therapy for Premenstrual Syndrome?" in *Medical Month* 2.2 (1984): 25–31.

### DISCUSSION QUESTIONS

1. Do you believe the benefits of progesterone therapy for PMS are worth the risks?

2. Do you think physicians and clinics should use progesterone therapy for PMS despite the fact that it has not been approved by the FDA?

**ECTOPIC PREGNANCY** An **ectopic pregnancy** is a pregnancy outside of the uterus, usually in the fallopian tubes. On rare occasions ectopic pregnancies can occur in the abdominal cavity, cervix, vagina, or even on the ovaries. About 0.5 to 1 percent of all pregnancies are ectopic, 90 percent of which are tubal. The rate of ectopic pregnancies increased by 300 percent from 1970 to 1980.[12] The risk of death from an ectopic pregnancy is ten times greater than childbirth, and fifty times greater than a legal abortion.[13]

The classic symptoms of an ectopic pregnancy are a missed period followed by dull, crampy abdominal pain, menstrual spotting, and pregnancy symptoms such as breast tenderness, fatigue, increased appetite, and nausea. Fortunately ultrasonography can detect an ectopic pregnancy as early as the sixth week of pregnancy. Ectopic pregnancies need to be diagnosed quickly because left untreated they can be fatal. Also, if tubal ectopics are diagnosed early, it may be possible for the physician to save the fallopian tube. Otherwise the usual course of action is to surgically remove the tube.

**MENOPAUSE** Many symptoms have been associated with menopause including nervousness, excitability, depression, giddiness, headaches, insomnia, palpitations, night sweats, vaginal dryness, and hot flashes. There is no clear set of symptoms for menopausal women, with the possible exception of hot flashes. The signs and symptoms of menopause usually subside within two years, or no longer elicit any concern on the part of the female. There are also females who do not experience any menopausal signs or symptoms.

A small proportion of the women who do experience symptoms will seek medical advice or drug therapy. The usual drug therapy is estrogen replacement, which is an artificial means to maintain the depleting estrogen levels in the menopausal female. Some women continue estrogen replacement therapy for ten years or more.

There are both pros and cons of estrogen replacement therapy. Some menopausal symptoms may be controlled by estrogen therapy. Additionally, some physicians believe that estrogen replacement prevents osteoporosis, the gradual loss of bone mass. In order to arrest osteoporosis, however, it is necessary for the estrogen therapy to continue for the remainder of the female's lifetime;[14] short-term estrogen therapy can provide minimal results at best. A woman taking estrogen for whatever reasons (birth control, hot flashes) assumes the health risks of estrogen. Menopausal females taking estrogen increase their risk of cardiovascular disorders and endometrial cancer.

## External Female Reproductive Structures

The external female reproductive structures are the vulva and the breasts.

**VULVA** The external female genitals (see figure 8.9) are all referred to as the **vulva.** The **labia majora** (Latin for "major lips") are paired folds that surround the clitoris, urethral opening, and vaginal opening. The labia minora (Latin for "small lips") are paired folds which extend along the vestibule. The labia minora and labia majora merge to form a clitorial hood. The **clitoris** is similar to the penis in structure and function. It is composed of erectile

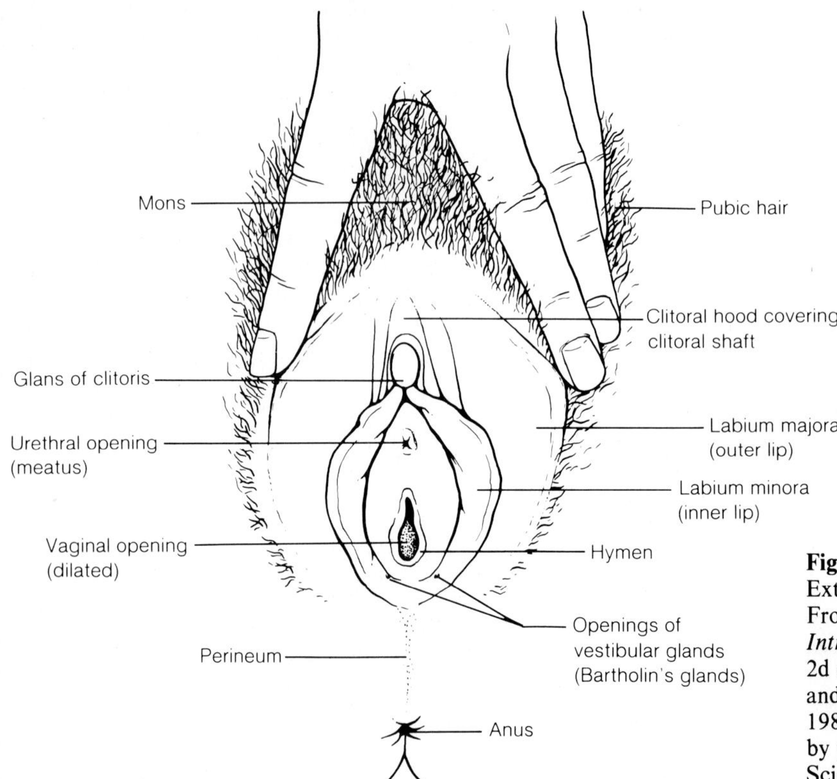


**Figure 8.9**
External female genitals. *Source:* From *Sexual Choices: An Introduction to Human Sexuality,* 2d ed., by Nass, G. D., R. W. Libby, and M. P. Fisher. Copyright 1984, 1981 by Wadsworth, Inc. Reprinted by permission of Wadsworth Health Sciences Division. Monterey, Calif. 93940.

tissue that swells with blood and becomes erect when stimulated. The shaft of the clitoris is referred to as the glands. All of the external female genitals are sensitive to touch, especially the clitoris.

The **vestibule** is the area enclosed by the labia minora. The **introitus** is the opening of the vagina. An imaginary line from the introitus to the anus is the area called the **perineum.** This area is sometimes surgically cut during childbirth in an operation called an **episiotomy.** The episiotomy is done to prevent tearing of the perineum during childbirth.

The **hymen** partially covers the introitus. The hymen oftentimes remains intact until the female's first experience of sexual intercourse. Although the intact hymen has been used as proof of virginity over the centuries, there are several problems with such an assumption. Some females are born with partially torn hymens, while others may tear their hymens prior to first intercourse (e.g., by the insertion of tampons).

The **Bartholin's glands** lie inside the labia minora, one on each horizontal side of the introitus. They secrete a mucus which appears prior to female orgasm. The exact function of the Bartholin glands and their secretions is unknown.

**BREASTS** Although the breasts are not directly responsible for reproduction, they are responsible for nurturing the product of reproduction, the infant. Each **breast** contains fifteen to twenty milk ducts, all of which open to the external nipple. The

8.1 ACTIVITY FOR WELLNESS 8.1

## Kegel Exercises for Women

Following the physical stress of childbirth, many women find that they have lost muscle tone in the muscles beneath the perineum and surrounding the vaginal opening. Loss of muscle tone in this area makes it more difficult for these women to control urination, and they often lose urine when they cough or sneeze.

In 1952, Arnold Kegel developed a series of exercises that were designed to restore this lost muscle tone and thereby help women to redevelop control of urination after childbirth.

To perform these exercises, a woman must first locate the pelvic muscles that support the vagina by voluntarily stopping and starting the flow of urine during urination. The muscles that stop the flow of urine also tighten the vagina around an inserted object, such as a finger or penis. These are the muscles to be strengthened by the Kegel exercises.

Once a woman has learned which muscles to concentrate on, she should contract those muscles, hold the contraction for two or three seconds, and then release. She should perform this exercise for ten repetitions five or six times a day, gradually working up to more.

Women who practice Kegel exercises on a daily basis should have much improved control of these muscles (and their urination) in six weeks. But it has also been found that Kegel exercises have some interesting advantages other than mere urinary control. Many of the women who strengthen these pelvic muscles also discover an increasing sensitivity of the vaginal area, which they find can result in increased sensations during intercourse and at orgasm. In addition, some women report that performing Kegel exercises makes it possible for them to stimulate their sex partners more because of the increased vaginal pressure they can apply to an inserted penis.

Source: Kenneth L. Jones, Louis W. Shainberg, and Curtis O. Byer, *Dimensions of Human Sexuality.* 

nipple is highly sensitive to stimulation. The action of hormones (prolactin, progesterones, and estrogens) cause a female to produce milk after childbirth; breast size has no relation to the quantity of milk produced by lactating females. The overwhelming majority of females are capable of breastfeeding following childbirth.

# HUMAN SEXUAL RESPONSE

Until 1966 relatively little was known about the physiological events involved in human sexual arousal. William Masters and Virginia Johnson opened the door to this kind of research by publishing their observations of humans during sexual arousal.[15]

Masters and Johnson described two major physiological events that occur during sexual response: vasocongestion and myotonia. **Vasocongestion** occurs when blood fills the sexual organs such as the penis or vulva. **Myotonia** refers to the muscles becoming tight and rigid. Masters and Johnson also separated the human sexual response cycle into four consecutive phases: excitement, plateau, orgasm and resolution.

## Excitement Phase

The first phase of sexual response is termed **excitement.** During this phase the female begins to secrete vaginal fluids. These fluids make the vagina more supple and less sensitive to friction. The vagina, cervix, and vulva expand due to vasocongestion, and the nipples become erect.

The male excitement phase begins with the penis becoming erect due to vasocongestion. The scrotal skin becomes smooth and the testes are drawn closer to the body. (See figures 8.10 and 8.11.)

## Plateau Phase

The **plateau phase** follows the excitement phase. During the plateau phase the female's vagina continues to swell until it reaches the "orgasmic platform," which causes the opening of the vagina to narrow by 30 percent or more. Additionally, the clitoris withdraws into its hood. The inner vaginal lips display color changes indicating that orgasm is imminent. Changes in skin color may occur in other parts of the female's body as well. There may also be an increase in breast size.

For the male the head of the penis and the testes increase in size. A male may also experience a skin color change around his penis. A small amount of seminal fluid, which may or may not contain viable sperm, may drip from the penis.

## Orgasmic Phase

The **orgasmic phase** is the third phase of sexual response. **Orgasm** for humans is the sudden release of sexual tension resulting in pleasurable feelings. Orgasm is a feeling of physical satisfaction unlike any other moment of the sexual response cycle.

Female orgasm involves anywhere from three to fifteen quick rhythmic muscular contractions of the uterus and vagina. Other muscle groups of the female's body may contract during orgasm as well.

Orgasm for the male begins with the pooling of semen into the urethra. Two sphincter muscles close off the urethra to the bladder during this stage. One sphincter muscle opens to the penis allowing semen to exit, propelled by several short muscular contractions. The release of semen (ejaculation) does not necessarily occur simultaneously with orgasm. Males can release semen without experiencing an orgasm, or experience the pleasurable sensations of orgasm without releasing average quantities of semen.

## Resolution Phase

The final stage of sexual response is **resolution.** During this phase both males and females return to their pre-excited state. Blood is pumped away from the sexual organs and muscles begin to relax. Heart beat, respiration, and brain wave patterns also return to their pre-excited state. In males, a recovery period, often referred to as a **refractory period,** must take place before a second orgasm can be experienced. The length of time needed for recovery varies with different men.

Many factors can affect the sexual response cycle, including the circumstances of sexual arousal

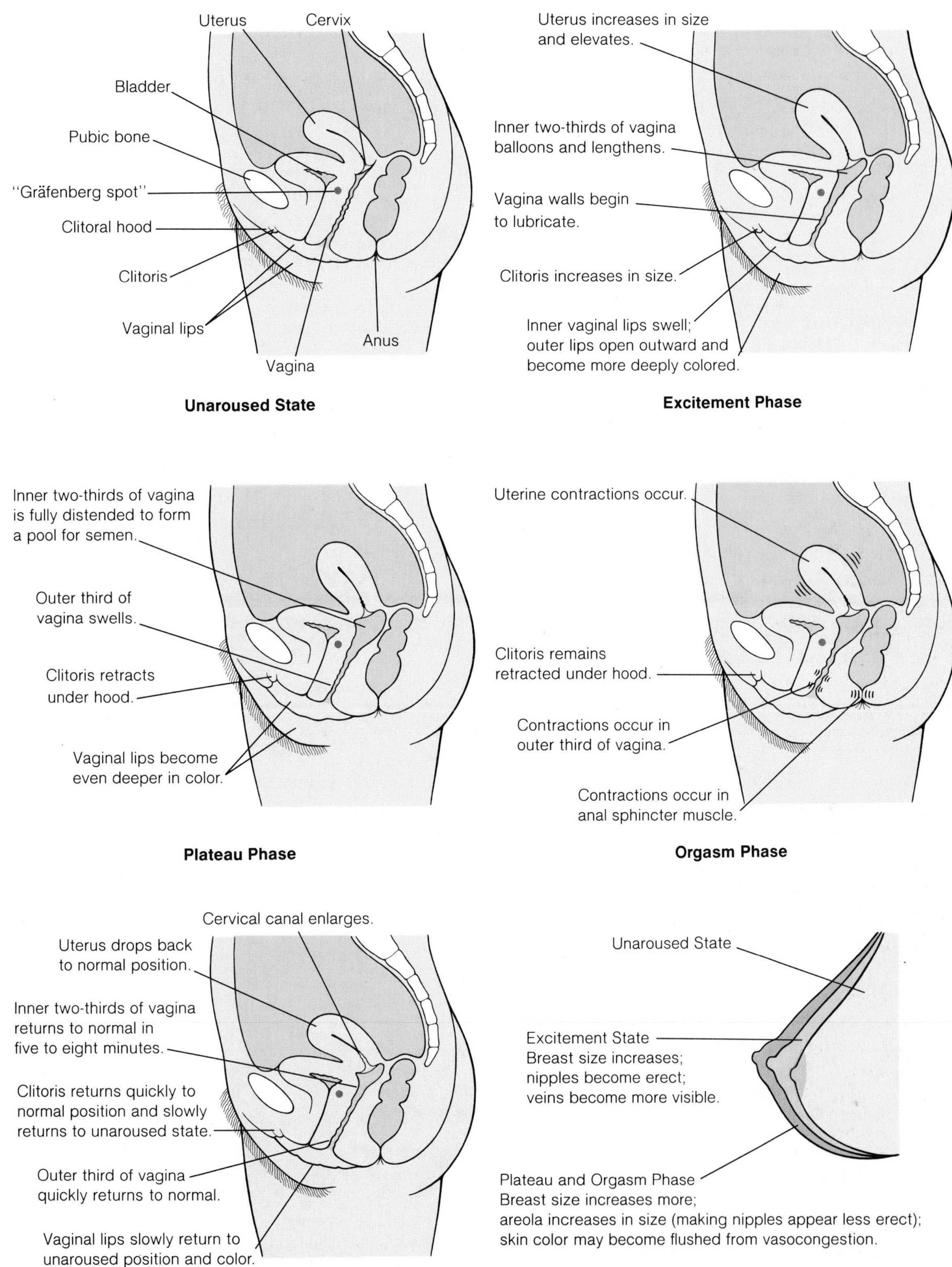
Uterus
Cervix
Bladder
Pubic bone
"Gräfenberg spot"
Clitoral hood
Clitoris
Vaginal lips
Anus
Vagina
Unaroused State
Uterus increases in size and elevates.
Inner two-thirds of vagina balloons and lengthens.
Vagina walls begin to lubricate.
Clitoris increases in size.
Inner vaginal lips swell; outer lips open outward and become more deeply colored.
Excitement Phase
Inner two-thirds of vagina is fully distended to form a pool for semen.
Outer third of vagina swells.
Clitoris retracts under hood.
Vaginal lips become even deeper in color.
Plateau Phase
Uterine contractions occur.
Clitoris remains retracted under hood.
Contractions occur in outer third of vagina.
Contractions occur in anal sphincter muscle.
Orgasm Phase
Cervical canal enlarges.
Uterus drops back to normal position.
Inner two-thirds of vagina returns to normal in five to eight minutes.
Clitoris returns quickly to normal position and slowly returns to unaroused state.
Outer third of vagina quickly returns to normal.
Vaginal lips slowly return to unaroused position and color.
Resolution Phase
Unaroused State
Excitement State
Breast size increases;
nipples become erect;
veins become more visible.
Plateau and Orgasm Phase
Breast size increases more;
areola increases in size (making nipples appear less erect);
skin color may become flushed from vasocongestion.
Breast Changes

**Figure 8.10**
Physical changes in the female during sexual response cycle. *Source:* From *Sexual Choices: An Introduction to Human Sexuality,* 2d ed., by Nass, G. D., R. W. Libby, and M. P. Fisher. Copyright 1981, 1984 by Wadsworth, Inc. Reprinted by permission of Wadsworth Health Sciences Division, Monterey, Calif. 93940.

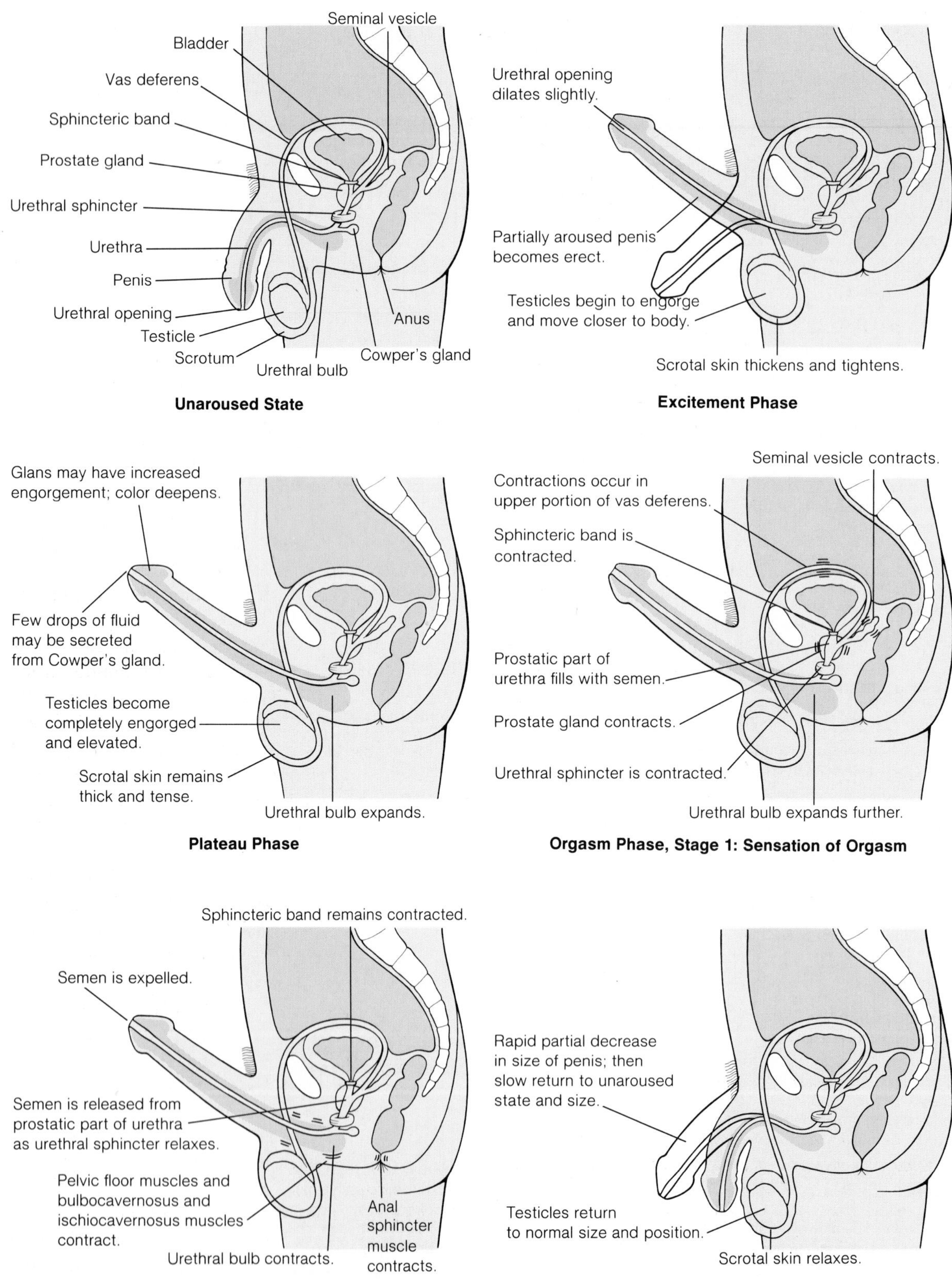


**Figure 8.11**
Physical changes in the male during the sexual response cycle. *Source:* From *Sexual Choices: An Introduction to Human Sexuality,* 2d ed., by Nass, G. D., R. W. Libby, and M. P. Fisher. Copyright 1981, 1984 by Wadsworth, Inc. Reprinted by permission of Wadsworth Health Sciences Division, Monterey, Calif. 93940.

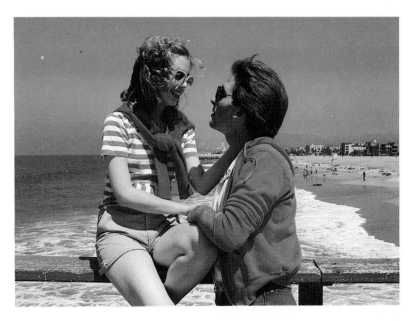

**Figure 8.12**
Communication is a crucial component of human sexuality.

(erotic literature, fantasies), drugs (legal and illegal), and age. The brain is an integral part of this cycle. Keep in mind that individuals go through the sexual response cycle in different ways. Even the same individual may experience sexual arousal in many ways, under different circumstances. (See figure 8.12.)

## Common Sexual Performance Issues

People view sexual performance and orgasm from different perspectives, and in terms of their definitions of sexuality. In addition, each culture has its own guidelines for how males and females should perform sexually. Gender roles also affect the way two people approach sexual intercourse, and how they rate their sexual performance.[16]

In the last thirty years Americans have been learning more and more about human sexual dysfunctions. People have been given labels such as frigid or impotent. An industry blossomed seemingly overnight using treatment approaches which have included physical exercises, communication skills, psychological counseling, hypnosis, and surgery.

There are several concerns regarding the definitions of sexual dysfunctions. The term dysfunction implies that something is not working right or to its full potential. When the word dysfunction is used with "sexual" it implies something is not working right sexually. But how do we define "right"?

For example, one sexual dysfunction often treated is premature or rapid ejaculation. The terms premature and rapid are subjective. Premature ejaculation has been defined in many ways including not enough male penile thrusts prior to ejaculation, not enough penis time (one minute) inside the vagina, and the lack of voluntary control over ejaculation.[17] Such definitions, if used in their strictest sense, would mean that the majority of all American males have a sexual dysfunction. Such criteria have caused sharp criticism of the definitions used in measuring human sexual performance.[18]

When an individual or couple perceives they are having a sexual performance problem, this is something that certainly should be addressed. For example, if they believe that the male's inability to have an erection in 10 percent of their sex play episodes is a problem, then this is their standard. The couple's standard is the beginning point of addressing their concern.

One of the first steps in addressing a sexual performance problem is to determine whether the cause is physiological. There are many physiological factors that can affect how people perform sexually. Diseases such as diabetes, drugs such as alcohol, and injuries, especially to the central nervous system, can result in a male or female being unable to perform sexual intercourse or reach orgasm. It is estimated that 10 to 20 percent of all sexual dysfunction cases are caused by physiological factors.[19] The remaining 80 percent of cases result from educational or psychological factors.

With this in mind we can examine some common behaviors which are considered sexual dysfunctions. All of these dysfunctions can be situational. They can occur with certain sexual partners, or only under certain conditions. For example, a male may be unable to gain an erection with one particular sexual partner and experience no erectile difficulties with another. A female may readily reach orgasm by masturbating, but not during intercourse.

**ANORGASMIA** **Anorgasmia** is the inability to reach orgasm. This is often situational. There are adult males and females who have never experienced orgasm in their lifetimes. Anorgasmia is usually associated with females, but males can also experience situational anorgasmia. In most cases of anorgasmia, males and females are sexually responsive. They simply do not reach orgasm.

Males and females may disguise "situational anorgasmia" by faking an orgasm. They may do this to prevent their partner from feeling they are sexually inept. They may also fake an orgasm because they are simply exhausted from sex play and want to rest. Or, they may be trying to hide their anorgasmia from their partner.

**ERECTILE DYSFUNCTION** The term **erectile dysfunction** has begun to replace the term impotence. Erectile dysfunction describes the male's inability to have an erection of sufficient strength and duration to perform intercourse. There are few adult males who have not experienced, at one time or another, the inability to have or maintain an erection. Often the problem is situational.

**PREMATURE EJACULATION** This dysfunction concerns the duration of intercourse. One way of defining **premature ejaculation** is in terms of the couple's satisfaction.[20] Premature ejaculation implies that one or both partners are not satisfied with the duration of their episodes of sexual intercourse due to the male's loss of erection following orgasm. The male may feel an obligation to satisfy his partner's sexual wishes. The female may feel slighted romantically or physically because of the short duration of the entire sexual episode. This may cause them to seek counseling.

**DYSPAREUNIA** **Dyspareunia** is the term for painful intercourse, which may occur in any of the four sexual response phases. Both males and females can experience dyspareunia. Antihistamines and vaginal infections can cause dyspareunia in females. Sexually transmitted diseases in both males and females can cause dyspareunia. People who experience dyspareunia should seek medical advice. Sometimes just the fear of painful intercourse can cause discomfort during sexual arousal.

Most people will probably experience one or more of these dysfunctions in their lifetime. Any time sexual performance is perceived as a problem it is prudent for the individual or couple to seek expert advice.

The more knowledgeable you are about the human reproductive system and the personal and social influences that affect human sexual performance, the better you will be able to assess your own sexual performance.

## SUMMARY

1. Males and females contribute their genes to their offspring. The genes combine and form a single cell called a zygote. The zygote will develop into a new adult member of the human race.
2. The testes and ovaries produce sperm and eggs, both of which carry chromosomes. They also produce hormones which are responsible for development of secondary sex characteristics and maintainence of the reproductive organs.
3. The formation of a zygote is called fertilization.
4. The hormone used by the hypothalamus to stimulate the testes and ovaries is called the gonadotropin-releasing hormone, or GnRH.
5. Implantation occurs when the zygote attaches itself to the uterus.
6. Females should be aware of what is normal for them regarding their reproductive cycles. When a female is experiencing a cycle which is unusual for her, the prudent action is to contact her physician by telephone.
7. Premenstrual syndrome (PMS) refers to chronic menstrual symptoms which are cyclic and subside at the beginning of menstruation. There is no consensus as to what causes PMS or how to treat it.

8. Menopause is the natural loss of fertility. There is no clear set of symptoms for menopause, with the possible exception of hot flashes.

9. An ectopic pregnancy is a pregnancy outside of the uterus, usually in the fallopian tubes. The rate of ectopic pregnancies increased by 300 percent from 1970 to 1980.

10. Masters and Johnson separated the human sexual response cycle into four consecutive phases: excitement, plateau, orgasm, and resolution. They also described two major physiological events that occur during sexual response: vasocongestion and myotonia.

### Recommended Readings

Boston Women's Health Book Collective. *Our Bodies Ourselves.* 3rd ed. New York: Simon & Schuster, 1979.

Brecker, R. and Brecker, E., eds. *An Analysis of Human Sexual Response.* New York: New American Library, 1974.

Castelman, M. *Sexual Solutions.* New York: Simon & Schuster, 1981.

Weideger, P. *Menstruation and Menopause: The Physiology and Psychology, the Myth and the Reality.* New York: Knopf, 1976.

Zilbergold, B., and Ullman, J. *Male Sexuality: A Guide to Sexual Fulfillment.* New York: Bantam, 1978.

### References

1. W. Witters and P. Jones-Witters, *Human Sexuality* (New York: Van Nostrand, 1980).

2. Witters, *Human Sexuality;* M. F. Campbell and J. H. Harrison, eds., *Urology 1* (Philadelphia: W. B. Saunders Co., 1970).

3. Kenneth L. Jones, Louis W. Shainberg, and Curtis O. Byer, *Dimensions of Human Sexuality* (Dubuque, Iowa: Wm. C. Brown Publishers, 1985), 117.

4. "Do You Recommend My Newborn Son Be Circumcised?" *Patient Care,* 18.4 (1984): 181.

5. Jones, et al., *Dimensions of Human Sexuality,* 507.

6. F. Hanson and J. Overstreet, "The Interaction of Human Spermatozoa with Cervical Mucus in Vivo," *American Journal of Obstetrics and Gynecology* 140 (1981): 173–77.

7. David M. Neuman, "Causes of Genitourinary Symptoms in Women," *Journal of the American Medical Association* 252.13 (1984): 1683; A. O. Berg, F. E. Heidrich, S. D. Fihn, et al., "Establishing the Cause of Genitourinary Symptoms in Women in a Family Practice: Comparison of Clinical Examination and Comprehensive Microbiology," *Journal of the American Medical Association* 251 (1984): 620–25; I. Elegbe and M. Botu, "A Preliminary Study on Dressing Patterns and Incidence of Candidiasis," *American Journal of Public Health* 72 (1982): 176–77.

8. Mary Laughlin and Ramona Johnson, "Premenstrual Syndrome," *American Family Physician* 29.3 (1984): 265.

9. Daniel Friedman, "Premenstrual Syndrome," *The Journal of Family Practice* 19.5 (1984): 674.

10. Reni L. Witt, "A Dangerous Fad Therapy for Premenstrual Syndrome?", *Medical Month* 2.2 (1984): 311.

11. Center for Disease Control, "Toxic Shock Syndrome: United States 1970–1982," *Morbidity and Mortality Weekly Review* 32.16 (1982): 201–204.

12. S. F. Dorfman, "Deaths from Ectopic Pregnancy, United States, 1979 to 1980," *Obstetrics and Gynecology* 62.3 (1983): 334–38.

13. S. A. LeBolt, D. A. Grimes, and W. Cates, Jr., "Mortality from Abortion and Childbirth: Are the Populations Comparable?", *Journal of the American Medical Association* 248.2 (1983): 188–91.

14. Bruce M. Rothschild, "Understanding and Preventing Osteoporosis," *Geriatric Consultant* 3.3 (1984): 22–24.

15. W. H. Masters and V. E. Johnson, *Human Sexual Response* (Boston: Little, Brown, 1966).

16. J. H. Gagnon and W. E. Simon, *The Social Sources of Human Sexuality* (Chicago: Aldine, 1973).

17. H. Kaplan, *The New Sex Therapy: Active Treatment of Sexual Dysfunction* (New York: Brunner/Mazel, 1974); E. Mozes, "Premature Ejaculation," *Sexology* (November 1963): 274–76; D. Reuben, *Everything You Always Wanted to Know about Sex but Were Afraid to Ask* (New York: Bantam, 1969).

18. A. Ellis, "A Review of Disorders of Sexual Desire by E. S. Kaplan," *Archives of Sexual Behavior* 10 (1981): 395–97; P. R. Kilmann, "The Treatment of Primary and Secondary Orgasmic Dysfunction: A Methodological Review of the Literature since 1968," *Journal of Sex and Marital Therapy* 4 (1978): 155–76; B. Zilbergeld and M. Evans, "The Inadequacy of Masters and Johnson," *Psychology Today* (August 1980): 29–43.

19. R. Kolodny, W. Masters, and V. Johnson, Textbook of Sexual Medicine. (Boston: Little, Brown, 1979); O. Munjack and L. Oziel, *Sexual Medicine and Counseling in Office Practice* (Boston: Little, Brown, 1980).

20. L. Derogatis, "Etiologic Factors in Premature Ejaculation," *Medical Aspects of Human Sexuality* 14 (1980): 32–47.

CHAPTER NINE

# Birth Control: Fertility Options



Sexual intercourse has traditionally been viewed as an act of personal commitment: economically, socially, spiritually, physically, and emotionally. A man and a woman, by having intercourse, automatically became responsible for any offspring resulting from their union. This was a practical approach, since birth control was unpopular and mostly ineffective in the past. The age-old way produced a family of at least two adults who would bear, rear, support, and socialize their offspring. Hence, marriage was for centuries the building block of society and sexual intercourse was associated with the consummation of marriage and the responsibility for children.

In the last thirty years the sense of urgency and responsibility to marry and have children early in life has waned. Increased life expectancy has largely contributed to this change in life-style. Today people in developed countries anticipate living past the age of seventy. Because of this it is easy, and sometimes more practical, to postpone marriage and parenthood until people reach their midtwenties.

Effective birth control has made the decision to adopt such a life-style possible and socially acceptable. Given effective birth control, people can choose to remain sexually active yet childless.Both childless single and married life-styles are increasing in popularity today.

Behind peoples' desire to manipulate their own fertility are their dreams, needs, and personal convictions. The fertility options you use, or avoid, will have a considerable effect on your level of wellness.

In this chapter you will be given the opportunity to examine which fertility products and services are compatible with your needs and personal convictions. You will learn what birth control is possible and then you can decide what is desirable in terms of your wellness goals.

## WHEN DOES LIFE BEGIN?

Before we discuss birth control, we must first address the question of "when does life begin?" The answer to this question is not a matter of science, but of personal conviction. Science can describe for us the events of human reproduction, but science cannot tell us when a cell or a network of cells becomes a human "life."

There are several common viewpoints people take regarding the beginning of life. Each of these views either accepts or rejects fertilization, implantation, and gestational age as the benchmark of new human life. "The Unresolvable Question" highlights these viewpoints. (See Exhibit 9.1.)

Which view you choose to accept, if any, has an impact on which birth-control methods you might find acceptable. For example, if you believe that the **zygote** (fertilized egg) is the beginning of new life, then you would reject abortion as a birth-control method. People who view zygotes as human lives would also theoretically have to reject some types of birth-control pills and all intrauterine devices (IUDs), because these methods do not prevent fertilization, but rather prevent implantation of the zygote in the uterus.

As an example, let's examine the birth-control decisions of a woman who is strongly opposed to abortion yet uses other birth-control devices. This woman will not have an abortion because she believes that abortions end the life of the developing zygote. This same woman who is opposed to abortion, however, might use an intrauterine device (IUD), which is a plastic device that is inserted into the uterus as a contraceptive. The IUD is designed not to prevent fertilization, but to end implantation. The IUD works as an automatic scraping tool to irritate the uterus and dislodge an implanted zygote. Abortion techniques used in the first several weeks of pregnancy call for the physician to mechanically dislodge the zygote from the uterine wall. Neither the abortion or the IUD prevent fertilization; they both are designed to prevent or end implantation.

There are many reasons why people do not understand how birth-control methods work. One major reason why people may be confused about birth-control methods is terminology. The word contraceptive has become a generic term describing methods that prevent fertilization, prevent implantation, or end implantation. The term contraceptive means "against conception." Many, if not most, people interpret "against conception" as meaning "preventing conception." They therefore conclude that if one uses a contraceptive, then one is preventing a pregnancy. As you have discovered, some "contraceptives" were never designed to prevent a zygote from forming. For this reason the term contraceptive will not be used in this text.

## BIRTH-CONTROL CATEGORIES

Birth-control methods can be grouped into four categories according to the way they work: natural, mechanical, chemical, and invasive. They are also sometimes used in combination with each other.

### Natural

The **natural birth-control** category involves techniques that do not prevent fertilization or end implantation. Some examples of natural birth-control methods are the calendar method and the basal-thermometer method. These methods utilize devices and techniques that estimate when the female is ovulating, but do not in any way attempt to alter ovulation, prevent fertilization, or end implantation.

9.1 EXHIBIT

## The Unresolvable Question

When does a human being begin to exist? That question is at the very heart of the abortion debate, yet it is far from susceptible to a sure answer. This much is beyond serious dispute: biological life begins at fertilization, when the female's egg is united with the male's sperm. But does a collection of cells constitute a human being? Some biologists believe that fertilization does mark the beginning of humanity, since the fertilized egg is a distinct and unique genetic entity. This belief shores up the antiabortion argument of Catholic bishops as well as those of secular pro-life groups. John T. Noonan, a professor of law at the University of California at Berkeley, explains the church's theological position this way: "Once conceived, the being was recognized as man because he had man's potential. The criterion for humanity, thus, was simple and all-embracing: if you are conceived by human parents, you are human."

Others argue that human life does not start until a week or so after conception, when the fertilized egg has traveled through the fallopian tube and implanted itself in the wall of the uterus. "We are able to discern [the embryo's] presence and activity beginning with implantation," wrote Dr. Bernard Nathanson, former chief of obstetrical services at New York City's St. Luke's Hospital, in his 1979 book *Aborting America.* "If this is not 'life,' what is?"

Others pinpoint the beginning of human life when the heart of the embryo begins beating, around the fourth week of pregnancy, or when the central nervous system has developed to the stage where simple reflexes are evident, around the sixth week. By the eighth week, the embryo is undergoing the transition to a fetus and is definitely recognizable as a human being—a stage that some defend as the beginning of human life. Says Dr. Maurice J. Mahoney of the Yale University School of Medicine: "For me, humanness requires that some process of development has taken place which gives the embryo a human form, so that it has a nervous system, a heart and circulatory apparatus, and indications of human shape."

Protestant theologian Paul Ramsey, a professor of religion at Princeton, declines to identify the precise moment when life begins. But he argues that science now offers evidence of human characteristics in the fetus far earlier than once believed. "I do not say human life begins with conception," says Ramsey, "but science has given us

### Mechanical

**Mechanical birth-control** devices can prevent fertilization or end implantation. Mechanical devices that prevent fertilization do so by mechanically blocking sperm from entering the fallopian tubes during intercourse. Examples of such devices include the condom, diaphragm, and cervical cap. One mechanical device, the intrauterine device (IUD), ends implantation.

### Chemical

**Chemical birth-control** methods employ chemicals that either prevent fertilization or end implantation. Examples of chemical methods include spermicides, which kill sperm, and hormones, such as birth-control pills, which attempt to prevent ovulation or end implantation.

### Invasive

**Invasive birth-control** methods involve a physician entering the body in order to surgically alter the internal reproductive organs or to end a pregnancy. Examples of these methods include sterilization and abortion.

These four basic categories of birth-control methods each consist of a variety of techniques. It is not unusual for an individual or couple to use more than one method from different categories. For example, a woman may utilize a diaphragm and a spermicide simultaneously. A couple may practice

## EXHIBIT 9.1

ample factual grounds for believing that the unborn child is an independent human being within the time span [that is, six months] in which the law now says this unborn child can be killed."

Some pro-choice biologists counter that human life does not begin until the fetus becomes viable, by which they mean sufficiently developed to survive outside the uterus. In 1973, when the Supreme Court gave women the legal right to have abortions up to the moment of viability, that age was placed at between twenty-four to twenty-eight weeks. Since then the age at which a fetus is considered viable by medical experts has slowly dropped. Doctors are now able to keep alive fetuses as young as twenty weeks and weighing 500 grams (1.1 pounds). Indeed, Dr. Norman Fost of the Medical School of the University of Wisconsin–Madison believes that the day will eventually arrive when all fetuses can be kept alive—in the laboratory if not in a nursery.

But is any of this relevant? Some experts argue that it is futile to rely on biological data at all in trying to determine when life begins. "Most biological data can never be decisive," says Lisa Cahill, a Catholic and assistant professor of theology at Boston College. "Any particular biological line that might be drawn, such as implantation or viability, is relative to the individual fetus, and each fetus reaches each stage at a slightly different time." Yet even if every fetus developed at precisely the same rate, a consensus would never be reached on when human life begins. "The question is unresolvable," says Fost, "It's not a question that doctors or religious authorities can be helpful on because it's not certifiable. It is just a matter of individual opinion."

Source: From Isaacson, Walter, "The Battle over Abortion," *Time* (April 6, 1981). 

### DISCUSSION QUESTIONS

1. When do you believe that human life begins? What has influenced your belief?

2. Has (or will) your view of the beginning of life influenced your decision making regarding birth control?

rhythm and use a condom. A woman may use an IUD that is also designed to release hormones. Two or more birth-control methods used simultaneously are usually more effective than just one.

## PERSONAL AND SOCIAL INFLUENCES

The decision about which birth-control method, if any, to use is complicated. In addition to understanding how each method prevents pregnancy, it is important to consider additional factors such as the effectiveness, safety, cost, and reversibility of each method. These factors should be weighed in light of personal circumstances as well as the social environment in which we interact.

### Effectiveness

**Effectiveness** measures the chances of procreating if you use a particular method of birth control. Birth-control effectiveness can be divided into two categories, theoretical effectiveness and use effectiveness. **Theoretical effectiveness** is the maximum effectiveness of a method if there is no human error. For example, in theory some birth-control pills are 98 percent effective in preventing fertilization or ending implantation. This theoretical effectiveness assumes that the pills are of the right quality, the user follows directions, and the user has been prescribed the correct type and dose of hormone(s). In other words theoretical effectiveness rates reflect the method's effectiveness under ideal conditions.

**Use effectiveness** is derived from a sample of people who have used a particular birth-control

**Table 9.1 First-Year Failure Rates of Birth-Control Methods**

| Method | Lowest Observed Failure Rate*(%) | Failure Rate in Typical Users†(%) |
|---|---|---|
| Tubal ligation | 0.04 | 0.04 |
| Vasectomy | 0.15 | 0.15 |
| Injectable progestin | 0.25 | 0.25 |
| Combined birth-control pills | 0.5 | 2 |
| Progestin-only pill | 1 | 2.5 |
| IUD | 1.5 | 5 |
| Condom | 2 | 10 |
| Diaphragm (with spermicide) | 2 | 19 |
| Sponge (with spermicide) | —†† | 10–20 |
| Cervical cap | 2 | 13 |
| Foams, creams, jellies, and vaginal suppositories | 3–5 | 18 |
| Coitus interruptus | 16 | 23 |
| Fertility-awareness techniques (basal body temperature, mucus method, calendar, and "rhythm") | 2–20 | 24 |
| Douche | — | 40 |
| Chance (no method of birth control) | 90 | 90 |

*Designed to complete the sentence: "In 100 users who start out the year using a given method and who use it correctly and consistently, the lowest observed failure rate has been ________."

†Designed to complete the sentence: "In 100 typical users who start out the year using a given method, the number of pregnancies by the end of the year will be ________."

††There are inadequate data to know the lowest observed failure rate of this new method of birth control.

Source: From Hatcher, Robert A., et al., *Contraceptive Technology 1984–1985,* 12th ed. © 1984 Irvington Publishers, New York. Reprinted by permission.

method. Use effectiveness rates are often lower than theoretical effectiveness rates. Use effectiveness rates reflect the human error involved in using a particular birth-control method and are usually based on the experience of typical users during the first year of use.

Both theoretical and use effectiveness rates are useful to consider if you are contemplating using a particular birth-control method. The human error involved in a particular method may not always be within the control of the user. People may follow the directions to the letter, but may have purchased a faulty birth-control chemical or device, or one that is not compatible with their body chemistry or reproductive cycle. Generally, the correct use of a method and the motivation to use it conscientiously are the most important variables related to achieving maximal effectiveness.

Table 9.1 presents estimates of first-year failure rates for major birth-control methods. These rates are estimates compiled from various sources, and, unless otherwise specified, are for a particular method when used as the only form of birth control. These rates are *only* estimates.

## Safety

Assessing both the health risks and benefits of birth-control methods should be an important component of your birth-control decision-making process. Each birth-control method is accompanied by health risks ranging from minor nuisance side effects to more severe effects such as infection, hospitalization, or perhaps even death. Studies of birth control have helped identify certain groups of people who are at a high risk for particular methods. **Contraindications** for a birth-control method indicate the conditions under which it should not be used. For example, diabetics should not use birth-control pills because the pills have an adverse effect on a diabetic's blood-sugar levels.

Fortunately, some birth-control methods also decrease the risk of certain health problems. It has long been recognized, for instance, that condoms are one of the better protections against many sexually transmitted diseases (STDs). It is important that you weigh the risks and benefits of each method, especially as they relate to your personal wellness levels and your susceptibility to certain health problems.

## Cost

There are several costs to consider when selecting a birth-control method. The most obvious cost is monetary. Many of the most effective birth-control methods involve the purchase of materials, either over-the-counter (OTC) or by physician's prescription. There may also be the expense of a physical examination. Monetary costs can be viewed as short term and long term. Some methods may cost more money in the short term due to the cost of seeing a physician and purchasing a major birth-control device. An IUD is a good example of a birth-control device with greater start-up costs. Other methods have their costs spread out over time, such as the regular purchase of condoms or spermicides. Some birth-control methods have high start-up costs as well as ongoing costs.

A second important cost to consider is that of inconvenience or dissatisfaction. If a birth-control method causes you or your partner great embarrassment or decreased pleasure, this may be a high cost to your sexual well-being.

## Reversibility

**Reversibility** estimates refer to the ability of an individual to procreate after discontinuing the use of a particular birth-control method. Reversibility estimates are recorded in terms of percentages. A 100-percent-reversibility estimate means that the individual's ability to procreate will be fully restored after discontinuing the use of a method. A 10-percent reversibility estimate indicates that one out of ten individuals will be able to procreate after discontinuing the use of a method.

The reversibility of a birth-control method may discourage or encourage individuals from using that particular method. For example, a young married couple who presently do not want children but do want children in the future will find certain birth-control methods unacceptable. On the other hand, a married couple with two children may decide that a nonreversible birth control method is acceptable.

There are circumstances in which an individual may regret selecting a method with little or no reversibility. For instance, a couple experiencing a tragedy in which their child is lost in a fire or traffic accident or a divorced person who remarries and then desires to procreate with their new spouse may regret their selection of a nonreversible birth-control method. Decisions regarding irreversible methods of birth control should therefore be made only after careful consideration of the alternatives.

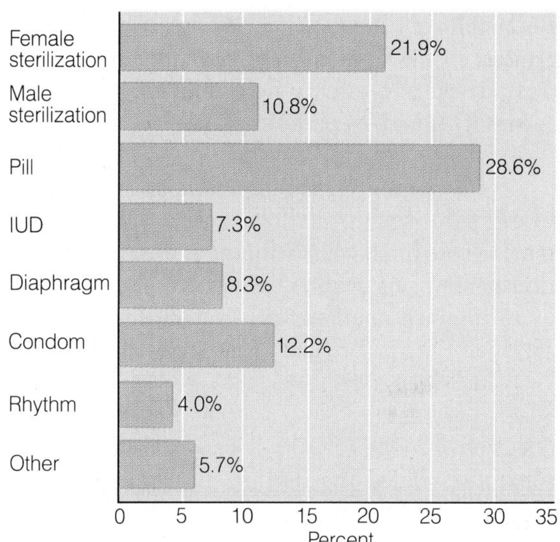


**Figure 9.1**
Contraceptive use. *Source: Understanding U.S. Fertility* (December 1984). National Center for Health Statistics (NCHS).

# BIRTH-CONTROL PROFILES

It has been estimated that over 50 percent of U.S. women aged fifteen to forty-four use some method of birth control. (See figure 9.1.) The common birth-control methods profiled in this chapter should help you make informed decisions regarding birth-control choices.

## Natural Family Planning

**Category:** Natural
**Theoretical Effectiveness:**
Calendar method: 87 percent
BBT: 93 percent
Mucus method: 98 percent
**Use Effectiveness:**
Calendar method: 53–80 percent
BBT: 80 percent
Mucus method: 75 percent

**Reversibility:** 100 percent
**Source:** Instructions from physician or clinic
**Cost:** Twenty to seventy-five dollars including consultation and/or paraphernalia.

**Natural family-planning** methods are designed to estimate when ovulation is occurring in the female. These birth-control methods prevent fertilization by requiring couples to refrain from intercourse or to practice another birth-control method for a specified time before and after ovulation.

**CALENDAR METHOD** The **calendar method,** sometimes called the rhythm method, is probably the simplest of the natural family-planning methods. The calendar method requires the female to record her reproductive cycles using the first day of menstruation as day one and the day before her next menstruation as the last day. After accurately recording eight consecutive cycles, the shortest cycle and the longest cycle are used to determine the period in which the female is ovulating. Table 9.2 shows one way in which couples using the calendar method can calculate the "unsafe" period during the female's reproductive cycle. For example, if the female's shortest cycle was twenty-six days and the longest cycle was thirty-three days, then the unsafe period is from day eight to day twenty-two of her reproductive cycle.

There are several ways to calculate the unsafe period; this is just one example. Most formulas take into consideration: (1) that ovulation varies from cycle to cycle; (2) that viable sperm can be found in the reproductive tract seventy-two hours after being deposited; and (3) that the unfertilized egg may be viable for as long as forty-eight hours.

**TEMPERATURE METHOD** **Basal body temperature** is defined as the lowest body temperature naturally reached by a healthy person. The **basal body temperature (BBT) method** calculates ovulation by plotting when the female's body temperature decreases slightly, followed by a sharp rise of 0.4 degrees F or more. The female is instructed to take her body temperature, orally or rectally, with a special thermometer for several cycles. A rise in

**Table 9.2 How to Figure the "Safe" and "Unsafe" Days for the Calendar Method of Rhythm**

| Length of Shortest Period | First Unsafe Day after Start of Any Period | Length of Longest Period | Last Unsafe Day after Start of Any Period |
|---|---|---|---|
| 21 days | 3rd day | 21 days | 10th day |
| 22 days | 4th day | 22 days | 11th day |
| 23 days | 5th day | 23 days | 12th day |
| 24 days | 6th day | 24 days | 13th day |
| 25 days | 7th day | 25 days | 14th day |
| 26 days | 8th day | 26 days | 15th day |
| 27 days | 9th day | 27 days | 16th day |
| 28 days | 10th day | 28 days | 17th day |
| 29 days | 11th day | 29 days | 18th day |
| 30 days | 12th day | 30 days | 19th day |
| 31 days | 13th day | 31 days | 20th day |
| 32 days | 14th day | 32 days | 21st day |
| 33 days | 15th day | 33 days | 22nd day |
| 34 days | 16th day | 34 days | 23rd day |
| 35 days | 17th day | 35 days | 24th day |
| 36 days | 18th day | 36 days | 25th day |
| 37 days | 19th day | 37 days | 26th day |
| 38 days | 20th day | 38 days | 27th day |

Source: From Hatcher, Robert A., et al., *Contraceptive Technology 1984–1985*, 12th ed. © 1984 Irvington Publishers, New York. Reprinted by permission.

the female's body temperature occurs between twenty-four and seventy-two hours after ovulation. Unsafe days for intercourse are the day the temperature drops slightly until three days after it rises.[1]

**CERVICAL MUCUS METHOD** The **cervical mucus method** estimates ovulation by the change in consistency of the female's cervical mucus. During pre-ovulation and post-ovulation times the mucus is thick and cloudy. During ovulation the cervical mucus is clear, slippery, and elastic. The mucus can be obtained by the female using one or two fingers to collect a sample from her cervix. The third consecutive day following peak slipperiness of the cervical mucus marks the end of the unsafe period.[2]

**SYMPTOTHERMAL METHODS** **Symptothermal methods** combine the calendar, BBT, and cervical mucus methods. Such combinations should logically yield improved use-effectiveness rates.

**WEIGHING THE BENEFITS AND RISKS** When making the decision of whether you or your partner should use natural family-planning methods, it is important to weigh both the advantages and disadvantages of these methods for your particular circumstances. The following summary should help you weigh the benefits and risks of natural family-planning methods.

Advantages:

- Health risks to the user are limited.
- No drugs or devices are needed.
- Natural family-planning methods may be more compatible with certain religous convictions.

Disadvantages:

- Natural methods require the user to make diligent, accurate measurements and to keep prolonged records.
- Natural methods require abstinence or additional birth-control methods during unsafe times.
- Females may have unsafe periods as long as twenty-one consecutive days, requiring prolonged abstinence.
- The BBT method estimates when ovulation has occurred, not when ovulation is about to occur.
- Females cannot use foams, diaphragms, deodorants, antihistamines, or douches while using the mucus method, because these methods may change the mucus reading.

Contraindications:

- Women who have a history of irregular reproductive cycles should not use natural family planning.[3]

## Diaphragm

**Category:** Mechanical
**Theoretical Effectiveness**
Diaphragm with spermicide: 95–98 percent
**Use Effectiveness:**
Diaphragm with spermicide: 81 percent
**Reversibility:** 100 percent
**Source:** Physician
**Cost:** Twenty-five to one-hundred dollars, including diaphragm and consultation.

The **diaphragm** is a shallow rubber dome two to four inches in diameter stretched over a flexible spring in its outer ring. The diaphragm is inserted over the cervix, preventing fertilization by trapping the sperm in the vaginal tract and not allowing it to enter the uterus and fallopian tubes. (See figure 9.2.) A spermicide should always be used along with the diaphragm to increase effectiveness. Diaphragms can be inserted as long as six hours prior to intercourse and must remain in place for six to eight hours after intercourse. If intercourse is repeated within that time, additional spermicide should be inserted into the vagina. Upon removal, the diaphragm should be washed with warm water and mild soap, rinsed, dried, and stored away from heat and light.

Women are fitted for diaphragms by a physician. The fitting will be preceded by a consultation that includes a medical examination and directions on how to insert, remove, maintain, and use the diaphragm. The diaphragm should be checked for proper fit and quality by a physician once a year. If a woman has a weight gain or loss of ten pounds, an abortion, or a pregnancy, she should be reexamined before using her diaphragm. Women need to check the diaphragm regularly, carefully looking for cracks and small holes. In addition, the diaphragm should be replaced with a new one every two to three years.

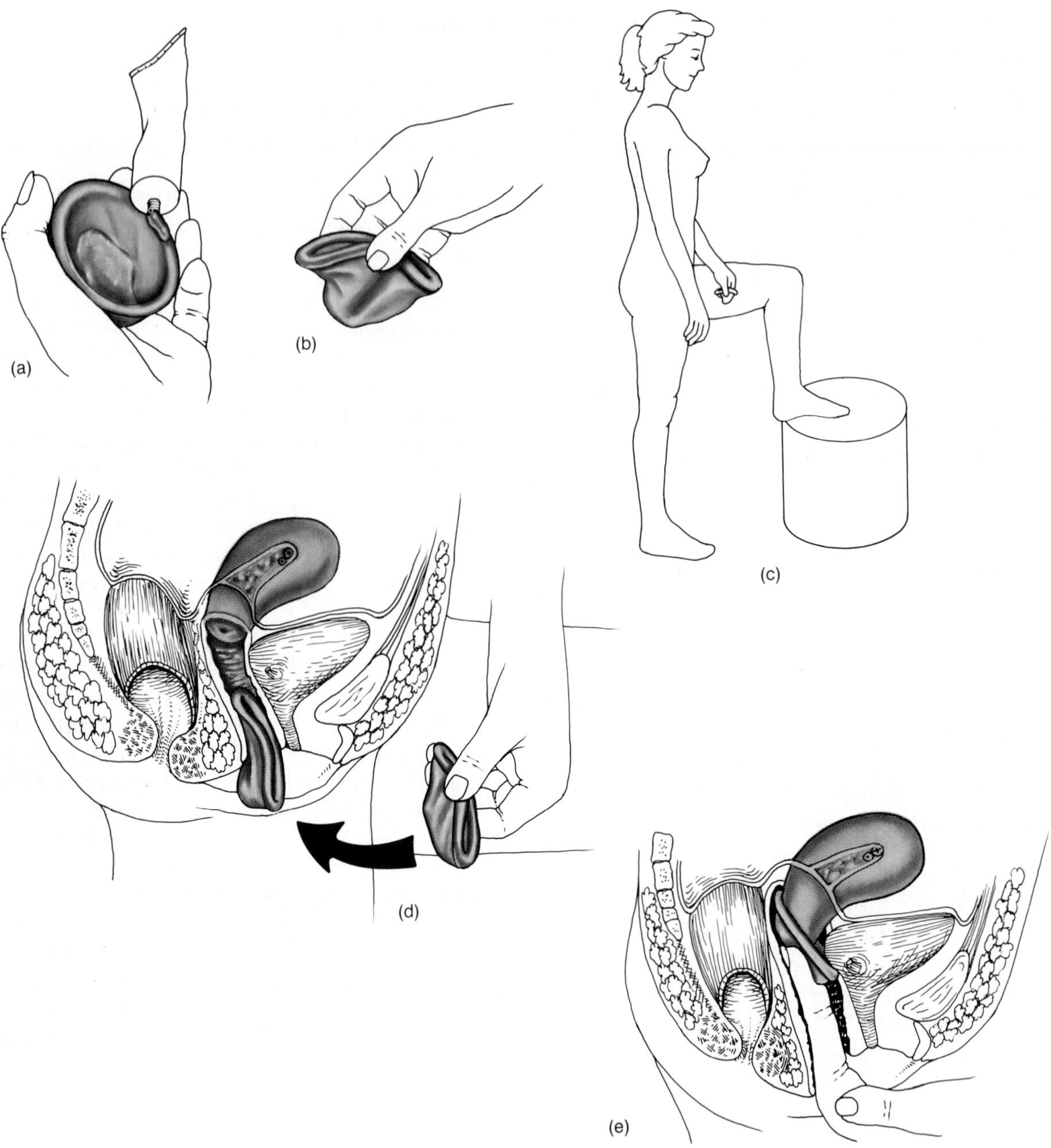


**Figure 9.2**
Insertion of the diaphragm: (a) spermicide is applied around the rim and in the dome; (b) the diaphragm ready for insertion; (c) the correct posture for insertion; (d) insertion before intercourse; (e) placement with dome covering cervix for correct positioning during and following intercourse. *Source:* From Jones, Kenneth L., Louis W. Shainberg, and Curtis O. Byer, *Dimensions of Human Sexuality.* © 1985 Wm. C. Brown Publishers, Dubuque, Iowa. All rights reserved. Reprinted by permission.

**Table 9.3 Danger Signs of Toxic-Shock Syndrome**

- Fever (temperature of 101° or more)
- Diarrhea
- Vomiting
- Muscle aches
- Rash (like sunburn)

Source: From Hatcher, Robert A., et al., *Contraceptive Technology 1984–1985*, 12th ed. © 1984 Irvington Publishers, New York. Reprinted by permission.

### WEIGHING THE BENEFITS AND RISKS

When making the decision of whether you or your partner should use a diaphragm it is important to consider both the advantages and disadvantages of this method for your particular situation. The following summary should help you weigh the benefits and risks of the diaphragm.

Advantages:

- No serious health risk to the user.
- May decrease the risk of cervical cancer.[4]
- May offer some protection against sexually transmitted diseases (STDs).
- This method is 100 percent reversible.

Disadvantages:

- User may forget to insert the device.
- User may have an allergic reaction to the rubber in the diaphragm or to the spermicide.
- Diaphragm use may increase the risk of **toxic-shock syndrome (TSS).**[5] (See table 9.3.)

Contraindications:

Women experiencing the following conditions should not use the diaphragm:[6]

- Certain abnormalities of the uterus or vagina
- A history of toxic-shock syndrome
- Repeated urinary tract infections

## Cervical Cap

**Category:** Mechanical
**Theoretical Effectiveness:** 98 percent
**Use Effectiveness:** 82–92 percent
**Reversibility:** 100 percent
**Source:** Physician
**Cost:** Twenty-five to one-hundred dollars, including consultation and cervical cap.

The **cervical cap** is a thimble-sized and -shaped device made of rubber or plastic. The cervical cap is placed over the cervix and is held in place by suction. Often used simultaneously with a spermicide, the cervical cap prevents fertilization by not allowing sperm to enter the uterus. The female, after a medical examination, is fitted for the cervical cap. At the time of fitting she will be instructed on the insertion, removal, and care of the cap. The cap must remain inserted for six to eight hours after ejaculation. Investigations are currently underway to determine if the cervical cap can safely be left in the vagina for several weeks at a time.[7]

Studies on the effectiveness of the cervical cap are also underway.[8] It appears that the cervical cap may be as effective as the diaphragm. Presently, the cervical cap is only available as an investigational device in a few clinics around the country, as FDA approval is still pending.[9]

### WEIGHING THE BENEFITS AND RISKS

When making the decision of whether you or your partner should use a cervical cap it is important to consider both the advantages and disadvantages of this method for your particular circumstances. The following summary should help you weigh the benefits and risks of the cervical cap.

**Table 9.4 Danger Signs of Pelvic Inflammatory Disease (PID)**

- Abdominal pain
- Back pain
- Leg pain
- Pelvic pain
- Fever
- Chills
- Vomiting
- Abnormally profuse menstrual flow
- Painful urination
- Painful intercourse
- Bleeding following intercourse

Source: From Hatcher, Robert A., et al. *Contraceptive Technology 1984–1985,* 12th ed. © 1984 Irvington Publishers, New York. Reprinted by permission.

Advantages:

- Presents no serious health risk to the user.
- Does not have to be removed after each episode of intercourse; thus, spontaneity is not interrupted.
- May reduce the risk of cervical cancer.[10]
- This method is 100 percent reversible.

Disadvantages:

- Can irritate the cervix after prolonged use.
- Requires more skill for insertion than the diaphragm.
- Females may develop an allergic reaction to the rubber or plastic that is used to make the cervical cap.
- Because the cervical cap may remain in place for long periods of time, it is advisable for the female to be alert for early signs of **pelvic inflammatory disease** (**PID**) and toxic-shock syndrome (TSS). (See table 9.4.)

Contraindications:

Women experiencing the following conditions should not use a cervical cap:[11]

- Cervical, vaginal, or pelvic infections
- Abnormal Pap smear
- Full-term delivery within the past six weeks
- History of toxic-shock syndrome

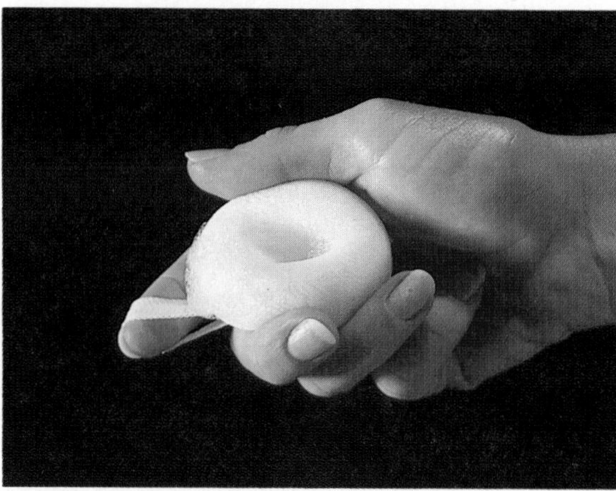

**Figure 9.3**
The contraceptive sponge is one of the newer birth control devices on the American marketplace.

## Vaginal Contraceptive Sponge

**Category:** Chemical
**Theoretical Effectiveness:** 92 percent
**Use Effectiveness:** 80–90 percent
**Reversibility:** 100 percent
**Source:** OTC
**Cost:** One dollar per sponge

The **vaginal sponge** is a soft, polyurethane pad containing a spermicide. (See figure 9.3.) The sponge must be moistened before insertion in order to activate the spermicide (nonoxynol-9). The sponge is then inserted into the vagina, covering the cervix. Intercourse may take place right after the sponge is properly inserted. The sponge must remain inserted for at least six hours after intercourse, and may be left in the vagina for as long as twenty-four hours. It is discarded after use.

The manufacturer of the sponge reports that it works by killing sperm, blocking the cervix, and absorbing sperm into its polyurethane foam. In general it acts to prevent fertilization. It should be noted that the sponge is a new entry to the American marketplace. In addition, this birth-control device employs a new delivery system for introducing a spermicide into the female reproductive tract. There is relatively little data on its effectiveness and safety.

### WEIGHING THE BENEFITS AND RISKS

When making the decision of whether you or your partner should use the contraceptive sponge it is important to consider both the advantages and disadvantages of this method for your particular circumstances. The following summary should help you weigh the benefits and risks of the contraceptive sponge.

Advantages:

- Appears to present no serious health risks to the user.
- May improve vaginal lubrication.
- May provide some protection against STDs and PID.
- Remains effective during multiple acts of intercourse.
- Absorbs vaginal secretions during intercourse.
- This method is 100 percent reversible.

Disadvantages:

- May produce a vaginal discharge.
- May produce a vaginal odor or itching.
- May discourage cunnilingus which some partners may view as disadvantageous.
- May be torn or shredded by unsuccessful attempts to remove it from the vagina.
- There have been a few cases of TSS among women using the sponge. These cases are rare. Risk of TSS can be decreased by leaving the sponge in place no longer than thirty hours and avoiding its use during menstruation.[12]

Contraindications:

If a woman (or her partner) experiences the following conditions, she should not use the sponge:[13]

- Allergic reaction to the spermicide or sponge
- History of TSS

## Condoms

**Category:** Mechanical
**Theoretical Effectiveness:**
Condom: 96–98 percent
Condom and diaphragm: 99 percent
Spermicidal condom: 99 percent

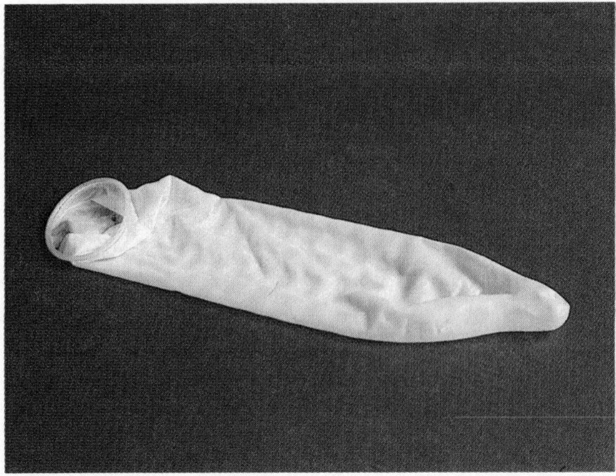

**Figure 9.4**
Some condoms are equipped with a reservoir tip to prevent tearing and sperm leakage.

**Use Effectiveness:**
Condom: 80–95 percent
Condom and diaphragm: 95–97 percent
Spermicidal condom: 98 percent
**Reversibility:** 100 percent
**Source:** OTC
**Cost:** Twenty-five cents to one dollar per condom.

The **condom** is a cylindrical sheath made of rubber or animal skin, which is unrolled over the erect penis. The condom prevents fertilization by trapping the semen in its tip. In order to prevent tearing of the condom and leakage of sperm, a one-half-inch space must be left at the tip of the condom to collect sperm. Some condoms are manufactured with a reservoir tip for this purpose. (See figure 9.4.)

Condoms are marketed in various shapes, colors, and with or without lubrication. Unlubricated condoms can be lubricated with saliva or K-Y jelly (not Vaseline) before being inserted into the vaginal tract. One condom is used for each ejaculation and must be removed prior to the loss of erection. The condom is held at the base of the penis as the penis is withdrawn from the vaginal tract.

Spermicidal condoms are now available in America. They are standard condoms laced with a spermicide. There have not been extensive studies on spermicidal condoms, but early reports indicate that they have a higher use effectiveness than standard condoms.

#### WEIGHING THE BENEFITS AND RISKS

When making the decision of whether you or your partner should use a condom it is important to consider both the advantages and disadvantages of this method for your particular situation. The following summary should help you weigh the benefits and risks of using condoms.

Advantages:

- Presents no serious health risk to the couple.
- Decreases the risk of either partner contracting an STD.
- Decreasing the risk of females contracting an STD may in turn reduce their chances of developing cervical cancer.[14]
- The condom is currently the only available male birth control method which is reasonably effective and 100-percent reversible.
- Condoms used during pregnancy may decrease the chances of amniotic-fluid infections and intrauterine infections that can lead to a miscarriage.[15]
- This method is 100 percent reversible.

Disadvantages:

- Reduces penis sensitivity, which may be negatively viewed by both the male and female.
- Some couples view the placement of the condom as an interruption of foreplay. (Others, however, incorporate the placement of the condom in their sex play.)
- The male or the female may be allergic to the rubber condom. Switching to a natural condom may alleviate this problem.
- Heat or cold can damage condoms. Condoms should not be left in automobile glove compartments, airplane luggage compartments, or hip wallets.
- Failure of the male to maintain an erection for proper placement and removal of the condom will dramatically reduce the condom's effectiveness.

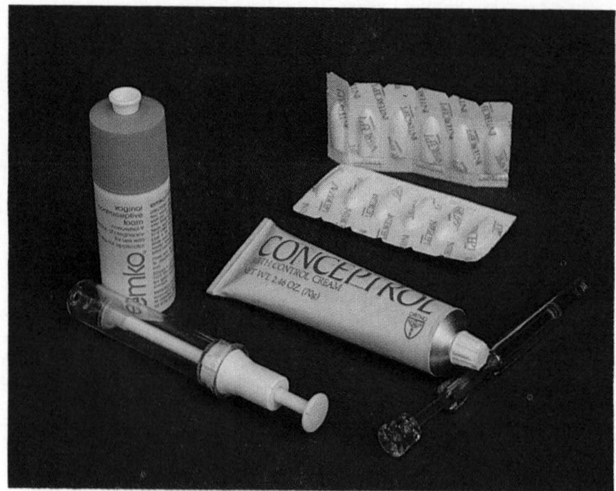


**Figure 9.5**
The various spermicidal products currently on the market differ in their application and effectiveness.

## Spermicides (Foams, Creams, Jellies, Suppositories)

**Category:** Chemical
**Theoretical Effectiveness:** 90–97 percent
**Use Effectiveness:** 82 percent
**Reversibility:** 100 percent
**Source:** OTC
**Cost:** From twenty-five cents to two dollars per application.

**Spermicides** are chemicals placed at the opening of the uterus prior to intercourse, preventing fertilization by destroying sperm or preventing them from passing through the uterus. There are a variety of spermicidal products on the market, which differ in their application and effectiveness. (See figure 9.5.) Foam spermicides are the most effective and easy to use. For maximum effectiveness spermicides should be inserted no longer than thirty minutes prior to intercourse. One chemical application is required for each act of intercourse. The product should not be removed from the vaginal tract for six to eight hours following intercourse.

#### WEIGHING THE BENEFITS AND RISKS

When making the decision of whether you or your partner should use spermicides it is important to consider both the advantages and disadvantages of this method for your particular circumstances. The following summary should help you weigh the benefits and risks of spermicides.

Advantages:

- No serious health risks for the user.
- Foams may improve vaginal lubrication.
- Foams provide some protection against STDs and PID.
- This method is 100 percent reversible.

Disadvantages:

- Usually result in a vaginal discharge after intercourse.
- May discourage cunnilingus, which some couples may view as a disadvantage.
- Some spermicidal products require a thirty-minute waiting period after insertion (tablets and suppositories).
- After prolonged use of a spermicide, females may experience vaginal infections.

Contraindications:

- Men or women who experience an allergic reaction to spermicides should not use them.[16]

## Intrauterine Device (IUD)

**Category:** Mechanical or chemical
**Theoretical Effectiveness:**
Mechanical: 95–99 percent
Mechanical and hormonal: 99 percent
**Use Effectiveness:**
Mechanical: 90–99 percent
Mechanical and hormonal: 97–98 percent
**Reversibility:** Theoretically 100 percent
**Source:** Physician
**Cost:** Fifteen to one-hundred-fifty dollars, including the IUD, consultation, and insertion.

The **IUD** is a plastic device one to one and one-half inches long, which is inserted into the uterus through the vaginal tract by a physician. There are two types of IUDs, nonmedicated and medicated. (See figure 9.6.) The nonmedicated IUD is made of plastic (e.g., Lippes Loop) and works mechanically to prevent implantation. Medicated IUDs (e.g., Copper 7, Progestasert T) leak chemicals (e.g., copper, hormones) to prevent implantation.

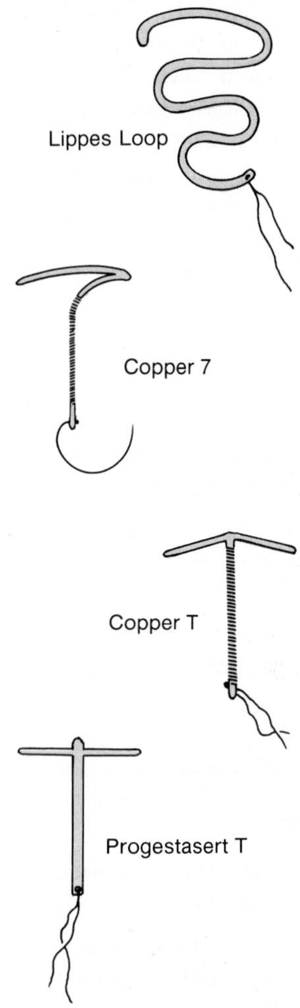


**Figure 9.6**
Types of IUDs. *Source:* From Jones, Kenneth L., Louis W. Shainberg, and Curtis O. Byer, *Dimensions of Human Sexuality*. © 1985 Wm. C. Brown Publishers, Dubuque, Iowa. All rights reserved. Reprinted by permission.

IUDs do not prevent fertilization of the egg, but rather prevent its implantation in the lining of the uterus.[17] It is not known exactly how the IUD prevents implantation.

If a female and her physician decide the IUD is indicated, a series of preliminary exams are required before its insertion. These exams will include a medical history and tests for sexually transmitted diseases and pregnancy. After the IUD is inserted the physician will teach the female how to check for the string that is attached to the IUD. Periodic checking is required to assure that the IUD has not been expelled.

Women with an IUD should have a medical examination three months after insertion and yearly pelvic examinations thereafter. Medicated IUDs need to be replaced at regular intervals. IUD users should immediately consult a physician if they suspect they are pregnant, have contracted a sexually transmitted disease, develop a pelvic inflammatory disease, or experience unusual vaginal bleeding, abdominal discomfort, or pain.

### WEIGHING THE BENEFITS AND RISKS

When making the decision of whether you or your partner should use an IUD it is important to consider both the advantages and disadvantages of this method for your particular situation. The following summary should help you weigh the benefits and risks of the IUD.

Advantages:

- Requires no pre-intercourse planning.

Disadvantages:

- As many as 20 percent of IUD users will expel the IUD in the first year of use. The IUD can be expelled without the female's knowledge.[18]
- Some IUD users experience symptoms such as anemia, cramping, spotting, and backaches.
- For the first three cycles immediately following insertion, the IUD user is required to use a back-up birth-control method.
- There is substantial evidence that IUDs increase the female's risk of pelvic inflammatory disease (PID). The string of the IUD may act as a passageway for bacteria to enter and infect the reproductive tract. Studies have indicated that PID occurs 50 percent more often in women using IUDs than in females using no birth-control method. Just one or two cases of PID can cause sterility in women.[19]
- In 1 percent of all IUD insertions the uterus is perforated. In rare cases the IUD can pass through the tear in the uterus and fall into the abdominal cavity requiring surgical removal. IUDs can also cause cervical perforations.
- There is a 1 to 2 percent chance that pregnancy will occur while the IUD is in place and this can lead to medical complications such as miscarriage,[20] PID, and maternal death.
- Increased risk of tubal pregnancy. One in thirty IUD-user pregnancies is **ectopic** (the fertilized egg implants outside the uterus). Users with IUDs that release hormones have an even greater risk of ectopic pregnancies than regular IUD users.[21]
- Females with the Dalkon Shield IUD should have them immediately removed because of their health risks. The Dalkon Shield has been recalled by its manufacturer, A. H. Robbins.

Contraindications:

Women experiencing the following conditions should not use an IUD:[22]

- Pregnancy
- PID (recent or chronic)
- History of gonorrhea
- Multiple sexual partners
- Abnormal Pap smears
- Abnormal uterine bleeding
- Use of anticoagulant drugs
- History of ectopic pregnancies
- Diabetes

## Birth-Control Pills

**Category:** Chemical
**Theoretical Effectiveness:**
Estrogen/Progestin: 99.7 percent
Progestin only: 98–99 percent
**Use Effectiveness:**
Estrogen/Progestin: 98 percent
Progestin only: 90–95 percent
**Reversibility:** Nine out of ten females desiring pregnancy after using birth-control hormones become pregnant within one year.
**Source:** Physician
**Cost:** Consultation, twenty to seventy-five dollars, plus three to eighteen dollars per month for packets.

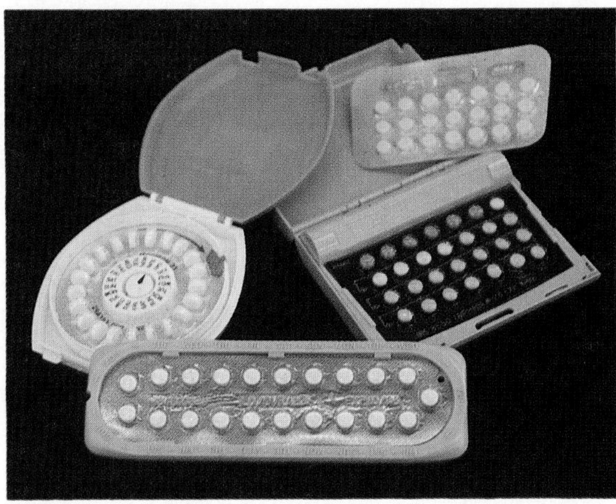

**Figure 9.7**
Despite the proliferation of brands, most birth-control pills now available are one of two types: either the combination pill or the mini-pill.

There are two major types of birth-control pills currently available to U.S. women. (See figure 9.7.) The first, a **combination birth-control pill,** contains estrogen and progestin (synthetic hormones that are similar to natural hormones produced by women). It is believed that the estrogen in the combination pill prevents the ovaries from releasing an egg, thereby preventing fertilization and pregnancy.[23]

The second available type of birth-control pill is known as the **"mini-pill."** It contains progestin only. Mini-pills change the quality of cervical mucus, making it difficult for sperm to survive, slowing down the egg's journey through the fallopian tube, and inhibiting implantation.

Women taking the combination or mini-pill usually take a monthly series of pills, one pill a day for twenty-one days or twenty-eight days, depending on the brand prescribed. Birth-control pills are most effective when taken at about the same time each day; this helps to maintain a steady level of hormones in the body.[24] The female should experience normal menstruation at the end of her monthly cycle. It is common for women on the birth-control pill to miss a period occasionally. If no pills have been forgotten during that month, the likelihood of pregnancy is small. If, however, a woman has forgotten to take one or more pills and misses a period, she should contact her physician and use another form of birth control until a pregnancy test can be completed.

## WEIGHING THE BENEFITS AND RISKS

When making the decision of whether you or your partner should use birth-control pills it is important to consider both the advantages and disadvantages of this method for your particular situation. The following summary should help you weigh the benefits and risks of birth-control pills. (See figure 9.8.)

Advantages:

- One of the most effective noninvasive means of birth control.
- Does not require pre-intercourse planning or cause interruption of the sexual act.
- In certain cases birth-control pills eliminate **mittelschmerz** (pain experienced during ovulation) and reduce menstrual duration, flow, and cramps.[25]
- May provide protection against endometrial and ovarian cancer.[26]
- Progestin may provide protection against PID.[27]

Disadvantages:

- May produce pseudo-pregnancy signs and symptoms such as nausea, water retention, breast enlargement, breast tenderness, spotting, and increased vaginal discharge.
- Increase the female's risk of heart attacks, stroke, blood clots, gall-bladder disease, and liver tumors.
- Increase the risk of hypertension in nonblack females.
- Increase the female's risk of yeast infections (this may be controlled by reducing or eliminating estrogen).
- May increase the growth of existing cancers.
- May cause hair loss.
- May cause jaundice, rash, darkened skin, and depression.
- Females using progestin-only pills increase their risk of an ectopic pregnancy.[28]
- May cause a false-negative reading (negative result when you really have the disease) for the tuberculin skin test.
- Can alter the results of medical-laboratory tests (e.g., thyroid, vitamin, and sodium tests).

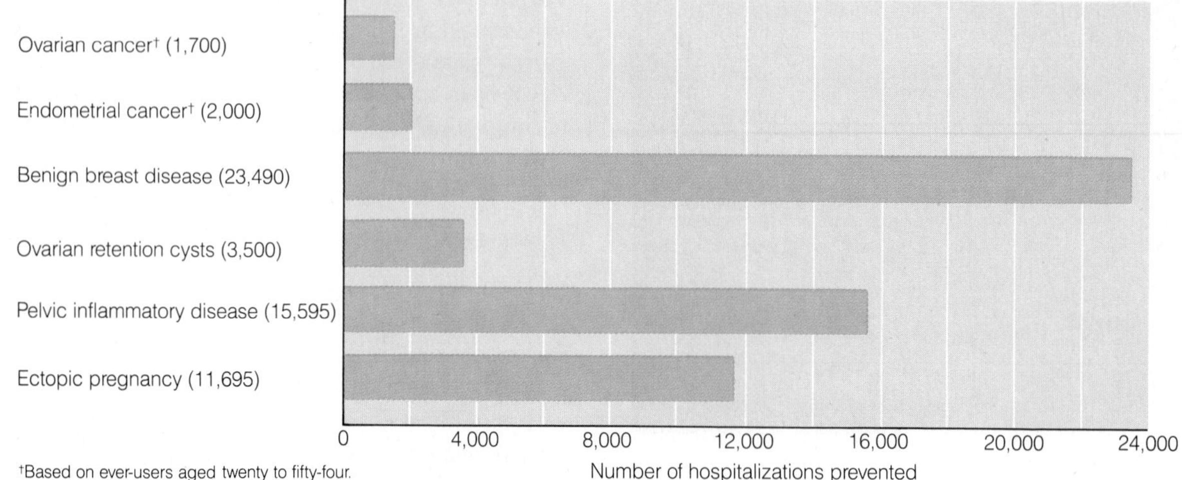


**Figure 9.8**
Estimated annual number of hospitalizations prevented by the use of oral contraceptives. *Source:* Reprinted with permission from *Making Choices: Evaluating the Health Risks and Benefits of Birth Control Methods,* by Howard Ory, M.D., Jacqueline Darroch Forrest, Ph.D., and Richard Lincoln, The Alan Guttmacher Institute, 1983.

- Because birth-control pills affect body metabolism, the use and excretion of vitamins and minerals can be altered, especially for vitamins A, $B_2$, $B_6$, $B_{12}$, C, folic acid, and the minerals iron and copper.

Contraindications:

Women experiencing the following conditions should not use birth-control pills.[29]

- Smoke more than fifteen cigarettes per day
- Have a history of heart attacks, strokes, angina, blood clots, cancer in the reproductive system, irregular menses, migraine headaches, clinical depression, acute mononucleosis, sickle-cell disorders, kidney disease, asthma, hypertension, diabetes, epilepsy, or liver disorders
- Pregnancy
- Thirty-five years of age or older
- Anticipate surgery in the next month

## Voluntary Sterilization

**Sterilization** is a permanent method of birth control. Voluntary sterilization is accomplished by cutting and closing off the tubes in men through which the sperm travel (vas deferens), and in women the tubes through which the egg travels (fallopian tubes). Voluntary sterilization is the most popular method of birth control, especially for married couples over age thirty.[30] Presently, operations for reversing voluntary sterilization have low success rates. Therefore, voluntary sterilization procedures should be considered permanent when making the decision on which method of birth control to use.[31]

### VASECTOMY (MALE STERILIZATION)

**Category:** Invasive
**Theoretical Effectiveness:** Almost 100 percent
**Use Effectiveness:** 99.85 percent
**Reversibility:**
*Reappearance of sperm in ejaculate: 40–90 percent
*Pregnancy rate: 5–70 percent
**Source:** Physician
**Cost:** Seventy-five to five-hundred dollars or more.

A **vasectomy** involves the cutting and tying of the vas deferens. (See figure 9.9.) The first human vasectomy was performed in 1894, nearly one hundred years ago.[32] A vasectomy prevents fertilization by blocking sperm from entering the vas deferens during ejaculation. A vasectomy operation takes about twenty minutes and is usually performed in a physician's office. Most males can return to normal sexual activity within a few days. A back-up birth-control method should be used for

9.2 EXHIBIT 9.2

## The Man's Turn?

We generally think of the quest for a birth-control pill for men as being fairly recent. Actually, it goes back at least half a century. By the 1950s, successful experiments were being made with testosterone, the male hormone on which sperm production is dependent. The governing theory was that injections of the hormone would cause the pituitary to shut down its own production. And, indeed, the sperm count did decline markedly, but not without complications. The injections, decidedly unpleasant, had to be given frequently. And when a testosterone pill was finally developed, the high doses necessary caused liver disorders and other adverse consequences.

Since then, researchers have moved away from testosterone, trying other hormones, both natural and synthetic. Medications used to reduce sperm count include stilbestrol (a female hormone) and nitrofurantoin (a urinary antibiotic). In 1979 a newly synthesized male hormone, danazol, was introduced. When taken daily in pill form, danazol reduced fertility in 85 percent of test subjects. Unfortunately, after taking these and similar preparations, many men report a diminished sex drive or impotence.

Other methods being tested:

*Gossypol.* This compound, extracted from the cotton plant, has been given in pill form to thousands of men in China. There is no question that gossypol causes infertility. Questions remain about its health hazards, reversibility, and genetic effects.

*Nasal spray.* Swedish scientists have pioneered this as a means to affect body hormones and thereby suppress sperm production. It is easier than having to inject oneself daily and perhaps less blunting to the libido. At Vanderbilt University, researchers are trying to prepare a nasal spray from a hormone produced naturally in the hypothalamus.

*Ultrasound.* A high-frequency device is briefly placed in contact with the man's scrotum. The procedure is painless and the sperm count is lowered, sometimes for up to two years. The risk of testicular cancer and genetic damage is being investigated.

In all of these methods, the object has been to suppress the production of sperm. But even a drastic reduction in their number may not be good enough, since it takes only one to achieve fertilization—and millions are released with each ejaculation. Consequently, some scientists are taking a different tack: Rather than reduce the number of sperm, try to inhibit their movement.

Many researchers expect a male pill (and/or spray, injection, or whatever) to be on the market by 1990. A study appearing in the *Journal of Applied Social Psychology* in 1981 concluded that men are likely to resist oral contraceptives until their effectiveness, risks, cost, and convenience approach perfection.

Source: From Lederer, Joseph, "The Man's Turn," in *Psychology Today* (June 1983). Reprinted with permission from *Psychology Today* magazine.


### DISCUSSION QUESTIONS

1. Do you agree with the concluding statement that men will be likely to resist oral contraceptives until effectiveness, risks, and costs "approach perfection"?

2. Do you believe that men's responses to birth-control risks, costs, and effectiveness are different from women's responses?

3. Who should ultimately be responsible for birth control—men or women? What has influenced your position on this issue?

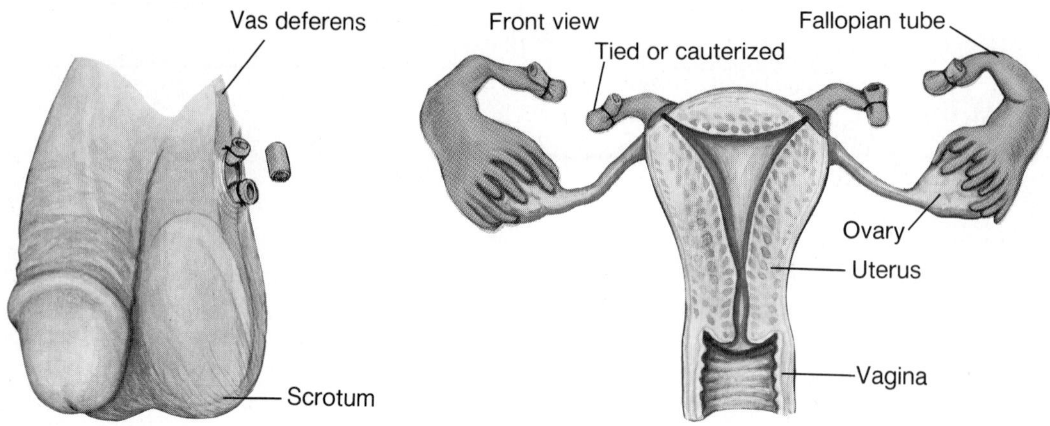


**Figure 9.9**
Vasectomy (at left) involves removal of a portion of each vas deferens; tubal ligation (at right) involves removal of a portion of each fallopian tube. *Source:* From Hole, John W., Jr. *Human Anatomy and Physiology,* 3d ed. © 1978, 1981, 1984 Wm. C. Brown Publishers, Dubuque, Iowa. All rights reserved. Reprinted by permission.

several months following the operation, because sperm may be present between the upper portion of the vas deferens and the urethra. A semen analysis will confirm if there are any sperm present in the male's ejaculate. If two consecutive semen analyses indicate sperm are not present then the male can engage in unprotected intercourse. Most vasectomized males cannot detect any change in the quantity or quality of their semen.

## WEIGHING THE BENEFITS AND RISKS

When making the decision of whether you or your partner should have a vasectomy it is important to consider both the advantages and disadvantages of this method for your particular situation. The following summary should help you weigh the benefits and risks of having a vasectomy.

Advantages:

- Very effective long-term male birth-control method.
- Seems to present no serious health risks to the male.[33]

Disadvantages:

- Some postoperative discomfort is possible.
- The male will be sexually incapacitated for twenty-four to forty-eight hours.
- The vasectomy itself or a reversal operation may not be covered by medical-insurance plans.
- Postoperative complications may include blood clots, infection, inflammation of the epididymis, and an inflammatory reaction to sperm that are absorbed by the body.
- Males may later regret their decision to have a vasectomy because of a child's death or a desire to have children with a new spouse.
- Males may feel emasculated because they can no longer procreate.
- One in 1,000 vasectomies will result in one vas deferens naturally repairing itself and allowing sperm to pass through the urethra once again.

Contraindications:

- Men who lack preoperative education regarding vasectomy as a birth-control option, including its reversibility, its risks, and the pre- and post-operative procedures should not have a vasectomy.

## TUBAL LIGATION (FEMALE STERILIZATION)

**Category:** Invasive
**Theoretical Effectiveness:** Almost 100 percent
**Use Effectiveness:** 99.96 percent
**Reversibility:** 0–60 percent range
**Source:** Physician
**Cost:** Seventy-five to thirteen-hundred dollars, depending on techniques and where the procedure is performed (e.g., hospital, physician's office).

**Tubal ligation** involves the blocking of the female's fallopian tubes. (See figure 9.9.) Tubal ligation prevents fertilization by preventing sperm from reaching an egg in the fallopian tube. There are several common ways in which tubal ligations are performed, ranging from an outpatient operation under general anesthesia to an operation requiring hospitalization and general anesthesia.

The most commmonly performed procedures are the minilaparotomy and the laparoscopy.[34] Both of these techniques can usually be performed on an outpatient basis, use a small incision, and take from twenty minutes to an hour to complete.

Tubal ligation is a popular form of birth control today. The National Center for Health Statistics reports that voluntary sterilization is the single most common birth-control method among women thirty years and older.[35]

## WEIGHING THE BENEFITS AND RISKS

When making the decision of whether you or your partner should have a tubal ligation it is important to consider both the advantages and disadvantages of this method for your particular situation. The following summary should help you weigh the benefits and risks of tubal ligation.

Advantages:

- Highly effective long-term female birth-control method

Disadvantages:

- The female will be incapacitated for twenty-four to seventy-two hours following the operation.
- Postoperative discomfort is possible.
- Tubal ligation and attempts to reverse the procedures are not usually covered by medical insurance plans.
- Postoperative complications such as bleeding, infection, or injury to organs adjacent to the fallopian tubes are possible.
- Females may experience postoperative depression resulting from their inability to procreate.
- Females may later regret their tubal ligation because of a child's death or a desire to have children with a new spouse.

Contraindications:

- Women who lack preoperative education regarding tubal ligation as a birth-control option, including its reversibility, its risks, and the pre- and post-operative procedures and events should not have a tubal ligation.

(See table 9.5 and Activity for Wellness 9.1.)

**Table 9.5 A Guide to the Pros and Cons***

| Type | Estimated Effectiveness | Risks | Noncontraceptive Benefits | Convenience | Availability |
|---|---|---|---|---|---|
| Condom | 64–97 percent | Rarely, irritation and allergic reactions | Good protection against sexually transmitted diseases, possibly including herpes and AIDS | Applied immediately before intercourse | OTC |
| Vaginal Spermicides (used alone) | 70–80 percent | Rarely, irritation and allergic reactions | May give some protection against some sexually transmitted diseases | Applied no more than one hour before intercourse; can be "messy" | OTC |

*Efficacy rates given in this chart are estimates based on a number of different studies. Methods which are more dependent on conscientious use and therefore are more subject to human error have wider ranges of efficacy than the others. For comparison, 60 to 80 percent of sexually active women using no contraception would be expected to become pregnant in a year. Because the contraceptive sponge has only been on the market a short time, effectiveness estimates for it are not based on as many studies as those for the other forms of contraception. This chart should not be used alone, but only as a summary of information in the accompanying text.

Source: Judith Willis, "Comparing Contraceptives," *FDA Consumer* 19.4 (1985), 30.

**Table 9.5** *Continued*

| Type | Estimated Effectiveness | Risks | Noncontraceptive Benefits | Convenience | Availability |
|---|---|---|---|---|---|
| Sponge | 80–87 percent | Rarely, irritation and allergic reactions; difficulty in removal; very rarely, toxic-shock syndrome | May give some protection against some sexually transmitted diseases | Can be inserted hours before intercourse, left in place up to twenty-four hours; disposable | OTC |
| Diaphragm with Spermicide | 80–98 percent | Rarely, irritation and allergic reactions, bladder infection, constipation; very rarely, toxic-shock syndrome | May give some protection against some sexually transmitted diseases | Inserted before intercourse; can be left in place twenty-four hours but additional spermicide must be inserted if intercourse is repeated | Rx |
| IUD | 95–96 percent | Cramps, bleeding, pelvic inflammatory disease; rarely, perforation of the uterus | None | After insertion, stays in place until physician removes it | Rx |
| Birth-Control Pills | 97 percent (Mini) 99 percent (Combination) | Not for smokers; blood clots, gall-bladder disease, noncancerous liver tumors, water retention, hypertension, mood changes, dizziness, nausea | Less menstrual bleeding and cramping, lower risk of fibrocystic breast disease, ovarian cysts, and pelvic inflammatory disease; may protect against cancer of the ovaries and of the lining of the uterus | Pill must be taken on daily schedule, regardless of the frequency of intercourse | Rx |
| Natural Family Planning or Rhythm | Very variable, perhaps 53–86 percent | None | None | Requires frequent monitoring of body functions and periods of abstinence | Instructions from physician or clinic |
| Vasectomy (Male Sterilization) | Over 99 percent | Pain; infection rarely; possible psychological problems | None | No care after surgery | Minor surgery |
| Tubal Ligation (Female Sterilization) | Over 99 percent | Surgical complications; some pain or discomfort; possibly higher risk of hysterectomy later in life | None | No care after surgery | Surgery |

9.1 ACTIVITY FOR WELLNESS 9.1

# Am I Going to Like This Method of Birth Control?

It is important to choose a method of birth control that works well to prevent pregnancy. It is also important to choose a method you will like! Ask yourself these questions so you can judge carefully.

What type of birth control are you thinking about? ____________________

Have you ever used it before? _____ yes _____ no If yes, how long did you use it? __________

________________________________________

| | Circle Your Answer | | |
|---|---|---|---|
| Are you afraid of using this method? | yes | no | don't know |
| Would you rather not use this method? | yes | no | don't know |
| Will you have trouble remembering to use this method? | yes | no | don't know |
| Have you ever become pregnant while using this method? | yes | no | don't know |
| Will you have trouble using this method carefully? | yes | no | don't know |
| Do you have unanswered questions about this method? | yes | no | don't know |
| Does this method make menstrual periods longer or more painful? | yes | no | don't know |
| Does this method cost more than you can afford? | yes | no | don't know |
| Does this method ever cause serious health problems? | yes | no | don't know |
| Do you object to this method because of religious beliefs? | yes | no | don't know |
| Have you already had problems using this method? | yes | no | don't know |
| Is your partner opposed to this method? | yes | no | don't know |
| Are you using this method without your partner's knowledge? | yes | no | don't know |
| Will using this method embarrass you? | yes | no | don't know |
| Will using this method embarrass your partner? | yes | no | don't know |
| Will you enjoy intercourse less because of this method? | yes | no | don't know |
| Will this method interrupt lovemaking? | yes | no | don't know |
| Has a nurse or doctor ever told you not to use this method? | yes | no | don't know |

Do you have any "don't know" answers? Ask your instructor or physician to help you with more information.

Do you have any "yes" answers? "Yes" answers mean you may not like this method. If you have several "yes" answers, chances go up that you might not like this method; you may need to think about another method.

Source: From Hatcher, Robert A., et al., *Contraceptive Technology 1984–1985,* 12th ed. © 1984 Irvington Publishers, New York. Reprinted by permission.

# ABORTION

The use of abortion is an important and hotly debated issue of the 1980s. The abortion debate, however, has been going on for some time. In 1962 the American Law Institute drafted the "Model Penal Code" which, among other things, called for abortion to be legalized under certain conditions.[36] In 1973 the U.S. Supreme Court (*Roe v. Wade*) established the conditions under which an abortion can be legally performed in America. In the first trimester (up to the sixteenth week) no state can outlaw a woman's right to an abortion. In the second trimester (up to the twenty-fourth week) states can control the circumstances under which a woman may have an abortion. In the third trimester states can outlaw abortion except in cases where the life or health of the pregnant woman is at stake. Since 1973 all fifty states under this ruling have legislated a whole host of regulations for second-trimester abortions. In subsequent cases the U.S. Supreme Court has ruled that a woman does not need parental consent for an abortion, nor does she need the consent of her spouse. These rulings are in line with the 1973 decision, which takes the position that a woman has the sole right to decide whether to continue or terminate her pregnancy.

## Types of Abortion

The medical definition of **abortion** is the termination of a pregnancy before the fetus is capable of extrauterine life. Abortions that occur naturally are termed miscarriages or spontaneous abortions. Voluntary abortions are termed induced abortions. There are several types of induced abortions. The timing of such an abortion will affect the abortion technique used.

**MENSTRUAL EXTRACTION** **Menstrual extraction** is a procedure that involves the use of suction to remove the lining of the uterus. Menstrual extraction is used in the first few weeks of pregnancy. Because it is used so early in the pregnancy it is difficult for the physician to be absolutely certain that the woman was indeed pregnant. Approximately 50 percent of the women receiving a menstrual extraction prior to the seventh day after a missed menses were actually pregnant.[37]

**VACUUM CURETTAGE** **Vacuum curettage,** a method that can be performed up until the thirteenth week, involves the insertion of a vacuum tool that suctions the contents of the uterus. There is little difference between a vacuum curettage and menstrual extraction. The philosophical difference is that the menstrual extraction is designed to prevent implantation while vacuum curettage is designed to end implantation. The menstrual extraction and vacuum curettage methods of abortion have the least amount of health risks of all abortions.

**DILATION AND CURETTAGE (D & C), AND DILATION AND EXTRACTION (D & E)** The **D & C** and **D & E** require the cervix to be dilated (expanded) to allow access to the uterus. Once the cervix is dilated, a physician can scrape the inner lining of the uterus (D & C) or use suction in addition to the scraping (D & E).

D & C and D & E are usually performed up until the sixteenth week of pregnancy. Eighty-four percent of abortions performed in America are D & E.[38] D & E is preferred because it reduces the chances of secondary infections, reduces blood loss, decreases the risk of uterine perforation, and requires less anesthetic.

**CHEMICAL ABORTIONS** In **chemical abortions** a toxic substance is introduced into the amniotic sac resulting in the premature delivery of a dead fetus. Saline, urea, and prostaglandins are the most common substances used to induce chemical abortions. These methods are used during the second trimester or up until the twenty-fourth week of gestation.

**HYSTEROTOMY** The **hysterotomy** is identical to a small cesarean section. An incision is made in the female's lower abdomen and then her uterus; the fetus is then removed. This procedure is usually done between twenty and twenty-four weeks of gestation. Hysterotomy is considered major intrauterine surgery and carries with it the inherent risks of such major surgery.

## Complications of Abortion

Abortions are an expensive method of birth control; they also carry substantial health risks, both physical and emotional.

**PHYSICAL-HEALTH RISKS** The physician's skill and abortion experience are factors in the effectiveness and subsequent health risk of the procedure. Some of the major physical-health concerns of abortion include the following:

- The female may develop a secondary infection as a result of an abortion.
- Females having abortions may experience uterine blood clots, injury to the intestines, hemorrhage, perforation of the uterus, and laceration of the cervix.
- Females with past abortions have a greater risk of future pregnancy failures and infant mortalities.[39]
- Females with past abortions may be more likely to have future pregnancy complications including low birth weight and premature births.[40]
- The death rate for abortions performed before the ninth week is one per 400,000 and after the sixteenth week is one per 10,000.[41]

**EMOTIONAL-HEALTH RISKS** There are also important emotional-health issues related to abortion. Guilt, anger, and sadness are only a few of the many emotions that may be experienced by a woman and her partner upon consideration of or use of an abortion. It is very important that women considering abortion receive unbiased professional counseling so that their feelings, values, and needs can be fully considered.[42]

Decisions about conception and birth control are often complex and emotional issues. Having a sound knowledge base regarding the wide range of birth-control options available is a starting point for wise decision making. Communication between sexual partners of their birth-control preferences and needs will add a valuable dimension to this process, and increase the chances for experiencing high levels of wellness. (See Exhibit 9.3)

9.3 EXHIBIT 9.3

# Beyond the Pill

A surprising number of new contraceptive techniques are at various stages of development. Some methods are available only outside the United States; such as *Depo-Provera,* a progesterone-like synthetic compound manufactured by the Upjohn Company. One injection prevents ovulation and conception for at least three months. It has been used by eleven million women in more than eighty countries, but is banned as a contraceptive in the U.S. Its possible licensing is currently the nation's primary contraception controversy. Several consumer and feminist groups are in the forefront of the opposition. Among their arguments: Under research conditions, Depo has caused tumors in some animals; women using it may experience weight gain, mood changes, and loss of libido; if a woman does not know that she is pregnant at the time of her injection, Depo could produce a defective fetus. Proponents (including the International Planned Parenthood Federation, the American College of Obstetricians and Gynecologists, and the World Health Organization) point out that Depo has been used in some countries for twenty years and that 100,000 women have used it for ten years or more, with no recorded deaths. Supporters and opponents agree that its most common side effect is a disturbed menstrual pattern.

Other methods are currently being tested in clinical trials, including RU-486 and Levonorgestrel.

*RU-486.* Now being tested in several countries, this is a menstruation-inducing pill taken two or three times a month. If pregnancy has already occurred, RU-486 will terminate it. Unlike the Pill, this protein compound does not affect the pituitary gland, and is therefore free of many of the Pill's side effects.

*Levonorgestrel.* This is a synthetic-hormonal compound that inhibits ovulation, discourages the uterine lining from accepting a fertilized egg, and impedes the passage of sperm by thickening the cervical mucus. It contains progestin but not estrogen, which causes several of the Pill's adverse side effects. Tests conducted abroad show the drug to be nearly 99 percent effective. It can be applied in two ways: an implant (six tiny silicone tubes in the arm) that lasts for up to five years, or a ring that fits around the cervix.

Source: From Lederer, Joseph, "The Man's Turn," in *Psychology Today* (June 1983). Reprinted with permission from *Psychology Today* magazine. 

## DISCUSSION QUESTIONS

1. Do you think there is a need for continuing research and development in contraceptive technology?

2. Would you (or your partner) be interested in using any of the birth-control methods described above?

3. What do you think are some of the cost, safety, effectiveness, and reversibility issues related to these experimental birth-control methods?

# SUMMARY

1. The birth-control options you use or avoid will have a considerable effect on your level of wellness.

2. There are several views regarding when life begins, each either accepting or rejecting fertilization, implantation, and gestational age as the benchmark of new human life.

3. Birth-control methods can be grouped into four categories: natural, mechanical, chemical, and invasive. These are often used in combination.

4. When deciding on a method of birth control it is important to consider the effectiveness, safety, cost, and reversibility of each available method.

5. Natural family-planning methods are designed to estimate when ovulation is occurring in the female.

6. The diaphragm, cervical cap, and contraceptive sponge are mechanical methods of birth control, often used with chemical spermicides, that prevent fertilization by trapping the sperm in the vagina, so the sperm cannot enter the uterus.

7. The condom is a mechanical method of birth control that prevents sperm from entering the vagina.

8. Spermicides are chemicals that prevent fertilization by destroying sperm.

9. IUDs are either a medicated or nonmedicated method of birth control; they are thought to end implantation of a fertilized egg.

10. Birth-control pills containing estrogen are thought to prevent pregnancy by inhibiting ovulation. Progestin-only pills change the quality of cervical mucus making it difficult for sperm to survive, slowing down the egg's journey through the fallopian tube, and inhibiting implantation of a fertilized egg.

11. Voluntary sterilization is an invasive method of birth control. Vasectomy, or male sterilization, involves the cutting and tying of the vas deferens. A vasectomy prevents fertilization by blocking sperm from entering the vas deferens during ejaculation. Tubal ligation, or female sterilization, involves the blocking of the fallopian tubes, thus preventing fertilization by preventing sperm from reaching the unfertilized egg.

12. The many types of abortion are used to terminate pregnancies at different stages of development.

### Recommended Readings

Djeassi, C. *The Politics of Contraception.* San Francisco: W. A. Freeman and Company, 1981.

Hatcher, Robert A.; Guest, Felicia; Stewart, Felicia; Stewart, Gary; Trussell, James; and Frank, Erica. *Contraceptive Technology 1984–1985,* 12th rev. Ed. New York: Irvington Publishers, 1984.

Jones, Kenneth L.; Shainberg, Louis W.; and Byer, Curtis O. *Dimensions of Human Sexuality.* Dubuque, Iowa: Wm. C. Brown Publishers, 1985.

Willis, Judith. "Comparing Contraceptives," *FDA Consumer* 19.4 (1985): 28–35.

### References

1. Robert A. Hatcher, Felicia Guest, Felicia Stewart, Gary Stewart, James Trussell, and Erica Frank, *Contraceptive Technology 1984–1985.* 12th rev. Ed. (New York: Irvington Publishers, 1984), 148.

2. Hatcher et al., *Contraceptive Technology,* 145.

3. Hatcher et al., *Contraceptive Technology,* 148.

4. M. Smith and B. Barwin, "Vaginal Contraceptive Devices," *Journal of the Canadian Medical Association* 129 (1983): 699–701.

5. "Virus, Diaphragm May Contribute to TSS," *Modern Medicine* 51.9 (1983): 67.

6. Hatcher et al., *Contraceptive Technology,* 109.

7. Judith Willis, "Comparing Contraceptives," *FDA Consumer* 19.4 (1985): 31.

8. Smith and Barwin, "Vaginal Contraceptive Devices."

9. Willis, "Comparing Contraceptives," 31.

10. Smith and Barwin, "Vaginal Contraceptive Devices."

11. Hatcher et al., *Contraceptive Technology,* 122.

12. Philip D. Darney, "New Developments in Barrier Methods of Contraception," *Sexual Medicine Today* 9.3 (1985): 8.

13. Hatcher et al., *Contraceptive Technology,* 118.

14. A. C. Richardson and J. B. Lyon, "The Effect of Condom Use on Squamous Cell Cervical Intraepithelial Neoplasia," *American Journal of Obstetrics and Gynecology,* 140 (1981): 909–13.

15. Richard L. Naeye, "Coitus and Associated Amniotic-Fluid Infections," *New England Journal of Medicine* 301 (1979): 1198–1200; R. Snowden, M. Williams, and D. Hawkins, *The IUD: A Practical Guide.* (London: Croom Helm, 1977).

16. Hatcher et al., *Contraceptive Technology,* 134.

17. Hatcher et al., *Contraceptive Technology,* 148.

18. S. C. Huber, "IUDs Reassessed—A Decade of Experience," *Population Reports* F.4 (Johns Hopkins Univ., 1974): F49–F64.

19. Laurie Liskin, "IUDs: An Appropriate Contraceptive for Many Women?" *Population Reports* B(4), (1982): B101–B135.

20. R. Kim-Farley et al., "Febrile Spontaneous Abortion and the IUD," *Contraception* 18 (1978): 561–70.

21. O. Liukko et al., "Ectopic Pregnancies during Use of Low-Dose Progestogens for Oral Contraception," *Contraception* 16 (1977): 575–80.

22. Hatcher et al., *Contraceptive Technology,* 80.

23. M. P. Bessey, M. Lawless, K. McPherson, and D. Yeates, "Fertility After Stopping Use of Interuterine Device," *British Medical Journal* 106 (1983): 286.

24. Hatcher et al., *Contraceptive Technology,* 64.

25. H. L. Judd and D. R. Meldrum, "Physiology and Pathophysiology of Menstruation and Menopause," in S. L. Romney, M. J. Gray, A. B. Little, J. A. Merrill, E. J. Quilligan, and R. W. Stander, *Gynecology and Obstetrics: The Health Care of Women,* 2d ed. (New York: McGraw-Hill, 1981), 886–907.

26. Willis, "Comparing Contraceptives," 33; M. Newhouse et al., "A Case Control Study of Carcinoma of the Ovary," *British Journal of Preventive and Social Medicine* 31 (1977): 148–53.

27. B. Hulka et al., "Protection against Endometrial Carcinoma by Combination-Product Oral Contraceptives," *Journal of the American Medical Association* 247 (1982): 475–77.

28. Liukko et al., "Ectopic Pregnancies."

29. Hatcher et al., *Contraceptive Technology,* 40–41.

30. Willis, "Comparing Contraceptives."

31. Willis, "Comparing Contraceptives."

32. D. Wolfers and H. Wolfers, *Vasectomy and Vasectomania* (St. Albans, England: Mayflower, 1974).

33. F. J. Massey et al. "Vasectomy and Health: Results from a Large Cohort Study," *Journal of the American Medical Association* 252 (1984): 1023–29.

34. Willis, "Comparing Contraceptives," 33.

35. Willis, "Comparing Contraceptives, 33.

36. C. Tietze, *Induced Abortion: 1979,* 3d ed. (New York: The Population Council, 1979).

37. T. Van der Vlought and P. T. Piotrow, "Menstrual Regulation Update," *Population Reports* F.4 (Johns Hopkins Univ., 1974): F49–F64.

38. Tietze, *Induced Abortion.*

39. C. Madore, W. Hawes, F. Many, and A. Hexter, "A Study on the Effects of Induced Abortion on Subsequent Pregnancy Outcome," *American Journal of Obstetrics and Gynecology* 139 (1981): 516–21.

40. New York State Department of Public Health, Office of Biostatistics, "Effects of Induced Abortion on Subsequent Reproductive Function" (Albany, N.Y.: 18 April 1980) (mimeo). Reviewed in *Family Planning Perspectives* 13 (1981): 80–81.

41. *Abortion Surveillance Report,* 1978. U.S. Department of Health and Human Services, Public Health Service, Centers for Disease Control, Bureau of Epidemiology, Family Planning Evaluation Division, Atlanta, Nov. 1980, 48.

42. Kenneth L. Jones, Louis W. Shainberg, and Curtis O. Byer, *Dimensions of Human Sexuality.* (Dubuque, Iowa: Wm. C. Brown Publishers, 1985), 463.

CHAPTER TEN

# Parenthood: Pregnancy and Parenting



Many decisions have been labeled "the most important decisions of your life"—who you marry, purchasing your first home, or choosing a career, to name a few. There is one life decision, however, that carries the ultimate responsibility—that of nurturing another human being. In the pages that follow we will explore the vocation of parenting.

You will be asked to consider seriously what it means to be a parent. Then you will see how the unborn child develops inside the mother's womb. You will learn about different options for assessing the mother's and unborn baby's health, as well as options for childbirth. In addition, the factors and options affecting couples who have difficulty procreating will be discussed. As you read this chapter take time to reflect on how the parenting experience can affect your level of wellness.

# SOCIAL AND PERSONAL INFLUENCES

In the "old days" procreating was a universal goal. In fact, one gauge of social status was the number of children a person had. People became parents because fertility technology was poor at best, and because children were an important cog in preindustrial societies. Some of the same preindustrial social rewards for procreating, such as heritage, mores, and tax incentives, have survived.

In the last thirty years several factors have contributed, either directly or indirectly, to the encouragement of small families and childless families. These factors include effective fertility technology, the rising divorce rate, an increase in women who work outside the home, overpopulation theories, and increased opportunities for self-satisfaction. Although cultures holding to traditional and contemporary philosophies of large family size can be found in America today, the national trend has seen a steady decrease in the size of families.

Children are a valued resource of most every society; they represent the vitality and immortality of both culture and person. Thus procreation is both a cultural and individual statement. Our ancestors had only to deal with the question of, "How many children?" You will be presented with much more complicated questions, such as "Should you become a parent?" and "How and when will you procreate?"

Many political, religious, cultural, and economic interests vie for the right to influence social mandates on natural and artificial procreation. By the end of this century, everyone will be wrestling with these issues; at the same time, people will cling to their own values, self-interests, and spiritual beliefs.

# PARENTHOOD

There are a variety of ways to become a parent: natural procreation, artificial procreation, through adoption, and by marrying into a family with children. Parents can be either married or single. Single parenthood can result from divorce, death, long separations due to occupational commitments, or from choosing parenthood without marriage.

The choice to become a parent is a momentous decision. Children have a profound and lasting effect on the lives of most parents who acquire ultimate responsibility for another human being.

First-time parents are often amazed how a child can dramatically and sometimes radically change their life-styles. For the first few years of a child's life, continuous adult supervision and nurturing are required. Parents find themselves adjusting their daily schedules in order to accommodate this new life. Children can make demands on their parents' occupational as well as recreational commitments. Parenting requires a great deal of time. (See figure 10.1.)

Many parents spend large amounts of energy and resources to locate apartments that allow children, neighbors with playmates for their child, and schools that meet their standards. Parents often find themselves in the baby-sitter market. In general, parents labor at establishing a social and physical environment which will support and enhance their child's wellness.

Although a child is an added expense on a family's budget, it almost seems sacrilegious to debate whether having a child is a financially sound decision. Nevertheless, some people do decide to postpone parenthood until they obtain a well-paying job, buy a house, or save up enough money. Whatever a couple's financial circumstances, it is reasonable for them to discuss the financial implications of parenthood. There is no magic figure under which a child should not be brought into the world, but future parents should work out a family budget.

## Making the Decision to Parent

The essential question to prospective parents is: Why do you want to become a parent? Do you need an excuse to go to Disney World each year, or attend Little League games? Do you want to carry on the family name, or provide grandchildren for your parents to spoil? Do you want to relive your childhood through your child? Do you want to have your child do and be what you could not accomplish and become? Or . . . Do you truly want to be part of some other person's life, joys, sorrows, and hopes? Do you want to be the first person a child loves and trusts? Do you want to experience the depths of your compassion and personal self-worth?

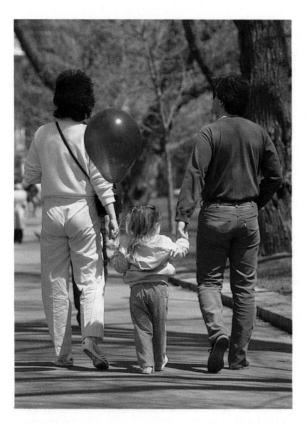

**Figure 10.1**
Small children require continuous adult supervision and nurturing.

Discovering the reasons why you want to become a parent will reveal some clues as to what kind of relationship will develop between you and your child. No one can predict who will be a good parent. You may explore your motives for wanting to be a parent by yourself and with your mate. Activity for Wellness 10.1 will help you in this exploration.

As you ponder the parenthood decision you will inevitably discover or rediscover your own motives and goals in life. Contemplating parenthood will cause you to review your priorities in life. Parenthood is one of the most important decisions any human being will make.

## Parenting

Since the 1950s Americans have been preoccupied with the art and science of parenting. The media tells American parents the "best" way to nurture their child, from toilet training to detecting drug consumption. The subject of parenting has been both popular and profitable. Still, there is no magic parenting formula that reduces parenting to a science, or guarantees the child will be all the parent hoped for.

America's preoccupation with parenting formulas has eroded some people's confidence in their ability to be successful parents. It is reasonable to assume that this lack of confidence can be detected by a child. This in turn can make parenting a difficult task. There are exceptions, but the vast majority of parents inherently have the necessary abilities and qualities to be successful in child rearing.

Rather than discussing "how to" parent, it is more enlightening to explore what parenting is. The vocation of parenting requires that the parent love his or her child. Without this love, parenting is reduced to caretaking.

The infant, and later the child, is molded by his or her environment. In other words, the parents and their environment become a model for the child. Early on, the child will emulate this model. Research suggests that this model is a good predictor of the child's future adult behavior.[1]

**PARENTAL EXPECTATIONS** All parents have expectations for their children. Some expectations are usually shared with the child, some are understood without verbal communication, and some are unknown to the child. These expectations include the values, life-styles, accomplishments, mannerisms, and personality a parent envisions for his or her child. Parents might want their male child to be, among other things, honest, hard working, and a professional athlete. Parents might want their female child to be, among other things, feminine, trustworthy, and a successful businesswoman. The virtues of such expectations are a matter of personal conviction. Such expectations will, however, affect the parent-child relationship and ultimately parenting.

Children who behave contrary to their parents' expectations may be unaware that their behavior is in conflict with their parents' expectations, unable to assume responsibility to fulfill their parents' expectations, or simply unwilling to fulfill these expectations. For example, a child may pursue playing the guitar as a possible occupation "unaware" that his parent would rather he become a gourmet chef.

10.1 ACTIVITY FOR WELLNESS

## Am I Parent Material?

For some people the answer to "Do I want to be a parent?" is obvious and unquestioned, but for others it is not. If we are uncertain, we can seek advice from others and try to learn from other people's experiences, but ultimately the decision is our own. Here is a sample of questions you might ask yourself in exploring your feelings about parenthood.

***Does having and raising a child fit the life-style I want?***

1. What do I want out of life for myself? What do I think is important?
2. Could I handle a child and a job at the same time? Would I have time and energy for both?
3. Would I be ready to give up the freedom to do what I want to do, when I want to do it?
4. Would I be willing to cut back my social life and spend more time at home? Would I miss my free time and privacy?
5. Can I afford to support a child? Do I know how much it takes to raise a child?
6. Do I want to raise a child in the neighborhood where I live now? Would I be willing and able to move?
7. How would a child interfere with my growth and development?
8. Would a child change my educational plans? Do I have the energy to go to school and raise a child at the same time?
9. Am I willing to give a great part of my life—at least eighteen years—to being responsible for a child? And spend a large portion of my life being concerned about my child's well-being?

***What's in it for me?***

1. Do I like doing things with children? Do I enjoy activities that children can do?
2. Would I want a child to be "like me"?
3. Would I try to pass on to my child my ideas and values? What if my child's ideas and values turn out to be different from my own?
4. Would I want my child to achieve things that I wish I had, but didn't?
5. Would I expect my child to keep me from being lonely in my old age? Do I do that for my parents? Do my parents do that for my grandparents?
6. Do I want a boy or a girl child? What if I don't get what I want?
7. Would having a child show others how mature I am?
8. Will I prove I am a man or a woman by having a child?

A parent may scold a child for talking during religious services, but the child may be "unable" to comprehend the request because of her young age. A young boy aware of his parents' expectations for him not to date girls, may be "unwilling" to comply because of his personal attraction to a special female friend.

Parenting becomes easier when children are aware of parental expectations. Parents who expect their child not to use profanity, not to talk to strangers, and to be respectful toward elders need to tell the child of these expectations. In cases where a child is unable or unwilling to fulfill such expectations, parents can either enforce their expectations, modify them to meet the abilities or desires of the child, or withdraw them totally.

The decision to enforce, modify, or withdraw an expectation is based on the parents' values and judgment. Children will inevitably not meet all of their

## ACTIVITY FOR WELLNESS 10.1

9. Do I expect my child to make my life happy?

***Raising a child? What's there to know?***

1. Do I like children? When I'm around children for a while, what do I think or feel about having one around all of the time?

2. Do I enjoy teaching others?

3. Is it easy for me to tell other people what I want, or need, or what I expect of them?

4. Do I want to give a child the love he or she needs? Is loving easy for me?

5. Am I patient enough to deal with the noise and the confusion and the twenty-four-hour-a-day responsibility? What kind of time and space do I need for myself?

6. What do I do when I get angry or upset? Would I take things out on a child if I lost my temper?

7. What does discipline mean to me? What does freedom, or setting limits, or giving space mean? What is being too strict, or not strict enough? Would I want a perfect child?

8. How do I get along with my parents? What will I do to avoid the mistakes my parents made?

9. How would I take care of my child's health and safety? How do I take care of my own?

10. What if I have a child and find out I made a wrong decision?

***Have my partner and I really talked about becoming parents?***

1. Does my partner want to have a child? Have we talked about our reasons?

2. Could we give a child a good home? Is our relationship a happy and strong one?

3. Are we both ready to give our time and energy to raising a child?

4. Could we share our love with a child without jealousy?

5. What would happen if we separated after having a child, or if one of us should die?

6. Do my partner and I understand each other's feelings about religion, work, family, child raising, future goals? Do we feel pretty much the same way? Will children fit into these feelings, hopes, and plans?

7. Suppose one of us wants a child and the other doesn't? Who decides?

8. Which of the questions listed here do we need to really discuss before making a decision?

Source: "Am I Parent Material?" National Alliance for Optional Parenthood, Washington, D.C.

parents' expectations. Parents need to assess the unique personality and feelings of their child when their expectations are not met. Is what they are requiring of or denying their child a self-serving indulgence on the part of the parent? One example might be a child who enjoys classical literature but whose parents believe he or she should take more business courses because the occupational outlook in classical literature is limited. In this case, a compromise is certainly possible. Another example might be a parent who denies his or her child permission to date because the parent believes this will increase the child's chances of an early marriage or an unwanted pregnancy. The child may find dating personally fulfilling, but want to remain a virgin, and not want to get married in the near future. In this case, the expectations of the parent and child may be identical, but this fact may be unknown to either of them.

10.1 EXHIBIT 10.1

## Mind Wrestling with Parental Expectations

**CHILDREN SHOULD NOT ENGAGE IN INTERCOURSE**

***Logic Debate***

Parent: You are not physically or financially ready for children.
Child: Birth control is quite effective today.

***Values Debate***

Parent: It is against my faith for unmarried people to have intercourse.
Child: I don't believe in your religion.

***Tradition Debate***

Parent: In my day young people were virgins until marriage.
Child: In your day people got married in their teens; today they are getting married in their twenties and thirties.

***Self-Respect Debate***

Parent: You lose your self-respect when you have intercourse with someone you are not married to.
Child: Not if that person loves you.

***Guilt Debate***

Parent: Your father would be crushed and so would I, if you lost your virginity.
Child: How would you feel if I lost the person I loved because of my virginity?

### DISCUSSION QUESTIONS

1. How many of the above types of debate do you use when dealing with parental expectations?
2. Do both sides of each debate have merit?

In any case, as children mature they have more influence on their parents' expectations. Children seek personal independence as they mature. Ultimately, children either reject or accept some, or many, of their parents' expectations. This process will find both parent and child using a variety of techniques to debate the merits of an expectation. Maybe that is the true purpose of parental expectations. Be that as it may, the child ultimately decides which expectations are reasonable and worthy of pursuit.

### ENFORCING PARENTAL EXPECTATIONS

Some parents believe that they have no control over their children. Such a view is an underestimation of their parental control. Parents possess the most powerful human intoxicant known . . . love. Parents can give or deny love to their children. This parental power can be more confining than a jail cell or more nurturing than a warehouse full of literary and art treasures. Parents may give their children love without question, they may hold their love for ransom, or they may deny their children love.

Parenting where parental love is in question can only be burdensome. The child soon learns that he or she is only lovable under certain conditions, or not lovable at all. Denying love to a child changes the kind of parenting experience that will develop. Children who are only shown love when they do chores or remain silent during adult conversation will in turn view love as a reward and punishment exercise. In practice these children may use love as a behavior modification tool to control other persons. There are few if any virtues to this practice. Parental love is "the" essential ingredient in human parenting. Love's omnipresence underlies all parent-child interactions. Children value their parents' love and this in turn makes them receptive to their parents' desires and needs. Most children accommodate their parents' expectations as best they can.

# PREGNANCY

There are numerous health concerns that affect wellness before and during a pregnancy. That is why **prenatal care** (before birth) is essential to the wellness of both mother and infant. Ideally, the female and her mate will begin prenatal care before pregnancy.

There are several health considerations a female should address before she becomes pregnant. One such consideration is her overall physical health. The female should not be infected with German measles (rubella) or a sexually transmitted disease (STD) just before or during pregnancy as these conditions may lead to pregnancy complications and birth defects. The prospective parents should determine whether there is a history of hereditary disease in their families. The couple may consider genetic counseling as a means of determining the likelihood of producing a child with a genetic disorder. Such counseling would educate the prospective parents on the nature of a particular disorder, and the medical options available to them and their future child.

Prenatal care increases the chances of the mother bearing a healthy baby. In addition, prenatal care will allow for the detection of potential and actual pregnancy problems. For example, one tool in prenatal care is ultrasonic fetal examinations. These ultrasound machines can produce an image of the fetus using relatively harmless sound waves. These tests can provide data about how the fetus is developing and whether any medical attention is required to treat the fetus while in the womb, or soon after birth. Prenatal care enables the parents to select options which will reduce the risk of pregnancy complications and congenital disorders. The physician becomes an important consultant during this time.

## Chemicals and Prenatal Development

Prospective parents should consider the female's drug use prior to and throughout her pregnancy. It may be as long as two to three weeks after a missed period when a pregnancy is confirmed. For women not planning a pregnancy the time lag may be greater. The day a woman is informed she is pregnant is not the day her pregnancy began. Confirming a pregnancy three weeks after a missed period may mean that the woman is five weeks pregnant. There is growing evidence that the first forty days of prenatal development are the most important.

Potentially harmful chemicals can be introduced to the fetus via the mother's blood. One such chemical is alcohol. Alcohol consumption during pregnancy has been linked to an increase in spontaneous abortions, as well as congenital heart defects, retardation, physical malformations, and other deformities.[2] The congenital defects produced by the mother's consumption of alcohol are referred to as **Fetal Alcohol Syndrome (FAS).** Chapter 12 provides greater detail on the health problems of FAS.

There are many other chemicals commonly used which may cause problems for the mother or fetus. The antibiotic tetracycline, if taken during pregnancy, can cause staining of the infant's teeth and stunt its long-bone growth.[3] Other antibiotics may cause congenital cataracts. Chemicals from tobacco smoke increase the risk of spontaneous abortion, stillbirth, and low birth weight.[4] Some evidence suggests that caffeine intake during pregnancy may result in lower birth weights and skeletal abnormalities.[5] Additionally, although it is not a drug, pregnant females should avoid X-ray radiation.

Although there is no definitive evidence in all cases, the prudent course of action is for the female to avoid the use of all prescription, over-the-counter (OTC), and illegal drugs from the first day of the reproductive cycle she chooses to become pregnant until after childbirth. (See table 10.1.) Mothers who breast-feed continue to abstain from drugs until the child is weaned (taken off the mother's milk).

Many women of childbearing age seem to be aware of the major risks chemicals pose to pregnancy. A 1981 U.S. survey of 1,499 people, conducted for the FDA by Louis Harris and Associates, revealed that 54 percent of the respondents acknowledged alcohol as a risk to pregnancy outcome.

**Table 10.1 OTCs and the Pregnant Woman**

| Medication/Substance | Adverse Effects on Fetus | Comments |
|---|---|---|
| Antacids | One report of a higher than usual incidence of congenital malformation | Avoid chronic ingestion of antacids containing a high sodium content, especially for those who have hypertension associated with pregnancy or fluid retention. |
| Antinauseants<br>Cyclizine (Marezine) Meclizine HCl (Antivert, Bonine) | Animal studies show teratogenicity. No evidence of teratogenicity in humans | Pregnancy is listed as a contraindication of these drugs.[2] |
| Bromides<br>In sleeping aids (i.e., Sominex, Nite-Rest Capsules, Quiet World, Sleep-Eze) | Neonatal hypotonic and neurologic depression; reports of infants manifesting irritability, difficulty in feeding, hypertonia, lethargy, and rash as signs of bromide intoxication; neonatal ileus and death have been suggested | Contraindicated in pregnant women; serum half-life of transplacentally acquired bromide is 8.5 days.[2–4] |
| Caffeine<br>Coffee, tea, cola, and internal analgesics containing caffeine, e.g., Excedrin; weight control products, e.g., Dexatrim; and stimulant products, e.g., Tirend and Double-E Alertness | Increased incidence of stillbirth, spontaneous abortion, and premature delivery | The adverse effects are associated with a caffeine consumption $>$ 600 mg/day, which is equivalent to about six cups/day.[2–4] |
| Cannabis<br>Marijuana | Increased incidence of anomalies in the newborn | Evidence is not conclusive.[5] |
| Ethanol<br>(Ethyl alcohol) | Fetal alcoholic syndrome—growth abnormalities, microcephaly, decreased IQ, central nervous system dysfunction; stillbirth; lower birth weight; acute alcohol withdrawal, and late hemorrhagic disease of the newborn; decreased unconjugated bilirubin; chromosomal defects; and transient muscular hypotonia of newborn when alcohol is ingested by the mother near labor | The amount of alcohol ingested by the mother to cause adverse effects is controversial; no absolutely safe level of ethanol consumption has yet been established.[2] |
| Laxatives | Purgatives, e.g., castor oil, may induce labor and should be avoided | Constipation should be relieved by fluids and laxative foods, e.g., fruits, vegetables, or a mild stool softener.[2] |
| Iodides<br>In cough medicines (e.g., containing potassium iodide) | Congenital goiter; hypothyroidism; mental retardation; and neonatal death | Teratogenesis associated with maternal ingestion of iodides is well documented. Early diagnosis with proper treatment is crucial in minimizing usually reversible adverse effects.[2–4] |
| Mineral oil | Regular use during pregnancy may reduce absorption of vitamin K, causing hypoprothrombinemia and hemorrhagic disorder in newborn; may also impair absorption of fat-soluble vitamins (A, D, E) and essential fatty acids | Contraindicated in pregnancy.[2] |

| Medication/Substance | Adverse Effects on Fetus | Comments |
|---|---|---|
| Nicotine (Tobacco) | Decrease in birth weight; increased incidence of abortion and premature birth; stillbirth, decrease in fetal breathing time; hyperkinesis; hyperirritability; and delayed crying time | Although smoking is clearly associated with many side effects, more data are needed to substantiate the claim that it increases the incidence of major malformations.[2-4] |
| Salicylates (Aspirin, Empirin, Anacin, etc.) | Decreased birth weight, prolonged gestation by inhibiting prostaglandin synthesis; increased stillbirth and perinatal mortality; inhibit fetal and neonatal platelet function, causing hemorrhagic tendency in newborn; and may cause hyperbilirubinemia | Congenital anomalies are more common in women taking salicylates in first trimester, but no cause and effect relationship has been proved. They should be avoided during the week before delivery.[2-4,6] |
| Vitamin A | Hypervitaminosis A may cause cleft palate, bone, and skull deformities, increased intracranial pressure, exophthalmos, papilledema, drying and cracking of skin, increased pigmentation, and jaundice | Recommended daily allowance (RDA) for normal pregnant woman is 5,000 IU.[2,3,7] |
| Vitamin $B_6$ | Large maternal doses of pyridoxine (vitamin $B_6$) have subjected neonates to withdrawal seizure after birth | RDA for normal pregnant woman is 2.6 mg.[2,7] |
| Vitamin C | The fetus may adapt to a high level of vitamin C in the mother and induced scurvy may occur shortly after birth when the intake of the vitamin drops to normal levels | RDA for normal pregnant woman is 80 mg.[2,7] |
| Vitamin D | Large doses during pregnancy may result in congenital supravalvular aortic stenosis, mental retardation, vasculotoxicity, and hypercalcemia | RDA for normal pregnant woman is 400 IU.[2,3,7] |
| Vitamin K | Has been implicated in causing hemolytic anemia, hyperbilirubinemia, and kernicterus in the newborn, especially premature infants | Menadione should not be given to women during the last few weeks of pregnancy. Phytonadione has not been shown to produce similar adverse effects.[2,3,7] |

References

[1]T. M. Shepard and A. G. Fantel, "Teratogenicity of Therapeutic Agents," in: L. Iffy, H. A. Kaminetzky, eds. *Principles and Practice of Obstetrics and Perinatology,* vol 1 (New York: John Wiley & Sons, 1981), 461–97.
[2]C. J. Latiolais, R. Schad, P. Schneider, "OTC Medications and Other Substances Hazardous to Use during Pregnancy," in: M. M., Houston, ed., *Modern Medicine OB-GYN Pocket Guide* (New York: Harcourt Brace Jovanovich, 1981), 54–56.
[3]J. E. Knoben, P. O. Anderson, A. S. Watanabe, eds., *Handbook of Clinical Drug Data* (Hamilton, Ill.: Drug Intelligence Publications, 1979), 119–31.
[4]R. H. Levin, "Teratogenicity and Drug Excretion in Breast Milk (Maternogenicity)," in: E. T Herfindal and J. L. Hirschman, eds., *Clinical Pharmacy and Therapeutics* (Baltimore: Williams & Wilkins, 1979), 22–36.
[5]R. C. Benson, *Current Obstetric and Gynecologic Diagnosis Treatment* (Los Angeles: Lange Medical Publications, 1980), 604.
[6]W.K.V. Tyle, Internal Analgesic Product," in: L. I. Corrigan, J. Welsh, M. T. Rasmussen, eds., *Handbook of Non-Prescription Drugs* (Washington, D.C.: APhA, 1979), 132–33.
[7]E. K. Kastrup, ed., *Facts and Comparisons* (St. Louis, Mo.: J.B. Lippincott, 1981): 4–41, 163.

Additional references

M. M. Nelson, J. O. Forfar, "Association between Drugs Administered during Pregnancy and Congenital Abnormalities of the Fetus, *Br Med J* 1 (1971): 523.
S. K. Clarren, D. W. Smith, "The Fetal Alcoholic Syndrome," *New Engl J Med* 298 (1978): 1063–67.

Source: This table is adapted from the Cook County Hospital Pharmacy Newsletter. Mr. Wong is a staff pharmacist and Dr. Chen is associate director, department of pharmacy services, Cook County Hospital, Chicago.

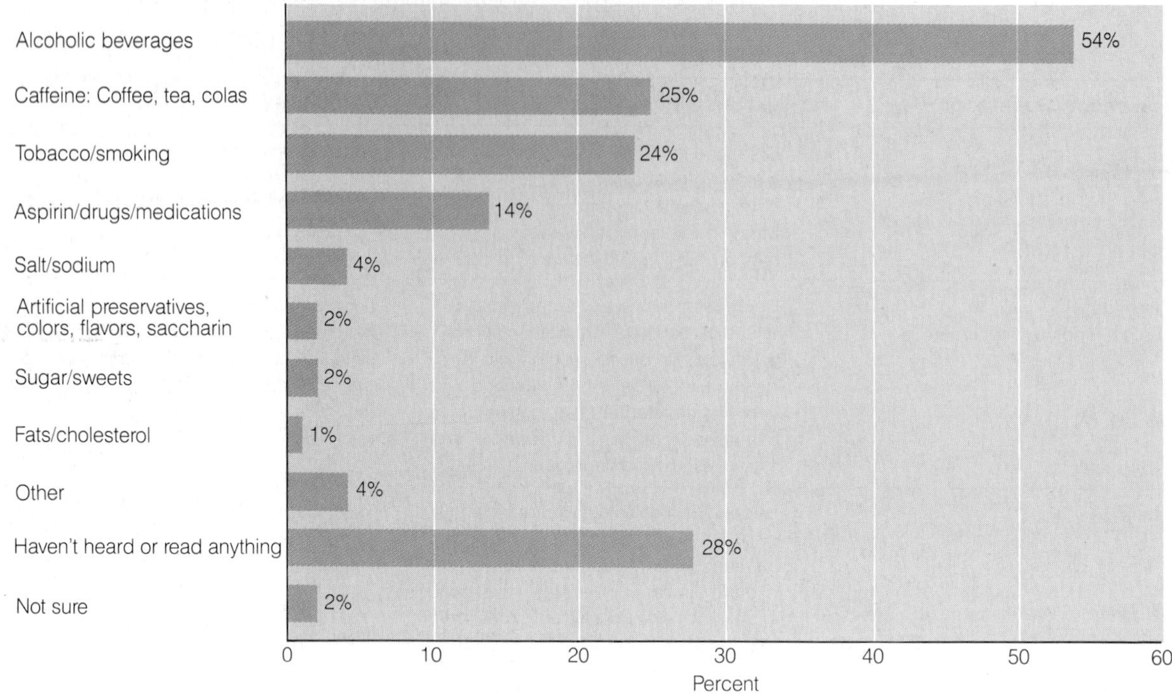


**Figure 10.2**
What have you recently read or heard of that pregnant women should not eat or drink, or eat or drink too much of?

A quarter of the respondents (25 percent) identified caffeine consumption as a risk and 24 percent mentioned smoking. Additionally, 14 percent were aware that other drugs and medications were also a risk when consumed during pregnancy.[6] (See figure 10.2.)

## Nutrition during Pregnancy

The nutritional needs of women increase significantly during pregnancy. The Recommended Dietary Allowances reflect this greater need. The average pregnant woman needs to increase her intake of calories by about 15 percent so that her minimum daily count is 2,400 calories.[7] Physicians recommend that during pregnancy a woman gain twenty-two to twenty-six pounds. This weight gain will vary somewhat during a pregnancy, with the greatest weight gain occurring during the last six months. A pregnant woman should average a gain of slightly less than one pound a week during the last six months.

In addition to more calories, the need for protein, vitamins, and minerals also increases. Although many physicians prescribe a vitamin/mineral supplement for pregnant women, this does not negate the need for a well-balanced diet. Pregnant women need to pay special attention to their food intake regarding protein, iron, calcium, sodium, and B-complex vitamins. (See table 10.2.)

**Table 10.2 Daily Food Guide During Pregnancy**

| The Five Food Groups | How Much Each Day—Servings and Sources |
|---|---|
| *Fruits and Vegetables*<br>Fruits and vegetables contain vitamins, minerals, and fiber, a natural laxative. The dark green leafy vegetables and deep yellow vegetables are rich in vitamin A. The dark green leafy vegetables are also valuable for iron, vitamin C, magnesium, folacin, and riboflavin. | Eat *at least one* serving of a good source of vitamin A *every other day:*<br>Apricots; Broccoli; Cantaloupe; Carrots; Dark-green leafy vegetables—beet greens, chard, collards, kale, mustard greens, spinach, turnip greens; Pumpkin; Sweet potatoes; Winter Squash<br><br>Eat *at least one* serving of a good source of vitamin C *every day:*<br>Broccoli; Brussel sprouts; Cantaloupe; Cauliflower; Green or sweet red pepper; Grapefruit or grapefruit juice; Orange or orange juice; Tomatoes; Dark-green leafy vegetables—chard, collards, kale, mustard greens, spinach, turnip greens; Cabbage; Strawberries; Watermelon<br><br>Select *two* servings of other vegetables and fruit *each day:*<br>Beets; Corn; Eggplant; Green and wax beans; Lettuce; Peas; Potatoes; Squash; Apples; Bananas; Cherries; Grapes; Pears; Pineapple; Plums |
| *Meat, Fish, Poultry, Eggs, Dried Beans and Peas, Nuts*<br>Meat, fish, poultry, eggs, dried beans and peas, seeds, nuts, and peanut butter supply protein as well as vitamins and minerals. Protein is needed to help build new tissues for you and your baby. | Eat *three* servings of protein food *daily:*<br><br>These amounts equal one serving:<br>• 2 or 3 ounces lean meat (Remove the extra fat when possible). Some examples: 1 hamburger, 2 thin slices of beef, pork, lamb or veal, 1 lean pork chop, 2 slices luncheon meat, 2 hot dogs.<br>• 2 or 3 ounces of fish. Some examples: 1 whole small fish, 1 small fish fillet, ⅓ of a 6½ ounce can of tuna fish or salmon.<br>• 2 or 3 ounces of chicken, turkey, or other poultry. Some examples: 2 slices light or dark meat turkey, 1 chicken leg, ½ chicken breast.<br><br>These amounts equal one-half serving:<br>• ½ to ¾ cup cooked dried beans, peas, or lentils, garbanzos (chick peas);<br>• 2 to 3 tablespoons peanut butter;<br>• 1 or 2 slices cheese;<br>• 1 egg;<br>• 1 cup tofu;<br>• 4 to 6 tablespoons nuts or seeds. |

Source: Adapted from *Prenatal Care,* U.S. Department of Health and Human Services, Public Health Service, Publication No. (HRSA) 83–5070. (Washington D.C.: U.S. Government Printing Office, 1983.)

**Table 10.2** *Continued*

| The Five Food Groups | How Much Each Day—Servings and Sources |
|---|---|
| *Milk and Milk Products*<br>You need four 8-ounce glasses of milk or milk products daily to give you and your baby the calcium and other nutrients needed for strong bones and teeth. Choose milks that have vitamin D added. You may select whole milk, buttermilk, lowfat milk, or dry or fluid skim milk. Lowfat milk and skim milk have fewer calories than whole milk. Milk or cheese used in making soup, pudding, sauces, and other foods count toward the total amount of milk you use. | Eat *four* 8-ounce glasses of milk or milk products *daily:*<br>These amounts equal the calcium in one 8-ounce glass of milk:<br>• 1 cup liquid skim milk, low fat milk, or buttermilk;<br>• ½ cup evaporated milk (undiluted);<br>• 2 one-inch cubes or 2 slices of cheese;<br>• ⅓ cup instant powdered milk;<br>• 1 cup plain yogurt, custard, or milk pudding.<br>These amounts equal the calcium in ⅓ cup of milk:<br>• ⅔ cup cottage cheese;<br>• ½ cup ice cream. |
| *Whole Grain or Enriched Breads and Cereals*<br>Breads and cereal foods provide minerals and vitamins, particularly the B vitamins and iron, as well as protein. Whole grain breads and cereals provide essential trace elements such as zinc, and also fiber, a natural laxative. Check the labels on breads and cereals to make sure that they are made with whole wheat or whole grain flour or are enriched with minerals and vitamins. | Eat *four or five* servings of whole grain or enriched breads, cereals, and cereal products *every day.*<br>These amounts equal one serving:<br>• 1 slice of bread;<br>• 1 muffin;<br>• 1 roll or biscuit;<br>• 1 tortilla or taco shell;<br>• ½ to ¾ cup cooked or ready-to-eat cereal, such as oatmeal, farina, grits, raisin bran, shredded wheat;<br>• 1 cup popcorn (1½ tablespoons, unpopped);<br>• ½ to ¾ cup noodles, spaghetti, rice, bulgur, macaroni;<br>• 2 small pancakes;<br>• 1 section waffle;<br>• 2 graham crackers or 4 to 6 small crackers.<br>These amounts count as two servings:<br>• 1 hamburger bun or hotdog roll;<br>• 1 English muffin. |
| *Fats and Sweets*<br>This group of other foods includes margarine, butter, candy, jellies, sugars, syrups, desserts, soft drinks, snack foods, salad dressings, vegetable oils, and other fats used in cooking. Most of these foods are high in fat, sugar, or salt. Use them to meet additional caloric needs after basic nutritional needs have been met. Eating too much fat and too many sweets may crowd out other necessary nutrients. | No specific number or types of servings are recommended for fats and sweets. |

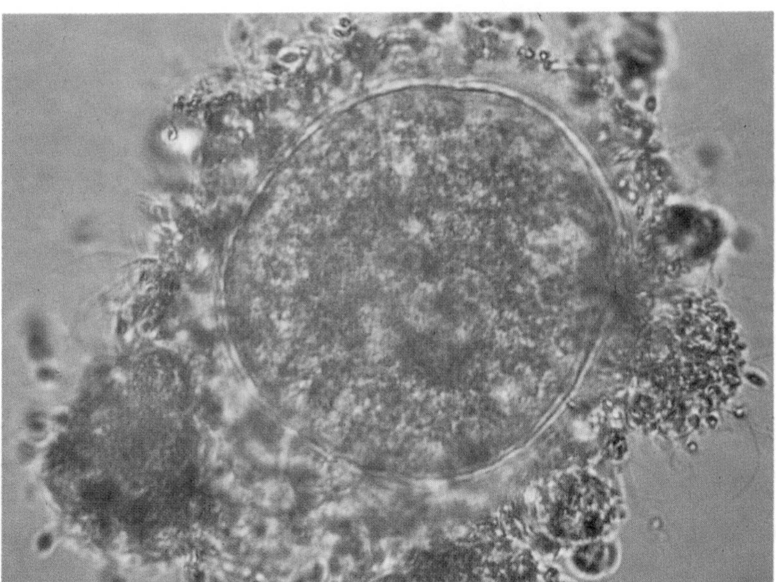

**Figure 10.3**
Pregnancy begins when an egg is fertilized.

## Prenatal Development

Pregnancy begins when an egg is fertilized (see figure 10.3), and ends with childbirth. It takes approximately 266 days (or thirty-eight weeks)—about nine calendar months—for a baby to develop fully. Pregnancy is divided into three phases called trimesters. The **first trimester** begins at the point of fertilization and continues to the end of the third month. The **second trimester** begins at the beginning of the fourth month and continues to the end of the sixth month. The **third trimester** begins at the beginning of the seventh month and continues until childbirth. Pregnancies that last until the ninth month are called **full-term** pregnancies.

**IMPLANTATION** By the sixth or seventh day after fertilization the fertilized egg will have traveled through the fallopian tubes where fertilization occurred, and implanted itself in the uterus. The female does not experience any physical sensation resulting from implantation. Sometimes implantation may cause "spotting" or bleeding, and this bleeding could be misdiagnosed as the onset of menstruation.

**TWINS** Identical twins, which come from the same fertilized egg, are formed sometime between fertilization and implantation, when the fertilized egg separates into two masses. Identical twins will be exact duplicates of each other in every way, from their physical appearance to their blood type.

Fraternal twins are created from two eggs that were fertilized independently. Thus fraternal twins do not share identical chromosomes. Fraternal twins are not identical in appearance or physiology. Approximately 70 percent of all twin births are fraternal and the remainder identical. Multiple births of three or more can be fraternal, identical, or both.

**EMBRYONIC PERIOD** For the first eight weeks after fertilization the developing baby is called an **embryo.** By the end of the first month the embryo is two-tenths of an inch long. The brain, eyes, spinal cord, nose, limbs, liver, pancreas, and gallbladder have begun to develop. The tube that will become the heart begins to pulsate.

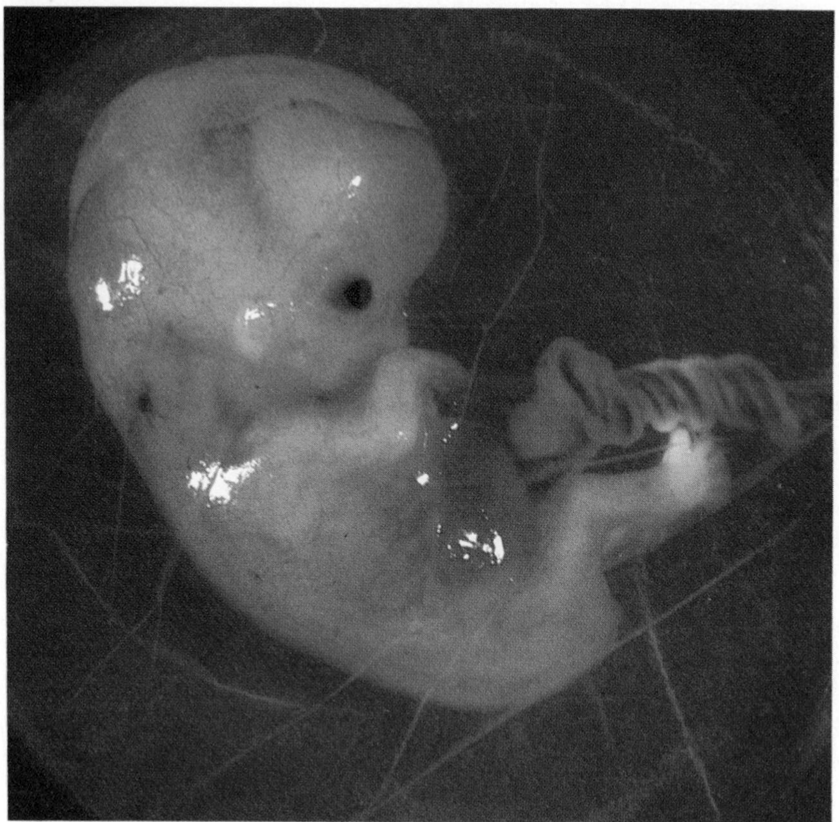

**Figure 10.4**
By the end of the second month, an embryo has fingers, toes, and many other attributes.

By the end of the second month the embryo has fingers, toes, blood vessels, lips, ears, eyelids, and a nose. (See figure 10.4.) Testicular tissue appears in male embryos, but female embryos will not begin to develop their reproductive organs until the following month. The embryo is now 1.2 inches long and weighs 1 gram (0.04 ounces).

**Amniotic Sac** During the embryonic period, important membranes will begin to form. The outer membrane, the **chorion,** and the inner membrane, the **amnion,** are tissue sacs which enclose the developing embryo, and later the fetus, until childbirth. These sacs hold amniotic fluid in which the embryo is submersed. The **amniotic fluid** acts as a barrier to physical shock and also serves to maintain the proper temperature.

**Placenta** The **placenta** will also begin to form during the embryonic period. The placenta is a temporary organ that transfers nutrients and oxygen to the embryo, and later to the fetus. The placenta secretes hormones in order to maintain pregnancy. The placenta is expelled by uterine contractions after childbirth.

**Umbilical Cord** The embryo, and later the fetus, is connected to the placenta by an **umbilical cord.** The umbilical cord contains two arteries and one vein. The maternal blood is circulated through the uterine side of the placenta. Although the two circulatory systems never physically mix, the placenta allows nutrients and oxygen to pass from the maternal blood to the embryo/fetal blood. The placenta also allows the waste products of the embryo/fetal blood to pass through to the maternal blood.

**FETUS** During the third month of pregnancy the embryo becomes a **fetus.** At the end of the third month the fetus has toenails, fingernails, fingerprints, and an excretory system. The fetus will demonstrate breathing motions by moving amniotic fluid in and out of its lungs. The fetus is able to move its fingers, arms, and neck. Additionally, the fetus will weigh two-thirds of an ounce and be four inches long.

By the end of the fourth month, the fetus weighs about six ounces and is about eight to ten inches long. During the fourth month **quickening** usually occurs. Quickening is the first fetal movement felt by the mother. The fetus will move its arms and legs and also demonstrate a swallowing reflex.

By the end of the fifth month the fetus weighs about one pound and will be about twelve inches long. The fetal heartbeat can now be heard with an ordinary stethoscope, and beats approximately 150 times per minute. The fetus will respond to lights and sounds and will spend part of its time awake and part asleep. The youngest fetus to survive outside its mother had an estimated gestation age of nineteen weeks.

By the end of the sixth month (second trimester) the fetus weighs about one-and-one-half pounds, is about fourteen inches long, and is very active. Mothers will regularly feel the movement of the fetus from then on. Ninety percent of the final fetal birth weight is yet to be gained.

By the end of the seventh month the fetus will usually turn upside down, head first into the birthing position. Babies not born in the head-first position are called breech. **Breech births** include buttocks first, legs first, or shoulder first presentations. Breech births can cause medical complications for both mother and infant. During the seventh month the fetus is covered with lanugo, a downy hair that will be shed before birth. The eyelids, which fused closed in the third month, will reopen. The fetus may begin to suck its thumb during the seventh month. The brain and nervous system are completely developed. The chances are 50 percent that the fetus will survive childbirth if born in the seventh month. The fetus weighs about four pounds.

By the end of the eighth month the fetus can taste sweet substances.[8] The fetus has a 95 percent chance of surviving childbirth. By the ninth month (full-term pregnancy) the survival rate in childbirth is better than 99 percent. The fetus is less active because of its cramped environment. All fetal eyes are blue and will change to another color (if genetically predetermined) when exposed to light following childbirth. The same is true of fetal skin color, which is pink or blue-pink. The genetically predetermined skin color will not fully appear until after its exposure to light. A full-term infant will weigh from six to nine pounds and measure about twenty inches.

## Pregnancy Indicators

There are several bodily changes that are caused by the hormones produced during pregnancy. The first such signs include the absence of menstruation, tingling nipples, enlarged or sensitive breasts, increased pigmentation around the nipples, increased urination, fatigue, and morning sickness. **Morning sickness** refers to the nausea and vomiting a pregnant female may experience throughout the day or night. These signs and symptoms are said to be "presumptive indicators" of pregnancy.

When presumptive indicators of pregnancy appear most women choose to have a pregnancy test. Pregnancy tests are based on the detection of a hormone in the female's blood or urine. This hormone is produced by the implanted embryo. The hormone is called **human chorionic gonadotropin (HCG).**

Laboratory pregnancy tests that use urine as the medium to detect HCG can be used as early as the first week after a missed menstrual period.

There are over-the-counter (OTC) pregnancy-test kits which the woman herself can perform. In general, these tests are less accurate than the ones performed by laboratory technicians. Many OTC pregnancy-test kits use a process which detects any protein contained in the urine, including HCG. Thus they have a 20 percent rate of false positive results (results which indicate that the female is pregnant, when she is not).[9] Other OTC kits test specifically for HCG; these are more accurate.

The most sensitive pregnancy blood test is the radioimmunoassay which can detect HCG as early as twenty-three days after the last menstrual period or one week "before" a missed menstrual period. This test is performed by a medical laboratory, takes about twenty-four hours, and is between 95 and 99 percent reliable.[10]

## Physiological Maternal Changes

During the first trimester the pregnant woman's breasts will swell and tingle. Her nipples may darken and broaden. She will urinate more frequently and her bowel movements may become irregular. She may experience nausea, and desire or be revolted by particular foods. During the second trimester the pregnant woman may experience hemorrhoids, nosebleeds, and edema. **Edema** is the swelling of arms and legs caused by the retention of water. The second trimester is also the time when the woman usually experiences the first movements of the fetus. During the third trimester there is increased pressure on several organs including the uterus, stomach, bladder, and lungs. These conditions may result in shortness of breath and heartburn. Nulliparous women (those who have never given birth) may experience "dropping," when the head of the fetus drops into position within the pelvis.

**Table 10.3 Pregnancy-Related Alterations in Sexual Response**

| Stage | Changes |
|---|---|
| Excitement and plateau | Breasts—tenderness, discomfort, enhanced erotic response; milk let-down after orgasm in late pregnancy<br>Labia—feeling of fullness<br>Vagina—increased secretions, feeling of fullness<br>Cervix—may bleed more easily at coitus, may be more sensitive |
| Orgasm | Tonic uterine contractions, transient fetal bradycardia, greater intensity (or first orgasm) |
| Resolution | Often poor or inadequate in late pregnancy |

Source: George W. Dameron, Jr., "Helping Couples Cope with Sexual Changes Pregnancy Brings," *Ortho Forum* 3.3 (1983): 8.

## Intercourse during Pregnancy

Most obstetrical physicians currently support the idea that intercourse during a normal pregnancy is quite safe for the fetus and the mother.[11] However, physical changes during pregnancy may affect sexual behavior. An expecting couple that understands these physiological changes may prepare for and cope with them. Many couples thus enjoy intercourse throughout the pregnancy.

Physiological changes will vary between the three trimesters. Table 10.3 presents the major alterations in sexual response during pregnancy. During the first trimester women may experience fatigue and morning sickness, both of which may decrease interest in sex. During that same time, however, congestion of blood vessels in the breasts and pelvic area may cause an enhanced erotic response. It is not uncommon for women to experience greater intensity of orgasm during the first two trimesters. In the third trimester the congestion of blood in the pelvic area is not well relieved during the resolution stage of sexual response, and may be a cause of discomfort. Also during the third trimester abdominal size may preclude intercourse in the male superior position, but alternative positions may be used.[12]

Certain problems of pregnancy may contraindicate intercourse and orgasm during specific phases of the pregnancy. A physician's consultation is important in determining if such problems exist. If there are no contraindications, it is safe for a couple to continue intercourse throughout the pregnancy as they may desire.[13] (See table 10.3.)

## Amniocentesis

**Amniocentesis** is a test used to discover genetic disorders, chromosomal abnormalities, sex-linked diseases, gender, and other information about the developing fetus. The physician who performs an amniocentesis obtains a sample of the amniotic fluid. This is accomplished by first using a noninvasive test (ultrasound) to map the position of the fetus inside the uterus. A local anesthetic is then used on the female's abdomen, after which an extremely fine tube is inserted through the abdominal wall and a sample of amniotic fluid is withdrawn. The results of the test can take from two to four weeks. Amniocentesis needs to be performed sometime between the fourteenth and sixteenth week of pregnancy. The timing of amniocentesis allows the option of abortion to parents who choose to terminate a pregnancy based on the results of the test.

The complication risk for mother and fetus from amniocentesis is less than 1 percent.[14] Thus there is a chance that a healthy fetus may be spontaneously aborted as a result of amniocentesis. Candidates for amniocentesis are parents with a family history of genetic disorders, women who have borne children with birth defects, and pregnant women over the age of thirty-five.

The option of amniocentesis with subsequent abortion has led to an ethical debate as to whether there is a personal responsibility on the part of the parents to bear and raise children with congenital disorders. Is it morally irresponsible to abort a fetus who is marginally or minimally handicapped as a result of a genetic disorder? Should the government force parents to bear children with certain disorders? If so, which disorders? If so, should the parents, government, or both pay for the additional medical and personal expenses incurred by giving birth to a handicapped child?

What if amniocentesis revealed that a woman was pregnant with twins, one having Down's syndrome and the other perfectly healthy? Parents would be faced with a perplexing decision of whether to abort a healthy fetus along with its genetically deficient sibling or to raise a healthy child along with its Down's syndrome sibling. When such a situation arose in 1980, the parents decided to abort the Down's syndrome fetus immediately and continue the pregnancy for the healthy fetus. Both procedures were successful.[15] The ethical issues, however, remain and cannot be solved by medical science alone.

## CHILDBIRTH

The physiological changes responsible for bringing about childbirth are not fully understood. There is strong evidence that prostaglandins produced by the uterus and fetal membranes are responsible for initiating labor. The childbirth process causes the delivery of the infant, placenta, and fetal membrane. This is accomplished by regular rhythmic uterine contractions which push the fetus toward the vulva.

There are several early signs that childbirth is about to begin. One sign is the expelling of the mucus plug that had closed off the cervix during pregnancy, offering protection against fetal infection. The mucus plug often has bloody streaks. Childbirth usually begins a few hours or days after this sign.

Another early sign is the rupturing of the amniotic sac (sometimes called the bag). The sac will break before labor begins in one out of ten childbirths. The expectant mother will feel the warm fluid exit the vagina. Childbirth will usually commence within twenty-four hours after the amniotic sac breaks.

The process of childbirth consists of three stages of labor. All three stages are usually longer for a woman's first baby. The entire childbirth process usually lasts from four to twenty-four hours or longer.

### First Stage of Labor

The **first stage of labor** begins with the onset of uterine contractions, and lasts until the cervix is completely dilated. During this stage of labor uterine contractions will become progressively stronger and arrive in shorter time intervals. When the contractions are two minutes apart and last forty-five seconds or longer, the birth of the baby is imminent. This is when the amniotic sac usually ruptures. Just prior to this time a physician or licensed midwife can introduce optional medications to reduce any discomfort or pain. (See figure 10.5.)

### Second Stage of Labor

The **second stage of labor** begins when the cervix is fully dilated and ends with the birth of the infant. During this stage, the strong uterine contractions push the fetus through the birth canal (vagina).

Before crowning, which is when the infant's head is at the vulva, an episiotomy may be performed. An **episiotomy** is the surgical cutting of some of the tissue between the anal and vaginal openings. This tissue is stitched together after childbirth. An episiotomy is performed to prevent this tissue from tearing during labor. This surgical incision widens the vaginal opening. An episiotomy after crowning is a risky procedure because of the close proximity of the infant's head.

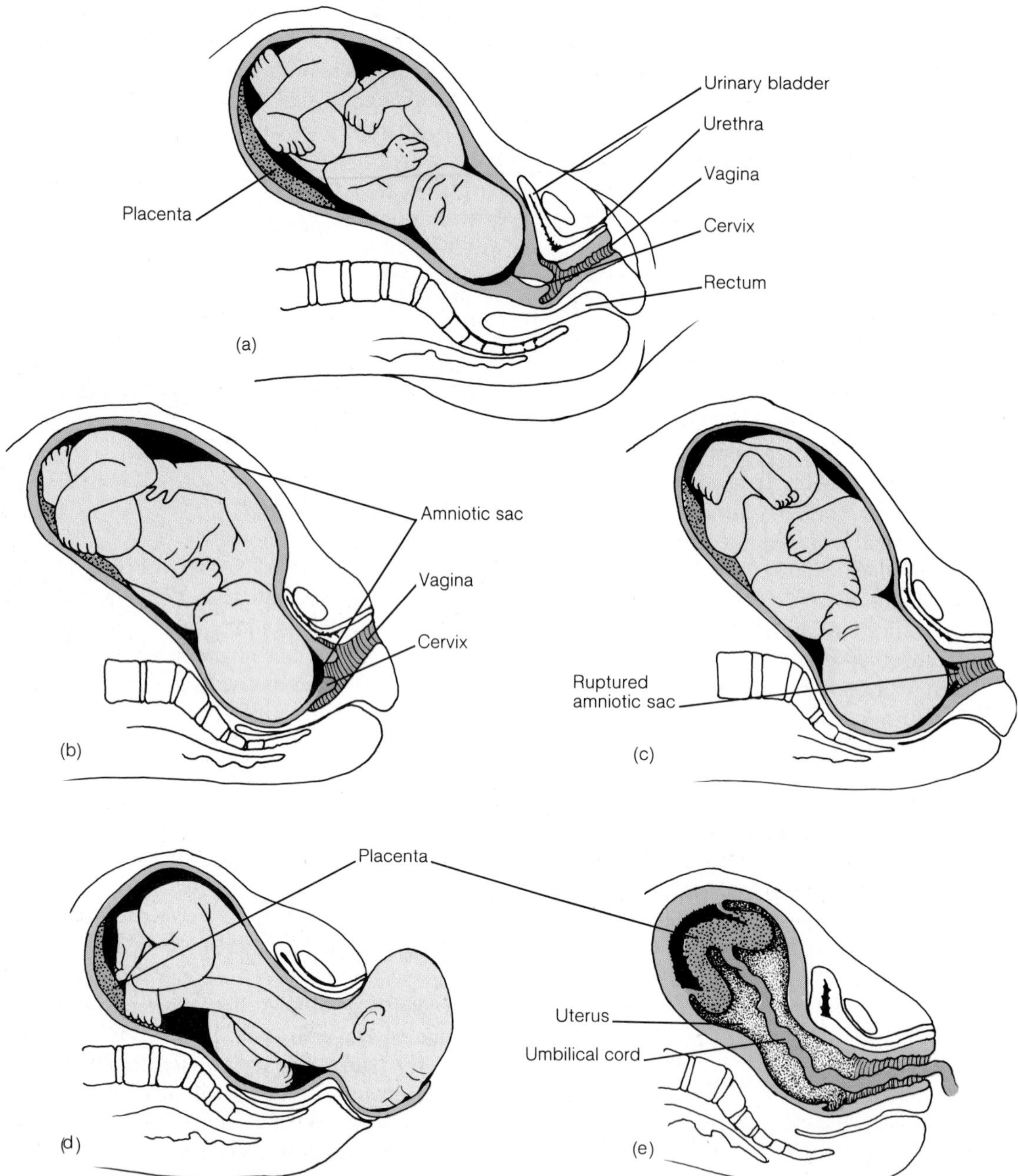


**Figure 10.5**
Birth. (a) Fetal position prior to birth; (b and c) stage of dilation; (d) stage of expulsion; (e) placental stage. *Source:* From Jones, Kenneth L., Louis W. Shainberg, and Curtis O. Byer, *Dimensions of Human Sexuality.* © 1985 Wm. C. Brown Publishers, Dubuque, Iowa. All rights reserved. Reprinted by permission.

Episiotomies in the U.S. have been criticized as unnecessary procedures. The physician usually performs an episiotomy before crowning as a preventive measure, so it is difficult to determine whether the episiotomy was really needed. Critics of the procedure cite studies indicating that considerably fewer episiotomies are performed, or considered necessary, for European women. Feminists have called episiotomies "husband stitches" because the procedure tightens the vaginal opening which in turn may make future intercourse more pleasurable for the male.[16] Since the episiotomy is usually a preventive measure, expectant parents should discuss with their childbirth supervisor the circumstances in which they would approve the procedure.

As soon as the infant's head is accessible, the oral and nasal openings are drained of fluids and mucus. The procedure is repeated until the infant draws its first breath of air. When the infant is stable and responsive, the umbilical cord is usually cut. The physician often places silver nitrate into the infant's eyes to prevent infection.

## Third Stage of Labor

Following the birth of the infant the uterus continues to contract in order to expel the placenta and the remains of the fetal membranes. The placenta and fetal membranes are referred to as the **afterbirth.** It is essential that no remnants of the afterbirth remain in the uterus, since they could lead to increased bleeding or infection.

## Apgar Score

At one minute after delivery the infant's health status is rated via an Apgar score. The **Apgar score** is a checklist of body functions used to determine if the infant's health or life is in jeopardy. The Apgar score ranges from zero to ten, where ten is the best score. The physical tests that comprise the Apgar score include heart rate, respiration, vigorous crying, muscle contractions, reflexes, and skin color. Eighty percent of newborn infants in the U.S. have a one minute Apgar score of seven or more.

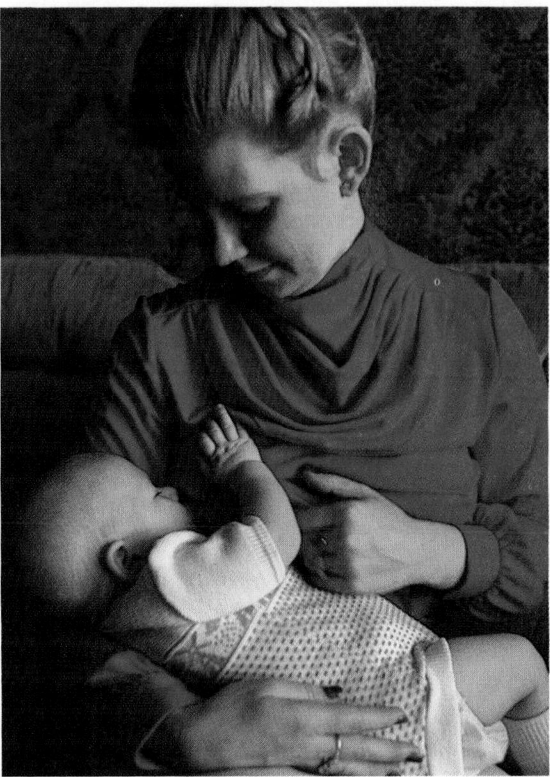

**Figure 10.6**
More American women are opting to breast-feed their babies.

## Breast-Feeding

After childbirth a yellowish fluid called **colostrum** will be secreted by the breasts. Colostrum contains several antibodies which can protect the newborn from illness, allergies, respiratory diseases, and diarrhea. Two to three days after childbirth the breasts will be able to secrete milk. Human milk contains sugar, protein, calcium, and water. Animal milks such as cow's milk, and products made from these animal milks (formulas), are not chemically or nutritionally equivalent to human milk.[17] Human milk helps the newborn's digestion. There is some evidence that the milk from mothers of premature infants may be especially suited to the premature infant.[18] Breast milk can meet the nutritional needs of the infant for the first four to six months of life.[19] In 1980 approximately 25 percent of American newborns were breast-fed until their sixth month of life.[20] (See figure 10.6.) Milk production subsides within a few days if the mother does not begin nursing, or stops nursing.

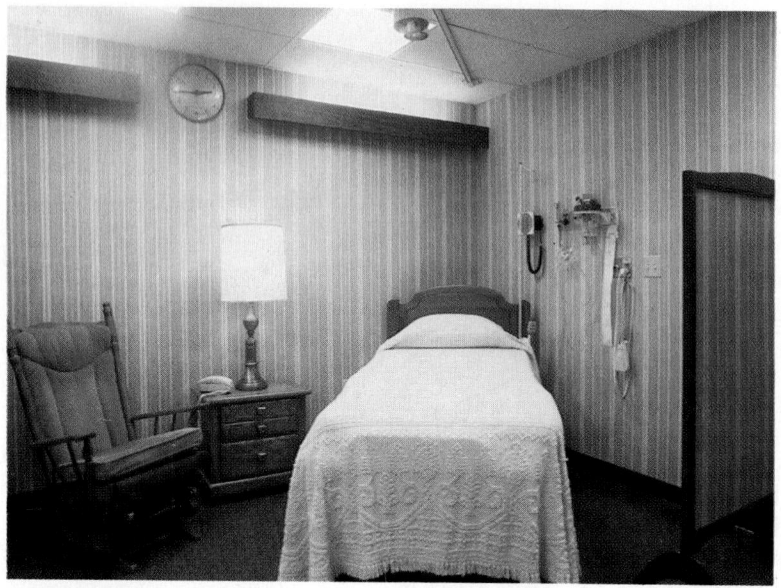

**Figure 10.7**
Birthing clinics (such as this one at Mercy Health Center in Dubuque, Iowa) provide a home setting, although they are often attached to hospitals.

There are several drawbacks to breast-feeding. Drugs taken by the mother, knowingly or unknowingly, could be passed on to the newborn by breast-feeding.[21] Regular breast-feeding can also be restrictive on both mother and family. Additionally, the breasts may leak milk, requiring the use of special bras. Some mothers report that their breasts are tender, or find the infant's sucklings painful.

To assist in breast-feeding there are special bras, and more and more public "nursing rooms" for privacy. In addition, the mother's milk can be pumped and stored for use at a later time.

## Childbirth Options

There are several childbirth options available to expectant parents. These options can be grouped into five categories: childbirth supervisors, childbirth facilities, childbirth courses, childbirth techniques, and childbirth witnesses. Parents may choose any combination from this array of options.

**CHILDBIRTH SUPERVISOR** The person in charge of childbirth, the childbirth supervisor, may be the physician, nurse midwife, lay midwife or a layperson. The childbirth supervisor is a key person during childbirth, but each of these supervisors has a different level of childbirth skills. Because every childbirth episode carries a degree of risk, it is prudent to consult a physician to assess the medical risks and health of both mother and future child.

There are physicians who will refuse to take part in childbirth if the parents opt for a particular assistant, place, or technique. On the other hand there are some physicians who will agree to be on call in case of a medical emergency during childbirth. Parents may opt for a medicated childbirth, in which case they may desire additional medical personnel who specialize in medicated deliveries. These matters should be clarified before, or soon after, pregnancy is confirmed.

**CHILDBIRTH FACILITIES** It is important that future parents select a childbirth facility which meets both their birthing and emotional needs. Some facilities emphasize medical services while bypassing family needs in terms of togetherness and bonding. Some facilities do just the opposite. There are also a few that combine both medical care and family care during childbirth.

Childbirth facilities include hospitals, birthing clinics, and home deliveries. With few exceptions, hospitals offer the emergency care and equipment needed when the mother or infant experience medical complications during or soon after childbirth. Eighty to 90 percent of all deliveries do not require extraordinary medical care or equipment. **Birthing clinics** specialize in childbirth and attempt to provide a "home setting" rather than a hospital setting. (See figure 10.7.) Birthing clinics are often physically or professionally attached to hospitals. They may have the same level of childbirth emergency care and equipment as a comprehensive hospital.

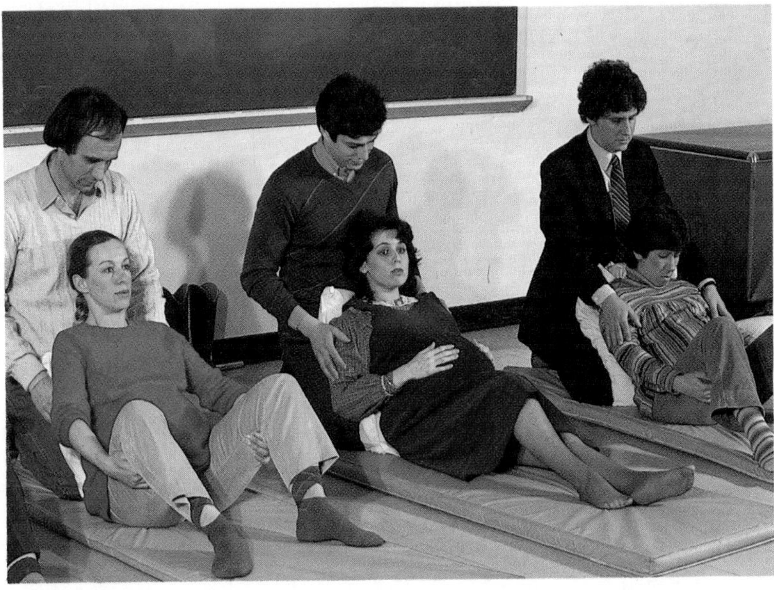

**Figure 10.8**
In the Lamaze birthing method each mother-to-be has a coach to aid in the childbirth process.

Home delivery usually occurs in the parents' residence, so it provides the most familiar and convenient setting for the family. However, home deliveries increase the distance (and time) between emergency care and the mother and infant.

**CHILDBIRTH COURSES** In prepared childbirth courses, expectant family members, prior to delivery, learn about the process and skills of childbirth. This method usually involves familiarizing the parents with the childbirth process, facilities, personnel, and equipment that will be involved in their child's delivery. Some courses prepare the entire family, including brothers and sisters, for the childbirth process. There are scores of childbirth courses, which use a variety of approaches. Most courses are helpful in preparing the family for the events of childbirth and the days that follow.

**CHILDBIRTH TECHNIQUES** There are a variety of childbirth techniques, with the lying-flat, physician-directed method most often used in the U.S. Physician-directed methods do not require any prior education or skills training on the part of the parents. The physician simply instructs the mother and the other participants on what course of action to take. It is essential, however, that the physician inform the parents of all delivery options, such as the use of electronic fetal monitoring (EFM) devices. EFM devices are sometimes inserted into the vagina to monitor the fetus's vital signs prior to delivery. There is controversy over whether the risks of EFM devices outweigh their benefits. In any event, such options should be explained and consent obtained prior to the delivery.

There are also birthing options regarding the position of the mother. There is the lying-flat position with the option of using stirrups. There is also the birthing chair in which the mother sits upright and the law of gravity assists her in the delivery. Some studies have reported that the birthing chair reduced the duration of the second stage of labor by one-half.

In the Lamaze method of childbirth, the mother is taught to relax and to control her breathing during labor. In Lamaze, the childbirth supervisor acts as the mother's coach during the delivery.[22] (See figure 10.8.)

The Leboyer method of delivery is an example of a delivery option which focuses on the infant. Frederick Leboyer promotes birthing techniques which introduce the infant into the world with the least amount of trauma. Leboyer methods include the use of dim lights, low noise levels, and warm baths for the infant after delivery. Leboyer recommends that the umbilical cord not be cut until after it has stopped pulsating.[23]

The Leboyer method, and other methods, encourage the mother and infant to make immediate skin contact in order to bring about bonding. Bonding is a recently popularized term defining the experiences which bring about the mother's emotional bond to her infant. Bonding occurs with other family members as well. Prospective parents who are interested in enhancing the bonding experience should select a childbirth facility which will accommodate their family's needs.

After taking a particular childbirth course the parents may be eager to use their new skills. It may turn out, though, that the parents never get a chance to use their birthing skills due to the need for a cesarean section, for medication during delivery, or other medical complications. In any case, many parents feel more comfortable and confident during pregnancy and childbirth after the completion of a childbirth course, even if specific skills cannot be used.

Another method of delivery is the **cesarean section,** a surgical procedure in which an incision is made in the mother's abdomen and the uterus. The infant is then removed through the abdominal cavity. The rate of cesarean births has more than doubled in the last ten years. The National Institute of Health has concluded that many cesarean sections performed in the U.S. are unnecessary.[24] The cesarean section is not the medically preferred method of delivery because of the increased risk of maternal mortality. However, there are instances in which a cesarean section is medically indicated to prevent maternal and/or infant injury or death. For instance, a cesarean section is often performed to prevent the infant from contracting an infectious disease (AIDS, herpes, hepatitis B, or gonorrhea) while passing through the vagina. The phrase "once a cesarean section, always a cesarean section" is not true for all women. A considerable proportion of women follow a cesarean birth with a normal vaginal birth.

Some people are confused by the terms natural and medicated childbirth. **Natural childbirth** implies that the mother used no drugs during delivery. In **medicated childbirth,** one or more drugs are given to the mother during childbirth. The kinds of drugs that are commonly used during childbirth in the U.S. range from mild tranquilizers like Valium to general anesthetics like nitrous oxide. The parents and the childbirth supervisor should decide, prior to delivery, which medications, under which circumstances, are to be administered during childbirth. The parents should understand that most drugs administered during childbirth will cross the placental barrier. The risk of birth complications depends on the drug, the dose, and when and how it is administered.

Some mothers or parents are disappointed if they had a medicated delivery after taking a prepared childbirth course which emphasized a natural delivery. This disappointment may prove to be temporary when the parents learn that the delivery was successful and the prognosis for mother and child is good.

**CHILDBIRTH WITNESS** Expectant parents will want to decide whether they want anyone to witness the childbirth. Witnesses can include the husband, children, immediate family, or friends. Parents may also choose to have present only the childbirth supervisor or team. Additionally, some parents may want to use a camera to document the birth.

Parents need to decide how much time they and their loved ones will spend with the newborn during the delivery and the days that follow. Some childbirth facilities place severe restrictions on who may visit with the newborn child and its mother, and when.

The parents also need to decide who will see, touch, and care for the infant right after birth, and in the days to follow. Hospitals tend to place the most restrictions on the parents' access to their newborn child. Expectant parents should select a facility which will meet their physical as well as family needs.

Not all childbirth supervisors and facilities will accommodate all childbirth options. In addition, medical insurance companies are often very selective in the kinds of childbirth facilities and practitioners they will cover.

All these options and details should be worked out prior to delivery. Mother, father, and other children can use this time to prepare to welcome the family's newest member. In this way every family member will have a chance to play a role in this momentous event.

## INFERTILITY

Ten to 15 percent of American married couples are involuntarily childless, and an additional 10 percent have fewer naturally conceived children than they desire.[25] A couple is considered **infertile** when they are unable to maintain a pregnancy after attempting for a year or more. A specific physiological cause can be diagnosed in approximately 85 percent of all infertile couples. A couple's infertility can be a result of male, female, or some combination of male and female factors. (See figure 10.9.)

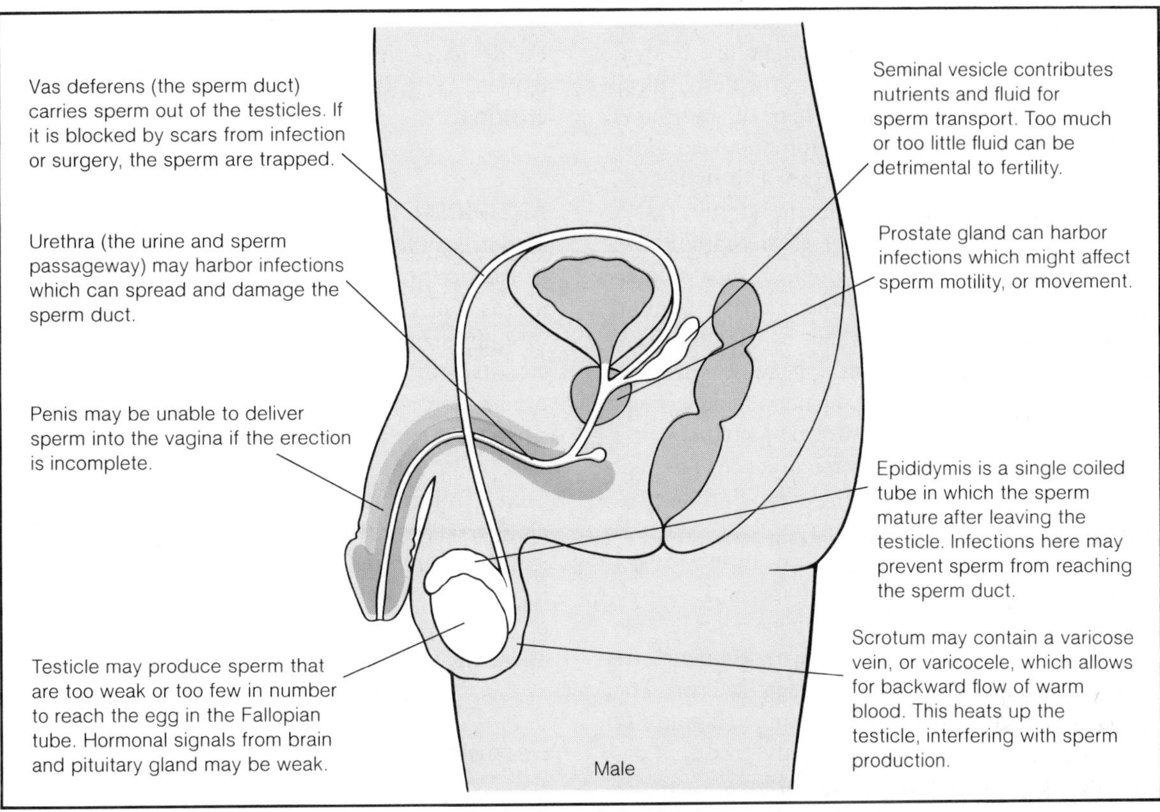

Vas deferens (the sperm duct) carries sperm out of the testicles. If it is blocked by scars from infection or surgery, the sperm are trapped.
Urethra (the urine and sperm passageway) may harbor infections which can spread and damage the sperm duct.
Penis may be unable to deliver sperm into the vagina if the erection is incomplete.
Testicle may produce sperm that are too weak or too few in number to reach the egg in the Fallopian tube. Hormonal signals from brain and pituitary gland may be weak.
Seminal vesicle contributes nutrients and fluid for sperm transport. Too much or too little fluid can be detrimental to fertility.
Prostate gland can harbor infections which might affect sperm motility, or movement.
Epididymis is a single coiled tube in which the sperm mature after leaving the testicle. Infections here may prevent sperm from reaching the sperm duct.
Scrotum may contain a varicose vein, or varicocele, which allows for backward flow of warm blood. This heats up the testicle, interfering with sperm production.
Male


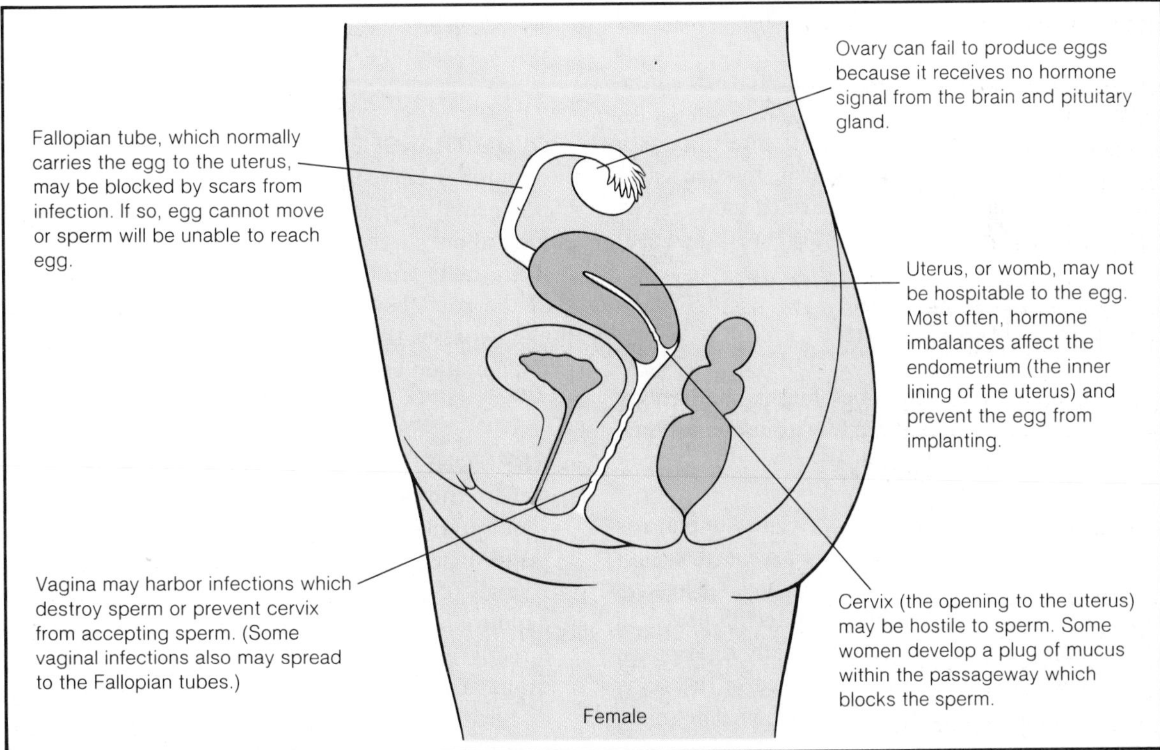

Fallopian tube, which normally carries the egg to the uterus, may be blocked by scars from infection. If so, egg cannot move or sperm will be unable to reach egg.
Vagina may harbor infections which destroy sperm or prevent cervix from accepting sperm. (Some vaginal infections also may spread to the Fallopian tubes.)
Ovary can fail to produce eggs because it receives no hormone signal from the brain and pituitary gland.
Uterus, or womb, may not be hospitable to the egg. Most often, hormone imbalances affect the endometrium (the inner lining of the uterus) and prevent the egg from implanting.
Cervix (the opening to the uterus) may be hostile to sperm. Some women develop a plug of mucus within the passageway which blocks the sperm.
Female


**Figure 10.9**
Where the problems are.

Common causes of female infertility are blocked fallopian tubes, endometriosis, and failure to ovulate. **Endometriosis** is a condition in which a piece of the endometrium in the uterus tears off and grows in the pelvic cavity on adjacent reproductive organs, such as the fallopian tubes or ovaries. This tissue acts exactly as endometrial tissue in the uterus, thickening during certain stages of each reproductive cycle and then attempting to slough off excess tissue at the time of menstruation. Endometrial tissue in the pelvic cavity, however, cannot be expelled from the body. It therefore continues to increase with each cycle, causing severe abdominal pain in some women. "Hostile mucus" has been identified as another cause of female infertility. Hostile cervical mucus does not allow sperm to pass through the cervix into the vagina.

Common causes of male infertility are low sperm counts and low mobility of sperm. Low mobility of sperm is a condition in which a considerable proportion of the total sperm in a male's ejaculate is not active enough to accomplish fertilization. The male may also develop an autoimmune response to his own sperm. In this case his body produces antibodies which destroy sperm or prevent their development. Another cause of male infertility is erectile inhibition, or the inability of the male to have and maintain an erection. Erectile inhibition is common among diabetic males, due to their circulatory difficulties.

A common combined cause of infertility is a woman's allergic reaction to sperm. In such cases she produces antibodies which attack and destroy sperm, in effect producing a natural spermicide.

## Male Infertility Options

Infertile males can sometimes father children by using erectile enhancers or artificial insemination.

**ERECTILE ENHANCERS** A penile implant is a surgical technique that has been somewhat successful in overcoming erectile inhibition.[26] The surgeon can implant semirigid rods into the penis, so that the male constantly has a partially rigid penis. Another device that can be implanted in the penis is an inflatable, cylinder-shaped balloon. The male, using a pump implanted in the scrotum, pumps up the device with fluid stored in a bag inside the abdomen. With this device the male can control his erection.

**ARTIFICIAL INSEMINATION** **Artificial insemination** occurs when some means other than the penis is used to introduce semen into the vaginal tract or uterus. For example, a physician can use a syringe to squirt semen into the vaginal tract. The first successful birth from artificial insemination in the U.S. occurred in 1884. The first successful birth from artificial insemination using frozen sperm occurred in 1953. The majority of artificial inseminations use semen from a paid or unpaid donor. About 15,000 children a year are born in the U.S. as a result of artificial insemination. The inheritance and other legal rights of those children, and the substantiation of who is the legal father, remain debatable legal questions in America.

## Female Infertility Options

Infertile women can sometimes produce genetic offspring through ovum transfer, hormone therapy, surrogate mothers, and in vitro fertilization.

**OVUM TRANSFER** Blocked fallopian tubes can sometimes be repaired with microsurgery. An experimental method called "low tubal ovum transfer" may allow surgeons to capture a Graafian follicle from the ovaries and insert it in the fallopian tube at the point beyond the blockage. In this way the egg bypasses the blocked tube and fertilization and implantation can take place naturally.

**HORMONE THERAPY** Females who do not ovulate can be prescribed clomiphene, an oral drug which stimulates the secretion of FSH and LH (gonadotropins). If clomiphene proves unsuccessful then a series of injections using human menopausal gonadotropins (HMG) may be tried. This drug acts directly on the ovaries to induce ovulation. These drugs are not without side effects; a couple should discuss the health risks with their physician. If pregnancy occurs with the use of HMG there is one chance in five that it will be a multiple birth.

**SURROGATE MOTHERS** Some infertile couples have contracted with surrogate mothers to bear their babies. **Surrogate mothers** are paid or unpaid volunteers who make their reproductive organs available for procreation and pregnancy.

Surrogate mothers can be artificially inseminated by the male of an infertile couple, in which case the male becomes the baby's genetic father, and the surrogate female its genetic mother. However, the three "parents" agree, usually with the assistance of a lawyer, that the surrogate mother will lay no claim to parent the baby once it is born. This allows the infertile female to become the baby's familial mother.

There is currently no legal standard for these contractual arrangements. Many events could occur that would place surrogate contracts in legal limbo. The surrogate mother, for example, may refuse to give up the baby. Or, what happens if a surrogate mother is accused of consuming alcohol and thereby damaging the baby? In such a case, who is legally and financially reponsible for that child if any or all of the "parents" refuse custody?

**IN VITRO FERTILIZATION** The technique that results in "test-tube babies" is called **in vitro fertilization (IVF).** IVF solves some fertility problems while creating other social issues. IVF involves removing the egg from the ovaries, fertilizing it artificially in a laboratory dish, incubating it for several days, and then implanting it inside the uterus.[27] This technique enables females with blocked fallopian tubes or no fallopian tubes to be the genetic parents of their children.

The first successful animal IVF took place in 1947, and the first successful human IVF was performed in 1972. There are now over forty medical centers in the U.S. who perform this service. Worldwide, 1,000 children are born each year as a result of IVF.

IVF also makes it possible for a female without a uterus to become the genetic parent of her child by using the services of a surrogate mother. In such a case the egg is removed from the female without a uterus, artificially fertilized by her mate's sperm in a laboratory dish, incubated, and then implanted in a surrogate mother. An infant produced this way would be the genetic product of the infertile couple with the surrogate mother acting as a human incubator. Here the surrogate or birth mother is not the genetic mother of the child she bore.

Of course IVF raises numerous legal and ethical questions. For example, most physicians administer hormones and cause the ovaries to produce several eggs. All of these eggs are retrieved from the ovaries and fertilized. Only those fertilized eggs that appear healthy and comprise only four cells will be placed into the uterus. Subsequently, there are leftover fertilized eggs. If they are sold to someone else, is that "baby selling," which is illegal? If they are destroyed, is that an abortion? How can a female have an abortion when she is not pregnant? Are IVF embryos orphans of the state?

Animal breeders have used a technique called twinning to produce identical offspring from a prize animal. Twinning involves a relatively simple technique of splitting one embryo into two or more masses. Each newly formed embryo could be an identical twin. By using IVF and twinning, it is possible for a couple to order identical twins, have them both immediately, or even freeze one or two for a later pregnancy.

## Infertility Issues

Test-tube babies and reimplantation techniques offer reproductively healthy couples pregnancy options. Some females might desire to be the genetic and familial parents of their children, but also desire to forgo pregnancy. Careers such as modeling, entertainment, or professional sports may be a factor in the prospective mother's desire to retain her figure. Pregnancy may be viewed as a handicap by some females who choose to remain in their professions during and following pregnancy. Reimplantation using surrogate mothers is an option that would allow such individuals to be the genetic and familial mother of their children, without experiencing the rigors of pregnancy or childbirth. It is possible today for a female to be the genetic mother of her child without ever having intercourse, going through pregnancy, or giving birth.

Fertility procedures such as artificial insemination, surrogate mothers, and reimplantation techniques have produced options for both fertile and infertile people. It will be interesting to follow the development of criteria for persons desiring to utilize these procedures.

As these procedures become more commonplace there will be an ever-increasing interest in and medical necessity for children to know the identity of their genetic parents and siblings. First, people often want to know their genetic roots and ancestry. Also, in matters of illness, medical emergency, and procreation it may be imperative to obtain a genetic history. Currently, there is no national consensus on whether or not records of a child's genetic parents should be kept or destroyed, or whether a child has a right to those records.

The next generation of Americans may consider pregnancy an optional form of procreation. In any event, artificial procreation procedures and products are becoming a legal nightmare. Legal issues include the responsibilities, liabilities, and rights of everyone involved, including doctors, donors, parents, and children.

## SUMMARY

1. Parents because they are parents inherit the ultimate responsibility—providing for their child's wellness.

2. Parental love is "the" essential human ingredient in parenting. Love's omnipresence underlies all parent-child interactions.

3. Prenatal care increases a mother's chances of bearing a healthy baby. In addition, prenatal care allows for the detection of potential and actual pregnancy problems.

4. Although there is no definitive evidence in all cases, it seems that the prudent course of action is for the pregnant female to avoid the use of all prescription, over-the-counter, and illegal drugs from the first day of the reproductive cycle she chooses to become pregnant until after childbirth. In cases where the mother chooses to breast-feed, this period of drug abstinence should continue until the child is weaned (taken off the mother's milk).

5. Pregnancy is divided into three phases called trimesters. The first trimester is from the point of fertilization to the end of the third month. The second trimester is from the beginning of the fourth month to the end of the sixth month. The third trimester is from the beginning of the seventh month and continues until childbirth.

6. Amniocentesis is a prenatal test used to discover genetic disorders, chromosomal abnormalities, sex-linked diseases, and the like.

7. The childbirth process causes the delivery of the infant, placenta, and fetal membrane. Childbirth is divided into three stages of labor.

8. Expectant parents have several childbirth options. These options can be grouped into five categories: childbirth supervisors, childbirth facilities, childbirth courses, childbirth techniques, and childbirth witnesses.

9. It is important that future parents select a childbirth facility which meets both their birthing and emotional needs.

10. Ten to 15 percent of American married couples are involuntarily childless; an additional 10 percent have fewer naturally conceived children than they desire. A couple's infertility can be a result of male, female, or a combination of male and female factors. Common causes of female infertility are blocked fallopian tubes, endometriosis, and failure to ovulate. Common causes of male infertility are low sperm counts and low mobility of sperm.

### Recommended Readings

Andrews, Lori. *New Conceptions.* New York: St. Martin's Press, 1984.

Klaus, M., and Kennel, J. *Parent-Infant Bonding,* 2d ed. St. Louis: C.V. Mosby, 1982.

### References

1. Godfrey Hochbaum, *Health Behavior* (Belmont, Calif.: Wadsworth Publishing Co., 1970).

2. Richard W. Erbe, "Drugs and Pregnancy: What Are the Dangers?" *Consultant* 23.11 (1983): 191, 195.

3. Erbe, "Drugs and Pregnancy," 195.

4. Erbe, "Drugs and Pregnancy," 195.

5. Chris Lecos, "Caution Light on Caffeine," *FDA Consumer* (October, 1980): 6–9.

6. Chris Lecos, "Pregnant Women Heed Advice," *FDA Consumer* 16.2 (1982): 25–26.

7. The National Foundation March of Dimes, *Food and Pregnancy* (White Plains, N.Y.: 1979).

8. Margaret Jensen and Irene Bobak, *Maternity and Gynecologic Care*, 3d. ed. (St. Louis: C.V. Mosby, 1985).

9. Mary Carpenter, "Physicians Ponder Popularity of Pregnancy Self-Test Kits," *Medical News* 3.14 (24 September 1979): 18.

10. Robert A. Hatcher et al., *Contraceptive Technology 1984–1984,* 12th ed. (New York: Irvington Press, 1984).

11. George W. Dameron, "Helping Couples Cope with Sexual Changes Pregnancy Brings," *Ortho Forum* 3.3 (1983): 7.

12. Dameron, "Helping Couples Cope."

13. Gordon S. Walbroehl, "Sex and Pregnancy: Advising the Patient," *Sexual Medicine Today* 9.1 (1985): 20.

14. Jensen and Bobak, *Maternity and Gynecologic Care.*

15. Thomas Kerenyi and Usha Chitkara, "Selective Birth in Twin Pregnancy with Discordancy for Down's Syndrome," *New England Journal of Medicine* 304.25 (1981): 1525–27.

16. S. R. Hahn and K. E. Paige, "American Birth Practices: A Critical Review," in J. E. Parsons, ed., *The Psychobiology of Sex Differences and Sex Roles* (New York: McGraw-Hill, 1980).

17. D. B. Jelliffe, and E. E. P. Jelliffe, "Breast Is Best: Modern Meanings," *The New England Journal of Medicine* 297 (1977): 93–106.

18. S. A. Atkins, G. H. Anderson, and M. H. Bryan, "Human Milk: Comparison of the Nitrogen Composition in Milk from Mothers of Premature and Full Term Infants," *American Journal of Clinical Nutrition* 33 (April 1980): 811–15; R. Schanler and W. Oh, "Composition of Breast Milk Obtained from Mothers of Premature Infants as Compared to Breast Milk Obtained from Donors," *Journal of Pediatrics* 96 (1980): 679–81.

19. American Public Health Association, "Infant Feeding in the United States," *American Journal of Public Health* 71.2 (1981): 207–11.

20. G. A. Marinez and J. P. Nalezienski, "1980 Update: The Recent Trend in Breast-Feeding," *Pediatrics* 67.2 (1981): 260–63.

21. A. C. Platzker, C. D. Lew, and D. Stewart, "Drug Administration via Breast Milk," *Hospital Practice* (September 1980): 111–22.

22. Fernand Lamaze, *Painless Childbirth: The Lamaze Method* (Chicago: Henry Regnery Co., 1970).

23. Frederick Leboyer, *Birth without Violence* (New York: Knopf, 1975).

24. G. B. Kolata, "NIH Panel Urges Fewer Cesarean Births," *Science* 210 (1980): 176–77.

25. Barbara Menning, *Infertility: A Guide for Childless Couples* (Englewood Cliffs, N.J.: Prentice-Hall, 1977).

26. J. J. Kaufman, R. J. Boxer, B. Boxer, and M. Quinn, "Physical and Psychological Results of Penile Prostheses: A Statistical Survey," *The Journal of Urology* 126 (1981): 173–75.

27. R. Mars et al., "A Modified Technique of Human in Vitro Fertilization and Embryo Transfer," *American Journal of Obstetrics and Gynecology* 147 (1983): 318–22.

# UNIT THREE

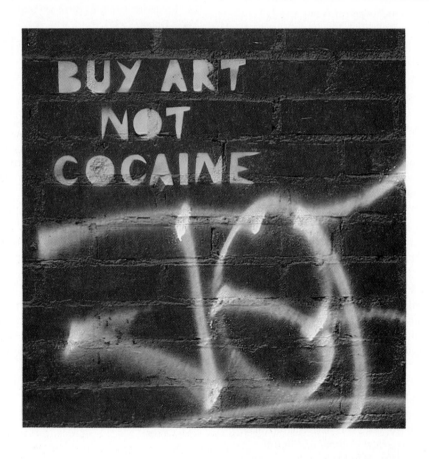

# Self-Responsibility: Minimizing Negative Life Habits

As we have seen in earlier chapters, you can choose to live a wellness life-style. Taking personal responsibility for achieving wellness involves minimizing negative life habits.

Virtually everyone uses drugs of some kind, but many of the drugs we ingest are not typically called drugs. In and of themselves, drugs are neither good nor bad; responsible patterns of drug use may be possible for almost all drugs now being used. However, drugs that are misused or abused can be very dangerous. Whether or not people use various drugs responsibly depends on many factors, including advertising, social attitudes, the influence of family and peers, and availability.

In unit 3, we will pay particular attention to the responsible use of alcohol and tobacco. Because they are so widely available, alcohol and tobacco can threaten wellness. In addition, alcohol and tobacco, though legally obtainable for much of the population, still account for the largest amount of illegal use among all drugs in our society.

Unit 3 will also introduce you to five other categories of drugs—herbal drugs, over-the-counter drugs, prescription drugs, unrecognized drugs, and illicit drugs. We will pay special attention to psychoactive drugs (those affecting the mind and behavior).

Unit 3 also presents the important noncommunicable diseases that may be roadblocks to high-level wellness. Cardiovascular disease, cancer, diabetes, emphysema, and other noncommunicable diseases pose significant threats to wellness. You will learn ways to moderate the risk factors that contribute to the disease process.

Sexually transmitted diseases, which include all the disorders that are transmitted through sexual contact of some kind, also threaten wellness. STDs are communicable diseases; there are no vaccines and no acquired immunities to them. In unit 3, you will learn ways to minimize the chances of contracting an STD.

CHAPTER ELEVEN

# Drugs and Drug Use: The Dynamics of Drug Taking



Drugs are everywhere in our environment. It is hard to imagine a day that goes by in which a person does not ingest a drug. Yet many of the drugs that we ingest are not typically called drugs. Everyone would agree that penicillin is a drug, as are morphine, heroin, cocaine, and PCP. However, many other substances that we commonly ingest (such as alcohol and tobacco products) also contain active ingredients that should properly be called drugs.

The cola beverages that we readily consume contain the drug caffeine, as do coffee and tea. Cocoa and some chocolates contain a drug called theobromine and caffeine as well. Both theobromine and caffeine are very potent drugs that stimulate the central nervous system. Many of our relatively common household spices also contain substances that can have profound effects on our consciousness and thought.

Herbs, in the forms of teas, poultices, spices, and medicines, are becoming more and more popular today. Herbs have been used for these purposes for many thousands of years. In fact, perhaps the best-known spice trader was the founder of Islam—Muhammed. The relatively recent resurgence in the popularity of herbs can be traced to many reasons, not the least of which is that a great many herbs directly affect the mood and behavior of individuals. By 1974, Norman Farnsworth had published a list of more than 200 herbal plants whose active ingredients directly affect consciousness and behavior.[1]

Drugs are a common and important aspect of American life. This chapter will introduce you to many basic concepts of drug use and abuse. Decision making for responsible use of drugs will be highlighted.

## WHAT IS A DRUG?

Since drugs are readily available to all of us, and since we use them in so many ways, it is important that we look at the dynamics of drug taking in a holistic way. There is no individual who is completely drug free, yet most of us do not have a clear definition of the term "drug." Defining the term itself to everyone's satisfaction is difficult to accomplish because we all have different frames of reference. Some people define drugs in terms of their effects, while others think mostly in social terms. For the purposes of this book, however, the term **drug** will be used to describe any substance, other than food and water, which by virtue of its chemical nature has a direct effect on the structure or function of an individual. A special subcategory of drugs, the **psychoactive drugs,** refers to only those drugs that directly affect a person's mood and/or behavior. In this regard, penicillin is a drug because it directly affects our ability to function in the presence of an infection. However, it does not directly affect our mood or cause behavioral changes. Alcohol, on the other hand, is not only a drug according to our definition, but it is also a psychoactive agent in that when we drink alcohol in sufficient quantities, direct effects on both our mood and behavior will be observable.

A definition this broad enables us to include virtually everything that we put into our bodies as drugs—and that is the way all such substances should be viewed. At this point, however, do not assume that we are necessarily labeling all of these substances as "good" or "bad" or "dangerous." We are merely using the term drug in a descriptive sense. As you will see later, the determinant of whether a drug is "good" or "bad" is how that drug is used—and that responsible patterns of drug use may be possible for almost all drugs now being used.

## CATEGORIES OF DRUGS

Drugs are categorized in many ways, but it is helpful to classify drugs according to their availability and sources.[2] These categories include:

1. **Herbal drugs,** which are not generally regulated by law, such as sassafras, tea, or catnip.
2. **Over-the-counter** (**OTC**) **drugs,** which are legally available without a prescription for self-medication, such as aspirin, some vitamins, and a variety of cough medications.
3. **Prescription drugs,** which require a physician's written order, such as tranquilizers, potent cough medications, and sleeping pills.
4. **Unrecognized drugs,** which are widely available products, some of which have clearly psychoactive effects but are generally not considered to be drugs. Some examples include caffeine-containing soft drinks and psychoactive spices such as mace and nutmeg.
5. **Tobacco** and related products such as cigarettes, cigars, snuff, and chewing tobacco.
6. Alcohol, including such **alcoholic beverages** as beer, wine, and distilled liquors.
7. **Illicit drugs,** which cannot be legally sold, purchased, or in many cases used, such as heroin, marijuana, cocaine, and PCP.

These seven categories then represent the broad spectrum of drugs with which we come into contact. You should recognize, however, that these seven categories include literally many thousands of drug substances. For instance, there are certainly more than 100,000 OTC drugs readily available in today's marketplace. Add to that perhaps 30,000 to 40,000 prescription medications that can be prescribed legally by physicians and dentists for human consumption. In addition, we can add several thousand herbal preparations containing one or more combinations of the 217 psychoactive ingredients now known, as well as innumerable foods and beverages that have psychoactive properties. We have not yet even touched the illicit drug preparations and perhaps the two most important drugs from the standpoint of health—alcohol and tobacco products.

11.1 EXHIBIT 11.1

# Real Targets: Doctors, Drug Firms

The new [1980] FDA Commissioner, Dr. Jere Goyan, has quickly identified the problem of "overmedication" as one of his top priorities in the drug area.

Patient package inserts and teaching Americans that "there is not a pill for every ill" are approaches that focus on the consumer. Coupled with this patient-directed strategy must be equally strong efforts by FDA to attack the roots of the problem: the drug companies and—for prescription drugs at least—those doctors who are agents of overmedication.

There are at least three major categories of drugs which contribute to the problem of overmedication. First, drugs which do not work or, in more refined terms, lack evidence of effectiveness. Second, drugs used for problems better treated by nondrug therapies. And, third, dangerous drugs used when safer and equally or more effective alternatives are available.

One out of ten prescriptions filled by Americans are for drugs that are ineffective, costing the public over $1 billion a year and causing thousands of avoidable adverse drug reactions. In addition, the majority of ingredients in over-the-counter drugs on the market have been found by FDA to lack effectiveness, thus causing the public to waste money and endanger its health.

This form of overmedication will only be changed when FDA orders these 400 plus prescription drugs off the market and when the thousands of over-the-counter drugs with ineffective ingredients are either reformulated or banned. In the meantime, FDA could warn doctors and patients—by leaflets—that "these drugs (or ingredients) don't work and are potentially harmful."

Drugs for problems better treated by nondrug therapy include oral diabetes pills, antiobesity pills, estrogens for menopause, tranquilizers, sleeping pills, and many others. Patient package inserts and strong warnings to doctors not to use these drugs unless all other measures have been thoroughly tried would reduce much of this form of overmedication. Doctors who inappropriately prescribe such drugs, despite warnings to the contrary, would likely be subject to malpractice suits. In addition to slowness in removing the ineffective drugs, FDA is also negligent because it has not warned doctors and patients about the oral (diabetes) and psychoactive drugs, and because it has not moved against all antiobesity drugs rather than just amphetamines.

Examples of overmedication with dangerous drugs, when safer alternatives would do just as well, include the use of Darvon, and antibiotics, such as Ilosone (erythromycin estolate), clindamycin, and chloramphenicol. Until Ilosone is removed from the market, doctors and patients should be urged by FDA not to use this liver-damaging drug, but to use the other safer erythromycins. As for Darvon—killer of more Americans than any prescription drug—banning or putting it into Schedule II—as a narcotic with no refills—would sharply reduce the number of prescriptions and deaths.

Drug companies are primarily in business to sell drugs. Overmedication is an important part of the strategy. Spending well over a billion dollars a year to push drugs, many of which are ineffective or are inferior to others that serve the same therapeutic purpose, is the clearest message the drug industry can send about its role in overmedication.

If FDA is to reduce this waste of money and lives, called overmedication, it will have to go much harder against its source—drug companies and doctors—rather than focusing mainly on its victims.

Source: Sidney M. Wolfe, M.D., Director, Public Citizen Health Research Group, "Real Targets: Doctors, Drug Firms." *FDA Consumer* (February 1980), 13.

## DISCUSSION QUESTIONS

1. Do you agree with Dr. Wolfe when he states that the FDA should impose greater sanctions on drug companies and physicians?

2. Dr. Wolfe implies that the major concern of drug companies is to make money. Do you agree with this view? What possible humanitarian concerns may also motivate drug companies?

11.2 EXHIBIT 11.2

# AMA: Don't Limit Doctors' Options

Are the American people overmedicated?

The answer to this question cannot be an unqualified yes or no, but depends a good deal upon one's bias, one's approach to the use of drugs. For example, a recent committee of the National Academy of Sciences' Institute of Medicine reviewed the management of insomnia and the use of sedative-hypnotic drugs. A Los Angeles survey was quoted which revealed that about 30 percent of the respondents complained of some difficulty sleeping, although only half considered the matter serious. Other studies have reported that about 15 percent of the middle-aged population complain of insomnia, 6 percent actually consult a physician for it, and about half that number receive a prescription. Thus, one biased against drug use could say that half of those patients who consult a doctor for insomnia get a drug prescribed, whereas someone else could say that only one in ten people who have difficulty sleeping use prescription drugs for it.

Of course, there are drug addicts and drug abusers who present social problems, so that there certainly are individuals who "overmedicate" themselves; to this group could be added those hypochondriacs who depend upon over-the-counter drugs for their own solution to problems. Whether the United States is more afflicted with these forms of overmedication than any other western country has not been established. The American Medical Association has collaborated with and encouraged the Federal agencies in their efforts to limit and control drug abuse.

At the same time that ponderous statements against the too frequent use of drugs are echoed about the land, the conscientious physician has to cope with the problem of drug compliance in the management of many chronic diseases. It is now possible to control virtually all hypertension with a schedule of one to three drugs, but physicians working in even the best organized clinics are succeeding in less than half of the hypertensive patients. This has been attributed to poor drug compliance or "under-medication" and was improved in one instance with an intensive educational effort to two-thirds of the patients. This example is only one of many, and it can be multiplied by the number of common chronic diseases that are susceptible to drug management and account for a large share of our adult-patient population.

The practicing physician carries the responsibility to alleviate pain and prolong life. These are difficult goals which are not always achieved and which can easily be inhibited rather than facilitated by misguided regulations. The physician needs as many options as possible in pursuing this charge. The risk of a feared untoward effect may be acceptable for one patient and the lack of untoward effects may make a second or third choice drug desirable for another. The American Medical Association has maintained repeatedly that the prescription drug options of the physician should not be unduly restricted. A good drug should not be made less available just because of abuse potential, because another drug is more often successful, or because remote or occasional adverse effects are known. The patient population of this country deserves the widest possible selection of therapeutic agents commensurate with reasonable estimates of safety and efficacy.

Source: Richard J. Jones, M.D., Director, Division of Scientific Activities, American Medical Association. *FDA Consumer* (February 1980), 14.

## DISCUSSION QUESTIONS

1. Do you agree with the position of the American Medical Association (AMA) that the prescription-drug options of physicians should not be unduly restricted?

2. Do you think undermedication (or lack of compliance with physician's instructions for drug use) is a major problem in the United States?

# POLYDRUG USE

Not only is no person drug free from day to day, but virtually everyone is a multidrug user. The use of several different drug substances at the same time is called **polydrug use.**

## Drug Interactions

When considering some of the potential hazards of drug use, it is important to consider more extensively the difficulties that may be encountered when more than one drug is taken at the same time. Remember, however, that within the context of our definition of the term drug, many substances that we do not consider to be drugs really are. More than that, it is important to remember that we are all multiple-drug users. However, there are some potentially hazardous outcomes when we mix drugs of different kinds. Some of these outcomes are due to one or more of the following ways in which drugs interact. First, drugs may interact in an additive sense; that is, the total effect of the drugs taken is equivalent to the sum of the effects of the individual drugs. Second, one drug may inhibit the actions of another. Third, drugs may have a **synergistic effect** on one another; that is, the total effects of the two or more drugs are multiplied because of the influence one may have on the actions of the other.

To give you some idea of the magnitude of the potential problems, table 11.1 contains a partial listing of some of the more common drug interactions. However, you should know that this list is not complete, in part because a complete list would be a book in itself. Yet perhaps the most important reason is that all of the potentially hazardous combinations of drugs are simply not known.

**Table 11.1 A Guide to Common Drug Interactions**

**This is only a sampling of some of the most common drug interactions. No action should be taken without checking with your own doctor.**

| *Tranquilizers* | *Combined with* | *Interaction* |
|---|---|---|
| Diazepam derivatives (Librium, Valium, Serax, etc.) and meprobamate (Miltown) | alcohol | increases effects of both |
| | barbiturate | increases effects of both |
| | MAO-inhibiting antidepressants (Nardil, Parnate, Marplan, Eutonyl) | oversedation |
| | phenothiazine tranquilizers (Thorazine, Compazine, etc.) | increases effects of both |
| | tricyclic antidepressants (Elavil, Aventyl, Tofranil, Pertofrane) | increases effects of both |
| Phenothiazines (Thorazine, Mellaril, Compazine, etc.) | alcohol | oversedation |
| | antihistamine | increases effects of both |
| | antihypertensive drugs | increases bloodpressure-lowering action |
| | barbiturate | increases sedation |
| | MAO-inhibiting antidepressants (Nardil, Parnate, Marplan, Eutonyl) | makes antidepressant less effective |
| | Demerol | increases sedation |
| | diazepam derivatives (Librium, Valium, etc.) | increases action of both |
| | thiazide diuretics (Diuril, Hydrodiuril) | causes shock |
| | tricyclic antidepressants (Elavil, Aventyl, Tofranil, Pertofrane) | increases action of both |

Source: U.S. Government Printing Office.

**Table 11.1** *Continued*

**This is only a sampling of some of the most common drug interactions. No action should be taken without checking with your own doctor.**

| *Analgesics* | *Combined with* | *Interaction* |
|---|---|---|
| Aspirin | anticoagulant | increases the blood-thinning effect and could cause bleeding |
| | para amonosalicylic açid (PAS) | makes PAS toxic |
| Meperidine (Demerol) | MAO-inhibitor antidepressants (Nardil, Parnate, Marplan, Eutonyl) | increases action of Demerol |
| | phenothiazine tranquilizers (Thorazine, Compazine, etc.) | increases sedation |
| Phenylbutazone | anticoagulant | increases the blood-thinning effect and could cause bleeding |

Oral antidiabetic drugs (Orinase, Diabenese) may make the blood sugar too low.

| *Antihistamines* | *Combined with* | *Interaction* |
|---|---|---|
| Diphenhydramine (Benadryl), chlorpheniramine (Chlor-Trimeton), dimenhydrinate (Dramamine), promethazine (Phenergan) and others | alcohol | increases sedation |
| | barbiturate | nullifies both |
| | hydrocortisone | lessens effect of hydrocortisone |
| | phenothiazine tranquilizers (Thorazine, Compazine, etc.) | increases effects of both |
| | reserpine | depresses central nervous system |
| | anticholinergics (slows intestinal movement) | makes the anticholinergic more potent |

| *Antidepressants* | *Combined with* | *Interaction* |
|---|---|---|
| MAO-inhibitors (Marplan, Nardil, Parnate, Eutonyl) | alcohol | increases depression of central nervous system |
| | amphetamine | increases effect of amphetamine |
| | barbiturate | makes barbiturate more potent |
| | Demerol | makes Demerol more potent |
| | diazepam tranquilizers (Librium, Valium, etc.) | increases effect of tranquilizer markedly |
| | thiazide diuretics (Diuril, HydroDiuril) | lowers blood pressure and increases action of MAO-inhibitor |
| | tricyclic antidepressants (Elavil, Aventyl, Tofranil, Pertofrane) | increases effects of both |
| Tricyclic antidepressants (Elavil, Tofranil, Aventyl, Pertofrane, etc.) | diazepam derivatives (Librium, Valium, etc.) | increases effects of both |
| | phenothiazine tranquilizers (Thorazine, Compazine, etc.) | increases effects of both |
| | reserpine | lessens effect of reserpine |

| *Antibiotics* | *Combined with* | *Interaction* |
|---|---|---|
| Tetracycline | penicillin, antacid, or milk | makes tetracycline less effective |
| Penicillin G | chloramphenicol (Chloromycetin), antacid, or tetracycline | makes penicillin less effective |
| Griseofulvin (Fulvicin, Grisactin, Grifulvin) | anticoagulant | may make the anticoagulant less effective |
| | phenobarbital | makes griseofulvin less effective |
| Sulfonamide | antacid | makes sulfa less effective |
| | anticoagulant | makes the anticoagulant more potent |
| | antidiabetics (Dymelor, Orinase, Diabenese) | makes antidiabetics too powerful |
| Furazolidone (Furoxone) | alcohol | lessens bacterial action of drug and could skyrocket blood pressure |
| | amphetamine | increases effect of amphetamine |
| | barbiturate | increases action of the barbiturate |
| | MAO-inhibitor antidepressants (Nardil, Parnate, Marplan, Eutonyl) | increases effects of both |
| | phenothiazine tranquilizers (Thorazine, Compazine, etc.) | increases effects of tranquilizers |
| | tricyclic antidepressants (Elavil, Aventyl, Tofranil, Pertofrane) | increases effects of antidepressant |

### *Drugs That May Interact with Alcohol*

Antibacterials—inhibits germ-killing action of antibacterials.
Antidiabetic agents (including insulin)—may lower blood sugar to dangerous levels. Insulin also increases the effects of alcohol.
Antihistamines—depresses central nervous system.
Antihypertensives—increases the blood-pressure-lowering effect of drugs.
Antidepressants—increases the effect of alcohol and depresses the central nervous system.
Tranquilizers—affects coordination and depresses the central nervous system.
Sedatives and hypnotics—causes oversedation and depression of the central nervous system.

### *Food Interactions*

Milk and dairy products combined with antibacterials (such as tetracycline) make the antibacterial less effective.
Aged cheese, broad beans, chocolate, bananas, passion fruit, pineapples, tomatoes, and lemon combined with MAO-inhibiting antidepressants cause blood pressure to increase to dangerous levels.
Soybean preparations, Brussels sprouts, cabbage, cauliflower, kale, turnips, peaches, carrots, and pears may enlarge thyroid glands in susceptible people and make thyroid tests inaccurate.

### *Drugs That May Cause Skin Eruptions when Patient Is Exposed to the Sun*

Antibacterial sulfas.
Antidiabetic drugs like Orinase and Diabenese.
Thiazide diuretics such as Diuril and HydroDiuril.
Tranquilizers, including Librium and Compazine, among others.
Antihistamines, particularly Benadryl.
Anti-toning preparations.
Antibiotics, including Aureomycin and Terramycin.
Antifungal agents.
Birth-control pills.

# DRUG-TAKING BEHAVIORS

## Use, Misuse, and Abuse

The terms drug use, misuse, and abuse raise many questions regarding the distinctions between them. Samuel Irwin proposed the following distinctions:

1. **Drug use** occurs when a sought-for drug effect is realized with minimal hazard.
2. **Drug misuse** occurs when a drug is used for its intended purposes in such a way as to significantly increase the potential hazard to a user or other individuals.
3. **Drug abuse** occurs when a person repeatedly misuses a drug or uses it for other than its intended effects.[3]

Although these distinctions seem clear, there is considerable overlap and some confusion regarding distinctions between these different drug-taking behaviors. For instance, Irwin does not base his distinctions on legality. It appears from his definitions that it is possible to use drugs that are apparently obtained illegally, while at the same time it is possible to abuse drugs that are obtained legally. There is certainly some controversy among professionals working in the drug-abuse area regarding these definitions.

## Patterns of Drug Taking

In 1973, the National Commission on Marijuana and Drug Abuse recommended the adoption of another classification system for describing drug-taking behavior.[4] In the Commission's report, five general patterns of drug-taking behavior were described, including:

1. **Experimental use,** which implies the short-term use of any one or a combination of drugs. Experimental use seems most often to be a function of individual curiosity or a reaction to peer-group pressure. Experimental use refers specifically to the relatively short-term use of any drugs, and is generally associated with low hazard potential.
2. **Social-recreational use** of drugs refers to the relatively low-risk use of any of a variety of drugs in a social setting to experience euphoria, increase enjoyment of other activities, or as a social lubricant. (See figure 11.1.)
3. **Circumstantial-situational use** refers to a pattern of drug taking that is characterized by short-term activity as a coping mechanism to deal with particular situations.
4. **Intensified use** of drugs refers to the regular long-term use of a drug or several drugs in combination, as a regular, daily pattern of behavior. Drug dependence is often a characteristic of intensified drug use.

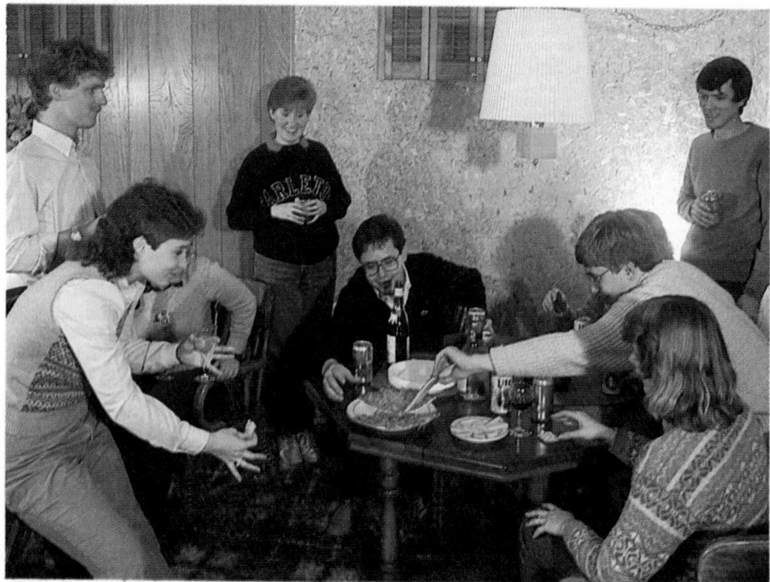

**Figure 11.1**
Drugs are used in a social-recreational context to increase enjoyment and encourage social participation.

5. **Compulsive use** of a drug or combination of drugs indicates that a person's patterns of use have changed substantially, and are no longer tied to pleasure, peer acceptance, or situational issues. This pattern of use reflects loss of control over the use of these drugs.

## Related Concepts

There are, of course, other terms that have been used historically to describe dependency states among drug users. The term **addiction** has been used to describe a state of chronic intoxication resulting from the repeated use of a drug. Addiction tends to be characterized by a compulsion to obtain and take a drug, the development of **tolerance** (the need to increase dose levels to obtain the same desired effects from a drug), and both a physical and psychological dependence on the drug. **Drug habituation** also refers to a state of chronic consumption based on a desire to experience the effects of the drug. Habitual users rarely feel a sense of overwhelming compulsion to use a particular drug, but there is a psychological dependence on the drug. (See table 11.2.)

**Table 11.2 Comparison of Addiction and Habituation**

| Drug Addiction | Drug Habituation |
|---|---|
| Drug addiction is a state of periodic or chronic intoxication produced by repeated consumption of a drug. Its characteristics include: | Drug habituation is a condition resulting from the repeated consumption of a drug. Its characteristics include: |
| 1. An overpowering desire or need (compulsion) to continue taking the drug and obtain it by any means. | 1. A desire (but not a compulsion) to continue taking the drug for the sense of improved well-being it engenders. |
| 2. A tendency to increase dose (tolerance). | 2. Little or no tendency to increase the dose. |
| 3. A psychic (psychological) and generally a physical dependence on the drug. | 3. Some degree of psychic dependence on the effect of the drug but absence of physical dependence. |
| 4. A detrimental effect on the individual and on society. | 4. Detrimental effect, if any, primarily on the individual. |

Source: Expert Committee on Addiction-Producing Drugs of the World Health Organization (1957). *WHO Technical Report Series no. 116, 1957.*

Both of these terms are often used interchangeably by people working in the field of drug abuse, and this has led to some confusion in the past. However, in 1965, the World Health Organization recommended that the term **drug dependence** be used in place of either addiction or habituation.[5] Eddy and others defined drug dependence as follows:

> Drug dependence is a state of psychic or physical dependence, or both, on a drug, arising in a person following administration of that drug on a periodic or continuous basis. The characteristics of such a state will vary with the agent involved, and these characteristics must always be made clear by designating the particular type of drug dependence in each specific case; for example, drug dependence of the morphine type, of the barbiturate type, of the amphetamine type, etc.[6]

Therefore, the term drug dependence is the preferred term to describe the results of chronic administration of a drug or combination of drugs.

When talking about drugs today, however, there are several other critical concepts that demand some attention. Richard Schlaadt and Peter Shannon refer to a "gray" area with respect to drug messages, and in fact define at least five aspects that relate to some of the confusion that we have about drugs today.[7] These areas include differences in the reactions to drugs by a variety of individuals, lack of quality control of the substances that we administer to ourselves, the effects of user expectations on drug outcomes, the influence of the setting in which drugs are taken, and the relationship between legality of a drug and its effectiveness and treatment.

The term **set** is an extremely important term related to drug use. In the broadest perspective, set refers to the total internal environment of an individual at the time that a drug is taken. This refers to an individual's mental, emotional, and physical state at that time. When you consider the complexity of describing the state of an individual at any given time, you realize that a great deal is involved, including an individual's physical-health status, mental and emotional state, nutritional status, mood, expectations, and experiences. Of particular importance are the user's expectations regarding a drug's effects. (See Exhibit 11.3.)

11.3 EXHIBIT 11.3

## The Love Drug of the Incas

The Incas possessed a drug that was such a powerful aphrodisiac that its use was restricted to those noblemen who could afford to support many wives. A man who drank this beverage could not possibly be satisfied by one woman or even by several but must have numerous wives available. The Spanish *conquistadors* found the drug to be equally potent, and many incidents of rape resulted from its use. The Catholic church tried to ban it as a destroyer of morals, but those who had become slaves to the habit could not give it up.

What was this potent aphrodisiac? It was hot chocolate! Admittedly the recipe was somewhat different from the hot chocolate your mother used to serve you when you came in from building a snowman, but the active ingredient was the same. Cocoa, with its caffeine and theobromine, gave the Inca's royal beverage its psychoactive kick. The Incan version contained no milk and, in place of marshmallows, contained crushed peppers, but these played no part in its aphrodisiac effects.

Some authorities suggest that the *cacao* plant of the Incas may have been bred for a higher concentration of caffeine and theobromine than the modern cacao plant but, even if this is true, it is not likely that the Incan hot chocolate was any more psychoactive than modern coffee. The difference was in the mind of the user. If we believed today that chocolate was an aphrodisiac, for most of us it would work as well as it did for the Incas.

Source: From *Drugs and the Whole Person,* by D. F. Duncan and R. S. Gold. (New York: Macmillan, 1982). Reprinted with permission of the publisher.

### DISCUSSION QUESTIONS

1. In what other ways can our expectations affect our experiences?
2. Are there any drugs today that people feel have aphrodisiac properties?
3. How do expectations play a role for these drugs?

**Setting** refers to the external environment of an individual when a drug is taken. Where a person is, what that person is doing, and who that person is with are all factors affecting the setting of a drug experience. (See figure 11.2.)

Set and setting play an extremely important role in determining exactly what a person will experience when taking a drug. When you consider the complexity of these factors, and how they constantly change for each of us, you may readily conclude that the likelihood of any individual's set and setting being the same at two different times is very small. Even less likely is the chance that all the variables that affect drug outcomes would be the same in two different individuals at any given time. Because of these differences, individuals may react differently to the same drug, and an individual may have somewhat different experiences when taking the same drug at different times. Differences in set and setting explain individual variation in drug experiences. In fact, when we talk about drug effects, we can only refer to likely effects in many cases, and these likely effects are based on averages and probabilities. When we talk about psychoactive drugs, there are few guaranteed effects. You have probably experienced some of these differences. You have seen or heard of times when a person could drink a great deal of a particular alcoholic beverage and appeared to tolerate it very well; yet at other times, an equivalent amount would result in drunkenness. This was probably due to differences in set and setting at the two different times. Table 11.3 illustrates some of the factors that are related to individual variation in drug experiences.

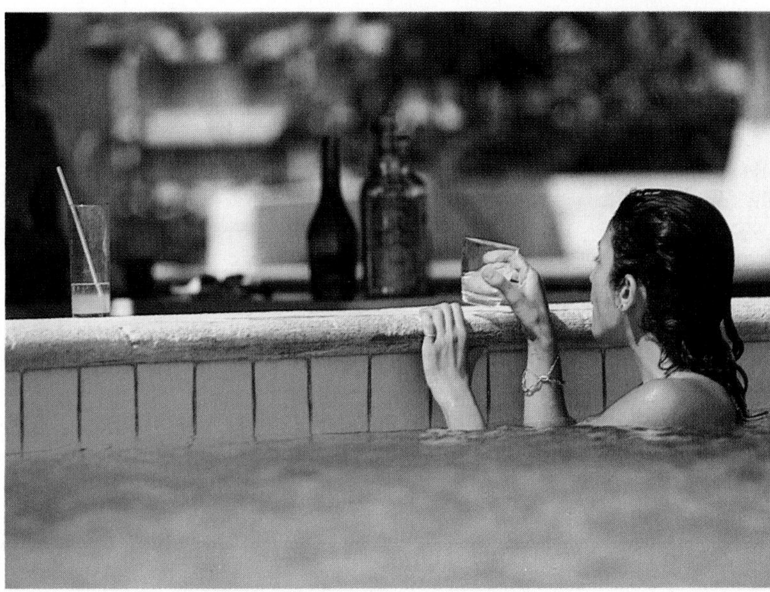

**Figure 11.2**
Setting strongly influences the experience of a drug user.

**Table 11.3 Some Factors Affecting the Outcome of a Drug Experience**

| Drug-Related | Set | | Setting |
|---|---|---|---|
| | *Physical* | *Mental* | |
| Which drug | Age | Motivation | Physical environment |
| Route of administration | Sex | Mood | What a person is doing |
| Dose level | Body size | Previous experience | Who a person is with |
| | Basal metabolism | Expectation | |
| | Heart rate | | |
| | Respiration rate | | |
| | Blood pressure | | |
| | General health | | |
| | Tolerance | | |
| | Genetic endowment | | |

Source: Adapted from: R. S. Gold and W. H. Zimmerli, *Drugs: The Fact. A Handbook for Helping Professionals.* Reprinted by permission and copyright © 1973 by Kendall/Hunt Publishing Company.

As can be seen from table 11.3, there are several drug-related variables that contribute to the effects experienced, including the drug taken, the dose level, and the route of administration of the drug. There are two very important terms related to dose level that should be considered carefully when talking about drugs. The **effective dose level** of a drug is the minimal dose required to elicit the desired response. Drug use implies the use of a drug with minimal hazard. All drugs can be dangerous when taken in too-large quantities. Therefore, in order to minimize the potential danger associated with drug taking, it is important that the smallest possible dose be taken that will result in the desired effects. As dose levels increase, the potential for side effects does as well.

The **lethal dose level** of a drug is that quantity which is sufficient to result in the death of the user. Clearly, dose levels approaching these quantities should be avoided. All drugs have lethal dose levels; overdose is a possibility with any drug.

# SOCIAL BARRIERS TO APPROPRIATE DRUG USE

Using recreational drugs such as alcohol can be an exciting and pleasurable social activity. Self-medication can be a source of relief from many unpleasant symptoms associated with illness and injury. However, responsible use in either case is important. The greater responsibility we take for our own actions, the greater the likelihood that the outcomes will be favorable. These responsibilities should not be taken lightly or given to others by default. We need to be responsible consumers of drugs as well as responsible users. This refers to both medicinal and recreational situations and settings. However, there are some barriers to appropriate use of some drugs. Most often, these barriers appear related to a lack of knowledge about responsible use, but there are many factors other than this that might explain inappropriate use. Among them are the influences of advertising, the attitudes and pressures from peers and family, and the availability of the drugs themselves. (See figure 11.3.)

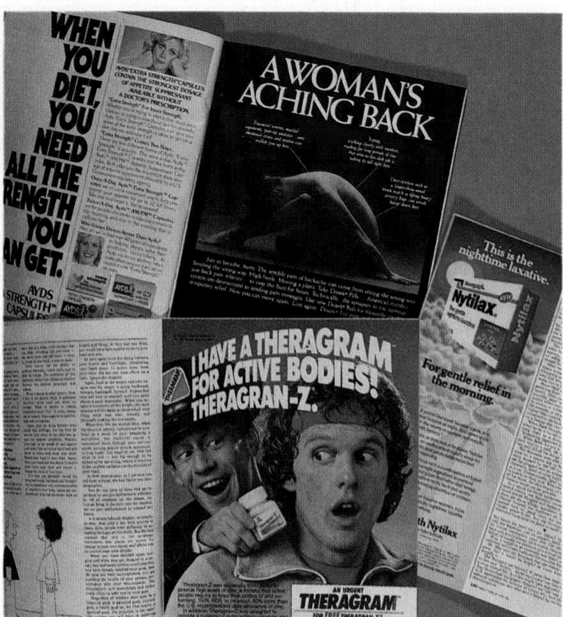


**Figure 11.3**
Advertisements for drugs are an attempt to sell better living through chemistry.

## Advertising

It is no secret that advertising is an important part of our everyday lives, helping to shape public opinion and consumer behavior in many ways. Advertising related to drugs has had many critics. Our concern here is whether or not the legitimate advertising of legal over-the-counter and prescription medications may in some ways shape our overall drug-taking behaviors. Arthur Berger has stated that "Although the act of taking drugs may be an individual one, the motivation that leads to this act is socially conditioned." Berger goes on to say that drug taking is "a learned behavior. Advertising which tells us of a better life through chemistry is doing some of this teaching. The climate of opinion that facilitates taking drugs is social, and not simply the result of individual decisions."[8] Similarly, Norman Johnson states that: "we manufacture a desire along with products. . . . It is a logical leap to say that because advertising is encouraging us to use some drugs, we tend to be more lenient with ourselves in using other drugs as well. It seems to me that this is a fairly obvious common sense conclusion to draw."[9]

The fact that we live in a drug-oriented society seems to be an important part of the following report. James Inciardi states that mass-media advertising of products has made the American public a puppet, especially: "in the areas of public health and physical fitness, since advertisements have traditionally stimulated feelings of anxiety which they say can be relieved by the consumption of various chemicals. And this notion of taking 'magic pills' is a phenomenon that has endured in the United States for over a century."[10]

In a study of the impact of televised over-the-counter drug advertisements and subsequent patterns of drug use, Chorsie Martin did an extensive review of the literature and found a great deal of controversy on the issue of whether or not advertising affected drug use, misuse, and abuse.[11] This may have been the result of faulty research designs rather than a clear statement about the relationship. It is clear, however, that advertising shapes our decisions, and our ability to make rational decisions is directly related to the safety and appropriateness of our drug use.

There are other important and related factors to be considered when examining cultural phenomena related to drug use, including attitudes that we have toward the drugs themselves, the attitudes of our parents and friends, the influences of peers and others, and the availability of drugs.

## Attitudes toward Drugs

In a study of high-school-student drug use from 1975 to 1980 done for the National Institute on Drug Abuse by Lloyd Johnston et al.,[12] the following was reported regarding beliefs about the harmfulness of drugs:

1. A substantial majority of high-school seniors perceive regular use of any of the illicit drugs, other than marijuana, as entailing great risk of harm for the user; however, only 50 percent of the sample felt that regular use of marijuana involved great risk, and many fewer respondents felt that a person runs a "great risk" of harm by simply trying the drug once or twice. Very few students in 1980 thought there was much risk in using marijuana experimentally (10 percent) or even occasionally (15 percent). At that time, the experimental use of other illicit drugs was still viewed as risky by a substantial proportion of the students surveyed (depending on the drug, the proportion ranged from 30 percent for amphetamines and barbiturates to 52 percent for heroin).[13]
2. From 1975 to 1979 there had been a modest but consistent trend in the direction of fewer students associating much risk with experimental or occasional use of most of the illicit drugs. This trend, however, was not continued in 1980.[14] (See table 11.4.)

**Table 11.4 Trends in Perceived Harmfulness of Drugs**

| | Percent Saying "Great Risk"* | | | | | | |
|---|---|---|---|---|---|---|---|
| *Question: How much do you think people risk harming themselves (physically or in other ways), if they . . .* | *Class of 1975* | *Class of 1976* | *Class of 1977* | *Class of 1978* | *Class of 1979* | *Class of 1980* | *'79–'80 Change* |
| Try marijuana once or twice | 15.1 | 11.4 | 9.5 | 8.1 | 9.4 | 10.0 | +0.6 |
| Smoke marijuana occasionally | 18.1 | 15.0 | 13.4 | 12.4 | 13.5 | 14.7 | +1.2 |
| Smoke marijuana regularly | 43.3 | 38.6 | 36.4 | 34.9 | 42.0 | 50.4 | +8.4 sss |
| Try LSD once or twice | 49.4 | 45.7 | 43.2 | 42.7 | 41.6 | 43.9 | +2.3 |
| Take LSD regularly | 81.4 | 80.8 | 79.1 | 81.1 | 82.4 | 83.0 | +0.6 |
| Try cocaine once or twice | 42.6 | 39.1 | 35.6 | 33.2 | 31.5 | 31.3 | −0.2 |
| Take cocaine regularly | 73.1 | 72.3 | 68.2 | 68.2 | 69.5 | 69.2 | −0.3 |
| Try heroin once or twice | 60.1 | 58.9 | 55.8 | 52.9 | 50.4 | 52.1 | +1.7 |
| Take heroin occasionally | 75.6 | 75.6 | 71.9 | 71.4 | 70.9 | 70.9 | 0.0 |
| Take heroin regularly | 87.2 | 88.6 | 86.1 | 86.6 | 87.5 | 86.2 | −1.3 |
| Try an amphetamine once or twice | 35.4 | 33.4 | 30.8 | 29.9 | 29.7 | 29.7 | 0.0 |
| Take amphetamines regularly | 69.0 | 67.3 | 66.6 | 67.1 | 69.9 | 69.1 | −0.8 |
| Try a barbiturate once or twice | 34.8 | 32.5 | 31.2 | 31.3 | 30.7 | 30.9 | +0.2 |
| Take barbiturates regularly | 69.1 | 67.7 | 68.6 | 68.4 | 71.6 | 72.2 | +0.6 |
| Try one or two drinks of an alcoholic beverage (beer, wine, liquor) | 5.3 | 4.8 | 4.1 | 3.4 | 4.1 | 3.8 | −0.3 |
| Take one or two drinks nearly every day | 21.5 | 21.2 | 18.5 | 19.6 | 22.6 | 20.3 | −2.3 |
| Take four or five drinks nearly every day | 63.5 | 61.0 | 62.9 | 63.1 | 66.2 | 65.7 | −0.5 |
| Have five or more drinks once or twice each weekend | 37.8 | 37.0 | 34.7 | 34.5 | 34.9 | 35.9 | +1.0 |
| Smoke one or more packs of cigarettes per day | 51.3 | 56.4 | 58.4 | 59.0 | 63.0 | 63.7 | +0.7 |
| N = | (2,804) | (3,225) | (3,570) | (3,770) | (3,250) | (3,234) | |

Note: Level of significance of difference between the two most recent classes: s = 0.05, ss = 0.01, sss = 0.001.
*Answer alternatives were: (1) no risk, (2) slight risk, (3) moderate risk, (4) great risk, and (5) can't say, drug unfamiliar.
Source: L. D. Johnston, J. G. Bachman, and P. M. O'Malley, *Drug Use among High School Students 1975–1980* (Washington, D.C.: National Institute on Drug Abuse Report under Grant no. 3 RO1 DA 01411–06), 79.

**Table 11.5 Trends in Proportions Disapproving of Drug Use**

| | Percent Disapproving* | | | | | | |
|---|---|---|---|---|---|---|---|
| *Question: Do you disapprove of people (who are eighteen or older) doing each of the following?*** | *Class of 1975* | *Class of 1976* | *Class of 1977* | *Class of 1978* | *Class of 1979* | *Class of 1980* | *'79–'80 Change* |
| Try marijuana once or twice | 47.0 | 38.4 | 33.4 | 33.4 | 34.2 | 39.0 | +4.8 ss |
| Smoke marijuana occasionally | 54.8 | 47.8 | 44.3 | 43.5 | 45.3 | 49.7 | +4.4 ss |
| Smoke marijuana regularly | 71.9 | 69.5 | 65.5 | 67.5 | 69.2 | 74.6 | +6.4 sss |
| Try LSD once or twice | 82.8 | 84.6 | 83.9 | 85.4 | 86.6 | 87.3 | +0.7 |
| Take LSD regularly | 94.1 | 95.3 | 95.8 | 96.4 | 96.9 | 96.7 | −0.2 |
| Try cocaine once or twice | 81.3 | 82.4 | 79.1 | 77.0 | 74.7 | 76.3 | +1.6 |
| Take cocaine regularly | 93.3 | 93.9 | 92.1 | 91.9 | 90.8 | 91.1 | +0.3 |
| Try heroin once or twice | 91.5 | 92.6 | 92.5 | 92.0 | 93.4 | 93.5 | +0.1 |
| Take heroin occasionally | 94.8 | 96.0 | 96.0 | 96.4 | 96.8 | 96.7 | −0.1 |
| Take heroin regularly | 96.7 | 97.5 | 97.2 | 97.8 | 97.9 | 97.6 | −0.3 |
| Try amphetamines once or twice | 74.8 | 75.1 | 74.2 | 74.8 | 75.1 | 75.4 | +0.3 |
| Take amphetamines regularly | 92.1 | 92.8 | 92.5 | 93.5 | 94.4 | 93.0 | −1.4 |
| Try barbiturates once or twice | 77.7 | 81.3 | 81.1 | 82.4 | 84.0 | 83.9 | −0.1 |
| Take barbiturates regularly | 93.3 | 93.6 | 93.0 | 94.3 | 95.2 | 95.4 | +0.2 |
| Try one or two drinks of an alcoholic beverage (beer, wine, liquor) | 21.6 | 18.2 | 15.6 | 15.6 | 15.8 | 16.0 | +0.2 |
| Take one or two drinks nearly every day | 67.6 | 68.9 | 66.8 | 67.7 | 68.3 | 69.0 | +0.7 |
| Take four or five drinks nearly every day | 88.7 | 90.7 | 88.4 | 90.2 | 91.7 | 90.8 | −0.9 |
| Have five or more drinks once or twice each weekend | 60.3 | 58.6 | 57.4 | 56.2 | 56.7 | 55.6 | −1.1 |
| Smoke one or more packs of cigarettes per day | 67.5 | 65.9 | 66.4 | 67.0 | 70.3 | 70.8 | +0.5 |
| N = | (2,677) | (3,234) | (3,582) | (3,686) | (3,221) | (3,261) | |

Note: Level of significance of difference between the two most recent classes: s = 0.05, ss = 0.01, sss = 0.001.
*Answer alternatives were: (1) don't disapprove, (2) disapprove, and (3) strongly disapprove. Percentages are shown for categories, (2) and (3) combined.
**The 1975 question asked about people who are "20 or older."
Source: L. D. Johnston, J. G. Bachman, and P. M. O'Malley, *Drug Use among High School Students 1975–1980* (Washington, D.C.: National Institute on Drug Abuse Report under Grant no. 3 RO1 DA 01411-06), 82.

3. By 1980, the great majority of students surveyed did not condone the regular use of any of the illicit drugs. Even regular marijuana use was disapproved by 75 percent. This seemed to be a marked reversal of the trends between 1975 and 1979 which indicated greater approval each year for regular use of many of these drugs.[15]

4. When we look at tobacco and alcohol, we see a general increase in the levels of disapproval over the entire study period.[16] The significance of this will be examined in the next few chapters.

These attitudes seem to be saying that the illicit drugs are generally perceived as risky by the students surveyed. However, there appeared to be somewhat higher levels of acceptance for the experimental use of some of these drugs. (See table 11.5.) It is within this cultural milieu or peer group that responsible decisions regarding the use of all drugs must be made. Let us look now at some of the other factors that influence our decisions.

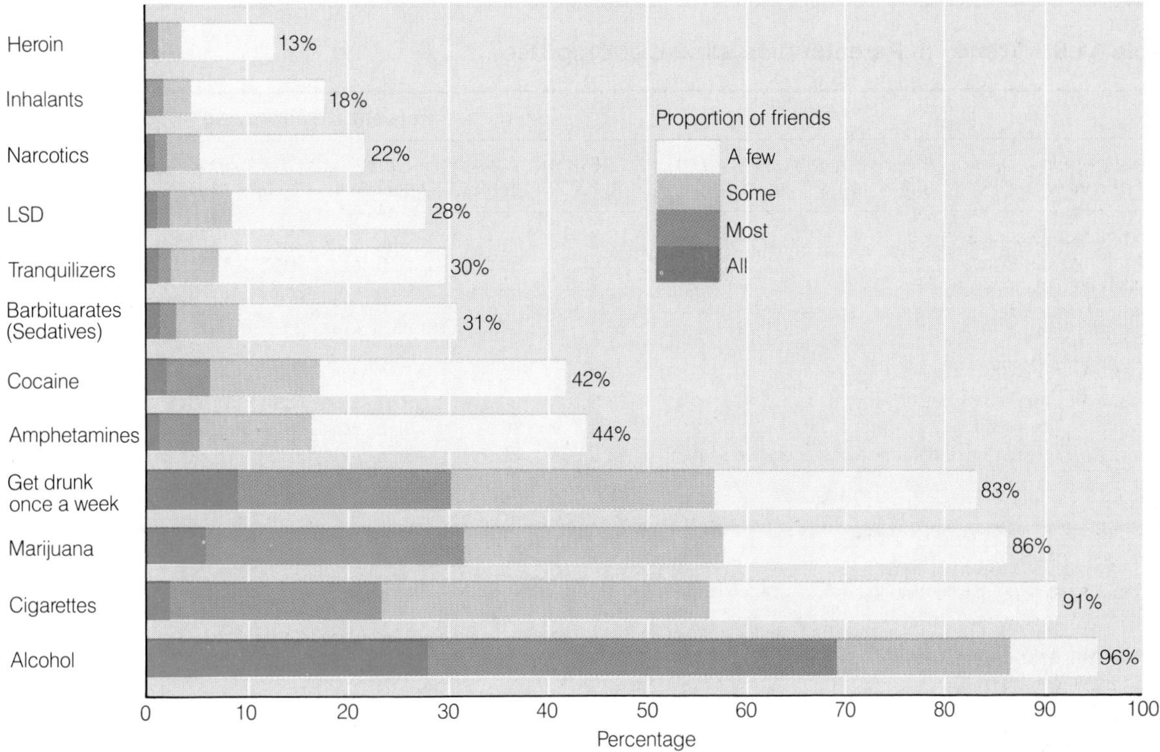


**Figure 11.4**
Proportion of friends using each drug as estimated by seniors, in 1980. *Source:* Johnston, Lloyd D., Jerald G. Bachman, and Patrick Y. O'Malley, *Drug Use Among High School Students* 1975–1980 (Washington, D.C.: National Institute on Drug Abuse under Grant no. 3 RO1 DA 01411–06), 99.

## Influence of Family, Peers, and Others

A good deal of research has indicated a relationship between the drug-taking behavior of an individual and the attitudes of his or her family and friends. With respect to friends, Johnston and others[17] report that such a relationship reflects several potential causal patterns. A person with friends who use a drug will be more likely to try the drug. Conversely, the individual who is already using a drug will be likely to introduce friends to the experience. Additionally, one who is already a user is more likely to establish friendships with others who also are users. Based on these potential relationships, several questions were asked in their study regarding exposure to drug use by friends and others. Figure 11.4 illustrates some of their results.

Johnston and others report the following summary of their results:

1. A comparison of responses about friends' use, and about being around people in the last twelve months who were using various drugs to get high, reveals a high degree of correspondence between these two indicators of exposure. For each drug, the proportion of respondents saying "none" of their friends use it is roughly equal to the proportion who say that during the last twelve months they have not been around anyone who was using that drug to get high. Similarly, the proportion saying they were "often" around people getting high on a given drug is roughly the same as the proportion reporting that "most" or "all" of their friends use that drug.[18]
2. Reports of exposure and friends' use closely paralleled the figures on seniors' own use. Highest levels of exposure involved alcohol and marijuana.[19]

The data concerning parental attitudes toward drug use by students indicates that the vast majority of parents disapprove of either experimental or regular use of most of the drugs. Table 11.6 illustrates the extent of that parental disapproval. Comparing table 11.6 with table 11.7, however, reveals quite a difference. In 1979 friends were perceived to be substantially more tolerant of drug use, although more than 40 percent disapproved all types of drug use. Compare 1979 with 1980 in table 11.7 and you will see that by 1980, significantly higher percentages of students disapproved of drug use.

## Table 11.6 Trends in Parental Disapproval of Drug Use

| | Percent Disapproving* | | | | | |
|---|---|---|---|---|---|---|
| *Question: How do you think your parents would feel about you . . .* | *Class of 1975* | *Class of 1976* | *Class of 1977* | *Class of 1978* | *Class of 1979* | *Class of 1980* |
| Trying marijuana once or twice | 90.8 | 87.4 | 85.8 | 83.2 | 84.9 | NA |
| Smoking marijuana occasionally | 95.6 | 93.0 | 92.5 | 90.8 | 93.2 | NA |
| Smoking marijuana regularly | 98.1 | 96.3 | 96.5 | 95.6 | 97.2 | NA |
| Trying LSD once or twice | 99.0 | 97.4 | 98.1 | 97.5 | 98.8 | NA |
| Trying an amphetamine once or twice | 98.0 | 97.1 | 97.2 | 96.7 | 97.9 | NA |
| Taking one or two drinks nearly every day | 89.5 | 90.0 | 92.2 | 88.9 | 91.8 | NA |
| Taking four or five drinks every day | 97.2 | 96.5 | 96.5 | 96.3 | 97.4 | NA |
| Having five or more drinks once or twice every weekend | 85.3 | 85.9 | 86.5 | 82.6 | 84.5 | NA |
| Smoking one or more packs of cigarettes per day | 88.5 | 87.6 | 89.2 | 88.7 | 91.3 | NA |
| Approx. N = | (2,546) | (2,807) | (3,014) | (3,054) | (2,748) | (NA) |

Note: NA indicates question not asked.
*Answer alternatives were: (1) not disapprove, (2) disapprove, and (3) strongly disapprove. Percentages are shown for categories (2) and (3) combined.
Source: L. D. Johnston, J. G. Bachman, and P. M. O'Malley, *Drug Use among High School Students 1975–1980* (Washington, D.C.: National Institute on Drug Abuse Report under Grant no. 3 RO1 DA 01411–06), 90.

## Table 11.7 Trends in Proportion of Friends Disapproving of Drug Use

| | Percent Saying Friends Disapprove* | | | | | | |
|---|---|---|---|---|---|---|---|
| *Question: How do you think your close friends feel (or would feel) about you . . .* | *Class of 1975* | *Class of 1976* | *Class of 1977* | *Class of 1978* | *Class of 1979* | *Class of 1980* | *'79–'80 Change* |
| Trying marijuana once or twice | 44.8 | NA | 42.3 | NA | 41.4 | 42.6 | +1.2 |
| Smoking marijuana occasionally | 54.0 | NA | 48.2 | NA | 47.4 | 50.6 | +3.2 |
| Smoking marijuana regularly | 70.4 | NA | 64.5 | NA | 65.6 | 72.0 | +6.4 sss |
| Trying LSD once or twice | 83.6 | NA | 84.6 | NA | 85.6 | 87.4 | +1.8 |
| Trying an amphetamine once or twice | 76.6 | NA | 78.1 | NA | 78.8 | 78.9 | +0.1 |
| Taking one or two drinks nearly every day | 59.4 | NA | 63.2 | NA | 63.2 | 70.5 | +7.3 sss |
| Taking four or five drinks every day | 79.9 | NA | 78.8 | NA | 79.2 | 87.9 | +8.7 sss |
| Having five or more drinks once or twice every weekend | 50.3 | NA | 48.7 | NA | 46.6 | 50.6 | +4.0 s |
| Smoking one or more packs of cigarettes per day | 55.3 | NA | 60.0 | NA | 65.1 | 74.4 | +9.3 sss |
| Approx. N = | (2,488) | (NA) | (2,971) | (NA) | (2,716) | (2,766) | |

Note: NA indicates question not asked.
*Answer alternatives were: (1) not disapprove, (2) disapprove, and (3) strongly disapprove. Percentages are shown for categories (2) and (3) combined.
Source: L. D. Johnston, J. G. Bachman, and P. M. O'Malley, *Drug Use among High School Students 1975–1980* (Washington, D.C.: National Institute on Drug Abuse Report under Grant no. 3 RO1 DA 01411–06), 91.

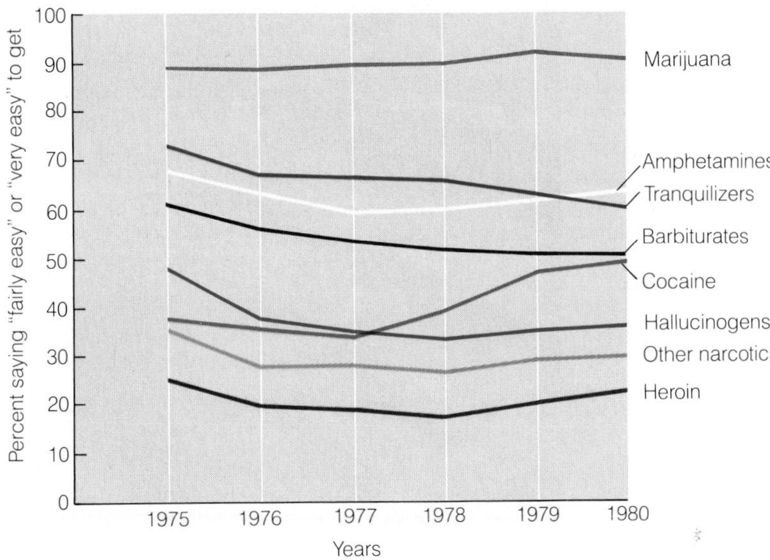


**Figure 11.5**
Trends in perceived availability of drugs. *Source:* Johnston, Lloyd D., Jerald G. Bachman, and Patrick Y. O'Malley, *Drug Use Among High School Students* 1975–1980 (Washington, D.C.: National Institute on Drug Abuse under Grant no. 3 RO1 DA 01411–06), 99.

### Availability of Drugs

Figure 11.5 contains the results of a set of questions regarding the perceived availability of drugs from the Johnston and others study of student drug use.[20] One set of questions asked for estimates of how difficult students thought it would be to obtain selected drugs. The results can be summarized as follows:

1. There were substantial differences in the reported availability of the various drugs. In general, the more widely used drugs were reported to be available by the highest proportion of respondents.[21]
2. Marijuana appeared to be almost universally available to these students, with almost 90 percent reporting that they thought it would be "very easy" to "fairly easy" for them to obtain.[22]
3. Amphetamines appeared to be available to 61.3 percent of the sample, followed by tranquilizers (59 percent), barbiturates (49 percent), and cocaine (48 percent).[23]

When comparing these data with previous years, there appeared to be no dramatic changes in the perceived availability of most of these drugs. The most substantial increase was for cocaine over the five-year period from 1975 to 1980.

## RESPONSIBLE DRUG USE

Drugs are clearly part of almost everyone's life-style and readily available to us in our environment. Not only are most people drug users, but more than that, most of us are polydrug users. It is possible for many reasons to slide from responsible use to misuse or abuse of any of the wide variety of drugs which we use. We have reviewed several different patterns of typical drug use, including experimental, social-recreational, circumstantial-situational, intensified, and compulsive drug use. For most of us, the choice of which drug to use and when is an individual choice and should not be taken lightly. An individual's ability to make decisions is important, and should be used appropriately when considering the use of drugs. Ruth Engs identifies several components of individual decision making that are relevant to choices concerning drug use.[24] When a situation is presented in which you should make a decision regarding drug use, you should:

1. Think about the situation and try to understand the reasons for using the drug.
2. Consider all the alternatives to using a drug by examining the reasons for use and thinking about alternatives for achieving your goals.

3. Attempt to identify potential difficulties associated with each of the alternatives identified.
4. Consider each alternative in the context of the situation you are in and select the one that seems best.
5. Take action on the alternative selected.
6. Assess the results so that you may have more information available to you the next time you are faced with a similar situation.

Choices regarding self-medication and recreational drug use lie with each person as an individual. However, in order to make reasonable decisions, we should understand the forces acting on us in each situation. Advertising may have an impact on our choices. Social forces such as parental and peer attitudes and availability of drugs also exert influences on our decisions regarding self-medication and recreational drug use. The issues specifically related to self-medication are important enough to deserve particular attention at this point.

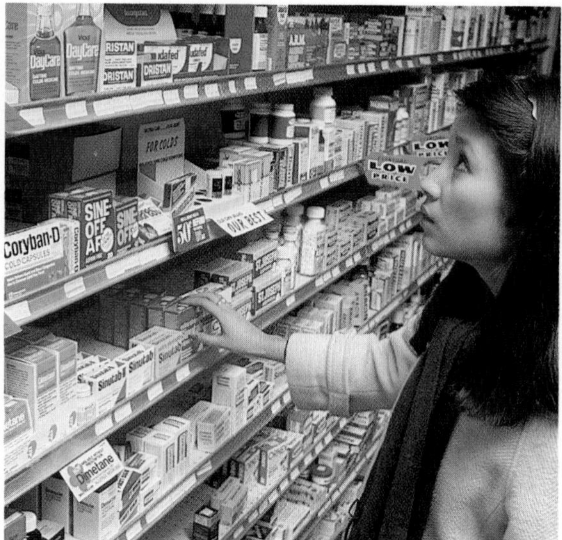


**Figure 11.6**
If used with care for short periods of time, OTC drugs can help relieve symptoms of discomfort or illness.

## Issues of Self-Medication

**Self-medication** refers to the self-selected or self-administered use of drug preparations to relieve symptoms of discomfort or illness. There are many times when we will legitimately want to use over-the-counter drugs or other medications for these purposes. The *Physician's Desk Reference for Non-Prescription Drugs* lists a great many afflictions that are more of an "inconvenience than a threat to everyday functioning."[25] It suggests, in fact, that if certain directions are followed, most people will be able to relieve the symptoms associated with these problems without harmful effects by the use of non-prescription medications. Among the conditions listed are acne, allergy, asthma, bronchitis, emphysema, burns and sunburn, the common cold, constipation, cough, dandruff, diarrhea, allergy or minor irritations of the eyes, fungal infections such as athlete's foot, hemorrhoids, indigestion, insomnia, menstrual problems, pain, skin irritations resulting from contact with poisonous plants, psoriasis, and a variety of vitamin and mineral deficiencies. Each of these conditions could legitimately be treated without a physician's supervision with over-the-counter preparations. (See figure 11.6.)

However, there are certain problems inherent in self-medication arising out of lack of knowledge concerning over-the-counter preparations, the belief many people hold that these preparations can be used safely without any potential for abuse or harm, and the potential of over-the-counter drugs to interact dangerously with other drugs we are taking and with some foods. These problems are magnified by the fact that many over-the-counter preparations are improperly or poorly labeled, that consumers often disregard the directions that are given, and that consumers are generally unaware of the potential problems arising from the warnings provided on many labels. However, the single most significant problem arising out of self-medication is the problem of delaying the diagnosis of a serious condition by masking its symptoms until it is too late. We sometimes forget that symptoms are the way that our body communicates to us that something is not right. If we choose to mask those symptoms by taking drugs to relieve them, we may be disregarding the messages we should be paying most careful attention to. Because of this, a medication should never be taken for a set of symptoms for more than a few days unless it has been recommended by a physician or someone else in a position to make a legitimate decision regarding the severity of the cause of those symptoms.

## Responsible Recreational Drug Use

In addition to the responsibility for appropriate self-medication for medicinal purposes, we must also recognize that we have certain responsibilities as recreational drug users. David Duncan and Robert Gold provide some general guidelines. They state that the recreational drug user:

> . . . has the responsibility of using the drugs with minimal hazard and of contributing to the pleasurable experience of being with friends in a social setting. These are important responsibilities that should not be overlooked. However, understanding those responsibilities and being able to live up to them requires knowledge about drugs and a commitment to their responsible use.[26]

Because of this, the responsibilities of recreational drug users are divided into three areas: (1) situational responsibilities; (2) health responsibilities; and (3) safety-related responsibilities.

**Situational responsibilities** arise out of circumstances in which drugs are used recreationally within a cultural or traditional context, such as social gatherings. Because psychoactive drugs are often made available in these circumstances, there are certain responsibilities that we should be aware of as a member of these groups, including:

1. Being prepared to provide a variety of acceptable models of behavior regarding the use of psychoactive drugs in recreational settings.
2. Respecting each individual's decision regarding the use of recreational drugs in a situation if it results in reasonable and responsible behaviors. It should be up to the group to define what is reasonable and responsible in these settings.
3. Recognizing that recreational drug use is not the only appropriate social lubricant in given situations.
4. Recognizing a responsibility for the health, safety, and pleasure of both the drug user and the abstainer by avoiding severe drug-induced intoxication and by helping others to do the same.
5. Having contingency plans ready to handle cases of severe intoxication if they occur in spite of the group's efforts at prevention. This means, of course, that each member of the group assumes some responsibility for the health and safety of other members of the group.
6. Being aware of the influences of set and setting on psychoactive drug experiences. You should recognize by now that this is quite a complex issue, but since set and setting are so important to the outcomes of recreational drug use, you should: (A) Only use recreational drugs when you want to use them. It is important not to be coerced into using potent psychoactive drugs you do not want to use, or when you do not want to use them. (B) Understand your own rationale for using any recreational drug. Make sure that your motivations and rationale are appropriate to the drug, yourself, and your situation. (C) Use psychoactive drugs recreationally only when you are in the company of others. We cannot take sole responsibily for the outcomes of drug use. If psychoactive drugs are used when you are alone, some of the outcomes are left to chance. Being with other people, especially those with whom we feel comfortable and sociable, reduces the potential for unanticipated negative experiences and tends to make the experience itself more pleasurable. (D) Provide or use recreational drugs only in an environment conducive to pleasant and rewarding experiences. This may well be different for each one of us, but consciously acting on this once again increases the potential for pleasure. Hazardous or threatening environments can negatively influence drug experiences.
7. Encouraging your peer group to set reasonable rules and rituals surrounding the use of recreational drugs. We typically find that when groups make a conscious effort to define the limits of responsible use of recreational drugs, there tend to be fewer difficulties associated with such drug use.

**Health-related responsibilities** are those that relate to our own health and the health of others. We can act responsibly for our own health and the health of others by:

1. Choosing to abstain from social-recreational drug use when it is appropriate for reasons of health or fitness.
2. Avoiding the frequent use of recreational drugs for the purpose of coping with problems.

3. Heeding the advice of a physician either to avoid the use of a particular recreational drug or to use it only as suggested.
4. Recognizing that social acceptability does not require drug use.
5. Using drugs in the manner intended, so as to reduce the potential hazards.
6. Recognizing that recreational drugs are DRUGS, and understand what that means. The outcomes of recreational drug use are substantially determined by the combined influences of set and setting, within the context of the quantity of the drug ingested and the circumstances under which it is taken. It is because of this that recreational drugs deserve as much of our respect as do other powerful psychoactive drugs.
7. Setting reasonable limits on the consumption of recreational drugs that are well within your own capacity, which can vary from time to time because of set and setting.
8. Being particularly careful of using combinations of drugs in recreational settings, because drug interactions can occur with these drugs as well as others.
9. Remembering that the use of some psychoactive drugs may mask signs and symptoms of serious illness or injury. It is thus important to avoid long-term continuous use of any psychoactive drug.

**Safety-related responsibilities** are an important consideration in any activity, including recreational drug use. Because of this, the following safety-related responsibilities are important to a recreational drug user:

1. Avoiding situations in which complex tasks must be performed while using recreational drugs. Most specifically, this means that motorized vehicles or large machinery should not be used at these times.
2. Avoiding situations in which we ride with a driver who is using recreational drugs, and discouraging that person from operating motor vehicles. (See figure 11.7.)

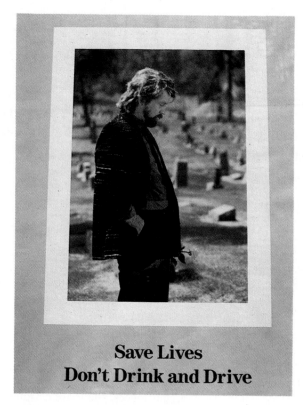


Save Lives
Don't Drink and Drive

**Figure 11.7**
Recreational drug users must always recognize their safety-related responsibilities.

3. Recognizing that our own drug-taking behavior can influence the behavior of others around us, especially the behavior of children. We should always consider carefully whatever actions are taken in the presence of children.
4. Using recreational drugs only in relaxed and responsible social situations.
5. Using recreational drugs in moderation, even if you think that your tolerance for these drugs is high. Remember that set and setting can influence behavioral tolerance to a drug as well as other characteristics of the drug experience.
6. Taking the smallest dose of a recreational drug that will produce the effects desired. Taking more than a minimally effective dose level of any recreational drug invites the potential for negative and unexpected side effects.

11.1 ACTIVITY FOR WELLNESS 11.1

## Deciding about Drug Use

List a drug you use now or are thinking about using. Dig out arguments for and against use of this drug. Some of these arguments are personal, others scientific in nature. Write your decision at the bottom of the page.

Drug: ______________________

| *For* (Positive Effects) | *Against* (Negative Effects) |
|---|---|
| 1. Effect on body ______ | Effect on body ______ |
| 2. Effect on mind ______ | Effect on mind ______ |
| 3. Effect on values ______ | Effect on values ______ |
| 4. Legality ______ | Legality ______ |
| 5. Effect on your human potential ______ | Effect on your human potential ______ |
| 6. Effect on family ______ | Effect on family ______ |
| 7. | |
| 8. | |
| 9. | |
| 10. | |

*Resolution:* Write down your decision. Will this decision change as you age? As your social situation changes? As you use other drugs? Or as the amount changes? ______________________

______________________

______________________

______________________

You may want to come back to this exercise after reading chapters 12 through 14.



7. Learning the usual side effects that can occur with the recreational drugs of your choice and being alert to any unexpected or expected side effects that may pose a potential threat to you or others around you.
8. Knowing basic first-aid techniques and taking responsibility for applying them appropriately in cases of drug emergencies.
9. Knowing your source of drugs, and only using sources you are confident you can trust.
10. Avoiding the use of unfamiliar drugs, especially when not in the company of others. This is even more important when we consider the consequences of mixing unfamiliar drugs.

(See Activity for Wellness 11.1.)

# DRUG USE AND PREGNANCY

Until now we have focused on some very broadly based issues related to drugs themselves and their use. We have tended to generalize these issues to all drugs. Before we go on, however, it will be worthwhile to examine one more general issue in regard to drug use—the relationship between drug use and pregnancy outcomes.

Poor pregnancy outcomes may result from disease, malnutrition, or lack of adequate prenatal care. Drug abuse, however, can be added as another potentially causative factor of poor pregnancy outcomes. As you remember from our discussion of set and setting, the specific effects of any drug taken by an individual cannot be predicted with precision. These factors are multiplied when we consider the difficulties associated with drug interactions, food/drug interactions, and the timing and dosage of drugs taken. In other words, nonmedical use of drugs during pregnancy is questionable and probably never justifiable. The Addiction Research Foundation of Ontario, Canada, lists three main ways in which a drug may influence the outcome of pregnancy:[27]

1. Prior to conception, a drug may alter the mother's bodily processes permanently or it may have a permanent effect on either of the parent's genes. Experiments on the effects of drugs on genes are generally limited to analysis of chromosomes in white blood cells, but it is only if the reproductive cells are damaged that the effect will be transmitted to a child.[28] Most of the current research has been done on such drugs as LSD and cannabis, but proof of their effects on genes is inconclusive. More important, a very defective fertilized egg will probably be spontaneously aborted shortly after being fertilized.[29]
2. During early pregnancy (embryonic stage), the use of some recreational drugs may be detrimental. It is especially dangerous during the first two months of pregnancy, since it is during this time that the organs are beginning to form. Drug use at this time may initiate deformities (teratogenic effects) in the developing neonate. Some critical periods of development include: the nervous system (fifteenth to twenty-fifth day); the eyes (twenty-fourth to fiftieth day); the heart (twentieth to fortieth day); and the legs (twenty-fourth to thirty-sixth day).[30] In the first week before cells begin to specialize, damage from a drug may lead to destruction of the ball of cells, or the unaffected cells might be able to compensate completely for the affected cells.[31]
3. During the later stages of pregnancy (fetal stage), when the fetus is growing and developing, drug use may be related to the potential for physical or mental retardation. We know that most drugs taken by a pregnant woman will reach an embryo or fetus. The placental link between the maternal and fetal blood supplies begins to develop within fourteen days of fertilization of the egg. This placental barrier has some of the same characteristics of other bodily barriers and membranes, that is, it allows the exchange of fat-soluble molecules between the two blood supplies. This, unfortunately, includes most recreational drugs and other drugs used for self-medication.[32]

Many problems are associated with drug use and pregnancy outcomes, regardless of whether drugs are taken prior to actual pregnancy or during the pregnancy itself. However, an embryo or fetus may face other drug-related problems during pregnancy. Perhaps the most important of these other possibilities is the potential for withdrawal from drugs to which the embryo or fetus became accustomed before birth. Such withdrawal, either during pregnancy or at birth, can be serious, especially with drugs such as barbiturates and opiates. We now know that this may also occur with some other common drugs such as alcohol,[33] and amphetamines.[34]

In the next few chapters we shall explore a variety of issues related to specific drugs. Additionally, we will take an in-depth look at alcohol, tobacco, and psychoactive drugs in the context of their use, misuse, and abuse.

# SUMMARY

1. We live in a drug-taking culture in which the availability of psychoactive agents is extensive.

2. There is no general agreement on a definition of the term "drug," but the soundest approach is to consider the term in its broadest context—as any agent which by its chemical action affects the structure or function of the body.

3. A useful way to categorize drugs is based on their availability and use. This scheme yields seven categories including herbal drugs, over-the-counter (OTC) drugs, prescription drugs, unrecognized drugs, tobacco, alcohol, and illicit drugs.

4. Many factors affect the outcome of a drug experience, particularly the set, setting, quantity, and route of administration of a drug.

5. Many cultural factors influence drug taking in our society, including advertising, attitudes toward drugs, and the availability of drugs.

6. Several guidelines for responsible recreational-drug use are provided, including situational responsibilities, health-related responsibilities, and safety-related responsibilities.

### Recommended Readings

Carroll, Charles. *Drugs in Modern Society.* Dubuque, Iowa: Wm. C. Brown Co., 1985.

Corry, James M., and Cimbolic, Peter. *Drugs: Facts, Alternatives, Decisions.* Belmont, Calif.: Wadsworth, 1985.

Duncan, David, and Gold, Robert. *Drugs and the Whole Person.* New York: John Wiley & Sons, 1982.

### References

1. Norman R. Farnsworth, "Psychotomimetic Plants II," *Journal of Psychedelic Drugs* 6.1 (1974): 83–84.

2. David F. Duncan and Robert S. Gold, *Drugs and the Whole Person* (New York: John Wiley & Sons, 1982), 5–6.

3. Samuel Irwin, "Drugs of Abuse: An Introduction to Their Actions and Potential Hazards," *Journal of Psychedelic Drugs* 3.2 (1971): 5–15.

4. National Commission on Marijuana and Drug Abuse, "Drug Use In America: Problem in Perspective." *Second Report of the National Commission on Marijuana and Drug Abuse* (Washington, D.C.: U.S. Government Printing Office, 1973), 95–97.

5. Nathan B. Eddy, J. Halbach, Harris Isbell, and M. H. Sievers, "Drug Dependence: Its Significance and Characteristics," *Bulletin of the World Health Organization* 32 (1965): 721–33.

6. Eddy et al., "Drug Dependence," 732.

7. Richard G. Schlaadt and Peter T. Shannon, *Drugs of Choice: Current Perspectives on Drug Use* (New York: Prentice-Hall, 1982), 1–2.

8. Arthur A. Berger, "Drug Advertising and the 'Pain, Pill, Pleasure' Model," *Journal of Drug Issues* 4.3 (1974): 208–12.

9. Norman Johnson, "Junkie Television," *Journal of Drug Issues* 4.3 (1974): 227–31.

10. James A. Inciardi, "Over-the-Counter Drugs: Epidemiology, Adverse Reaction, Overdose Deaths, and Mass Media Promotion," *Addictive Disease* 3.2 (1977): 253–72.

11. Chorsie E. Martin, "An Exploratory Study of the Relationship Between Commercial Television's Advertising of Over-the-Counter Drugs and Drug Use, Misuse, and Abuse Among Selected College Students," Ph.D. dissertation, Southern Illinois University, 1981.

12. Lloyd D. Johnston, Jerald G. Bachman, and Patrick O'Malley, *Highlights from Student Drug Use in America.* Department of Health and Human Services, Public Health Service, USDHHS publication no. (ADM) 81–1066 (Washington, D.C.: U.S. Government Printing Office, 1980), 78.

13. Johnston et al., *Highlights from Drug Use in America,* 78.

14. Johnston et al., *Highlights from Drug Use in America,* 80.

15. Johnston et al., *Highlights from Drug Use in America,* 81.

16. Johnston et al., *Highlights from Drug Use in America,* 81.

17. Johnston et al., *Highlights from Drug Use in America,* 89.

18. Johnston et al., *Highlights from Drug Use in America,* 100.

19. Johnston et al., *Highlights from Drug Use in America,* 100.

20. Johnston et al., *Highlights from Drug Use in America,* 103.

21. Johnston et al., *Highlights from Drug Use in America,* 104.

22. Johnston et al., *Highlights from Drug Use in America,* 104.

23. Johnston et al., *Highlights from Drug Use in America,* 104.

24. Ruth Engs, *Responsible Drug and Alcohol Use* (New York: Macmillan, 1979), 14–18.

25. *Physician's Desk Reference for Non-Prescription Drugs* (Oradell, N.J.: Medical Economics, 1980).

26. Duncan and Gold, *Drugs and the Whole Person,* 216.

27. Addiction Research Foundation, *Information Review: General Information on Psychoactive Drugs and Pregnancy* (Toronto: Alcoholism and Drug Addiction Research Foundation, 1979), 20.

28. N. Gray, *Everything You've Always Wanted to Know about Chromosome Damage* (Phoenix, Ariz.: Do it Now Foundation, 1975), 8.

29. Jerome M. Jaffe, *Prenatal Determination of Behavior* (New York: Pergamon Press, 1969).

30. Bernard L. Mirkin, "Effects of Drugs on the Fetus and Neonate," *Postgraduate Medicine* 47 (Jan 1970): 91–5.

31. Addiction Research Foundation, *Information Review,* p. 8.

32. Miriam F. Shore, "Drugs Can be Dangerous During Pregnancy and Lactation," *Canadian Pharmacology Journal* 103 (1970): 358–67.

33. M. M. Nichols, "Acute Alcohol Withdrawal Syndrome in a Newborn," *American Journal of Diseases in Children* 113 (June 1967): 714–15.

34. C. Ramer, "The Case History of an Infant Born to an Amphetamine-Addicted Mother," *Clinical Pediatrics* 13.7 (1974): 596–97.

CHAPTER TWELVE

# Alcohol: Risks and Responsible Usage



People use drugs for many reasons; virtually everyone uses drugs of some kind. Alcohol and tobacco, though legally obtainable for much of the population, still accounts for a large amount of illegal use among all drugs in our society. For example, more than 75 percent of the tenth graders surveyed reported having drunk alcohol though still under age to purchase it.[1] According to a survey done by Lloyd D. Johnston et al., nearly all students have tried alcohol by the time they graduate from high school (93 percent). The vast majority (72 percent) drank alcoholic beverages within thirty days of the time that the survey was conducted.[2] Moreover, nearly 6 percent of those high school students surveyed reported that they drink alcoholic beverages daily and 41 percent stated that during the prior two-week period they had more than five drinks on one occasion.

In the United States, the approximate average yearly consumption per person aged fourteen or older is: 29.78 gallons of beer, 2.60 gallons of distilled spirits, and 2.51 gallons of wine.[3] These beverages are not 100 percent alcohol, but in 1981 it was estimated that the yearly consumption of absolute alcohol was 2.77 gallons of alcohol per person, per year (beer 1.40 gallons; distilled spirits 1.01 gallons; and wine 0.35 gallons).[4] Per-capita alcohol consumption has been increasing yearly for the last few decades, with the largest increase in the consumption of beer. (See figure 12.1.)

Such large amounts of alcoholic beverages also account for a great deal of money spent in the United States. It is estimated that more than $43 billion is spent by Americans yearly on alcoholic beverages.[5] For comparison, the entire cost to the U.S. government for health care in 1978 was $192 billion. Alcohol expenditures equal approximately one-fifth of the total national expenditure for health care.

This chapter will introduce you to the effects of alcohol on the body, risks associated with misuse and abuse of alcohol, and suggestions for using alcohol responsibly.

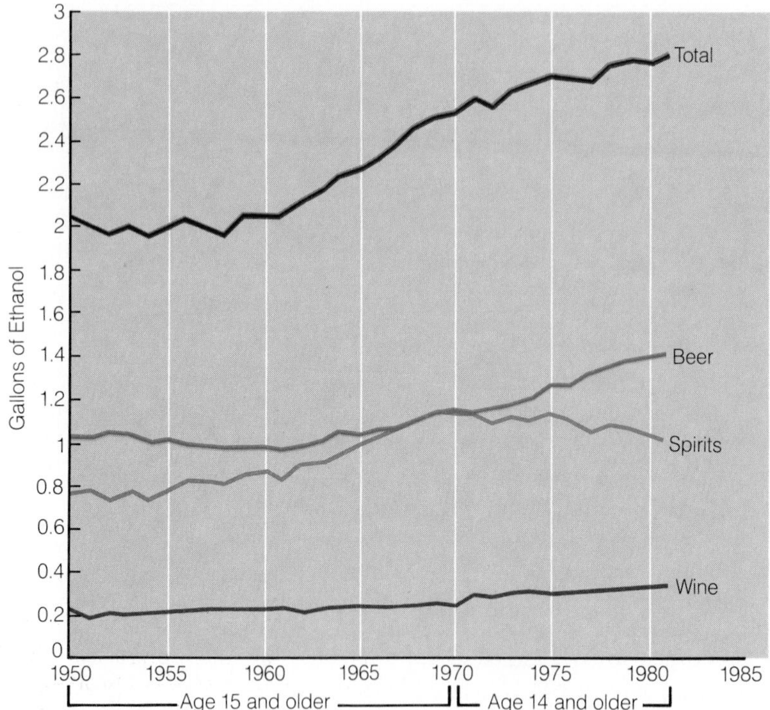


**Figure 12.1**
Apparent consumption of alcoholic beverages in gallons of ethanol per capita, 1950–1981. *Source:* Fifth Special Report to the U.S. Congress on Alcohol and Health, from the Secretary of Health and Human Services. DHHS, Washington, D.C. U.S. Government Printing Office (1983), 2.

## BASIC PHARMACOLOGY

There are many kinds of alcohols, but only three are commonly used. **Methyl alcohol,** sometimes called wood alcohol, is used in many industrial products such as antifreezes and fuels. It is very toxic to humans even in small quantities. **Isopropyl alcohol** (rubbing alcohol) is used as a disinfectant and a solvent. **Ethyl alcohol** (grain alcohol) is consumable. Ethyl alcohol can be produced either synthetically or naturally by a process called **fermentation.** Fermentation is a metabolic form of combustion of grains, with ethyl alcohol as one of the end products. Fermentation can occur in fruits, vegetables, or grains; therefore any one of these products can be used to produce drinking alcohol. (See table 12.1.) The process of fermentation will continue naturally until the concentration of alcohol is sufficiently high to kill the yeast organisms that are responsible for fermentation. Approximately 14 percent alcohol is the natural limit on production by yeast organisms. In order to get an alcohol concentration higher than 14 percent, additional action must be taken, such as distillation or fortification. With either of these two processes, the concentration of alcohol produced can be much higher than 14 percent.

In the U.S. today, there are four principal types of alcoholic beverages made from ethyl alcohol: beers (3–5 percent alcohol); wines (10–14 percent alcohol); fortified wines, such as sherry, port, and vermouth (14–20 percent alcohol); and distilled spirits, such as whiskey, rum, and gin (approximately 40 percent alcohol). Based on absolute alcohol, a 12-ounce bottle of beer, a 5-ounce glass of wine, 3 ounces of fortified wines, or 1.5 ounces of distilled spirits all contain the same quantity of alcohol—approximately 0.6 ounces of absolute alcohol. (See figure 12.2.)

Table 12.1 **Sources of Alcoholic Beverages**

| Beverage | Source | Percent Alcohol | Comments |
|---|---|---|---|
| Beer | Malted barley | 4–6 | — |
| Ale | Malted barley | 6–8 | — |
| Wine | | | |
| Dry | Grape juice | 12–14 | — |
| Sweet | Grape juice | 18–21 | Fortified |
| Whiskey | Malted grains | 40–50 | Distilled |
| Brandy | Grape juice | 40–50 | Distilled |
| Rum | Molasses | 40–50 | Distilled |
| Vodka | Various sources | 40–50 | Distilled |
| Gin | Various sources | 40–50 | Distilled |

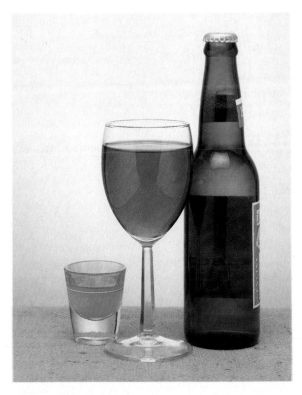

**Figure 12.2**
A bottle of beer, a glass of wine, and a shot of whiskey all contain the same quantity of absolute alcohol.

## Alcohol Absorption

Ethyl alcohol requires no digestion before it is absorbed into the bloodstream. Approximately 20 percent of the alcohol ingested is absorbed in the stomach while the remaining 80 percent is absorbed in the upper third of the small intestine (called the **duodenum**). Figure 12.3 illustrates some of the primary absorption sites.

Darwin Dennison, Thomas Prevet, and Michael Affleck have identified seven factors that influence the rate of absorption at the primary absorption sites.[6] These seven factors are: alcohol concentration, rate of consumption, amount of alcohol consumed, chemical present in the alcoholic beverage, condition of the stomach, pylorospasm, and emotional condition.

**ALCOHOL CONCENTRATION** The higher the concentration of alcohol, the more rapidly it is absorbed in the digestive tract to an upper limit of approximately 40 percent. After that limit is reached, absorption is slowed.

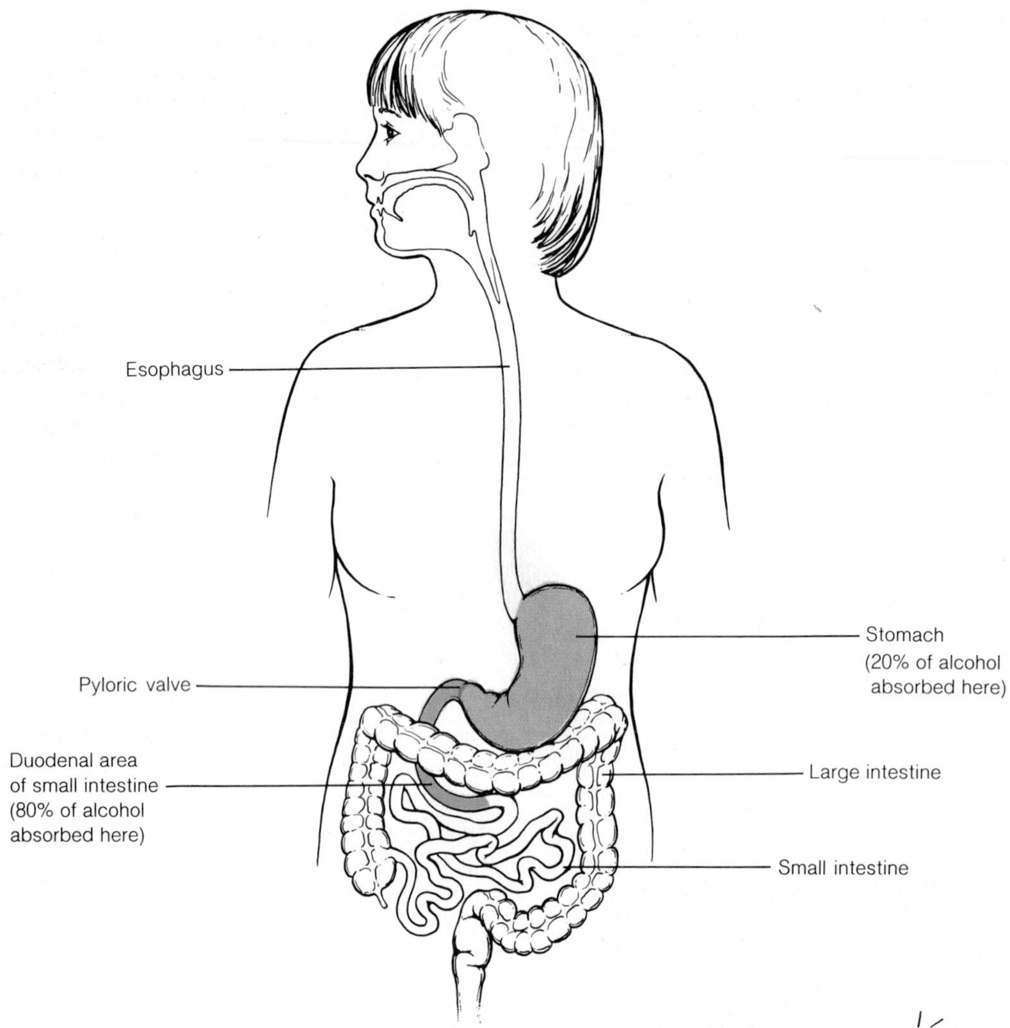


**Figure 12.3**
Sites of alcohol absorption. *Source:* Reproduced by permission from D. Dennison, T. Prevet, and M. Affleck, *Alcohol and Behavior.* St. Louis, 1980, The C. V. Mosby Company.

**RATE OF CONSUMPTION** The more rapidly a person drinks, the greater the quantity of absorption to a point. Overall, however, the rate of absorption is not affected by quantity consumed.

**AMOUNT OF ALCOHOL CONSUMED** The greater the quantity consumed, the longer absorption takes.

**CHEMICAL PRESENT IN THE ALCOHOLIC BEVERAGE** When nonalcoholic beverages are mixed with alcohol, the absorption process is generally slowed, unless the mixers contain carbonated beverages. Carbonated beverages cause the **pyloric valve** (the ring of muscle separating the stomach and the duodenum) to relax, thereby emptying the contents of the stomach more rapidly into the small intestine. Since the small intestine is the site of the greatest absorption of alcohol, carbonated beverages (such as champagne, other carbonated wines, and drinks mixed with carbonated mixers) increase the rate of absorption by causing a more rapid transition through the stomach. (See figure 12.4.)

**CONDITION OF THE STOMACH** Many people think that eating will slow absorption of alcohol because the stomach will be coated. It is not uncommon for people to drink milk or eat other related

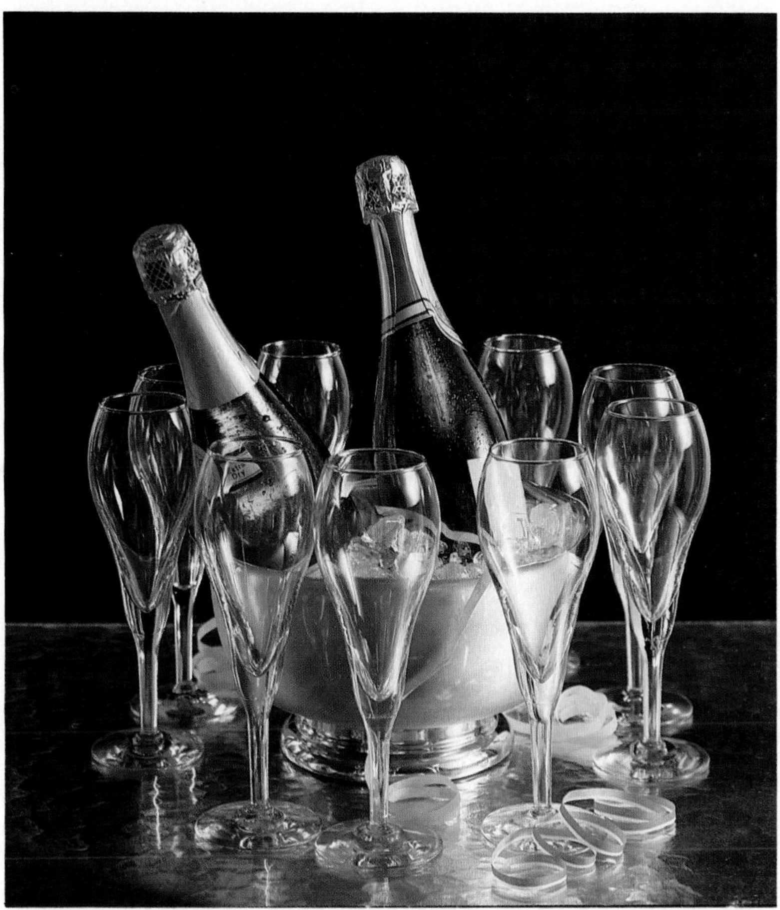

**Figure 12.4**
Carbonated beverages are absorbed more quickly into the bloodstream.

products before going drinking. This will slow absorption of alcohol, but it is not because the stomach is coated, but because the stomach will not empty its contents into the small intestine until digestion in the stomach is complete. The presence of food in the stomach will slow this emptying into the small intestine and slow down the absorption of alcohol. Not all foods remain in the stomach for the same length of time. Complex chemicals such as proteins remain in the stomach much longer than do carbohydrates, and therefore, proteins will slow absorption at a greater rate than carbohydrates.

**PYLOROSPASM** Alcohol can be an irritant to the lining of the digestive system. Occasionally, this irritation can cause the pyloric valve to go into a spasm (contraction) called **pylorospasm**. When the pyloric valve is closed, nothing can move from the stomach to the upper small intestine, and absorption is slowed. If the irritation continues, it can cause nausea and vomiting to occur.

**EMOTIONAL CONDITION** We have already seen in chapter 11 that set and setting are important factors in determining the outcomes of drug experiences. In the case of alcohol absorption, the emotions play an important role in the operation of the pyloric valve and therefore affect the rate at which alcohol is absorbed. Stress and tension cause more rapid emptying of the stomach, and therefore alcohol is absorbed much more rapidly when people are tense than when they are relaxed.

All of these factors taken together determine the absorption rate of alcoholic beverages by affecting transit time in the digestive system. Those factors that reduce transit time are associated with more rapid absorption of alcohol; those factors that increase transit time slow down the rate of absorption of alcohol.

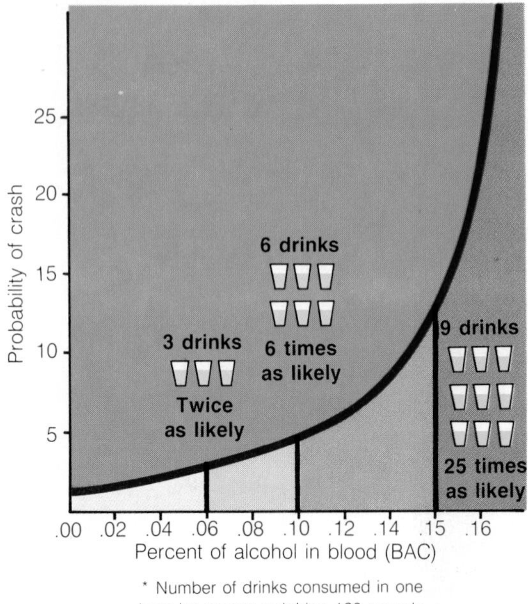


**Figure 12.5**
One drink can be too many—for safe driving. *Source:* Courtesy of AAA Iowa.

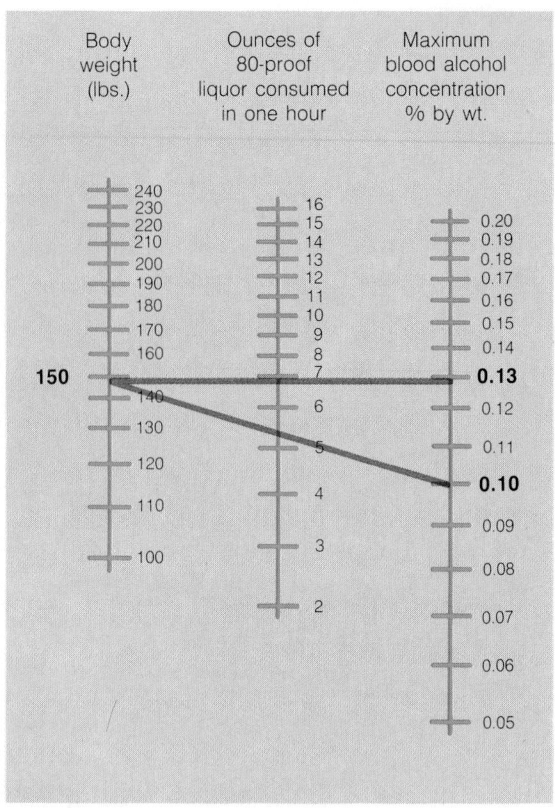


**Figure 12.6**
How drinking increases your chances of having a crack up. *Source:* Courtesy of AAA Iowa.

## Alcohol Distribution

Alcohol is water soluble and therefore, once it is absorbed, distribution to all bodily tissues is complete. Alcohol easily crosses all tissue barriers, including the **placental barriers.** Once in the bloodstream, metabolism of alcohol begins. In humans, the rate of metabolism of alcohol is relatively stable, with approximately 7–10 grams (0.31–0.44 ounces) of absolute alcohol metabolized per hour. Of all the alcohol consumed, 95 percent must be metabolized by the liver, with the remainder eliminated in the breath, urine, and perspiration.

## Blood Alcohol Levels

**BLOOD ALCOHOL CONCENTRATION** **Blood alcohol concentration** (**BAC**) can be defined as the ratio of alcohol to total blood volume. As an example, in an average male, (weighing approximately 150 pounds), one drink would produce a BAC of approximately 0.02 (two parts of alcohol to every one hundred parts of blood). At the 0.07 level, people are considered impaired and at the 0.1 level people are considered intoxicated.[7]

Figures 12.5 and 12.6 provide information regarding blood alcohol levels and number of drinks necessary to cause those levels, based on body weight. Larger people are generally able to maintain a lower BAC than smaller people who drink the same amount of alcohol at the same rate. However, this is not a hard-and-fast rule. Some people who weigh the same have different concentrations of muscle and fat, so blood alcohol concentrations may differ between them.

**PHYSIOLOGICAL AND PSYCHOLOGICAL EFFECTS** Of greater importance overall than absolute BAC are the immediate physiological and psychological effects of alcohol at these various levels and their subsequent impact on a person's behavior. Once again, we must recall the importance of the notion of individual variation when we consider the

**Table 12.2 General Behavioral Characteristics at Various Blood Alcohol Levels**

| Number of Alcoholic Beverages | Blood Alcohol Level (%) | Effects | Time to Wait Before Driving (Hours) |
|---|---|---|---|
| 1 | 0.02–0.03 | Slight elevation of mood; mild euphoria; sense of well-being; slight dizziness; some impairment of judgment and memory | — |
| 2 | 0.05–0.06 | Sense of warmth; lowered alertness; mental relaxation; mild sedation; exaggerated behavior; loss of restraints; disruption of judgment; slowed reaction time; decrease in fine-motor coordination | 1 |
| 3 | 0.08–0.09 | Speech impairment; visual and hearing perception impaired; loss of some motor skills; equilibrium reduced; exaggerated emotion; talkativeness; noisiness | 2 |
| 4 | 0.11–0.12 | Gross-motor coordination affected; clumsiness; impaired ability to drive a car; drowsiness; unsteadiness; depression of sensory functioning; mental faculties impaired | 3 |
| 5 | 0.14–0.15 | Major physical and mental impairment; severe impairment of perception and judgment; unsteadiness and staggering; difficulty in talking | 4 |
| 7 | 0.20 | Marked depression of sensory and motor capabilities; difficulty in maintaining standing position; visual distortions; poor judgment; confusion; high driving risk | 5 |
| 10 | 0.30 | Severe motor disturbances; poor comprehension; uninhibited behavior; stupor condition; may vomit; involved in accidents frequently | 9 |
| 14 | 0.40 | Almost complete loss of feeling and perception; may be unconscious, in a stupor, or coma | |
| 17 | 0.50 | Coma | |
| 20 | 0.60 | Death due to cardiac and respiratory failure | |

Source: Reproduced by permission from D. Dennison, T. Prevet, and M. Affleck, *Alcohol and Behavior*. St. Louis, 1980, The C.V. Mosby Company.

overall effects of alcohol. For instance, at a given level of BAC, two different people may exhibit differences in their degree of intoxication within some range. These differences are once again related to set and setting, that is the biological, psychological, and social differences between individuals. Therefore, two different people with a 0.05 BAC may exhibit quite different behavior. Table 12.2 contains a summary of the *general* behavioral characteristics of most individuals at given blood alcohol levels.

Alcohol is primarily a depressant. It acts on the central nervous system by decreasing its activity over time. The greater the BAC, the greater the effects on the central nervous system. Exactly how alcohol depresses the central nervous system is not yet known. However, the depression is progressive and continuous. At the lowest levels of BAC, the higher centers of the brain are affected first. (See figure 12.7.) As the number of drinks increases and BAC increases, the depression of the central nervous system continues until the deepest motor areas are affected. (See Exhibit 12.1.)

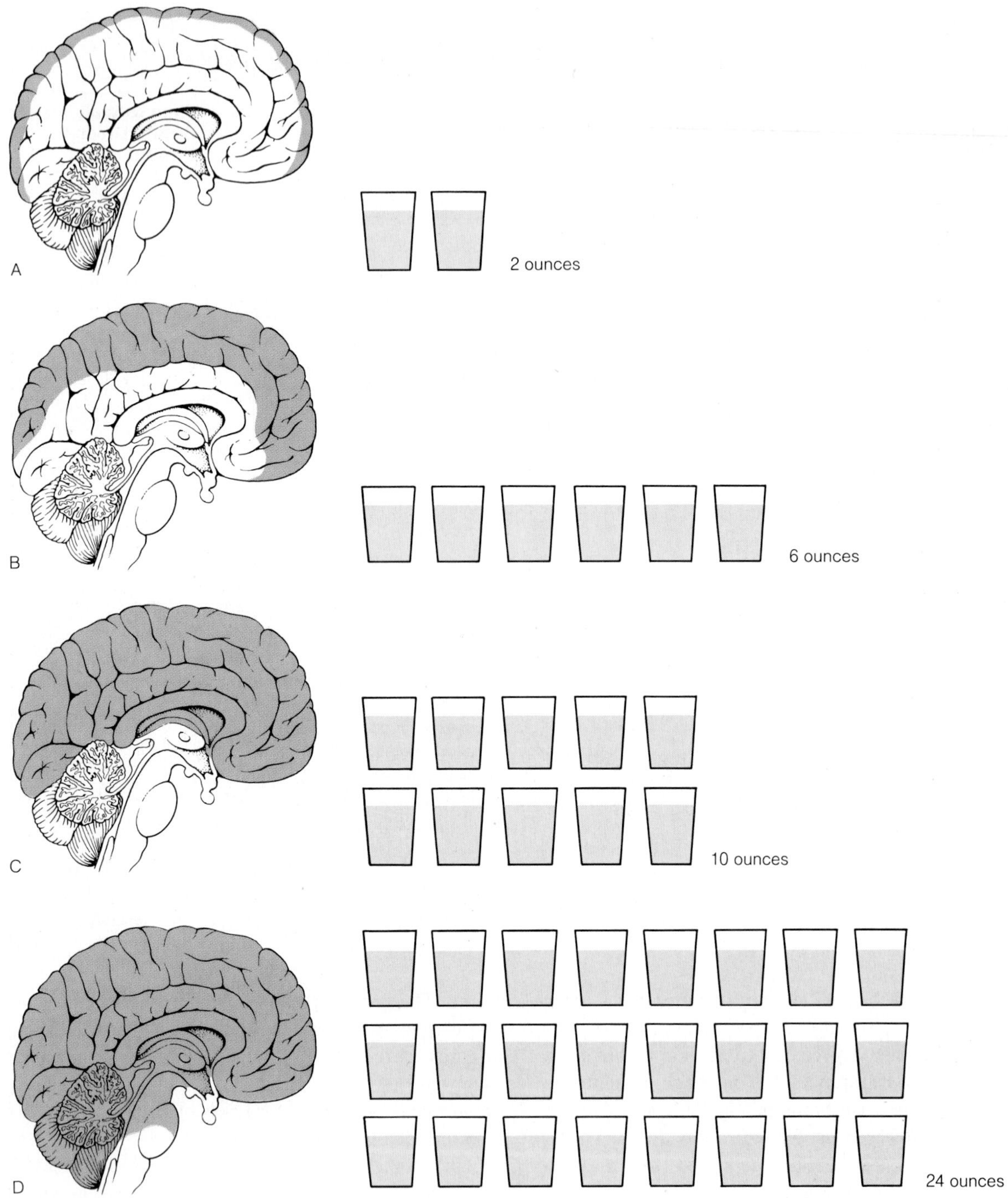


**Figure 12.7**
Alcohol and its effects on the brain. *Source:* Reproduced by permission from Betty S. Bergersen (in consultation with Andres Goth) *Pharmacology in Nursing,* 12th ed. St. Louis, 1973, The C.V. Mosby Company.

12.1 EXHIBIT 12.1

## Differences in Women

Substitute a 120-pound woman in these examples, and the weight differential would certainly speed up the process. With one drink in one hour, she would have a blood alcohol level of 0.03; two and a half drinks would mean a level of 0.07; five drinks, a reading of 0.14. Should she make it through a pint, she'd be in a coma with a level of 0.45. Tomorrow might not come as soon for her. Besides the differences in body weight, other factors can speed up or alter this process. Women and men differ in their relative amounts of body fat and water. Women have a higher proportion of body fat and correspondingly lower amounts of water. Alcohol is not fat soluble. Therefore, a woman and a man of the same body weight, both drinking the same amounts of alcohol, will have different blood alcohol levels. The woman's will be higher, since her body has less water than his in which to dilute the alcohol.

There is another critical difference between men and women in regard to how they handle alcohol. A woman's menstrual cycle significantly influences her rate of absorption. This difference presumably relates to the changing balances of sex hormones and appears to be the result of several interacting factors. During the premenstrual phase of her cycle, a woman absorbs alcohol much more rapidly than in other phases of the menstrual cycle. So premenstrually a woman will get a higher blood alcohol level than she would get from drinking an equivalent amount at other times. In practical terms, a woman may find herself getting drunk faster right before her period. There is also evidence that women taking birth-control pills also will absorb alcohol faster and thereby have higher blood alcohol levels.

Other differences may also exist between men and women in terms of alcohol's effects. Virtually all the physiological research so far has been conducted on men. Researchers have simply assumed that their findings are equally true for both men and women. Although the basic differences between absorption rates of men and women were reported as early as 1932, they were forgotten and/or ignored until the mid-1970s. Believe it or not, the impact of the menstrual cycle was first reported in 1976! This failure to examine the effects of the primary and obvious difference between males and females makes us wonder what more subtle areas have not been looked at.

Source: Reproduced from Jean Kinney and G. Leaton, *Loosening the Grip. A Handbook of Alcohol Information*, 2d ed. St. Louis, 1983. The C.V. Mosby Company.

### DISCUSSION QUESTIONS

1. If the effects of alcohol were not distinguishable between men and women for so long, what other differences might remain undiscovered?

2. What do you think are the reasons that virtually all physiological research to date has been conducted on men?

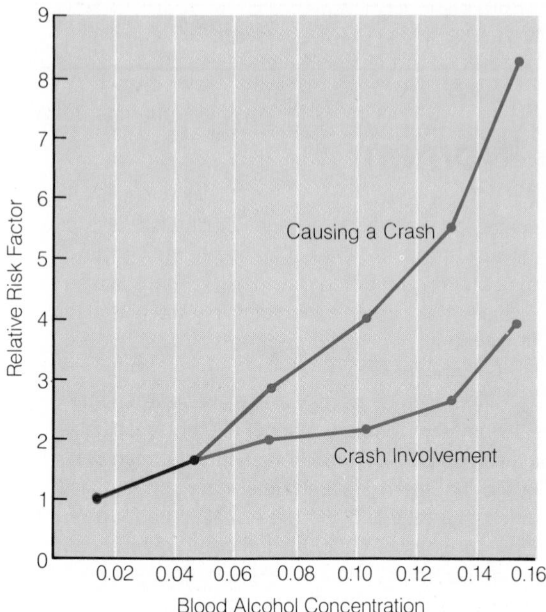


*Relative to the probability that a driver with a BAC of less than 0.03% is in or causes a crash.

**Figure 12.8**
Relative probability* that a driver causes and is involved in a crash as a function of blood alcohol levels. *Source:* Aarens, Marc, Tracy Cameron, Judy Roizen, Ron Roizen, Robin Room, Dan Schneberk, and Deborah Winegard, *Alcohol Casualties and Crime.* Special report prepared for National Institute on Alcohol Abuse and Alcoholism under Contract No. ADM 281–76–0027. (Berkeley, Calif.: Social Research Group, University of California, 1977.)

# IMPAIRMENT OF DRIVING SKILLS

Table 12.2 contains a summary of some of the more common behavioral consequences of selected BACs, as well as the amount of time to wait before driving. However, the influence of alcoholic-beverage consumption and driving performance needs somewhat more attention. Of the nearly 60,000 fatal automobile accidents yearly on U.S. highways, at least half can be attributed to alcohol. In addition to these fatalities, it is estimated that alcohol could be involved in more than 50 percent of the nearly fifteen million crashes and one million major injuries yearly on our nation's highways.[8] Many of these occur among drivers under twenty-one years of age. Brent Q. Hafen indicates several reasons why this may be so, including:

1. The young person who drinks lacks experience in compensating for the effects of alcohol.
2. The young driver is an inexperienced driver, hence necessary driving skills are less automatic and more inclined to deteriorate from alcohol's effects.
3. The inclination to take risks, especially strong in young people, may be accentuated by alcohol.
4. On the average, young people weigh less than adults and are therefore more susceptible to the effects of smaller amounts of alcohol.[9]

Figure 12.8 illustrates the direct relationship between the amount of alcohol in a driver's bloodstream and the likelihood of an accident occurring. At a BAC of 0.10, a driver has approximately ten times the likelihood of being involved in a car accident than a driver who has not been drinking alcoholic beverages. At a BAC of 0.15, the probability increases to twenty-five times. The specific effects of BAC concentration on our ability to drive are summarized in table 12.3.

# ALCOHOL AND PREGNANCY

In 1977, this statement was published in two sources:

> Recent reports indicate that heavy use of alcohol by women during pregnancy may result in a pattern of abnormalities in the offspring, termed Fetal Alcohol Syndrome (FAS), which consists of specific congenital and behavioral abnormalities. Studies undertaken in animals corroborate the initial observations in humans and indicate as well an increased incidence of stillbirths, resorptions, and spontaneous abortions. Both the risk and the extent of abnormalities appear to be dose-related, increasing with higher alcohol intake during the pregnancy period. In human studies, alcohol is an unequivocal factor when the full pattern of the Fetal Alcohol Syndrome is present. In cases where all of the characteristics are not present, the correlation between alcohol and the adverse effects is complicated by such factors as nutrition, smoking, caffeine, and other drug consumption. Given the total evidence available at this time, pregnant women should be particularly conscious of the extent of their drinking. While safe levels of drinking are unknown, it appears that a risk is established with ingestion above 3 ounces of absolute alcohol or six drinks per day. Between 1 ounce and 3 ounces [current thinking puts these figures at 2 ounces or four drinks a day], there is still uncertainty but caution is advised. Therefore, pregnant women and those likely to become pregnant should discuss their drinking habits and the potential dangers with their physicians.

Table 12.3 **Blood Alcohol Concentration and Driver Impairment**

| Blood Alcohol Concentration | Common Effects on Driving Ability | Approximate Amount of Liquor* |
|---|---|---|
| 0.02% | Mild changes occur. Many drivers may have slight change in feelings. Existing mood (anger, elation, etc.) may be heightened. Bad driving habits are slightly pronounced. | 1–2 ounces |
| 0.05 | Driver takes too long to decide what to do in an emergency. Inhibitions may be influenced. Shows a "so what" attitude, exaggerated behavior and what appears to be loss of finger skills. In most states this blood alcohol concentration may be considered with other competent evidence in determining whether the person is legally under the influence of alcohol. | 2–3 ounces |
| 0.10 | Driver exhibits exaggerated emotion and behavior—less concern, mental relaxation. Inhibitions, self-criticism, and judgment** are seriously affected. Shows impairment of skills of coordination. At this blood-alcohol level a driver is presumed "under the influence" in all states—and in many, .10% BAC is evidence of being "under the influence." | 5–6 ounces |
| 0.15 | Shows serious and noticeable impairment of physical and mental functions; clumsy, uncoordinated, should wait 9–10 hours before driving. | 7–8 ounces |
| 0.40 | At this point most drivers have "passed out" (unconsciousness, clammy skin, dilated pupils). | Approximately 15–20 ounces |

*Beverages 90–100 proof.
**The effect of alcohol on judgment, inhibitions, and self-control, even in the lower blood alcohol levels, is serious because (1) since self-criticism is affected early, the drinker often is unlikely to recognize any change in his behavior and (2) he often feels more perceptive and skillful and, therefore, is likely to take more chances in passing, speeding, or negotiating curves (self-confidence increases as skill decreases—the worst possible combination).
Source: Reprinted with permission from *Alcohol: The Crutch That Cripples,* by Jafen, B. Q. Copyright © 1977 by West Publishing Company. All rights reserved. Page 41.

Versions of this statement appeared in the 3 June 1977 *Morbidity and Mortality Weekly Report,*[10] and the November/December 1977 issue of the Food and Drug Administration's *Drug Bulletin.*[11] On 15 November 1977, the FDA Commissioner asked the Director of the Bureau of Alcohol, Tobacco, and Firearms to place a similar warning label on alcoholic beverages. Chapter 11 stressed that pregnant women should take drugs only with the utmost caution and only under the guidance or supervision of a physician. In this chapter, we will pay particular attention to the effects of alcohol on pregnancy because of the potential number of people involved.

In 1972, Dr. Christy Ulleland published the results of a study she had done as a pediatric resident. During that time, she found several cases of infants who would not respond to medical care. Their failure to thrive caused Ulleland to search their records in an attempt to identify a cause for their poor development. In each case, she found that the mothers of these infants had been alcoholics during pregnancy. In following up her suspicions in the medical histories of similar cases, she was able to identify twelve more cases with similar circumstances. Of these twelve babies, she found that ten were undersized at birth. Of ten that were tested for normal development, five were found to be retarded, three borderline, and only two were found to be normal.[12]

Problems associated with the consumption of alcohol during pregnancy have been confirmed by many other studies. The specific pattern of deformities associated with **Fetal Alcohol Syndrome (FAS)** was first described in France by Lemoine and others,[13] and subsequently confirmed and named Fetal Alcohol Syndrome by Jones and Smith in the United States.[14]

The three most commonly occurring physical features of FAS are small eye slits, small head circumference, and pre- and postnatal growth impairments expressed primarily in deficiency in length at birth and postnatal growth deficiency in length and weight.[15] The most common abnormal developmental characteristic of FAS is mental retardation, which may occur with or without the other associated physical abnormalities.

In the *Third Special Report to the U.S. Congress on Alcohol and Health* (1978), the current evidence on FAS was summarized as follows:

1. Research on the impact of maternal alcohol consumption on human infants has demonstrated that the fetal alcohol syndrome (FAS) is a clinically observable abnormality.
2. A high blood alcohol level during a critical time of embryonic development probably is necessary to produce the FAS. The average alcohol consumption may not be as important as the maximum concentrations obtained during binge drinking at critical periods during pregnancy.
3. The evidence from animal studies is quite compelling and clearly suggests a risk for human infants when daily alcohol consumption is three ounces or more of alcohol. Further animal experimentation and human prospective studies will be required to determine the risk from lower doses of alcohol.
4. Observations of alcohol's effects on physiology and metabolism, particularly as related to the central nervous system, support the view that placental alcohol exposure may impair morphological and neurological fetal development.
5. The projected incidence of fetal alcohol syndrome makes it the third leading cause of birth defects with associated mental retardation—following only Down's syndrome and spina bifida—and the only one of the three that is preventable.[16]

Clearly, drinking and pregnancy do not mix. The responsible use of alcohol precludes its use during pregnancy. (See figure 12.9.)

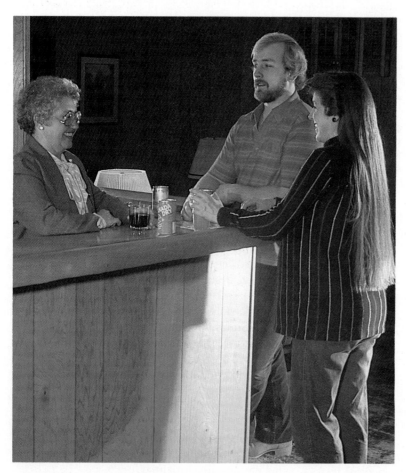

**Figure 12.9**
Pregnancy and drinking do not mix.

# ASSOCIATED DISEASE RISKS

Once alcohol is absorbed, it is distributed throughout the body. If alcohol is used over long periods of time in sufficient quantities, it can adversely affect the performance and health of every organ system in the body. Our focus here is on two specific disease risks associated with long-term abuse of alcohol—the risk of developing or aggravating heart disease and the association between alcohol and cancer.

A great many studies have been done on the relationship between consumption of alcohol and its subsequent impact on health. There is some conflict in the results of these studies and some of the evidence is inconclusive. However, when we look at the total health of a person, data from the Framingham study (a longitudinal study of the risk factors to health) indicate that the relationship between alcohol and health is not linear but rather U-shaped. In other words, zero intake of alcohol appears to be less healthful than small to moderate amounts. However, intakes higher than the equivalent of two drinks per day are associated with increased rates of nutritional, gastrointestinal, neurological, cardiological, hematologic, pulmonary, electrolyte, and cancer problems.[17] The paradox here lies in our inability to determine which individuals are prone to the development of alcoholism. Therefore, taking these data and making a blanket recommendation for the general public to change its drinking habits would be negligent. Recommending that everyone drink to improve their health would certainly result in an increase in the rates of alcoholism.

## Drinking and Coronary-Heart Disease

The results here appear to be the most inconclusive and difficult to determine. It appears that moderate amounts of alcohol may be protective against the subsequent development of coronary artery disease mostly because of the influence of alcohol on high-density lipoprotein (HDL) levels. (See chapter 15.) However, the mechanism of action is not yet known. Although these data appear to be encouraging, alcohol consumption may be positively related with the development of cardiac myopathies (a disease of the heart muscle that is associated with congestive heart failure and other muscle anomalies) and significant increases in blood pressure which may be associated with increased risk of stroke as well as increased risk of other coronary-related diseases. Once again, the mechanism of action of each of these outcomes is unknown and therefore we cannot tell whether they are a direct effect of the ingestion of alcohol or a result of some of the behavioral changes that may occur in individuals who consume large quantities of alcohol over time.

## Drinking and Cancer

Although there is a great deal of evidence linking smoking to subsequent cancers, the relationship between drinking and cancer is still being studied. Alcohol consumption is undeniably associated with both the development of cancers and the subsequent outcomes. Heavy drinkers have a greater risk of developing cancer and survival rates are substantially lower among heavy drinkers than among the general population.[18] The sites most often affected include the mouth, tongue, pharynx and larynx, esophagus, stomach, rectum, and liver. How alcohol may exert a carcinogenic effect is not yet known. However, in a review of health hazards associated with alcohol consumption, M. J. Eckardt and others list the following theories currently under study:

1. Alcohol-induced immunologic suppression.
2. Alcohol-induced irritation of tissues.
3. Alcohol as a cocarcinogen with tobacco or as a trigger mechanism for a possible viral cause.
4. Alcohol-induced outcomes (such as malnutrition and anemia) as a precursor to cancer.
5. Alcohol as a carrier of other carcinogens.[19]

## Other Disease Risks

There is a much greater incidence of several other disorders such as pneumonia, tuberculosis, and other respiratory-tract infections among heavy drinkers.[20] As with cancer, not only is the incidence rate higher among heavy drinkers than in the general population, but mortality associated with these conditions is also higher for heavy drinkers.

**Table 12.4 Estimated Core Costs for Alcohol Abuse, 1977 (in millions of dollars)**

| **Total Core Costs** | **$43,161** | | |
|---|---|---|---|
| *Direct* | $ 6,372 | *Indirect* | $36,789 |
| Treatment | 5,637 | Mortality | 10,715 |
| Alcohol-abuse-specific illness —specialty setting | 707 | Direct primary causes—alcohol psychosis, alcoholism, alcoholic cirrhosis of liver, alcohol poisoning | 2,617 |
| Alcohol-abuse-specific illness —general setting | 2,001 | Direct secondary causes—cirrhosis of liver (other), malignant primary liver neoplasms, other malignant neoplasms of gastrointestinal tract, pancreatitis, respiratory tuberculosis, other associated diseases | 1,063 |
| Alcohol-abuse-related-illness categories | 1,711 | Indirect causes—motor vehicle crashes, falls, fires, other accidents, homicides, suicides | 7,035 |
| Gastrointestinal tract | 220 | Morbidity | 26,074 |
| Liver disease | 181 | Lost productivity | 23,593 |
| Nervous system | 6 | Males | 20,178 |
| Heart | 17 | Females | 3,415 |
| Endocrine system | 608 | Lost employment | 2,481 |
| Nutritional deficiency | 108 | Trauma | 545 |
| Cancer | 171 | Residential treatment | 328 |
| Mental disorder | 293 | Long-term disability | 1,608 |
| Infectious disease | 107 | | |
| Alcohol-abuse-related trauma | 1,217 | | |
| Support | 735 | | |
| Research | 28 | | |
| Training and education | 225 | | |
| Construction | 193 | | |
| Health-insurance administration | 289 | | |

Source: Cruze, A. M.; Harwood, H. J.; Kristiansen, P. L.; Collins, J. J.; and Jones, D. C., *Economic Costs to Society of Alcohol and Drug Abuse and Mental Illness—1977* (Rockville, Md.: Alcohol, Drug Abuse, and Mental Health Administration, 1981).

## Secondary Consequences to Alcohol Use

There are many other medical, economic, and social consequences of irresponsible use of alcohol. In addition to automobile accidents, alcohol may play either a direct or indirect role in many other types of accidents and crimes of violence including assault, rape, and family abuse. These problems are tremendously costly to American society in terms of ruined and lost lives, as well as the enormous economic costs. Tables 12.4 and 12.5 summarize some of these costs.

Irresponsible use of alcohol carries with it an enormous cost in many ways. Since alcohol use is such a traditional part of American society, it is important that we become responsible users.

# RESPONSIBLE DRINKING BEHAVIORS

In chapter 11, we listed a great many responsibilities for recreational-drug users. These were originally outlined in Duncan and Gold, 1982.[21] Responsible drinking behavior includes the following. (See figure 12.10.):

1. When you are the host of a gathering in which alcohol will be served, you:
   a. Should provide some food as well as drink.
   b. Should not insist that everyone drink alcohol. Some will prefer other beverages, or none at all.
   c. Should provide alternative nonalcoholic beverages.
   d. Should make contingency plans for drunkenness.
   e. Should set reasonable rules regarding levels of consumption for each of your guests.

Table 12.5 **Estimated Other Related Costs for Alcohol Abuse, 1977 (in millions of dollars)**

| **Total Other Related Costs** | **$ 6,213** | | |
|---|---|---|---|
| *Direct* | $ 4,441 | *Indirect* | $ 1,772 |
| Motor vehicle crashes | 1,782 | Crime careers | - |
| Crime | $ 1,685 | Incarceration | 1,418 |
| Public criminal justice system | 1,479 | Homicide | 276 |
| Law enforcement | 313 | Felonious assault | 120 |
| Legal and adjudication | 139 | Robbery | 46 |
| Corrections | 1,027 | Burglary | 49 |
| Private criminal justice system | 191 | Drug laws | 0 |
| Law enforcement | 184 | Driving under the influence | 287 |
| Legal and adjudication | 7 | Liquor laws | 158 |
| Corrections | - | Public drunkenness | 461 |
| Property loss/damage | 15 | Other | 21 |
| Social welfare programs | 142 | Motor vehicle crashes | 354 |
| Fire losses | 319 | | |
| Fire protection | 482 | | |
| Highway safety | 31 | | |

Source: Cruze, A. M.; Harwood, H. J.; Kristiansen, P. L.; Collins, J. J.; and Jones, D. C., *Economic Costs to Society of Alcohol and Drug Abuse and Mental Illness—1977* (Rockville, Md.: Alcohol, Drug Abuse, and Mental Health Administration, 1981).

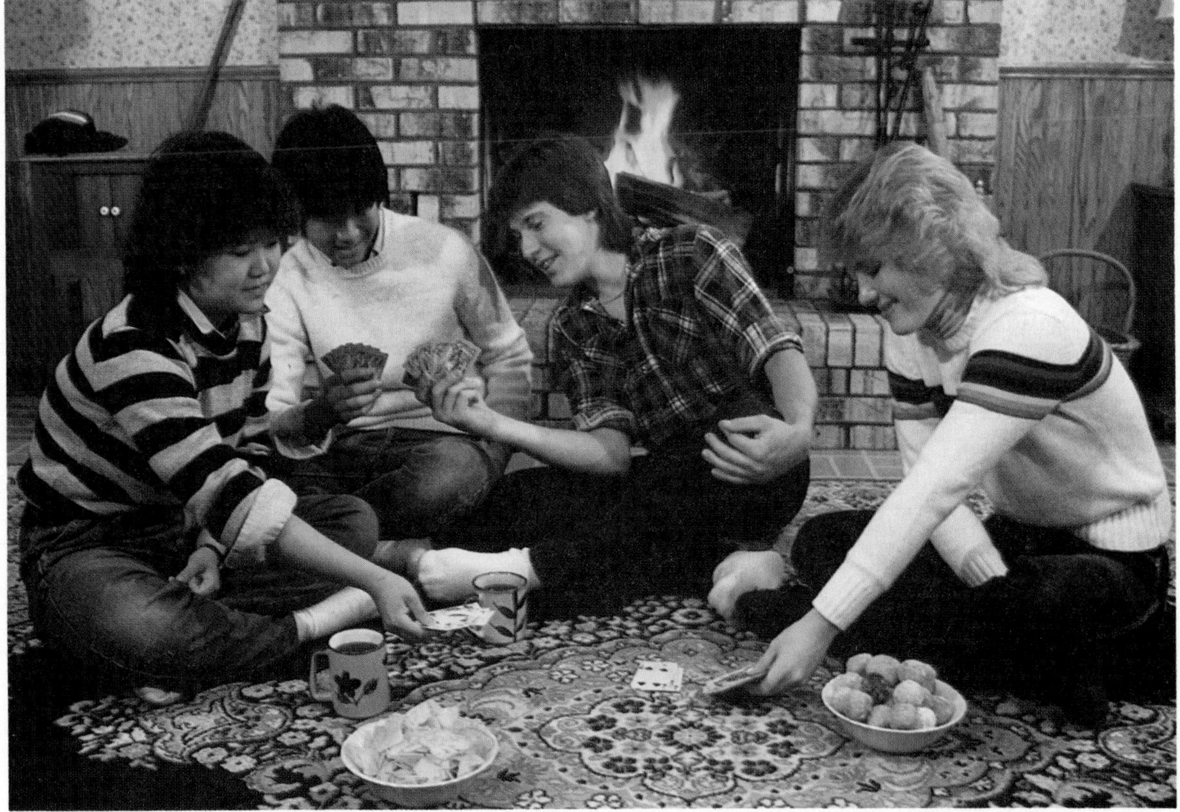

**Figure 12.10**
A party that offers various activities and doesn't focus on drinking encourages the responsible use of alcohol.

**Table 12.6 Potential Interactions of Alcohol with Other Common Drugs**

| Alcohol Combines with | To Produce | And May Result in |
|---|---|---|
| Barbiturates (all) | Supraadditive effects | Impaired motor performance, increased mortality rates, respiratory failure, avoidance behaviors |
| Minor tranquilizers (all) | | |
| Meprobamate | Additive effects | Decreased oculomotor control and body steadiness, increased drowsiness and fatigue, impairment of time estimation, attention, reaction time and alertness |
| Benzodinzepines | Additive effects | Severe hypertension, depressed cardiac functioning, and respiratory arrest |
| Major tranquilizers | Additive effects | Depression of respiratory center, impaired hepatic functioning, lowered seizure threshold, hypertension |
| Antidepressants | Antagonism with stimulants, potentiation with depressants | Nausea, severe headaches, hypertensive crisis, decreased motor coordination, lowered seizure threshold |
| Anticonvulsants | Potentiation | Increased tolerance level |
| Antihistamines | Additive, possible potentiation effects | Increased CNS depression, drowsiness |
| Anesthetics | Supraadditive effects | Greater threshold dose for narcosis, but deeper narcosis results, increased sleep time, possible death cross tolerance |
| Ethanol analogs (chloral hydrate, paraldehyde) | Supraadditive effects | Respiratory depression, cardiovascular changes, possible death |
| Opiates (morphine, heroin) | Potentiation | Increased CNS depression, sensitization to lethal effects of opiates |
| Marijuana | Additive effects | Increased difficulty with motor control |
| Stimulants | Varying levels of antagonism | Hyperexcitability, reduction of CNS depression |
| Oral antidiabetics | Intolerance | Alcohol intolerance like that produced by disulfiram |
| Antibiotics | Intolerance | Alcohol intolerance like that produced by disulfiram |
| Antihypertensives (methyldopa) | Additive effects | Hypotension |
| Tobacco | | Dissolving of tars, making them more available to body tissues—increased risk of cancer, especially of head, neck, and esophagus |

Source: From *Drugs and the Whole Person,* by D. F. Duncan and R. S. Gold (New York: Macmillan, 1982). Reprinted by permission of the publisher.

2. When you are some place where alcoholic beverages are being served, you:
   a. Should drink only when you want to, not when someone else thinks that you should.
   b. Should be aware of the influences of set and setting and establish reasonable limits for yourself when you choose to drink.
   c. Should recognize your responsibility for the health, safety, and pleasure of yourself and others.
   d. Should be aware of the potentially adverse effects of mixing alcohol and other drugs. (See table 12.6.)

You are responsible for your own behavior. Recreational use of alcoholic beverages is perfectly acceptable behavior if you remember to drink responsibly.

## SOCIAL BARRIERS TO RESPONSIBLE USE OF ALCOHOL

According to the *Third Special Report to the Congress on Alcohol and Health,* six factors are important determinants of youthful drinking behavior, including peer influences, familial and parental influences, sociocultural factors, environmental-contextual influences, personality, and behavioral influences.[22] Of these, peer and parental influences seem to be the most important because of the strong relationship between the drinking practices of young adults and those of their peers and parents.

### Parental and Peer Attitudes

We can find direct relationships between parental attitudes toward alcohol and alcohol-related behavior and the attitudes and behavior of their children. Problem drinking among parents is highly related to problem drinking in their children.[23] The pattern of drinking practiced in the home when children are growing up is often the same as the patterns displayed by young adults. Drinking behavior often conforms to what people think their peers find acceptable. The survey conducted by Johnston and others gives some indication of current parental and peer attitudes and beliefs about alcohol.[24] The following summary data has been abstracted from their final report:

1. Perceived harmfulness of alcohol. Only 20 percent of these adolescents associate much risk of harm with having one or two drinks almost daily. Only about a third (36 percent) think there is great risk involved in having five or more drinks once or twice each weekend. Considerably more (66 percent) think the user takes a great risk in consuming four or five drinks nearly every day.
2. Personal disapproval of alcohol use. Drinking at a rate of one or two drinks daily received disapproval from two-thirds of the high-school seniors surveyed, although weekend-binge drinking was deemed more acceptable than moderate daily drinking. This was found even though great risk was more often associated with binge drinking (36 percent) than with daily drinking (20 percent).
3. Current perceptions of parental attitudes. Approximately 85 percent of the adolescents surveyed thought their parents would disapprove of their having five or more drinks once or twice every weekend. At the same time, 88 percent thought their friends would disapprove of heavy daily drinking (which was the highest percentage of disapproval reported for more than fifteen other drugs in the survey). In the past five years, alcohol was one of two drugs in this survey on which there had been some discrepancy between the seniors' attitudes and their perceptions of their friends' attitudes. However, in 1980, the discrepancy narrowed.
4. Exposure to alcohol use. Almost 70 percent reported that most or all of their friends drink alcoholic beverages; 30 percent said that their friends get drunk at least once a week. Although the trend over the last five years has been increasing alcohol use by friends, the 1980 survey showed a decline of nearly 2 percent of those who reported that their friends get drunk at least once a week. (See figure 12.11 and Activity for Wellness 12.1.)

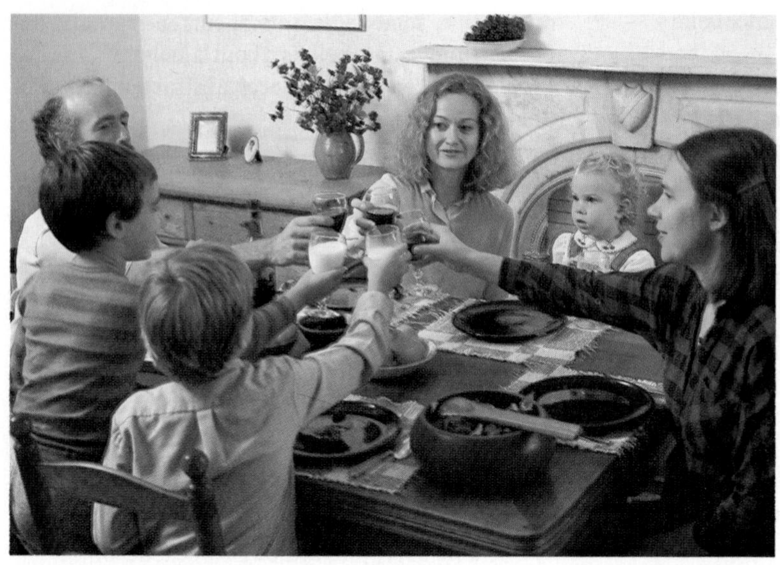

**Figure 12.11**
Children who are introduced early to the responsible use of alcohol tend to experience fewer alcohol-related problems as adults.

12.1 ACTIVITY FOR WELLNESS 12.1

## Social Self-Assessment

The National Institute on Alcohol Abuse and Alcoholism summarized the existing literature and found that the following factors were indicative of the fewest problems with alcohol as an adult. How do you stack up with these factors? Remember, these are associated with the lowest rates of problems associated with drinking.

You Are Least Likely to Have Problems with Alcohol if:

[ ] 1. You were exposed to alcohol in relatively small quantities early in life by your family or within the context of a religious or cultural group.

[ ] 2. Your family members viewed alcohol as a food and consumed small quantities primarily at mealtime.

[ ] 3. Your parents set a good example by practicing responsible drinking behaviors.

[ ] 4. Your family did not view drinking alcoholic beverages as a means of demonstrating maturity, adulthood, or masculinity/femininity.

[ ] 5. Abstinence was accepted as a legitimate choice with respect to the consumption of alcoholic beverages.

[ ] 6. Drunkenness was not an acceptable form of behavior.

[ ] 7. Alcohol was viewed as a beverage and not as the central focus of a group activity.

[ ] 8. Rules and rituals associated with drinking were known and understood by all group members; they were both reasonable and agreeable to those members.

Source: National Institute on Alcohol Abuse and Alcoholism.

# ALCOHOL ABUSE

In 1978, it was reported in the *Third Special Report to the Congress on Alcohol and Health* that ". . . alcohol abuse is a generic term, applied to the misuse of alcohol, which is manifested in one or more alcohol-related problems or alcohol-related disabilities."[25] These alcohol-related problems lie in three general areas: (1) Psychological—involving loss of control over drinking, alcohol dependence and depression, and suicidal states of mind; (2) Medical—involving both acute and chronic illness and injuries; and (3) Social—involving antisocial or socially unacceptable behaviors.

A great many alcohol-related problems may be the result of excessive use that should not be confused with alcoholism. Although alcoholism directly and indirectly affects many people, there is still considerable controversy over its definition. We will distinguish between alcohol-related disability, alcoholism, and problem drinker as follows:

**ALCOHOL-RELATED DISABILITY** is a broad term that includes alcoholism but doesn't require that alcoholism be present. An alcohol-related disability exists when there is an impairment in the physical, mental, or social functioning of an individual, so that it may be reasonably inferred that alcohol is part of that disability. Impairment includes actual health problems related to a specific drinking bout; offensive behavior caused by heavy drinking; injuries, death, and property loss caused by accidents related to drinking; failure of the chronic excessive drinker to fulfill his or her roles in the family or on the job; and mental problems, such as depression and anxiety, related to drinking.[26]

**ALCOHOLISM** is addiction to alcohol. It is also defined as alcohol-dependence syndrome by the World Health Organization (WHO) in the ninth revision of the *International Classification of Diseases* (ICD–9)[27] and by the American Psychiatric Association in the third revision of the *Diagnostic and Statistical Manual of Mental Disorders* (DSM-III).[28] Alcoholism is characterized by a compulsion to take alcohol on a continuous or periodic basis to experience its psychological and physical effects and sometimes to avoid the discomfort of its absence. Tolerance may or may not be present.[29]

**Table 12.7 Rates of Problem Drinking Among U.S. Drinkers, by Drinking Population, 1975**

| Drinking Population | Percentage of Problem Drinkers |
|---|---|
| All drinkers | |
| No problems | 63 |
| Potential problems | 26 |
| Problem drinkers | 10 |
| Males | |
| No problems | 57 |
| Potential problems | 31 |
| Problem drinkers | 13 |
| Females | |
| No problems | 73 |
| Potential problems | 21 |
| Problem drinkers | 6 |

Source: P. Johnson, D. Armor, S. Polick, and H. Stambul, *U.S. Adult Drinking Practices: Time Trends, Social Correlates and Sex Roles*, draft report prepared for NIAAA, Contract No. ADM 281-76-0020, July 1977. National Institute for Alcohol Abuse and Alcoholism, National Institutes of Health, Bethesda, Md.

A **PROBLEM DRINKER** is a person who drinks alcohol to an extent or in a manner that an alcohol-related disability is manifested. Therefore, the term problem drinker generally is applied to those who demonstrate problems in relation to drinking alcohol.[30]

There are probably between nine and twelve million problem drinkers in the adult population of the United States out of approximately 145 million adults aged eighteen and older.[31] This estimate includes alcoholics. Since as many as 95 percent of those nine to twelve million problem drinkers are not social isolates, it is quite feasible that the drinking of each one directly affects the lives of as many as four friends, family members, or coworkers. Between thirty and forty-eight million Americans are thus either directly or indirectly affected by problem drinking—clearly a public health problem of massive proportions. Table 12.7 contains a summary of the rates of problem drinking in the U.S. population.

12.2 ACTIVITY FOR WELLNESS 12.2

# Are You A Problem Drinker?

How can we spot early signs of potential problems? The U.S. Department of Health and Human Services's National Institute on Alcohol Abuse and Alcoholism suggests that honest answers to the following questions may provide clues. Check off those questions that apply to you. If you answer "yes" to as few as one-fourth of these (seven questions), you may have a problem with alcohol.

[ ] 1. Do you drink to feel better about yourself?
[ ] 2. Do you turn to alcohol when you have troubles?
[ ] 3. Do you make excuses for the reasons you drink?
[ ] 4. Do you feel guilty after drinking?
[ ] 5. Do you drink to help you fall asleep?
[ ] 6. Do you often have diarrhea, indigestion, or nausea due to drinking?
[ ] 7. Have you had other problems related to your drinking?
[ ] 8. Have you ever fallen down or burned yourself while you were drinking?
[ ] 9. Do you feel worried, anxious, or depressed most of the time?
[ ] 10. Do you find yourself not realizing you are repeating things while drinking?
[ ] 11. Have you ever been unable to remember what happened while you were drinking?
[ ] 12. Have you ever missed work or put off work because of your drinking?
[ ] 13. Have you put yourself or others in danger by driving after drinking?
[ ] 14. Have you had financial or legal problems in which drinking was involved?
[ ] 15. Do you drink alone?
[ ] 16. Do you drink less with others than you do when alone?
[ ] 17. Do you feel isolated and alone?
[ ] 18. Do you often feel the need to telephone people when you are drinking?
[ ] 19. Have you changed friends to be around people who drink like you do?
[ ] 20. Do you hide your drinking from your spouse or children?
[ ] 21. Have others told you that they think you drink too much?
[ ] 22. Is either parent, or your spouse or housemate a heavy drinker?
[ ] 23. Do you think you drink too much?
[ ] 24. Do you plan activities around being able to drink?
[ ] 25. Do you find yourself thinking of drinking in-between times?
[ ] 26. Have you failed in promises to yourself to cut down on your drinking?
[ ] 27. Are there times when you don't drink because you're afraid you'll lose control of yourself?
[ ] 28. Do you drink and use other drugs?

Source: U.S. Department of Health and Human Service's National Institute on Alcohol Abuse and Alcoholism, *For Women Who Drink.* USDHHS Publication No. ADM 82–1176, 1982.

Although a great many theories are under study in an attempt to identify the causes of problem drinking and alcoholism, a great deal of controversy remains. Hereditary factors seem to provide solid clues on causality, but research results are inconclusive.[32] At best, we can only explain alcoholism within a complex and multicausal framework, with both genetic and environmental factors influencing its development.

Alcohol is a drug which, when abused or misused, can cause great problems for individuals and society. But alcohol and wellness can coexist. Acting responsibly when you use alcohol and encouraging similar behavior in your friends will increase your chances of attaining high levels of wellness.

# SUMMARY

1. Alcohol and tobacco, though legally obtainable for much of the population, still account for the largest amount of illegal use among all drugs in our society.
2. The average yearly per capita consumption of pure alcohol in this country is 2.77 gallons.
3. Many factors influence the rate of absorption of alcohol in the body, including the concentration of alcohol, the rate of consumption, the amount of alcohol, other chemicals present with the alcohol, the condition of the stomach, pylorospasm, and the emotional condition of the drinker.
4. The effects experienced by an individual when drinking are related to the blood alcohol level reached and these levels are affected by individual characteristics such as age, height, weight, and percentage of body fat as well as quantity of alcohol consumed and the amount of time during which it is consumed.
5. Alcohol is primarily a depressant and therefore has potentially dramatic effects on the central nervous system. Drinking and driving should be particularly avoided. In more than half of all traffic fatalities, the driver had a blood alcohol level high enough to be considered legally intoxicated (0.10 BAC).
6. Alcohol has many effects beyond the initial consequences of intoxication. Also related to alcohol consumption are fetal alcohol syndrome, coronary-heart disease, cancer, other diseases, crimes of violence, and alcoholism.
7. Among the social barriers to responsible use of alcohol are parental and peer attitudes and alcohol's widespread availability.

## Recommended Readings

*Fifth Special Report to the U.S. Congress on Alcohol and Health from the Secretary of Health and Human Services.* USDHHS: Public Health Service, National Institute on Alcohol Abuse and Alcoholism: Washington, D.C. Sup't. of Documents, 1983.

## References

1. Fifth Special Report to the U.S. Congress on Alcohol and Health from the Secretary of Health and Human Services. U.S. Department of Health and Human Services, National Institute on Alcohol Abuse and Alcoholism. (Washington, D.C.: U.S. Government Printing Office, 1983), 4.

2. Lloyd D. Johnston, Jerald G. Backman, and Patrick M. O'Malley. *Highlights from Student Drug Use in America,* 1975–1980. U.S. Department of Health and Human Services, Public Health Service, DHHS Publication No. (ADM) 81–1066. (Washington, D.C.: U.S. Government Printing Office, 1980.)

3. M. M. Hyman, M. A. Zimmerman, C. Gurioli, and A. Helrich, "Drinkers, Drinking and Alcohol-Related Mortality and Hospitalizations: A Statistical Compendium," 1980 edition. (New Jersey: Rutgers University Center for Alcohol Studies, 1980.)

4. National Institute of Alcohol Abuse and Alcoholism, *For Women Who Drink.* USDHHS Publication No. ADM 82–1176, 1982, 14.

5. Ralph E. Berry, Jr., and James P. Boland, *The Economic Cost of Alcohol Abuse* (New York: The Free Press, 1977).

6. Darwin Dennison, T. Prevet, and M. Affleck, *Alcohol and Behavior: An Activated Education Approach* (St. Louis: C. V. Mosby, 1980).

7. Dennison et al., Alcohol and Behavior: An Activated Education Approach.

8. Brent Q. Hafen, *Alcohol: The Crutch that Cripples* (St. Paul, Minn.: West Publishing, 1977).

9. Hafen, *Alcohol: The Crutch that Cripples,* 38.

10. Morbidity and Mortality Weekly Report. U.S. Department of Health and Human Services, Center for Disease Control, Atlanta, GA, June 3, 1977.

11. Drug Bulletin. U.S. Department of Health and Human Services, Public Health Service, Food and Drug Administration, November 15, 1977.

12. Christy Ulleland. The Offspring of Alcoholic Mothers. Annals of the New York Academy of Sciences *197:* May 25, 1972, 167–69.

13. P. Lemoine, H. Harrousseau, J. P. Borteyru, and J. C. Manuet, "Les enfants des parents alcoliques anomalies observees. A propos de 127 cas," *Quest Medical* 21 (1968): 276–482.

14. K. L. Jones, D. W. Smith, C. N. Ulleland, and A. P. Streissguth, "Pattern of Malformation in Offspring of Chronic Alcoholic Mothers," *Lancet* 1 (1973): 1267–71.

15. K. R. Warren, *Critical Review of the Fetal Alcohol Syndrome.* Report for the National Institute on Alcohol Abuse and Alcoholism, 1977.

16. E. P. Noble, ed., *Third Special Report to the U.S. Congress on Alcohol and Health.* (Washington, D.C.: U.S. Government Printing Office, 1978.)

17. W. P. Castelli, "Editorial: How Many Drinks a Day?", *Journal of the American Medical Association* 242.18 (1979): 2000.

18. *Fifth Special Report on Alcohol and Health,* 59.

19. M. J. Eckardt, E. S. Parker, and E. Vanderveen, "Health Hazards Associated with Alcohol Consumption," *Journal of the American Medical Association* 246.6 (1981): 648–66.

20. *Fifth Special Report on Alcohol and Health,* 55.

21. David F. Duncan and Robert S. Gold, *Drugs and the Whole Person* (New York: John Wiley & Sons, 1982), 216–23.

22. Noble, *Third Special Report to the U.S. Congress on Alcohol and Health,* 19.

23. *Fifth Special Report on Alcohol and Health,* 15.

24. Johnston et al., *Highlights,* 91–104.

25. *Third Special Report on Alcohol and Health,* 7.

26. National Institute on Alcohol Abuse and Alcoholism, *Drinking Etiquette.* NIAAA Publication No. 77–305, U.S. Government Printing Office (Rockville, Md.: 1977). *Fifth Special Report to the U.S. Congress on Alcohol and Health.* USDHHS: National Institute on Drug Abuse. (Washington, D.C.: U.S. Government Printing Office, 1983.)

27. *International Classification of Diseases,* Ninth Revision with Clinical Modifications (Second Edition), U.S. Department of Health and Human Services. DHHS Publication No. (PHS) 80–1260. (Washington, D.C.: U.S. Government Printing Office, 1980.)

28. *Diagnostic and Statistical Manual of Mental Disorders,* Third Revision. (Washington, D.C.: American Psychiatric Association, 1980.)

29. *Third Special Report on Alcohol and Health,* 7.

30. *Third Special Report on Alcohol and Health,* 7–8.

31. O. Ray, *Drugs, Society and Human Behavior* (St. Louis: C. V. Mosby Co., 1978), 153.

32. *Fifth Special Report on Alcohol and Health,* 15.

*CHAPTER THIRTEEN*

# Tobacco: Seeking a Smoke-Free Life-Style



On 11 January 1964, the first Surgeon General's report on smoking and health was published.[1] That report represented an important scientific contribution to our knowledge regarding tobacco and health. Among other factors, it clearly established a link between cigarette smoking and morbidity and mortality. In 1979, another Surgeon General's report on smoking and health was published.[2] The 1979 report did much to add to our knowledge regarding smoking and health; in fact, it presented substantial evidence that cigarette smoking was even more dangerous than suggested in 1964. Among other things, the 1979 report presented information on a subject not extensively covered in 1964—women and smoking. Evidence was presented suggesting that women who smoke during pregnancy risk creation of long-term, irreversible effects on their babies. Moreover, as the amount women smoke increases, so does their morbidity and mortality. For the first time, evidence was presented that demonstrated that women who smoked as much as men were just as likely to die from smoking-associated causes as men were.

The 1979 report also provided new evidence on the occupational hazards that smokers face. Irrefutable evidence was provided indicating that working in certain environments and industries with materials such as asbestos, rubber, coal, textiles, uranium, and chemicals increases the potential for health hazards associated with smoking. Additionally, the 1979 report also suggested the enormity of a growing concern—smoking among children. The report suggests that 100,000 children under age thirteen in the U.S. are regular smokers.

The report also heralded the fact that more than thirty million Americans were ex-smokers in 1979. In addition, it stated that the number of cigarettes consumed per person in the U.S. declined from 4,345 in 1963 to 3,965 in 1978—the lowest per capita cigarette consumption in twenty years.

# FORMS OF TOBACCO CONSUMPTION

Although the focus of this chapter is on cigarette smoking, there are many other forms of tobacco consumption. Among them are the following:

**Snuff:** a powdered tobacco that can be sniffed or placed in the pouch of the mouth and sucked on. Here the active agents in the tobacco (e.g., nicotine) are absorbed through the mucous membrane linings of the nose or mouth. Snuff was much more heavily used in the eighteenth century in America, but recently has had a resurgence in popularity.

**Chewing Tobacco:** a preparation of tobacco leaves mixed with a variety of flavoring agents (e.g., molasses). As the tobacco is chewed, nicotine and other tobacco constituents are absorbed through the mucous membrane linings of the mouth. As with snuff, chewing tobacco has enjoyed a resurgence in popularity recently. Both are often called **smokeless tobacco.** (See figure 13.1.)

**Pipes and Cigars:** these are two other forms of tobacco that are smoked. As with cigarettes, the use of either pipes or cigars involves the inhalation of hot smoke containing the principal products of the combustion of tobacco into the smoker's mouth and lungs where these products are absorbed.

**Table 13.1 Estimated Percentage of Current, Regular Cigarette Smokers, Aged 12–18, in the U.S., 1970–1979**

| Year | Ages 12–14 | Ages 15–16 | Ages 17–18 |
|---|---|---|---|
| *Females* | | | |
| 1970 | 0.6 | 9.6 | 18.6 |
| 1979 | 4.4 | 11.8 | 26.2 |
| *Males* | | | |
| 1970 | 2.9 | 17.0 | 30.2 |
| 1979 | 3.2 | 13.5 | 19.3 |

Source: The *Health Consequences of Smoking for Women: A Report to the Surgeon General.* VSDHHS/PHS (Washington, D.C.: U.S. Government Printing Office, 1980), 36.

Most of the issues involved with cigarette smoking are also pertinent to these forms of tobacco. However, prospective epidemiologic studies show that individuals who smoke only pipes and cigars have mortality rates slightly higher than nonsmokers, but lower than cigarette smokers.[3] In addition, the mortality rates associated with smoking do not pertain to smokeless tobacco.

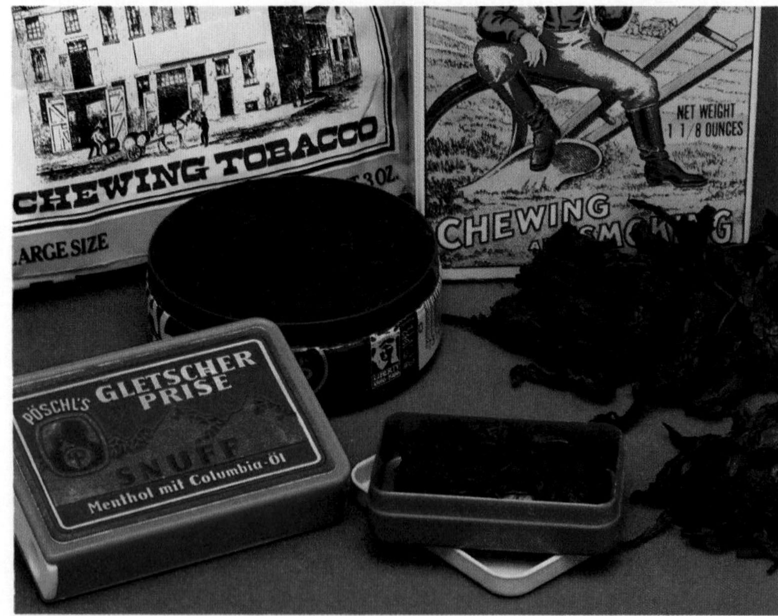


**Figure 13.1**
Smokeless tobacco products are becoming increasingly popular among adolescents and young adults.

# COMPOSITION OF TOBACCO SMOKE

Tobacco is an important crop, both economically and agriculturally. Some types of tobacco are grown in almost every country in the world and tobacco is used everywhere. The plant itself, Nicotiana tabacum, was originally found in the Americas. There are more than sixty-five species of tobacco and there are wide variations in the chemical characteristics between these species, types, varieties, strains, and grades.

Given these many differences between tobaccos, a lighted cigarette will generate more than 2,000 known compounds.[4] The chemical constituents found in the atmosphere, however, are derived from two different sources—**mainstream** and **sidestream smoke.** Mainstream smoke is produced when smoke is being drawn through the tobacco during puffing; sidestream smoke rises from the burning tobacco. We will compare mainstream and sidestream smoke later in this chapter.

Table 13.2 contains a summary of the composition of cigarette smoke, which contains a large number of chemical compounds, including gases, vapors, and small particles. When these particles are condensed, they form **tars** which account for approximately 8 percent of the total volume of cigarette smoke. The remaining 92 percent comes from the gases and vapors in the smoke. These tars contain **carcinogens** (cancer-producing chemicals), **cocarcinogens** (substances that can combine with some others to produce cancer), and various other chemicals, such as nicotine, that are suspected to be dangerous in many ways. (See table 13.3.)

During puffing, temperatures in the burning cone of a cigarette reach 900 degrees centrigrade, with some portions of the cone getting as hot as 1,050 degrees centrigrade. It is during these temperatures that mainstream smoke (smoke inhaled directly through the cigarette, pipe, or cigar) is produced. Sidestream smoke (smoke from the burning tobacco that enters the environment) is generated during smoldering of the tobacco at temperatures as high as 800 degrees centrigrade. It has been estimated that between 55 and 70 percent of the tobacco of a cigarette is burned between puffs and thus serves as a source for sidestream smoke and ash.[5]

**Table 13.2 Percent Distribution of Cigarette-Smoke Components**

| Material | Weight (mg) | Percent of Total |
|---|---|---|
| Particulate matter | 40.6 | 8.2 |
| Nitrogen | 295.4 | 59.0 |
| Oxygen | 66.8 | 13.4 |
| Carbon dioxide | 68.1 | 13.6 |
| Carbon monoxide | 16.2 | 3.2 |
| Hydrogen | 0.7 | 0.1 |
| Argon | 5.0 | 1.0 |
| Methane | 1.3 | 0.3 |
| Water vapor | 5.8 | 1.2 |
| Hydrocarbons | 2.5 | 0.5 |
| Carbonyls | 1.9 | 0.4 |
| Hydrogen cyanide | 0.3 | 0.1 |
| Other gaseous materials | 1.0 | 0.2* |

*Total 101.2 percent due to rounding error.
Source: Adapted from Keith, C. H., & Tesh, P. G., "Measurement of the Total Smoke Issuing from a Burning Cigarette," *Tobacco Science* 9 (1965): 61–64, with the approval of Lockwood Trade Journal Company.

**Table 13.3 Harmful Constituents of Cigarette-Smoke Particulate Matter**

1. Compounds judged most likely to contribute to the health hazards of smoking:

   Nicotine 50–2,500 micrograms/cigarette
   Tar 500–35,000 micrograms/cigarette
2. Compounds judged as probable contributors to the health hazards of smoking:

   Cresols 68–97 micrograms/cigarette
   Phenol 9–202 micrograms/cigarette
3. Compounds judged as suspected contributors to health hazards of smoking:

   DDT 0–0.77 micrograms/cigarette
   Hydroquinone 83 micrograms/cigarette
   Pyridine 25–218 micrograms/cigarette
   Endrin 0–0.06 micrograms/cigarette
   Nickel compounds 0–0.58 micrograms/cigarette

Source: U.S. Public Health Service, *The Health Consequences of Smoking: A Report of the Surgeon General: 1972,* USDHEW, PHS, HSMHA, DHEW Publication Number (HSM) 72-7516 (1972), 141–50.

Although it is generally possible to quantify the constituents of tobacco smoke by using smoking machines, it is important to remember that the actual content of the smoke that reaches the users of tobacco and the bystanders in a smoke-filled environment varies. There are many factors that influence the actual content of mainstream or sidestream smoke including the types of filters used, ventilation, the tobacco variety, the agricultural practices followed in producing the tobacco, the processing methods used in the manufacture of tobacco products, and the nature of the additives combined with the tobacco products (e.g., burning agents, flavoring agents).[6] Added to this are the complicating factors associated with the type of smoker a person is. Some patterns of behavior alter the amount and content of the smoke puffed. There are several ways to characterize these behaviors, including the type of cigarette smoked, the number of cigarettes smoked, the amount of cigarettes smoked, the number of puffs taken from a tobacco product, the depth of inhalation, and the length of inhalation.[7] Each of these factors will ultimately influence the makeup of smoke. Because of this complexity, we will focus here on three major constituents of tobacco smoke and their associated disease risks: nicotine, tars, and carbon monoxide.

## Nicotine

Although **nicotine** can be absorbed from tobacco smoke in the lungs, it can also be absorbed from the mouth cavity from either smoke or the juice of chewing tobacco or snuff.[8] The person who smokes one pack of cigarettes a day takes an estimated 70,000 puffs a year. This frequency of drug ingestion is unmatched by any other type of drug-taking.[9]

Nicotine is just one of many substances found in tobacco, but most would agree that it is the most powerful pharmacologic agent in tobacco. Once absorbed, nicotine rapidly enters all major organ systems, tissues, and body fluids. The initial effect of nicotine on the nervous system is principally early stimulation, followed by a more lasting depression.[10] Some of the immediate effects of nicotine include increased heart rate and blood pressure, an increase in the amount of blood pumped by the heart each minute, increased oxygen consumption and coronary-blood flow, increased arrythmias, constriction of peripheral blood vessels and bronchial tubes, and increased respiration. In addition to these effects, nicotine rapidly crosses the placental barrier causing a number of related effects on the fetus during pregnancy,[11] and can also be found in the milk of lactating women.

It does not take long for nicotine to be absorbed from the lungs, mouth cavity, or stomach. After absorption, nicotine is metabolized very rapidly in the liver. The half-life of nicotine in the human body is approximately thirty minutes; this might explain why regular smokers seek to replenish the levels of nicotine in their bodies about every half hour when they are awake.[12]

It is possible for smokers to experience **nicotine poisoning.** In fact, most people do experience some form of nicotine poisoning when they first begin to smoke or when they smoke too much. Nicotine poisoning causes dizziness, faintness, rapid pulse, cold clammy skin, nausea, and occasionally vomiting and diarrhea. As smokers develop a tolerance to nicotine, these symptoms are diminished. In severe cases, however, tremors can occur, followed by convulsions and death.[13] (See Exhibit 13.1.)

It appears certain that nicotine is the major active agent in tobacco that causes its addiction potential.[14] The third report of the Royal College of Physicians of London adds that "Tobacco smoking is a form of drug dependence different from but no less strong than that in other drugs of addiction."[15]

## Tar

Tar is defined as the total of the particulate matter found in smoke, other than moisture and nicotine. Tobacco smoke is composed of gases, vapors, and particles of material; it is these particles that we call tar. The tar content of cigarettes varies between brands, and each year the Federal Trade Commission determines and publishes these levels for both tars and nicotine. These two substances, tars and nicotine, exhibit a high degree of association, and therefore the specific effects that each has on the human body is somewhat unclear. As with nicotine, tars and carbon monoxide are obtained from the smoke of burning tobacco and therefore are found in the smoke from cigarettes, pipes, and cigars.

13.1 EXHIBIT 13.1

## Smoking: Habit or Addiction?

"In the 1950s people talked about cigarette smoking as a psychosocial habit," notes Lynn T. Kozlowski, Ph.D., clinical instructor at the Addiction Research Foundation in Toronto. "But now we believe that it is an actual drug dependence." In the American Psychiatric Associations latest diagnostic manual, DSM-III, tobacco dependence is classified as an addiction and an organic mental disorder. Tobacco dependence "clearly meets the criterion for addiction," says Robert L. Spitzer, M.D., chairman of the APA task force responsible for the manual.

Source: "Medical News," *Journal of the American Medical Association* 247.17 (1982) 2333–38. American Medical Association.

### DISCUSSION QUESTIONS

1. Do you think that the general public realizes that tobacco dependence is considered such a serious health problem that it is included in the DSM-III?
2. What does this addiction classification imply for people you know who smoke?

However, the same is not true for snuff and chewing tobacco. Neither of these two products produce tars or carbon monoxide and therefore the Surgeon General has suggested that these two products may be somewhat safer in terms of lung cancer mortality for users of smokeless tobacco products.[16] (See figure 13.2.)

The particulate matter found in tobacco smoke has been clearly shown to be related to increased morbidity.[17] Several mechanisms explain how tars are related to morbidity. Tars have been established as carcinogens or **tumor initiators** in a variety of sites in the human body, particularly the esophagus, the lungs, the pancreas, and the kidney and bladder. At the same time, they are also considered **tumor promoters** in that they help maintain the process of tumor formation when the process has already been established by some other mechanism. Finally, some tars have been shown to be cocarcinogens. A cocarcinogen is a substance that cannot by itself initiate the growth of a tumor, but when combined with other substances that are also cocarcinogens, can cause tumor growth.

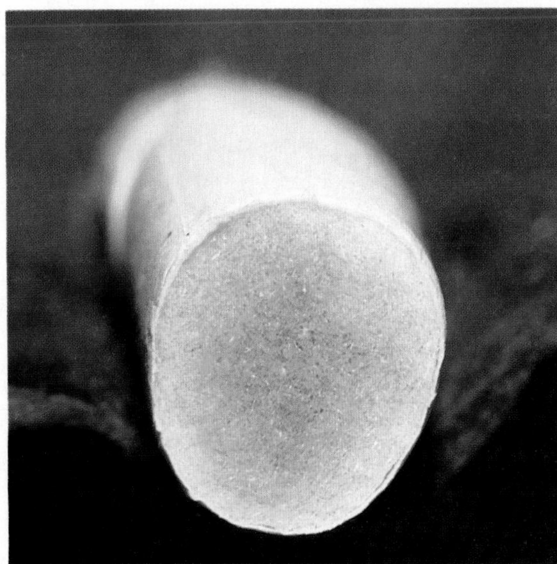

**Figure 13.2**
Tar from the smoke of cigarettes is believed by scientists to be capable of initiating and promoting tumor growth.

### Carbon Monoxide

Other than nicotine, it appears that **carbon monoxide (CO)** from tobacco smoke causes the most noticeable physiological effects. In doses of 10,000 to 50,000 parts per million (approximately 1 to 5 percent of the smoke), CO interferes with the ability of hemoglobin in the blood to carry oxygen. At the same time, CO may also have some ability to impair normal functioning of the nervous system.

The CO found in tobacco smoke probably has both acute and chronic effects on the smoker. There is some evidence that the CO levels in smoke are in part responsible for increasing the risk of heart attack and stroke, and that together with nicotine it increases the risks of all cardiovascular diseases. There are some who believe that CO may contribute to the risk of developing dependence on tobacco. However, there is little evidence to support this view.[18]

## RISKS ASSOCIATED WITH TOBACCO

Use of tobacco is associated with both mortality risks and morbidity risks.

### Mortality Risks

The following is a summary of the overall mortality risks identified by the Surgeon General.[19] Although there will be some differences in the mortality rates between men and women, these differences may be less significant than they seem. It has been hypothesized that women exhibit some lower rates than men principally because of differences in exposure to smoke. However, women whose smoking habits are comparable to those of men experience mortality rates that are comparable to men.[20]

The risk of death among the average smoker compared to the nonsmoker is 1.7 times greater for men and 1.3 times greater for women.[21] When a person smokes as much as two packs of cigarettes a day, this risk is increased to 2.0 times that of the nonsmoker for men and 1.7 for women. These ratios are called **mortality ratios.**

The life expectancy of a cigarette smoker is substantially shorter than the life expectancy of a nonsmoker. For someone thirty to thirty-five years of age and a regular smoker, the reduction in life expectancy is approximately nine years.

The *overall* mortality ratios for smokers are actually highest at younger ages and these ratios decline slightly with age.[22] This is a relative effect, because death rates from other causes increase significantly as we age. The actual number of excess deaths directly attributable to smoking increases with age for both men and women.[23] Mortality ratios for smokers (for all causes of death) are related to several specific factors for both men and women: (1) The longer a person has smoked, the higher the mortality ratios; (2) The earlier in life a person started smoking, the higher the mortality ratios; (3) The more someone inhales with each puff, the greater the mortality ratios; and (4) The higher the levels of tar and nicotine in the tobacco smoked, the higher the mortality ratios. Keep in mind, however, that even those who smoke low-tar and low-nicotine cigarettes (less than 1.2 milligrams nicotine and less than 17.6 milligrams tar) have mortality ratios more than 50 percent higher than their nonsmoking counterparts.[24]

The overall mortality ratios of ex-smokers decline with the number of years since smoking.[25] By the time someone has been an ex-smoker for fifteen years, the overall mortality ratio is comparable to someone who has never smoked. Regardless of how long a person has smoked, or how much, or what brand, quitting smoking reduces the associated disease risks (see table 13.4) unless the person is already ill when smoking is stopped.

### Morbidity Risks

Following is a summary of the data available on the morbidity risks associated with smoking. Once again, these risks appear to be comparable for both men and women given similar exposure to smoke.[26] Smokers tend to report both more acute and more chronic conditions than those who have never smoked. Specific examples include chronic bronchitis, emphysema, chronic sinusitis, peptic ulcer-diseases, influenza, and arteriosclerotic heart disease. There is a strong relationship between the amount smoked and the likelihood of reporting such

**Table 13.4 Diseases Related to Smoking**

- Cancer of the lung
- Chronic obstructive lung diseases (emphysema, chronic bronchitis)
- Cancer of the larynx
- Cancer of the oral cavity
- Cancer of the esophagus
- Ischemic heart disease
- Cancer of the bladder
- Cancer of the pancreas
- Aortic aneurysm
- Ulcers of the stomach and duodenum

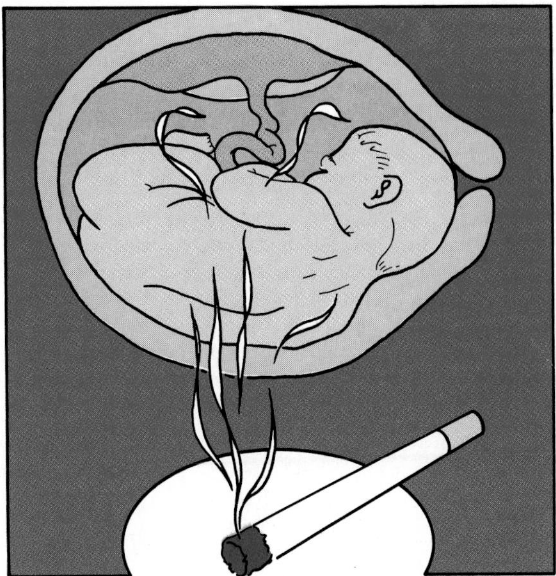

**Figure 13.3**
What does a fetus "inhale" when his or her mother smokes? *Source:* Reprinted from the *Journal of Cardiovascular Medicine* 4.7 (1979), with permission.

acute or chronic conditions.[27] The more smoked, the longer smoked, the higher the tar and nicotine content, and the more inhaled, the higher the morbidity rates. (See chapter 15 for a more detailed discussion of cardiopulmonary diseases.)

Both men and women who smoke report more days lost from work due to illness when compared with nonsmokers (33 percent excess for male smokers, 45 percent excess for female smokers), and more bed disability days (14 percent excess for male smokers, 17 percent excess for female smokers).[28] Both men and women who smoke report comparable increases in limitation of activity days due to chronic diseases when compared with nonsmokers. Current smokers report more hospitalizations than nonsmokers.

In a special report by the Surgeon General on the health consequences of smoking for women, some additional problems associated with women's smoking were raised. Babies born to women who smoke during pregnancy average 200 grams less in birth weight than babies born to women not currently smoking.[29] (See figure 13.3.) This relationship between smoking behavior and birth weight appears to be independent of all other factors that ordinarily influence birth weight (e.g., race, number of children previously borne, maternal size, socioeconomic status, sex of child, and gestational age). The relationship between smoking behavior and its influences during pregnancy is dose related—that is, the more smoked, the greater the influence on pregnancy.

The pattern of fetal-growth retardation that occurs with maternal smoking is a decrease in all dimensions including body length, chest circumference, and head circumference. The risk of spontaneous abortion, fetal death, and neonatal death increases directly with increasing levels of maternal smoking during pregnancy.[30] Although there seems to be little effect from smoking on mean gestation (average time from conception to birth), there does seem to be a higher proportion of fetal deaths and live births that occur before term among women who smoke during pregnancy.

An infant's risk of developing **"sudden infant death syndrome"** is increased with maternal smoking during pregnancy.[31] Additionally, infants and children born to smoking mothers may experience more long-term morbidity than those born to nonsmoking mothers.

There are many other risks associated with smoking. (See table 13.5.) Recent studies in both men and women indicate that smoking may impair fertility.[32] Additionally, women who use oral contraceptives and smoke are at a higher risk for fatal and nonfatal heart attacks when compared with women who use oral contraceptives but do not smoke.

### Table 13.5 Risks Associated with Smoking

| Risks of Smoking | Benefits of Quitting | Relative Risks: Filter-Tipped, Low T/N Brands | Risks of Smoking | Benefits of Quitting | Relative Risks: Filter-Tipped Low T/N Brands |
|---|---|---|---|---|---|
| **Risk: shortened life expectancy.** Twenty-five-year-old two-pack a day smokers have life expectancy 8.3 years shorter than nonsmoking contemporaries. Other smoking levels: proportional risk. | Benefit: reduces risk of premature death cumulatively. After ten to fifteen years, ex-smokers' risk approaches that of those who've never smoked. | Reduced risk of death from certain diseases (see below) implies increased life expectancy. | **Risk: coronary-heart disease.** Cigarette smoking is major factor; responsible for 120,000 excess U.S. deaths from coronary-heart disease (CHD) each year. | Benefit: sharply decreases risk after one year. After ten years ex-smokers' risk is same as that of those who never smoked. | Low T/N male smokers had 12 percent lower CHD rate, female low T/N smokers 19 percent lower than high T/N smokers. |
| **Risk: lung cancer.** Smoking cigarettes "major cause in both men and women." [SG 1979] | Benefit: gradual decrease in risk. After ten to fifteen years, risk approaches that of those who never smoked. | Filter tips reduce risk, but it is still five times that of nonsmokers. Low T/N brands reduce male risk by 20 percent, female risk by 40 percent. | **Risks: chronic bronchitis and pulmonary emphysema.** Cigarette smokers have four to twenty-five times risk of death from these diseases as nonsmokers. Damage seen in lungs of even young smokers. | Benefit: cough and sputum disappear during first few weeks. Lung function may improve and rate of deterioration slow down. | No identified benefit |
| **Risk: larynx cancer.** In all smokers (including pipe and cigar), it's 2.9 to 17.7 times that of nonsmokers. | Benefit: gradual reduction of risk after smoking cessation. Reaches normal after ten years. | Filter tips reduce risk 24 to 49 percent. | **Risks: stillbirth and low birth weight.** Smoking mothers have more stillbirths and babies of low birth weight—more vulnerable to disease and death. | Benefit: women who stop smoking before fourth month of pregnancy eliminate risk of stillbirth and low birth weight caused by smoking. | No identified benefit |
| **Risk: mouth cancer.** Cigarette smokers have three to ten times as many oral cancers as nonsmokers. Pipes, cigars, chewing tobacco also major risk factors. Alcohol seems synergistic carcinogen with smoking. | Benefit: reducing or eliminating smoking/drinking reduces risk in first few years; risk drops to level of nonsmokers in ten to fifteen years. | No identified benefit | **Risks: children of smoking mothers smaller, underdeveloped physically and socially, seven years after birth.** | Benefit: since children of nonsmoking mothers are bigger and more advanced socially, inference is that not smoking during pregnancy might avoid such underdeveloped children. | No identified benefit |

*Low T/N Brands = brands that are low in tar and nicotine.
Source: *Dangers of Smoking—Benefits of Quitting, and Relative Risks of Reduced Exposure.* American Cancer Society, 1980. Reprinted by permission of the American Cancer Society.

**Table 13.5** *Continued*

| Risks of Smoking | Benefits of Quitting | Relative Risks: Filter-Tipped, Low T/N Brands | Risks of Smoking | Benefits of Quitting | Relative Risks: Filter-Tipped Low T/N Brands |
|---|---|---|---|---|---|
| Risk: cancer of esophagus. Cigarettes, pipes, and cigars increase risk of dying of esophageal cancer about two to nine times. Synergistic relationship between smoking and alcohol. | Benefit: since risks are dose related, reducing or eliminating smoking /drinking should have risk-reducing effect. | No identified benefit | Risk: peptic ulcer. Cigarette smokers get more peptic ulcers and die more often of them; cure is more difficult in smokers. | Benefit: ex-smokers get ulcers but these are more likely to heal rapidly and completely than those of smokers. | No identified benefit |
| Risk: cancer of bladder. Cigarette smokers have seven to ten times risk of bladder cancer as nonsmokers. Also synergistic with certain exposed occupations: dyestuffs, etc. | Benefit: risk decreases gradually to that of nonsmokers over seven years. | No identified benefit | Risk: allergy and impairment of immune system. | Benefit: since these are direct, immediate effects of smoking, they are obviously avoidable by not smoking. | No identified benefit |
| Risk: cancer of pancreas. Cigarette smokers have two to five times risk of dying of pancreatic cancer as nonsmokers. | Benefit: since there is evidence of dose-related risk, reducing or eliminating smoking should have risk-reducing effect. | No identified benefit | Risks: alters pharmacologic effects of many medicines, diagnostic tests, and greatly increases risk of thrombosis with oral contraceptives. | Benefit: majority of blood components elevated by smoking return to normal after cessation. Nonsmokers on Pill have much lower risks of thrombosis. | |

## PERSONAL AND SOCIAL BARRIERS TO A SMOKE-FREE LIFE-STYLE

Public awareness of the dangers of smoking has steadily increased since the first Surgeon General's report. By 1978, more than 90 percent of all Americans believed that cigarette smoking was hazardous to their health.[33] This does not, however, necessarily translate into nonsmoking behavior. There are many factors to be considered when trying to understand smoking behavior. Such factors influence the likelihood of starting to smoke, continuing once started, and the possibility of cessation. Smokers differ in their choices of cigarettes (e.g., low versus high tar and nicotine content), the number of cigarettes smoked (which may range from none to a high of about one hundred cigarettes per day), the amount of the cigarette smoke (some people only smoke the first few millimeters of a cigarette while others smoke a cigarette down to the butt end), the number of puffs taken from each cigarette (ranging from one or two to a high of about twenty per cigarette), the depth of inhalation (from the noninhaler to the deep inhaler), and the length of inhalation. Given all of these differences, someone who smokes only ten cigarettes a day could absorb more nicotine, tars, and carbon monoxide than someone who smokes two or three times that amount. Many factors influence smoker's decisions and habits.

13.2 EXHIBIT 13.2

## What Does Advertising Do?

In the 1975 Adult Use of Tobacco Survey a majority of former smokers and nonsmokers of both sexes agreed with the statement "Cigarette advertising should be stopped completely." The percentages for men were 56.9 percent for nonsmokers and 56.4 percent for former smokers, and for women, 68.2 percent for nonsmokers and 62.5 percent for former smokers. However, only 42.6 percent of female smokers agreed with the statement. It appears that adult smokers value cigarette advertisements, but why they do—whether for information about brand characterization and availability, identification with the image portrayed, or some other reason—is not known. Martin Fishbein concluded that cigarette advertising influences the decision to smoke as well as the choice of brand. Furthermore, he points out that cigarette advertising may serve as a discriminative stimulus for smoking behavior. Advertising can influence the initiation of smoking, the choice of brand smoked, and the level of consumption. Commenting that the tobacco industry asserts that advertising serves only to influence brand choice and not initiation or consumption, Fishbein maintains that it is somewhat unrealistic to assume that an advertisement which can do one of these things is not also capable of doing the other.

Source: *The Health Consequences of Smoking for Women: A Report of the Surgeon General.* USDHHS, Public Health Service (Washington, D.C.: U.S. Government Printing Office, 1980).

### DISCUSSION QUESTIONS

1. Do you believe that advertising affects the decision to smoke, or just selection of brand?
2. What factors of advertisements affect you most?

## Advertising and the Media

In 1978, approximately $900 million was spent on advertising and promotion of cigarettes in the U.S., almost a 300 percent increase in expenditures for such advertising since 1970.[34] Recently, much of this cigarette advertising has been directed specifically at women, demonstrating such themes as the emancipation of women, romantic love, and the independent single woman.[35] Research indicates that most female smokers have a positive impression of the individuals pictured in these advertisements. Females surveyed who smoke view these images of women in advertisements as attractive (69 percent), enjoying themselves (66 percent), well dressed (66 percent), sexy (54 percent), young (50 percent), and healthy (49 percent).[36] (See Exhibit 13.2.) The Surgeon General's report stated that:

> . . . advertisers have been successful in creating a sense of mystery, sophistication, and power around the behavior of smoking. Although smoking was once frowned upon for women, people now respond less negatively to a woman smoking. There is evidence that, for some women, smoking is linked with attitudes and behaviors that comprise a socially valued and successful self-image, and that giving up smoking is a threat to that image.[37]

Although the general argument that advertising will influence tobacco-using behavior seems compelling, there is still some controversy in a number of areas. There is little empirical research to substantiate the claims of the effectiveness of prosmoking advertising to increase use or antismoking advertising to decrease use. Bans on television advertising for cigarettes in several other countries (United Kingdom, Denmark, Ireland, New Zealand, and Italy) seem to have had little impact on consumption.[38] On the other hand, Kenneth Warner has suggested that the reduction in media advertising coupled with the antismoking advertising seen in some media may have prevented even greater increases in consumption of tobacco products than we have seen.[39] Others seem to agree that

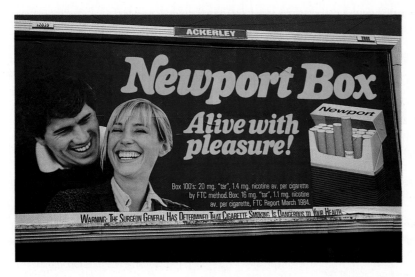


**Figure 13.4**
Cigarette advertising, and the nature of its influence, are controversial issues.

recent reductions in cigarette consumption can be attributed to antismoking ads on television.[40] In any case, the reduction in advertising in the media has been coupled with an increase in advertising at the point of sale and the specific influence of either change is difficult to determine by itself.

Martin Fishbein's arguments notwithstanding (see Exhibit 13.2),[41] the cigarette industry has stated that the major effect of cigarette advertising appears to be to shift brand preferences rather than to influence decisions whether or not to smoke.[42] It seems clear that advertising does exert some influence on decisions regarding use of tobacco products. However, there are other influences that are probably more important.

## Other Factors Influencing the Decision to Smoke

People decide whether or not they will smoke partly based on their parents' smoking habits and what their peers do.

**PARENTAL SMOKING HABITS** Parental behavior can have strong influences on the behavior of children—and smoking behavior is one of those areas in which clear empirical evidence of parental influence exists. In families where both parents smoke, 22.2 percent of the boys and 20.7 percent of the girls also become smokers. In families where neither parent smokes, those rates are reduced to 11.3 percent in boys and 7.6 percent in girls.[43] It appears that parental smoking behavior is the second best predictor of smoking among junior-high and high-school students, following the number of friends who smoke.[44]

**PEER PRESSURE** Perhaps the most important determinant of smoking behavior is the number of friends who smoke.[45] This relationship, however, is strongest at younger ages and seems to diminish with age.[46] Peer pressure seems only to work when an adolescent belongs to or would like to belong to a group in which smoking is part of the life-style. When the peer-group behavior does not include smoking, there may be little pressure on the adolescent to begin to smoke.[47]

These data suggest the importance of peer pressure and conformity in determining whether adolescents will begin smoking. Some studies, however, indicate that adolescents overestimate the number of their peers who smoke. If smoking were considered a behavior to emulate, these overestimates might increase the numbers who actually begin smoking.[48]

## Personal Self-Assessment

Many factors determine who is most likely to become, or continue to be a tobacco user. Many studies have attempted to determine how many different types of smokers there are. Included here is a short instrument designed to help smokers determine why they smoke. It is adapted from the Smokers Self Test.[49] (See also Activity for Wellness 13.1.)

13.1 ACTIVITY FOR WELLNESS

# Why Do You Smoke?

Here are some statements made by people to describe what they get out of smoking cigarettes. How often do you feel this way when smoking them? Circle one number for each statement.

IMPORTANT: Answer every question.

**HOW TO SCORE:**

1. Enter the numbers you have circled in the Part I questions in the spaces below, putting the number you have circled to Question A *over* line A, to Question B *over* line B, and so on.
2. Add together the number above each letter to get your totals. For example, the sum of your scores over lines A, G, and M gives you your score on Stimulation—lines B, H, and N gives the score on Handling, and so on.

| | | | | Totals |
|---|---|---|---|---|
| ___ + | ___ + | ___ = | ___ | |
| A | G | M | | Stimulation |
| ___ + | ___ + | ___ = | ___ | |
| B | H | N | | Handling |
| ___ + | ___ + | ___ = | ___ | |
| C | I | O | | Pleasurable Relaxation |
| ___ + | ___ + | ___ = | ___ | |
| D | J | P | | Crutch: Tension Reduction |
| ___ + | ___ + | ___ = | ___ | |
| E | K | Q | | Craving Psychological Dependence |
| ___ + | ___ + | ___ = | ___ | |
| F | L | R | | Habit |

Scores can vary from 3 to 15. Any score 11 and above is high; any score 7 and below is low.

| Question | Always | Frequently | Occasionally | Seldom | Never |
|---|---|---|---|---|---|
| A. I smoke cigarettes in order to keep myself from slowing down. | 5 | 4 | 3 | 2 | 1 |
| B. Handling a cigarette is part of the enjoyment of smoking it. | 5 | 4 | 3 | 2 | 1 |
| C. Smoking cigarettes is pleasant and relaxing. | 5 | 4 | 3 | 2 | 1 |
| D. I light up a cigarette when I feel angry about something. | 5 | 4 | 3 | 2 | 1 |
| E. When I have run out of cigarettes I find it almost unbearable until I can get more. | 5 | 4 | 3 | 2 | 1 |
| F. I smoke cigarettes automatically without even being aware of it. | 5 | 4 | 3 | 2 | 1 |

ACTIVITY FOR 13.1
# WELLNESS

| Question | Always | Frequently | Occasionally | Seldom | Never |
|---|---|---|---|---|---|
| G. I smoke cigarettes to stimulate me, to perk myself up. | 5 | 4 | 3 | 2 | 1 |
| H. Part of the enjoyment of smoking a cigarette comes from the steps I take to light up. | 5 | 4 | 3 | 2 | 1 |
| I. I find cigarettes pleasurable. | 5 | 4 | 3 | 2 | 1 |
| J. When I feel uncomfortable or upset about something, I light up a cigarette. | 5 | 4 | 3 | 2 | 1 |
| K. I am very much aware of the fact when I am not smoking a cigarette. | 5 | 4 | 3 | 2 | 1 |
| L. I light up a cigarette without realizing I still have one burning in the ashtray. | 5 | 4 | 3 | 2 | 1 |
| M. I smoke cigarettes to give me a "lift." | 5 | 4 | 3 | 2 | 1 |
| N. When I smoke a cigarette, part of the enjoyment is watching the smoke as I exhale it. | 5 | 4 | 3 | 2 | 1 |
| O. I want a cigarette most when I am comfortable and relaxed. | 5 | 4 | 3 | 2 | 1 |
| P. When I feel "blue" or want to take my mind off cares and worries, I smoke cigarettes. | 5 | 4 | 3 | 2 | 1 |
| Q. I get a real gnawing hunger for a cigarette when I haven't smoked for a while. | 5 | 4 | 3 | 2 | 1 |
| R. I have found a cigarette in my mouth without remembering putting it there. | 5 | 4 | 3 | 2 | 1 |

Although each smoker's habit is unique, the Smokers Self Test includes six categories of smokers, including:

1. **Stimulation:** those who smoke because smoking is stimulating. This accounts for approximately 10 percent of smokers.
2. **Handling:** those for whom the process of smoking is the most important issue. About 10 percent of smokers fall into this category.
3. **Pleasurable relaxation:** those who fall into this category smoke as a way to relax and enjoy a pleasurable experience. If this smoker is able to identify a satisfactory substitute, there is some indication of a high degree of ability to stop smoking.[50] This group accounts for 15 percent of all smokers.
4. **Crutch:** this group uses smoking as a means to reduce tension in their lives. Approximately 30 percent of all smokers fall into this category.
5. **Craving:** these smokers have a psychological dependence upon smoking, and may have some difficulty in quitting if they want to. About 25 percent of smokers are in this group.
6. **Habit:** for this group, smoking is done without thought—it becomes an automatic behavior. About 10 percent of regular smokers fall into this category.

# QUITTING SMOKING

Although the title of this section might sound like it is designed only for smokers who want to quit smoking, it is also for nonsmokers who are interested in helping others to quit.

## Some Concerns

Smokers vary in terms of the age when they began, the length of time they have been smoking, whether they inhale or not, their choice of cigarette, how much of each cigarette they actually smoke, and how many cigarettes they smoke each day. There are also differences in the motivations of smokers to continue smoking or quit. Because of all of these differences, there is no single technique for quitting or long-term maintenance of cessation that works for all smokers. Methods that are effective for some smokers may not be useful for others. Some smokers may be successful regardless of the technique used, while others will not be able to stop smoking with any method. A more realistic approach for the latter group is reduction of smoking, or preparation for cessation.[51] (See Exhibit 13.3.)

A. G. Christen and K. H. Cooper[52] raise several important questions regarding smoking: "(1) In light of the well-known, thoroughly publicized health hazards of smoking, why does this habit continue to have such widespread appeal? (2) Why is it so difficult for many persons to quit smoking once having become habituated? (3) Can a person really do anything to control this tenacious habit?"

In response, Christen and Cooper add two statements similar in nature to the issues raised in Activity for Wellness 13.1: "(1) Smoking provides powerful, immediate satisfactions for the individual—pharmacological, psychological, emotional, and social. (2) Millions of Americans have successfully quit smoking. It can be done." The following discussion is based on some of these ideas.

**QUITTING IS NOT FOR EVERYONE** Unlikely as it might seem, there are many individuals who should probably NOT consider quitting smoking at the current time. People who are experiencing some life crisis or emotional difficulties or who are severely depressed should not be considered prime candidates for smoking cessation. Smoking reduction might be a more realistic alternative in some cases than cessation.

**ALL OR NOTHING AT ALL** Many people feel that smokers consider quitting an all-or-nothing proposition. Heavy smokers might find a reduction in their intake a more appropriate course of action. About 50 percent of those who successfully quit smoking have done so gradually, with a graded reduction rather than abrupt cessation.[53]

13.3 EXHIBIT 13.3

## Sigmund Freud: The Cigarette Smoker

> Whoever understands the human mind, knows that hardly anything is harder for a man to give up than a pleasure he has once experienced. Actually, we can never give anything up; we only exchange one thing for another. What appears to be a renunciation is really the formation of a substitute or surrogate.*

When he was thirty-eight years old, Dr. Sigmund Freud's physician advised him to stop smoking because of some difficulties he was having with his health. Freud tried to stop and wrote the following:

> Soon after giving up smoking there were tolerable days . . . Then there came suddenly a severe affection of the heart, worse than I ever had when smoking . . . And with it an oppression of mood in which images of dying and farewell scenes replaced the more usual fantasies . . . The organic disturbances have lessened in the last couple of days; the hypomanic mood continues . . . It is annoying for a doctor who has to be concerned all day long with neurosis not to know whether he is suffering from a justifiable or a hypochondriacal depression.**

Seven weeks later, Freud began to smoke again. Soon after, he was diagnosed as having cancer of the jaw and oral cavity. Although he knew it was probably related to his smoking, Freud continued to smoke through more than thirty operations on his jaw including the construction of an entirely artificial jaw. He continued to smoke and developed chest pains related to his habit (angina). These pains stopped when he quit smoking, but he was only able to sustain this for twenty-three days before starting again. He finally died of cancer many years later.

Sources: *Sigmund Freud, *Creativity* (Middlesex: Penguin Books, 1970), 126–28.
**Dr. Ernest Jones, cited in R. C. Bone, J. R. Phillips, and P. Chowdhury, "The Smoking Habit: Physical Dependence on Nicotine," *The Journal of Respiratory Diseases* 2.5 (1981): 14–15.

### DISCUSSION QUESTIONS

1. Try to relate this story to your own attempts to change your behavior. What were the similarities? The differences?
2. Do you think this is a common occurrence?

**PHYSIOLOGICAL WITHDRAWAL** Nicotine and some other tars actually produce a physical dependence on tobacco products. Two types of withdrawal occur when a person quits smoking. The first is based on that physical dependence on nicotine (**physiological withdrawal**) and the other is based on the psychological dependence that smokers develop to the habit (**psychological withdrawal**). Of the two, physiological withdrawal is the easier to deal with. During this time, a person may experience many unpleasant symptoms related to the withdrawal, such as headaches, irritability, muscle aches, cramps, increased anxiety, some sleep disturbances, tingling in the fingers, and a craving for tobacco. These symptoms will peak in about three days and stop in about a week.[54] Although these symptoms may be different for each person, they are generally related to an attempt on the part of the body to eliminate nicotine. This is accomplished by flushing the bloodstream by the kidneys and can be helped by drinking lots of fluids—particularly fruit juices—during this time.[55]

**PSYCHOLOGICAL WITHDRAWAL** Of the two types of withdrawal experiences following cessation of drug use, psychological withdrawal is generally the more difficult to deal with. This can sometimes last for weeks or years. Some ex-smokers who have not had a cigarette for many years may still experience an occasional yearning for just one. Research seems to indicate that the first several months following cessation are the most critical and this is generally the time when someone will return to smoking.[56] This type of withdrawal is often characterized by changes in behavior and mood and sometimes by a severe craving for tobacco.

Figure 13.5 illustrates one view of some of the obstacles to quitting. As Christen and Cooper describe figure 13.5:

> The short-term quitter (X) can either return to his habit by the front door (A) by means of a conscious decision, or he can attempt to overcome numerous hidden and entrenched psychological obstacles (B). These obstacles provide strong unconscious mechanisms that can act forcefully upon the individual so that he is "off the hook" and free to enter the smoking habit via the rationalized back door (C). Long-term quitting (D) is a complicated, lengthy process, and coming to grips with the obstacles to quitting involves a great deal of unconscious, constructive and painful inner conflict.[57]

Smoking cessation is a continuous process that requires reinforcement and effort.

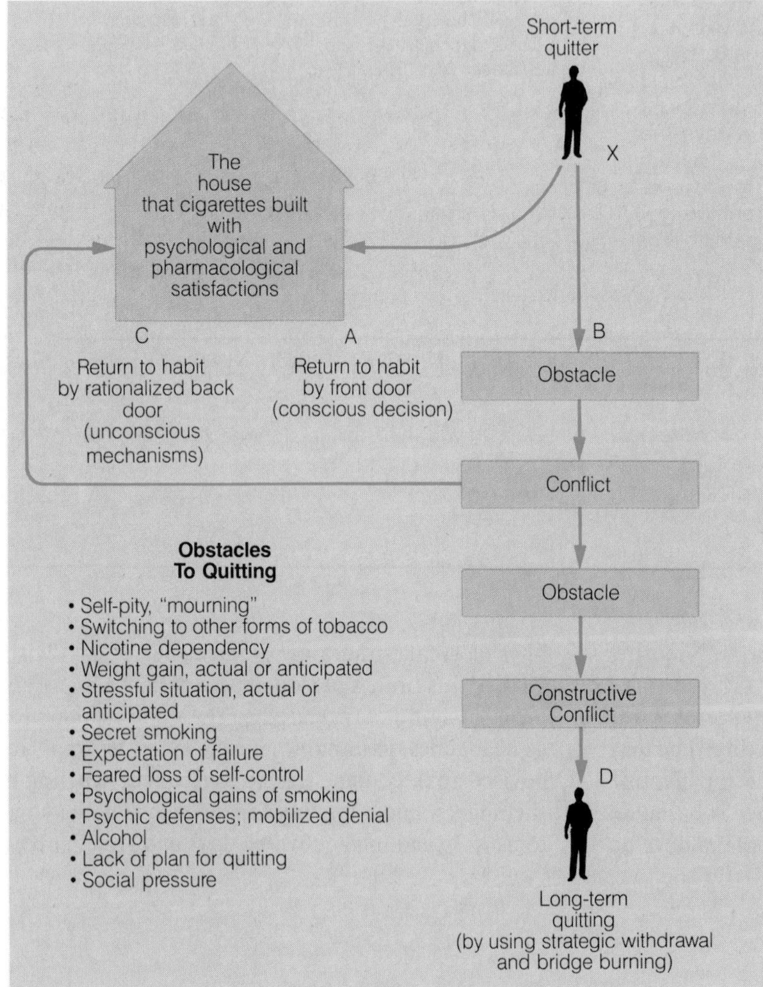


**Figure 13.5**
Diagrammatic presentation of the quit-smoking process as seen from a psychological vantage point. Note the obstacles that must be overcome and strong tendencies for the individual to resume smoking via unconscious mechanisms. Successful long-term quitting entails working through unconscious, constructive, and painful internal conflict over a prolonged period. *Source:* From Christen, Arden G., and K. H. Cooper, "Strategic Withdrawal from Cigarette Smoking," in *CA—A Cancer Journal for Clinicians* 29.2 (1979). © 1979 American Cancer Society, Inc. Reprinted with permission.

## Strategies for Smoking Cessation

Many different strategies have been tried in an effort to help people quit smoking. The strategies that have been studied most carefully are drug treatments, hypnosis, and social learning theory and behavior modification approaches.

**DRUG TREATMENTS** A good deal of research has been done in an attempt to find drugs that could minimize the distress of withdrawal and assist people in overcoming their dependence on nicotine and the smoking habit. There have been nicotine substitutes, such as Lobeline, which seem to be no more effective in long-term studies than the use of placebos.[58] Nicotine-containing chewing gum has been marketed as an aid to smoking cessation. Its use appears to be more effective than placebos in minimizing the distress during withdrawal, but has not yet been proven to be a major factor in cessation.[59] In addition, the person retains a dependence on the nicotine in the gum itself.

**HYPNOSIS** Although hypnosis was once thought to be a substantial aid to smoking cessation, the research is mixed and leaves some controversy regarding its potential for success.[60] Success rates have ranged from 20 percent to a high of almost 90 percent. It appears, however, that the most effective way that hypnosis can be used is in conjunction with counseling or other therapies.[61]

**SOCIAL LEARNING THEORY AND BEHAVIOR MODIFICATION APPROACHES** Research in social learning theory and behavior modification has been plentiful and has led to many approaches to smoking cessation.[62] Among the most popular are self-control strategies, such as stimulus control, contingency contracting, and adversive strategies.

**Stimulus control** provides the smoker with an increased awareness of the expected outcomes and tries to control stimuli and provide skills to deal with those situations in order to accomplish those outcomes. The research in this area has also been mixed, with the most successful programs combining several approaches.[63]

**Contingency contracting** involves the depositing of sums of money for later disbursement if certain goals are achieved. This has produced some encouraging results, but as with stimulus control, the most effective use of contingency contracting appears to be within the context of a much broader program.[64]

**Aversion strategies** attempt to change behavior by using aversive stimuli. There are three major forms of stimuli used in such approaches, including the use of electric shock, covert sensitization, and cigarette smoke. The first involves the application of electric shocks in order to link smoking with discomfort; covert sensitization involves the use of methods to produce aversion to smoking by linking smoking with nausea or other discomfort; and cigarette-smoke aversion involves either doubling or tripling consumption prior to withdrawal, or by forcing someone to rapidly puff a cigarette to produce unpleasant feelings during smoking. Of the three, it appears that cigarette-smoke aversion holds the most promise when used alone. These approaches are seldom used together, and again research results on their success rates are mixed.

Smoking-cessation programs often utilize many of these social learning theory and behavior modification techniques together to encourage and support the person trying to give up smoking. This multicomponent approach appears to hold the most potential for success when considering the general population of smokers.

Research indicates that 95 percent of those who have quit smoking have done so without the aid of any organized smoking-cessation program.[65] Moreover, surveys of most current smokers indicate a preference for quitting on their own and they tend to disfavor entrance into organized, comprehensive programs.[66]

## Maintenance of Cessation

Most current studies indicate that maintenance of nonsmoking behavior following quitting is a difficult process. W. A. Hunt and J. D. Matarazzo demonstrated that only about 25 percent of the participants of smoking-cessation clinics remain abstinent within three to six months following treatment.[67] These results were replicated by D. Evans and D. S. Lane.[68] There have been few studies demonstrating more than 30 percent abstinence six months following treatment.[69]

New emphasis on techniques to improve the maintenance phase of cessation promises to improve abstinence rates, with several reports of greater than 50 percent abstinence at follow-ups of six months or longer.[70] To improve maintenance of nonsmoking after intensive treatment programs have ended, reinforcement should be built into the natural environment. Smoking-cessation programs in the workplace may offer an opportunity for this. Social-support interventions are also promising.[71] Reliable findings link relapse to social cues and friends and spouses who smoke. The presence of group support, nonsmoking spouses, and professional contact decreases recidivism. Providing skills and support to maintain abstinence following treatment seems to be an important part of the treatment process itself.

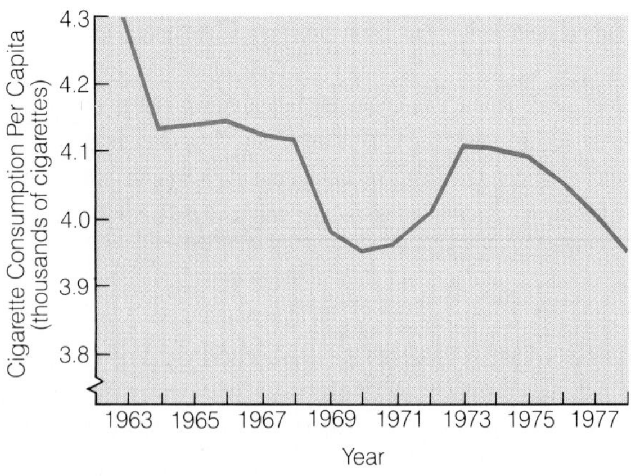


**Figure 13.6**
Annual per capita consumption of cigarettes in the U.S. for persons eighteen and older, 1963–1978. *Source:* "The Health Consequence of Smoking: The Changing Cigarette." *A Report of the Surgeon General.* U.S. Department of Health and Human Services, 1981.

## IS THERE A SAFE WAY TO SMOKE?

Despite the preponderance of evidence that smoking is hazardous to health, there are still many who smoke and are either not willing or not ready to give it up for their health. For these people, the apparent choices available include all those steps that can be taken to minimize the potential hazards associated with smoking. There appear to be at least four major areas[72] in which this can be accomplished: (1) smoke fewer cigarettes each day; (2) take fewer puffs on each cigarette; (3) reduce the depth of each inhalation; and (4) choose a brand low in tar and nicotine. All available evidence appears to indicate that some of these suggestions are being followed extensively by smokers. Figure 13.6 displays the average annual consumption of cigarettes per capita in the U.S. for the years 1963 to 1978. We can see clearly that average consumption has dropped substantially in those sixteen years.

Perhaps more important, however, are the data summarized in figure 13.7. Here we see a substantial drop in the average levels of tar and nicotine in cigarettes consumed in the U.S. during that same sixteen-year period. The data in these two tables seem to indicate that smokers are generally following some sound advice. That is, many are giving up smoking and those who do not give it up appear to be smoking cigarettes low in tar and nicotine. Some words of caution are provided by the Surgeon General:

1. There is no safe cigarette and no safe level of consumption.
2. Smoking cigarettes with lower yields of "tar" and nicotine reduces the risk of lung cancer and, to some extent, improves the smoker's chance for longer life, provided there is no compensatory increase in the amount smoked. However, the benefits are minimal in comparison with giving up cigarettes entirely. The single most effective way to reduce hazards of smoking continues to be that of quitting early.
3. It is not clear what reductions in risk may occur in the case of diseases other than lung cancer. The evidence in the case of cardiovascular disease is too limited to warrant a conclusion, nor is there enough information on which to base a judgment in the case of chronic obstructive lung disease. In the case of smoking's effects on the fetus and newborn, there is no evidence that changing to a lower "tar" and nicotine cigarette has any effect at all on reducing risk.
4. Smokers may increase the number of cigarettes they smoke and inhale more deeply when they switch to lower-yield cigarettes. Compensatory behavior may negate any advantage of the lower-yield product or even increase the health risk.
5. The "tar" and nicotine yields obtained by present testing methods do not correspond to the dosages that the individual smokers receive: in some cases they may seriously underestimate these dosages.
6. A final question is unresolved, whether the new cigarettes being produced today introduce new risks through their design, filtering mechanisms, tobacco ingredients, or additives. The chief concern is additives.[73]

You have all heard the advice. If you don't smoke, don't start; if you smoke, quit.

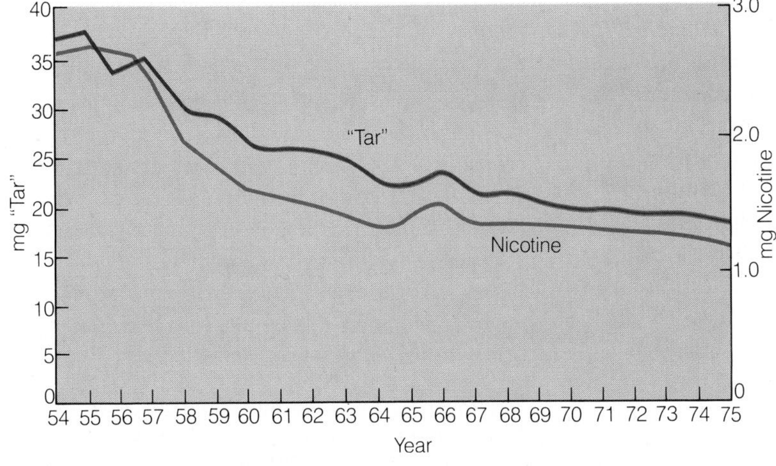


**Figure 13.7**
Sales-weighted averages of tar and nicotine per cigarette consumed in the U.S., 1954–1975. *Source:* Wakeman, H. "Sales-Weighted Average Tar and Nicotine Deliveries of U.S. Cigarettes from 1957 to Present," in Wynder, Ernst et al., *Lung Cancer.* International Union Against Cancer, UICC Technical Report Series 25 (1976):151–52.

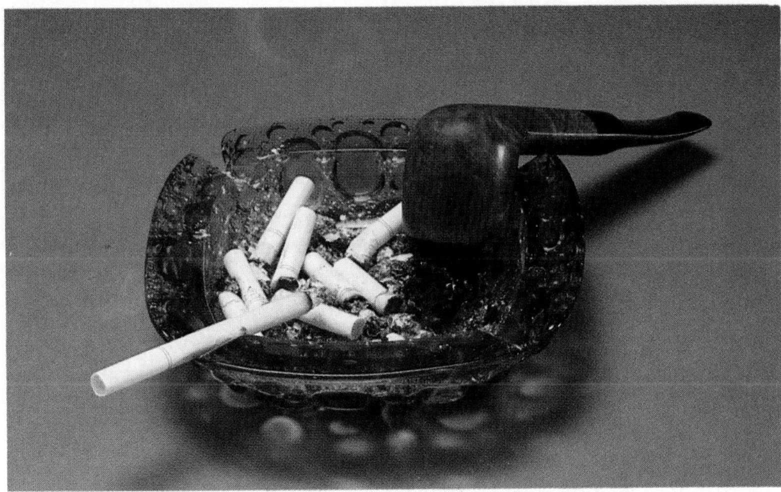

**Figure 13.8**
Research has only recently begun to focus on the dangers of sidestream smoke to the nonsmoker.

# RIGHTS OF NONSMOKERS

Our discussion so far has focused on the effects of tobacco on those who use it. What about its effects on nonusers?

## Mainstream versus Sidestream Smoke

Although the issues related to the health effects of smoking on the smoker have been thoroughly documented and are well known to the general population, this is not the case with the effects of smoke-filled environments on the nonsmoker. (See figure 13.8.) More information is beginning to be available in this matter.

Mainstream smoke is the smoke inhaled by the smoker while puffing burning tobacco and sidestream smoke is the smoke that enters the environment from the tip of a burning cigarette. We now know that many of the constituents of mainstream smoke are also found in sidestream smoke—including the carcinogens, cocarcinogens, and carbon monoxide. What was not known until relatively recently was that these constituents may be in even higher concentrations in sidestream smoke than in mainstream smoke. For example, sidestream smoke contains approximately eight times the levels of carbon dioxide, two and a half times the amount of carbon monoxide, and almost three times the nicotine content as mainstream smoke.[74] The impact of this issue needs some further clarification.

Mainstream smoke is inhaled directly into a smoker's body, but sidestream smoke enters the environment. Therefore, sidestream smoke is diluted in the ambient air. What is inhaled by the nonsmoker in a smoke-filled environment appears to be less in quantity than what a smoker gets from mainstream smoke. However, the strength of the content of the smoke is higher from sidestream than mainstream smoke. Inhaling sidestream smoke is called **involuntary smoking** or **secondhand smoke.** At issue is how dangerous involuntary smoking is.

## Health Risks to Nonsmokers from Involuntary Smoking

Substantial evidence exists to indicate that involuntary smoking has certain health-related effects on the nonsmoker. Among the most important points related to involuntary smoking are the following:

1. It is possible in a heavily smoke-filled environment during an eight-hour workday to be exposed to enough carbon monoxide to exceed maximum limits. Such exposure has been shown to produce slight deterioration in some tests of psychomotor performance, especially in the areas of attentiveness and cognitive function. These effects are increased when coupled with such factors as fatigue and the presence of other drugs.[75]
2. Unrestricted smoking on buses and planes is reported to be annoying to the majority of nonsmoking passengers.[76]
3. Children of parents who smoke are more likely to have bronchitis and pneumonia during the first year of life and this may be due in part to the presence of smoke in the environment.
4. The levels of carbon monoxide found in some smoke-filled environments have been shown to decrease the capacity of some people with cardiovascular diseases to exercise without chest pain. Similar deficits were found in other groups, such as those with chronic obstructive lung diseases.[77]
5. It has been reported that persons with a history of allergies are more likely to experience reactions to the presence of tobacco smoke in the environment.[78]
6. Although there is some doubt concerning the relationship between involuntary smoking and the potential risk of developing lung cancer, there is some evidence of substantial concern. At least two studies have reported an increased risk of lung cancer in nonsmoking wives of smoking husbands[79,80] while one other indicated no such increased risk.[81]

There are many issues and some controversy regarding involuntary smoking. There are some points about which we are sure: (1) the potential risk is dependent on many factors, including length and extent of exposure; (2) the most dramatic effects appear to be those related to the immediate exposure to the smoke itself and to carbon monoxide; and (3) involuntary smoking appears to be distasteful to most people.[82]

## Nonsmokers' Bill of Rights

With all of these issues regarding involuntary smoking and its potential effects on health, more people are beginning to demand what is called their dual rights: (1) the right to choose not to smoke and (2) the right not to have to breathe the smoke of those who choose to smoke.[83] Because of these issues, the following has been proposed:

The Nonsmokers' Bill of Rights*

*Nonsmokers help protect the health, comfort and safety of everyone by insisting on the following rights.*

1. The right to breathe clean air. Nonsmokers have the right to breathe clean air, free from harmful and irritating tobacco smoke. This right supersedes the right to smoke when the two conflict.

2. The right to speak out. Nonsmokers have the right to express—firmly but politely—their discomfort and adverse reactions to tobacco smoke. They have the right to voice their objections when smokers light up without asking permission.

3. The right to act. Nonsmokers have the right to take actions through legislative channels, social pressures, or any other legitimate means—as individuals or in groups—to prevent or discourage smokers from polluting the atmosphere and to seek the restriction of smoking in public places.

*Source: Courtesy National Interagency Council on Smoking and Health.

This nonsmokers' bill of rights has been proposed by several groups, including Group Against Smoker's Pollution (GASP) and Your Christmas Seals Association.

Smoking is a barrier to wellness that affects both smokers and nonsmokers alike. Advances toward a smoke-free society are also steps toward higher levels of wellness.

## SUMMARY


1. Since the first Surgeon General's Report on Smoking and Health in 1964, the link between smoking and health has been clearly established. Today, most people realize that smoking cessation is the one activity likely to have the largest impact on the health of our nation.

2. Tobacco smoke contains more than 2,000 chemical agents with the potential to affect our health negatively. The major constituents include tars, nicotine, and carbon monoxide.

3. Tars are made up of condensed particulate matter and may be both carcinogenic and cocarcinogenic.

4. Nicotine is an addicting drug and perhaps the most powerful agent in tobacco smoke.

5. Carbon monoxide affects our ability to absorb and use oxygen.

6. There are many health risks associated with the use of tobacco, including cancer, heart disease, emphysema, respiratory infections, and problems with pregnancy.

7. Among the prominent social barriers to a smoke-free society are advertising and the media, and parental and peer smoking habits.

8. Once begun, the tobacco habit proves difficult to stop. Educational efforts should be focused on preventing use before the habit becomes extrenched.

9. Involuntary smoking from sidestream smoke in the environment can be hazardous to the health of nonsmokers.


### Recommended Readings


American Cancer Society, *Cancer 1981 Facts and Figures* (New York: American Cancer Society, 1980).

American Cancer Society, *Dangers of Smoking—Benefits of Quitting and Relative Risks of Reduced Exposure* (New York: American Cancer Society, 1980).


### References


1. *Smoking and Health: A Report of the Advisory Committee to the Surgeon General of the Public Health Service.* U.S. Department of Health Education and Welfare, Public Health Service, Washington, D.C.: U.S. Government Printing Office, Publication No. 1103 (1964).

2. *Smoking and Health: A Report of the Surgeon General.* U.S. Department of Health Education and Welfare, Public Health Service, Washington, D.C.: U.S. Government Printing Office, Publication No. (PHS) 79–5006 (1979).

3. *Smoking and Health,* 1964.

4. *Smoking and Health,* 1979, 14–35.

5. *Smoking and Health,* 1979, 11–5.

6. *The Health Consequences of Smoking: The Changing Cigarette: A Report of the Surgeon General* U.S. Department of Health and Human Services, Public Health Service, DHHS Publication No. (PHS) 81–50156 (1981), 5.

7. *Smoking and Health,* 1979, 14–35, 14–36.

8. *Smoking and Health,* 1979, 14–85.

9. S. C. Glauser, E. M. Glauser, M. N. Reidenberg, et al., "Metabolic Effect in Man of the Cessation of Smoking," *Pharmacologist* 11.2 (1969): 283.

10. R. C. Bone, J. R. Phillips, and P. Chodhury, "The Smoking Habit: Physical Dependence on Nicotine," *The Journal of Respiratory Diseases* 2.5 (1981): 10–16.

11. *The Health Consequences of Smoking for Women: A Report of the Surgeon General,* U.S. Department of Health and Human Services, Public Health Service, Office of the Assistant Secretary for Health, Office on Smoking and Health, Washington, D.C.: U.S. Government Printing Office (1980).

12. Bone et al., "The Smoking Habit," 10–16.

13. David F. Duncan and Robert S. Gold, *Drugs and the Whole Person* (New York: John Wiley & Sons, 1982), 86.

14. *Smoking and Health,* 1979, 14–97.

15. Royal College of Physicians, *Smoking and Health* (London: Pitman Medical, 1977), 98–112.

16. *Smoking and Health,* 1979, 2–21.

17. *Smoking and Health,* 1979, 14–64.

18. *Smoking and Health,* 1979, 1-10–1-31.

19. *Smoking and Health,* 1979, 2–26.

20. *Smoking and Health,* 1979, 2–26.

21. *Smoking and Health,* 1979, 2–25.

22. E. Rogot, "Smoking and Life Expectancy Among U.S. Veterans," *American Journal of Public Health* 68.10 (1978): 1023.

23. *Smoking and Health,* 1979, 2–43.

24. *Smoking and Health,* 1979, 2–43.

25. *Smoking and Health,* 1979, 2–43.

26. *Smoking and Health,* 1979, 3–6.

27. *Smoking and Health,* 1979, 3–6.

28. *Smoking and Health,* 1979, 3–10.

29. *The Health Consequences of Smoking for Women: A Report of the Surgeon General,* U.S. Department of Health and Human Services, Public Health Service, DHHS Publication No. (PHS) 82–50179, 1982, vii.

30. *The Health Consequences of Smoking for Women,* vii–viii.

31. *The Health Consequences of Smoking for Women,* 225.

32. *The Health Consequences of Smoking for Women,* 178.

33. *The Health Consequences of Smoking: The Changing Cigarette,* 204.

34. *The Health Consequences of Smoking: The Changing Cigarette,* 202.

35. *The Health Consequences of Smoking for Women,* 325.

36. Yankelovich, Skelly, and White, Inc., *A Study of Cigarette Smoking among Teen-age Girls and Young Women: Summary of Findings,* U.S. Department of Health, Education, and Welfare, Public Health Service, National Institutes of Health, National Cancer Institute, DHEW Publication No. (NIH) 77–1203 (1977), 55.

37. *The Health Consequences of Smoking for Women,* 326.

38. E. E. Leavitt, "The Television Cigarette Commercial: Teenage Transducer or Paper Tiger?", *Yale Scientific Magazine* 45.1 (1970): 10–13.

39. K. E. Warner, "The Effects of the Anti-Smoking Campaign on Cigarette Consumption," *American Journal of Public Health* 67.7 (1977): 645–50.

40. E. Foote, "The Time Has Come: Cigarette Advertising Must Be Banned," in: M. E. Jarvik, J. W. Cullen, E. R. Gritz, T. M. Vogt, and L. J. West, eds., *Research on Smoking Behavior,* National Institutes on Drug Abuse Research Monograph 17, Public Health Service, Alcohol, Drug Abuse and Mental Health Administration, National Institute on Drug Abuse, DHEW Publication No. (ADM) 78–581 (December 1977): 339–46.

41. Martin Fishbein, "Consumer Beliefs and Behavior with Respect to Cigarette Smoking: A Critical Analysis of the Public Literature," in: Federal Trade Commission, *Report to Congress Pursuant to the Public Health Cigarette Smoking Act, for the Year 1976* (May 1977).

42. *Smoking and Health,* 1979, 18–23.

43. *Smoking and Health,* 1979, 17–13.

44. *Smoking and Health,* 1979, 17–13.

45. A. B. Palmer, "Some Variables Contributing to the Onset of Cigarette Smoking among Junior High School Students," *Social Science and Medicine* 4 (1970): 359–66; and J. P. Rudolph and B. L. Borland, "Factors Affecting the Incidence and Acceptance of Cigarette Smoking among High School Students," *Adolescence* 11.44 (1976): 519–25.

46. I. M. Newman, "Status Configurations and Cigarette Smoking in a Junior High School," *Journal of School Health* 40 (1970): 28–31.

47. National Institute of Education, *Teenage Smoking: Immediate and Long Term Patterns,* Department of Health, Education, and Welfare, National Institute of Education (November 1979).

48. Fishbein, "Consumer Beliefs and Behavior with Respect to Cigarette Smoking."

49. D. Horn, "An Approach to Office Management of the Cigarette Smoker," *Diseases of the Chest* 54.3 (1968): 203–209.

50. Bone et al., "The Smoking Habit: Physical Dependence on Nicotine."

51. J. K. Ockene and I. S. Ockene, "9 Ways to Help Your Patients Stop Smoking," *Your Patient and Cancer* 2.1 (1982): 47–61.

52. A. G. Christen and K. H. Cooper, "Strategic Withdrawal from Cigarette Smoking," *CA—A Journal for Clinicians* 29.2 (1979): 96–107.

53. E. Adams, "An Approach to Patients Who Can't Stop Smoking," *Preventive Medicine* 2 (1973): 313–17.

54. *Smoking and Health,* 1979, 16–14.

55. Christen and Cooper, "Strategic Withdrawal from Cigarette Smoking."

56. M. Dubitzky and J. L. Schwartz, "Ego-Resiliency, Ego-Control, and Smoking Cessation," *Journal of Psychology* 70 (1968): 27–33.

57. Christen and Cooper, "Strategic Withdrawal from Cigarette Smoking."

58. G. C. Davison and R. C. Rosen, "Lobeline and Reduction of Cigarette Smoking," *Psychological Reports* 31.2 (1972): 443–56.

59. N. G. Schneider, P. Popek, M. E. Jarvik, and E. R. Gritz, "The Use of Nicotine Gum During Cessation of Smoking," *American Journal of Psychiatry* 134.4 (1977): 439–40.

60. *Smoking and Health,* 1979, 19–17.

61. L. L. Pederson, W. G. Scrimgeour, and N. M. Lefcoe, "Comparison of Hypnosis plus Counseling, Counseling Alone, and Hypnosis Alone in a Community Service Smoking Withdrawal Program," *Journal of Consulting and Clinical Psychology* 43.6 (1975): 920.

62. *Smoking and Health,* 1979, 19–19.

63. J. C. Brengelmann, "Manual on Smoking Cessation Therapy: Facts and Suggestions for the Treatment of Smoking," *International Journal of Health Education* (1975).

64. H. A. Lando, "Successful Treatment of Smokers with a Broad-Spectrum Behavioral Approach," *Journal of Consulting and Clinical Psychology* 45.3 (1977): 361–66.

65. U.S. Department of Health, Education, and Welfare, *The Smoking Digest: Progress Report and a Nation Kicking the Habit,* U.S. Department of Health, Education, and Welfare, Public Health Service, National Institutes of Health, National Cancer Institute, Office of Cancer Communications (1977).

66. *The Health Consequences of Smoking: Cancer. A Report of the Surgeon General,* U.S. Department of Health and Human Services, Public Health Service, Office on Smoking and Health, DHHS Publication No. (PHS) 82–50179 (1982).

67. W. A. Hunt and J. D. Matarazzo, "Three Years Later: Recent Developments in the Experimental Modification of Smoking Behavior," *Journal of Abnormal Psychology* 81.2 (1973): 107–14.

68. D. Evans and D. S. Lane, "Long-Term Outcome of Smoking Cessation Workshops," *American Journal of Public Health* 70.7 (1980): 725–27.

69. *The Health Consequences of Smoking.*

70. *The Health Consequences of Smoking.*

71. *Smoking and Health,* 1979.

72. Bone et al., "The Smoking Habit."

73. *The Health Consequences of Smoking.*

74. *Smoking and Health,* 1979, 14–38.

75. I. Yabroff, E. Meyers, V. Fend, N. David, M. Robertson, R. Wright, and R. Braun, *The Role of Atmospheric Carbon Monoxide in Vehicle Accidents,* (Menlo Park, Calif.: Stanford Research Institute, 1974).

76. *Smoking and Health,* 1979, 11–26.

77. W. S. Aronow and M. W. Isbell, "Carbon Monoxide Effect on Exercise-Induced Angina Pectoris," *Annals of Internal Medicine* 79.3 (1973): 392–95.

78. N. Epstein, "The Effects of Tobacco Smoke Pollution on the Eyes of the Allergic Nonsmoker," in: J. Steinfield, W. Griffiths, K. Ball, and R. M. Taylor, eds., *Proceedings of the Third World Conference on Smoking and Health, New York, June 2–5, 1975, Volume II: Health Consequences, Education, Cessation Activities, and Social Action,* U.S. Department of Health, Education and Welfare, Public Health Service, National Institutes of Health, National Cancer Institute, DHEW Publication No. (NIH) 77–1413 (1977): 337–45.

79. T. Hirayama, "Non-Smoking Wives of Heavy Smokers Have a Higher Risk of Lung Cancer: A Study from Japan," *British Medical Journal* 282.6259 (1981): 183–85.

80. D. Trichopoulos, A. Dalandidi, L. Sparros, and B. MacMahon, "Lung Cancer and Passive Smoking," *International Journal of Cancer* 27.1 (1981): 1–4.

81. L. Garfinkel, "Time Trends in Lung Cancer Mortality among Nonsmokers and a Note on Passive Smoking," *Journal of the National Cancer Institute* 66.6 (1981): 1061–66.

82. *Smoking and Health,* 1979, 11–25.

83. Duncan and Gold, *Drugs and the Whole Person,* 91.

CHAPTER FOURTEEN

# Psychoactive Drugs: Impacts on Mind and Behavior



All drugs can be placed in seven categories—herbal drugs, over-the-counter (OTC) drugs, prescription drugs, unrecognized drugs, and illicit drugs. Since tobacco and alcohol present so substantial a health concern, they warranted chapters of their own. The remaining drug categories will be covered in this chapter. We will emphasize the psychoactive drugs (those affecting the mind and behavior) and their impact on wellness. All drugs have the potential to be misused or abused, so we have combined all of these categories so we can consider them in one chapter.

# HERBAL DRUGS

**Herbal drugs** are plant substances that possess drug effects; they can legally be grown or gathered in the wild by anyone. This is the oldest category of drugs. The first drugs used by humankind were various fruits, seeds, flowers, leaves, and roots with real or imagined drug effects.

In the past two decades, there has been a rebirth of interest in these drugs. Herbal preparations are not only on the shelves of health-food stores, but also on supermarket and drugstore shelves. Gold, Duncan, and Sutherland found that this was the category of drugs in which college students expressed the greatest interest.[1]

Various herbal drugs that have stimulant effects are available. Caffeine is to be found in a number of plants, not only the coffee, tea, and cocoa plants, but also in American holly, Dahoon holly (or cassina), Brazilian soapberry (or guarana), kola nut, and yerba maté. The Mormon tea plant contains the stimulant ephedrine and cinnamon has a stimulant effect through an active ingredient that has never been identified. Sassafras contains safrole, which is a stimulant; unfortunately it is also a carcinogen (a substance that can cause cancer).

Valerian contains chatinive and valerine which have depressant effects.[2] Snakeroot contains reserpine, which has a tranquilizing effect and also lowers blood pressure. Wild lettuce contains lactucarine, "lettuce opium," which has a narcotic effect.[3]

Psychedelic effects (affecting the mind) are produced by a number of mushrooms which contain psilocin and psilocybin,[4] and by the seeds of the Hawaiian wood rose and a number of varieties of morning glory which contain lysergic acid amide.[5] Lysergic acid amide can be found in some preparations that may be legal in some states and illicit in other states (e.g. morning glory seeds). The lysergic acid amide found in a number of flower seeds produces essentially the same effects as LSD, but a larger dose is required.[6]

Unfortunately, many people believe that herbal drugs are safe because they are "natural." This is nearly the opposite of the truth. Herbal drugs usually contain more than one active drug. Furthermore, the amount of drug present in an herbal preparation may be somewhat unpredictable. Poisoning due to the presence of arsenic or lead in a number of herbal preparations has occurred with increasing frequency as herbal drugs have become more popular.[7] (See figure 14.1.)

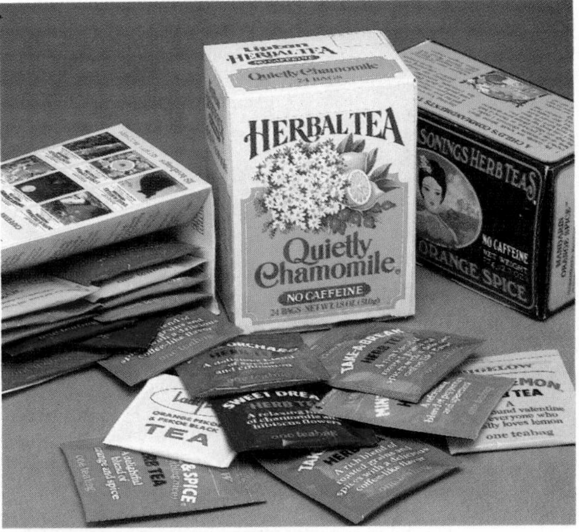


**Figure 14.1**
Herbal products often contain more than one active drug.

# OVER-THE-COUNTER DRUGS

**Over-the-counter** (OTC) drugs are big business in the U.S. today.[8] Americans spend more than four billion dollars every year on more than 200,000 different brand-name products.[9] Despite the large number of products (there may be more than 200,000), they are actually composed of different combinations of less than 200 basic drugs.

Until 1952, there was almost no regulation of OTC drugs. The 1952 Durham-Humphrey Amendment to the 1938 Pure Food and Drug Act required that all drugs being marketed should be placed in one of two categories: those that were unsafe for unsupervised use by individuals (prescription drugs) and those that could be used safely without medical supervision (OTC drugs). Ten years later, the 1962 Kefauver-Harris Amendment to the 1938 act mandated a review by the Food and Drug Administration of the safety and effectiveness of OTC drugs.

Since no one even knew how many OTC products were on the market (estimates ranged from 100,000 to 250,000), the FDA concluded that it could not conduct such a review product by

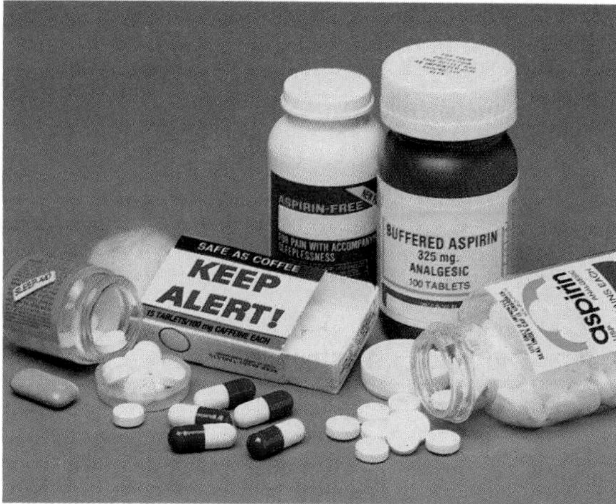


**Figure 14.2**
The F.D.A. has been investigating the safety and effectiveness of many drugs commonly found in OTC preparations.

product.[10] Instead the FDA would review the available research on the basic drugs from which the OTC products were compounded. Each of these drugs was to be categorized into one of three groups:

1. Those generally recognized as safe (**GRAS**) and effective (**GRAE**)
2. Those known to be either unsafe or ineffective
3. Those about which not enough was known.

Drugs in the second category would be removed from the OTC market. Those in the third group would be removed from the market unless the drug manufacturers could provide new evidence of their safety before a specific deadline. This review process began in 1972 and is only now nearing completion.[11]

Some OTC drugs contain belladonna or other substances capable of producing a state of delirious drunkenness and are occasionally misused for this purpose. The three major types of psychoactive OTC products, however, are the analgesics, sedatives, and stimulants. (See figure 14.2.)

## Analgesics

**Analgesics** are drugs that relieve pain. OTC analgesics may be classified into two groups depending on how they are taken. **Internal analgesics** are taken by mouth and **external analgesics** are rubbed or sprayed on the skin.

There are three basic types of OTC analgesics, including aspirin, acetaminophen, and salicilamide. The most common internal analgesic is aspirin, which not only relieves pain but also lowers fever and reduces inflammation and swelling in joints.[12] Aspirin, however, causes unpleasant side effects in some users, including upset stomach, allergic reactions, or irritation of ulcers. Many people (including some who do not suffer from these side effects) have switched from aspirin to acetaminophen, which does not produce these same side effects. Acetaminophen is an effective pain reliever and fever reducer, but does not have the antiinflammatory effect of aspirin. Thus, it is not satisfactory for arthritis pain or other pain resulting from inflammation.[13] Salicilamide is less widely used than either of these analgesics. It has effects much like aspirin, but with less likelihood of side effects.[14] It is also somewhat faster acting than aspirin products.

External analgesics are of three types. Some contain salicilamide which can be absorbed through the skin. Others contain a synthetic cocaine substitute such as benzocaine which causes numbness where it is applied. Counterirritant preparations, containing such substances as menthol, camphor, or methyl salycilate, produce sensations of warmth that may relieve musculoskeletal pain.

## Sedatives

Opium was the basic ingredient in many early OTC sedatives. Later OTC tranquilizers and sleeping pills were compounded with bromides or belladonna alkaloids as their prime active ingredients. A few of these are still on the market but their potential for overdose or cumulative poisoning is great enough that today only those containing diphenhydramine are approved.[15]

Most of the current OTC sedatives rely on the depressant side effects of antihistamines—antiallergy drugs—such as pyrilamine, doxylamine, and diphenhydramine. Some also contain aspirin or

**Table 14.1 Over-the-Counter Drug Interactions Potential Interactions Involving Common OTC Preparations**

| OTC Preparation | Combined with | Interaction Produced |
|---|---|---|
| Antacids: neutralize stomach acids (Alka-Seltzer®, Maalox®, and Mylanta®) | Antibiotics | Absorption of antibiotic decreased |
| | Anticoagulants | Absorption of anticoagulant decreased |
| | Aspirin | Absorption of aspirin reduced |
| | Digitalis | Action of digitalis inhibited |
| | Sulfonamides | Action of sulfonamide inhibited |
| Antihistamines: hay-fever preparations, antiasthmatics, cough suppressants, decongestants, sleeping aids (Allerest®, Nyquil®, Nytol®, Sleep-Eze®, and Sominex®) | Alcoholic beverages | CNS depression potentiated |
| | Anticoagulants | Anticlotting effects inhibited |
| | Anticholinergic | Anticholinergic potentiated |
| | Other CNS depressants | CNS action potentiated |
| | Hydrocortizone | Action of hydrocortizone inhibited |
| | Phenothiazines | Action of phenothiazines potentiated |
| | Reserpine | CNS depression |
| Aspirin-based products: reduce pain, fever, some inflammation (Anacin®, Bufferin®, Doan's Pills®, Empirin®, Midol®, Pamprin®, and Vanquish®) | Alcoholic beverages | Irritation of stomach wall increased |
| | Anticoagulants | Anticlotting effects potentiated |
| | Antidepressants | Potentially lethal combination |
| | Antidiabetics | Action of antidiabetics potentiated |
| | Antihypertensive | Action of antihypertensions may be counteracted by caffeine found in many aspirin products |
| | Para aminosalicyclic acid (PAS) | PAS toxicity |
| Cathartics: increase bowel movements (Ex-Lax®, Epsom Salts®, Milk of Magnesia®) | Digitalis | Absorption decreased by reducing transit time in intestines |
| | | Action of absorbed digitalis potentiated |
| Nasal decongestants: containing phenylpropanolanine and phenylephrine (Neosynephrine®) | Antihypertensives | Action of antihypertensive inhibited |

Source: From *Drugs and the Whole Person*, by D. F. Duncan and R. S. Gold (New York: Macmillan, 1982). Reprinted with permission of the publisher.

acetaminophen on the assumption that minor aches or pains are a common cause of tension or inability to sleep.

## Stimulants

OTC stimulants contain a dose of caffeine equivalent to one or two cups of coffee. Some also contain a small amount of vitamin $B_{12}$ for its mythical energizing effects. Large doses of caffeine, whether in the form of OTC products or of beverages such as coffee or tea, can produce the same psychological effects as other major central nervous system stimulants—increased alertness, excitement, nervousness, irritability, and, in very large doses, paranoia.[16] The effects of caffeine are more fully discussed in the section on unrecognized drugs.

Like many other drugs, OTC preparations should be regarded as potentially dangerous when mixed with other preparations. Table 14.1 contains a summary of some of the more common interactions between OTC preparations and other drugs.

## PRESCRIPTION DRUGS

**Prescription drugs** are those that can be administered or sold only by or on the order of a physician—or in some instances a dentist or veterinarian. Herbert Abelson and Ronald Atkinson found that 46 percent of all Americans have taken psychoactive prescription drugs for a medical purpose.[17] More women than men had used them and more whites than other racial groups. Nonmedical use was less common but far from rare. Nonmedical use of a sedative in order to get high was reported by 4 percent of the adults and 5 percent of the youths (aged twelve to seventeen). Nonmedical use of tranquilizers was reported by 3 percent of both age groups. Nonmedical use of stimulants was reported by 6 percent of the adults and 5 percent of the youths.

**Sedative-hypnotics** are drugs that have a calming effect in small doses and induce sleep in larger doses. If the user does not yield to the sleep-inducing effects, these drugs will produce a drunken state identical to that induced by alcohol.[18] The best known of the sedative-hypnotics include barbiturates such as Seconal, Nembutal, and Tuinal and methaqualone preparations such as Quaalude and Sopor.

**Minor tranquilizers,** such as Valium and Librium, relax the muscles and relieve anxiety. **Major tranquilizers,** such as Thorazine, Stelazine, and Haldol, relieve the symptoms of schizophrenia—the most severe of the psychotic mental illnesses. They also are used in smaller doses to control nausea and vomiting.

The term tranquilizer was originally coined to describe opium and the tranquil dreamy state it induced in users. Opium contains two active ingredients, morphine and codeine, which are now available, along with several related synthetic substances, as prescription drugs. Known as **opiates** or **narcotic analgesics,** they are used for relief of severe pain. They do not block the sensation of pain so much as they make the person less aware of and less concerned about the pain.[19]

**Amphetamines** and other stimulant drugs were once widely prescribed for weight control because of their effect of suppression of appetite.[20] Unfortunately, tolerance to amphetamines develops rapidly and appetite suppression can be sustained only if the dosage is regularly increased. Today, stimulants are prescribed mainly for the treatment of hyperactive children (because of their ability to increase attention span) and of narcoleptics (people who suffer from uncontrollable spells of falling asleep). Prolonged and unsupervised use of stimulants can result in a severe paranoid reaction known as "amphetamine psychosis."[21]

As consumers, we need to take a more active stance in terms of demanding more information from health-care professionals regarding the use of these drugs. If they are prescribed for you, you should be certain you know why and how to use these drugs. Your physician or pharmacist should be willing to answer all your questions in this regard.

## UNRECOGNIZED DRUGS

**Unrecognized drugs** are commercial products that have drug effects but that our culture does not consider to be drugs. These substances are produced, sold, and used by people who might well be offended if you suggested that they were involved with drugs. The unrecognized drugs are one of the major reasons why we may conclude that there are no drug-free individuals in our society—just people who do not realize they are using drugs.

Two of the unrecognized drugs—alcohol and tobacco—are so important in our society that they are covered in chapters of their own in this and other textbooks. (See chapters 12 and 13.) How many more unrecognized drugs there may be is impossible to estimate—it is simply too hard to rise above our cultural definitions and identify how many things we consider nondrugs are really drugs. In this chapter, we will look at just two examples of unrecognized drugs. One illustrates how widely used such substances may be and a second shows what unexpected things may be unrecognized drugs. (See figure 14.3.)

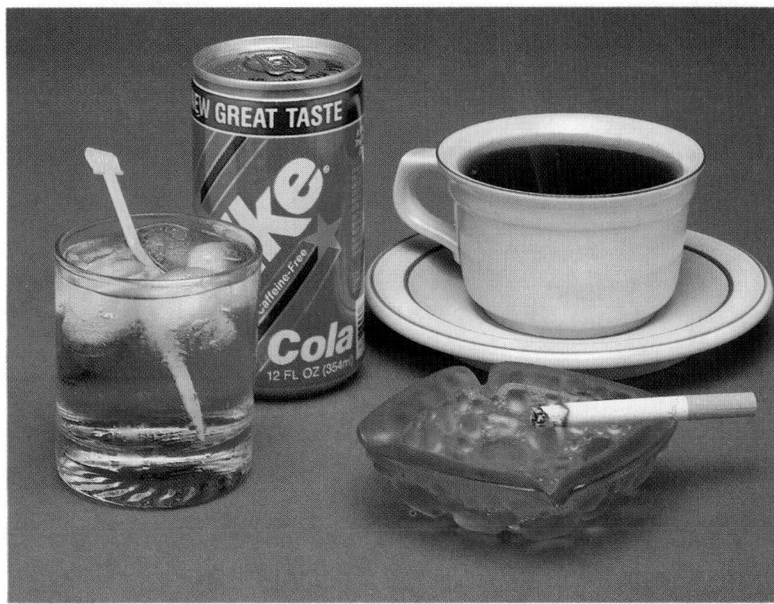


**Figure 14.3**
Many products that can be technically classified as drugs go unrecognized as such by the general public.

## Caffeine

Caffeine is probably the most widely used drug in our society.[22] Along with the similar drugs theophylline and theobromine, caffeine is found naturally in coffee, tea, and chocolate. Caffeine is added to other substances as well. Table 14.2 contains a summary of the levels of caffeine found in some commonly used beverages, drugs, and foods. Caffeine is an important part of many products.

A dose of 100 milligrams of caffeine will stimulate the central nervous system resulting in feelings of alertness and well-being. The voluntary muscles and heart muscle are stimulated by caffeine while the involuntary muscles,[23] especially the bronchial muscles, are relaxed by it. Heart rate, oxygen consumption, metabolic rate, blood pressure, secretion of acid by the stomach, and urinary output are all elevated by caffeine. Learning and recall of memories are enhanced by caffeine as are test performance, driving skills, and typing speed and accuracy.[24] Tasks requiring delicate muscular control or accurate timing, on the other hand, may be impaired by use of caffeine.

For most people, 400 milligrams of caffeine will produce nervousness, irritability, muscle tremors, and headache.[25] Twice that much is enough to cause hallucinations and possibly convulsions. The lethal dose of caffeine for most of the population is 10 grams, which causes death due to respiratory failure. Deaths have resulted from convulsions brought on by doses as low as 1 gram.[26]

Because of its effects on heart rate and blood pressure, caffeine has long been suspected of being a cause of heart disease. Several studies have, in fact, shown that regular coffee drinkers are more likely to suffer a heart attack than people who don't drink coffee.[27] However, the same studies found no association between use of tea and heart disease, which seems to indicate that caffeine was not the cause of the heart disease.

Caffeine has been found to cause chromosome breaks in white blood cells,[28] which has led to suspicions that it might cause birth defects, but studies have shown that mothers of babies with birth defects are no more likely to be coffee drinkers than are mothers in general.[29] Likewise, roasted coffee and black tea both contain small amounts of carcinogens, but there is no evidence so far that coffee or tea drinkers have higher rates of cancer.[30]

## Table 14.2 The Latest Caffeine Scorecard

### Caffeine Content of Beverages and Foods[1]

| *Item* | *Milligrams Average* | *Caffeine Range* |
|---|---|---|
| Coffee (5-oz. cup) | | |
| Brewed, drip method | 115 | 60–180 |
| Brewed, percolator | 80 | 40–170 |
| Instant | 65 | 30–120 |
| Decaffeinated, brewed | 3 | 2–5 |
| Decaffeinated, instant | 2 | 1–5 |
| Tea (5-oz. cup) | | |
| Brewed, major U.S. brands | 40 | 20–90 |
| Brewed, imported brands | 60 | 25–110 |
| Instant | 30 | 25–50 |
| Iced (12-oz. glass) | 70 | 67–76 |
| Cocoa beverage (5-oz. cup) | 4 | 2–20 |
| Chocolate milk beverage (8 oz.) | 5 | 2–7 |
| Milk chocolate (1 oz.) | 6 | 1–15 |
| Dark chocolate, semi-sweet (1 oz.) | 20 | 5–35 |
| Baker's chocolate (1 oz.) | 26 | 26 |
| Chocolate-flavored syrup (1 oz.) | 4 | 4 |

### Caffeine Content of Soft Drinks[2]

| *Brand* | *Milligrams Caffeine (12-oz. serving)* |
|---|---|
| Sugar-Free Mr. PIBB | 58.8 |
| Mountain Dew | 54.0 |
| Mello Yello | 52.8 |
| TAB | 46.8 |
| Coca-Cola | 45.6 |
| Diet Coke | 45.6 |
| Shasta Cola | 44.4 |
| Shasta Cherry Cola | 44.4 |
| Shasta Diet Cola | 44.4 |
| Mr. PIBB | 40.8 |
| Dr. Pepper | 39.6 |
| Sugar-Free Dr. Pepper | 39.6 |
| Big Red | 38.4 |
| Sugar-Free Big Red | 38.4 |
| Pepsi-Cola | 38.4 |
| Aspen | 36.0 |
| Diet Pepsi | 36.0 |
| Pepsi Light | 36.0 |
| RC Cola | 36.0 |
| Diet Rite | 36.0 |
| Kick | 31.2 |
| Canada Dry Jamaica Cola | 30.0 |
| Canada Dry Diet Cola | 1.2 |

### Caffeine Content of Drugs[3]

Caffeine is an ingredient in more than 1,000 nonprescription drug products as well as numerous prescription drugs. Most often it is used in weight-control remedies, alertness or stay-awake tablets, headache and pain relief remedies, cold products, and diuretics. When caffeine is an ingredient, it is listed on the product label. Some examples of caffeine-containing drugs are:

| *Prescription Drugs* | *Milligrams Caffeine* |
|---|---|
| Cafergot (for migraine headache) | 100 |
| Fiorinal (for tension headache) | 40 |
| Soma Compound (pain relief, muscle relaxant) | 32 |
| Darvon Compound (pain relief) | 32.4 |

| *Nonprescription Drugs* | *Milligrams Caffeine* |
|---|---|
| Weight-Control Aids | |
| Codexin | 200 |
| Dex-A-Diet II | 200 |
| Dexatrim, Dexatrim Extra Strength | 200 |
| Dietac capsules | 100 |
| Maximum Strength Appedrine | 140 |
| Prolamine | |
| Alertness Tablets | |
| Nodoz | 100 |
| Vivarin | 200 |
| Analgesic/Pain Relief | |
| Anacin, Maximum Strength Anacin | 32 |
| Excedrin | 65 |
| Midol | 32.4 |
| Vanquish | 33 |
| Diuretics | |
| Aqua-Ban | 100 |
| Maximum Strength Aqua-Ban Plus | 200 |
| Permathene H2 Off | 200 |
| Cold/Allergy Remedies | |
| Coryban-D capsules | 30 |
| Triaminicin tablets | 30 |
| Dristan Decongestant tablets and Dristan A-F Decongestant tablets | 16.2 |
| Duradyne-Forte | 30 |

[1]Source: FDA, Food Additive Chemistry Evaluation Branch, based on evaluations of existing literature on caffeine levels.
[2]Source: Institute of Food Technologists (IFT), April 1983, based on data from National Soft Drink Association, Washington, D.C. IFT also reports that there are at least 68 flavors and varieties of soft drinks produced by 12 leading bottlers that have no caffeine.
[3]Source: FDA's National Center for Drugs and Biologics.
Source: From *FDA Consumer* 18.2 (March 1984). U.S. Department of Health and Human Services.

## Myristicin

Most of us think of nutmeg and mace, if we think of them at all, as spices used to season baked beans or soufflés or as something to sprinkle on top of eggnog. For some, however, these common kitchen spices are the means to take a psychedelic "trip." Both spices contain the psychedelic drugs myristicin and elemicin. The amounts used in seasoning foods contain considerably less than the minimum effective dose of either drug, but one to two tablespoons of either spice will give an effective dose of myristicin.[31]

The first effects, experienced one to five hours after taking the drug, are dizziness and nausea, often with vomiting. These effects last about forty-five minutes and are followed by the "high" characterized by euphoria and alternating periods of tranquility and giddiness. In some cases, however, a "bad trip" occurs, with nervousness, fear, and panic taking the place of the usual "high." Other effects are floating sensations, rapid heartbeat, flushed skin, bloodshot eyes, dry mouth and throat, excessive thirst, constipation, and difficulty in urinating.[32] Difficulty in sleeping is commonly experienced during the next twenty-four hours following a myristicin "trip." Large quantities of these spices can be fatal.

Because of the unpleasantness of the side effects of myristicin, regular use of this drug is rare and chronic effects are therefore not generally a concern. In addition to myristicin and elemicin, nutmeg contains safrole, a weak carcinogen which could be a serious hazard for any frequent user of these substances.[33]

# ILLICIT DRUGS

The **illicit drugs** are those drugs which have been outlawed. It is generally illegal to produce, sell, possess, or use these drugs. This is the youngest and smallest group of drugs. On a nationwide level, there were no illicit drugs in America until 1914, when Congress in effect outlawed heroin (a form of opium used for smoking) and cocaine.[34] Since then, the number of illicit drugs has grown substantially.

## Heroin

**Heroin** is a semisynthetic drug produced from morphine. Its effects are the same as those of any other narcotic (such as opium, morphine, codeine, or methadone), but the dose necessary to produce these effects is smaller and the effects may be produced somewhat more rapidly.[35]

Heroin depresses brain activity producing a dreamy, mentally slow feeling and drowsiness. Experienced heroin users are more likely to experience it as a feeling of depression and unhappiness. A heroin user may, however, experience either reaction to this drug effect the first time or the hundredth time.[36]

Heroin slows the passage of food through the digestive tract, producing chronic constipation in regular users. It slows respiration, reduces urinary output, constricts the pupils of the eyes, and suppresses the cough reflex.[37] Heroin relaxes the muscular walls of the blood vessels in the skin, causing an increased flow of blood to the skin and a slight drop in blood pressure. The rush of blood to the skin may cause itching. It causes the skin to feel warm, but at the same time heat loss through the skin is increased. As a result, the user's body temperature will drop while the user may feel hot and perspire.

Like all narcotics, heroin suppresses aggression, hunger, and sex drives. Contrary to the myth of the sex-crazed dope fiend, heroin addicts are typically passive and uninterested in sex.[38] It is when heroin or a substitute narcotic cannot be obtained that the addict may become violent while trying to get the drug or the money to buy it.

Other than dependence itself, chronic use of pure heroin seems to have no ill effects.[39] However, heroin is rarely seen in its pure form by anyone but the chemist who makes it. The "heroin" that most users buy on the street contains less than 5 percent heroin. The remaining 95+ percent may be milk sugar, quinine, talc, or almost any other powder. Many chronic problems result from these impurities and from unsanitary injection practices. Impairment of lung and liver function is almost universal among heroin addicts for these reasons.[40]

Dependence is the most important of the chronic effects of heroin. Heroin produces both physical and psychological dependence. Despite the emphasis placed on physical dependence, the psychological dependence is probably much more important and certainly is far more persistent. (Compare the differences between physiological and psychological dependence on tobacco discussed in chapter 13.) Also commonly overlooked is the substantial number of heroin users who have used the drug for years without becoming addicted because they have not used it on a daily basis.[41]

Where an addiction to heroin has been established there is a distinct withdrawal syndrome. A heroin addict begins to crave another dose about four to six hours after the last dose.[42] About eight to twelve hours after the last dose the addict begins to experience nervousness, perspiration, watery eyes, runny nose, yawning, and a craving for sweets. Over the next thirty-six hours, additional symptoms of restlessness, irritability, loss of appetite, muscle aches and pains, tremors, dilated pupils, and "gooseflesh" develop. The withdrawal syndrome hits its peak forty-eight to seventy-two hours after the last dose. At this point, all of the preceding symptoms continue with the addition of nausea, abdominal cramps, vomiting, diarrhea, hot and cold flashes, rapid heartbeat and respiration, elevated blood pressure, sneezing and other cold symptoms, and spontaneous orgasms. Once this peak has passed, the symptoms gradually subside over the next week. Some symptoms may persist for as long as ten weeks.[43]

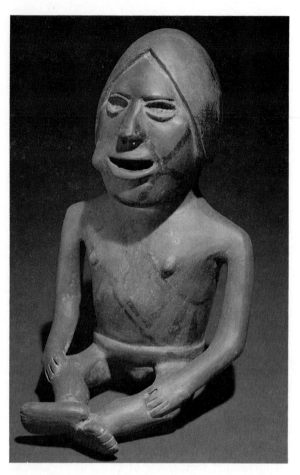

**Figure 14.4**
This ceramic of a coca chewer comes, like the coca plant that is the source of cocaine, from South America.

## Cocaine

**Cocaine** (also known as "coke") is a crystalline powder extracted from the leaves of the South American coca plant. Cocaine is both a powerful central nervous system stimulant and a local anesthetic. (See figure 14.4.) As an anesthetic its effects are essentially the same as those of novocaine or procaine. As a stimulant its effects are basically the same as the amphetamines or caffeine. In fact, mixtures of novocaine or procaine with caffeine or amphetamines have often been sold as cocaine in the illicit street market.

Physically, in addition to acting as a local anesthetic, cocaine increases heart and respiratory rates and blood pressure. It enhances alertness, relieves fatigue, and suppresses appetite. Psychologically, it produces euphoria, heightened self-confidence, and temporary relief from depression. Continued use of large doses leads to weight loss, insomnia, and anxiety. Paranoid delusions and full-blown psychosis may result from regular high-dosage usage.[44] A major problem experienced by users of cocaine relates to damage to the lining of the nose and nasal passages resulting from chronic snorting.

Psychological dependence on cocaine can be quite severe, especially where it has been used to cope with chronic depression. Such dependence was once relatively rare, probably because cocaine was too expensive for many people to use it regularly. As cocaine has gotten cheaper, dependence has become more common.

The increasing use of cocaine today is alarming to most authorities. Cocaine is perhaps our biggest illicit drug problem of the 1980s; its use appears to be spreading almost unchecked in all segments of society.[45] While the use of marijuana and LSD appears to be either checked at current levels or decreasing in popularity, the use of cocaine is increasing dramatically. From the most prominent members of society to the middle class, cocaine has become a drug of choice—yet there has been an enormous price paid for that popularity. Increasing numbers of people in our society are addicted to cocaine and many more are driven by a compulsion they don't understand to continue using the drug despite the health consequences. (See Exhibit 14.1.)

14.1 EXHIBIT 14.1

## A Fire in the Brain

Drug laws in the U.S. classify cocaine as a narcotic, along with opium, heroin and morphine. Yet the last three are "downers," which quiet the body and dull the senses, while coke is a stimulant, or "upper," similar to amphetamines. It increases the heartbeat, raises blood pressure and body temperature, and curbs appetite. Like a shot of adrenaline, coke puts the body into an emergency state.

Exactly how coke does that is something of a medical puzzle. But like other stimulants, even caffeine, it apparently intensifies the action of body chemicals called neurotransmitters. Firing off one nerve cell after another like a string of firecrackers, these chemicals help send tiny electric impulses coursing through the nervous system. (By contrast, narcotics tend to suppress these impulses.) As the signals multiply, they inundate the system's peripheral areas, which control such involuntary functions as the pulse and perspiration. They also flood at least three critical parts of the brain itself: the cerebral cortex, which governs higher mental activities like memory and reasoning; the hypothalamus (appetite, body temperature, and sleep, as well as such emotions as anger and fear); and the cerebellum (walking, balance, and other motor activities).

The consequences are inevitable. "Like an overburdened telephone switchboard," explains Dr. Walter Riker, Jr., chief of pharmacology at New York Hospital—Cornell Medical Center, "the brain cannot handle all the messages. There is too much information flowing in, and the user becomes hyper-aroused." With higher doses and chronic use, the alertness and exhilaration so prized by coke's connoisseurs quickly turn into darker effects, ranging from insomnia to fullfledged cocaine psychosis. Even a single overdose can cause severe headaches, nausea and convulsions—indeed, total respiratory and cardiovascular collapse. Says UCLA psychopharmacologist Ronald Siegel: "Extreme cocaine dosages light a kind of fire in the brain."

Ignition can occur in various ways. "Snorting," or sniffing the white powder, ensures absorption of the drug into the bloodstream through the mucous membranes. But it also constricts the myriad little blood vessels in these membranes, reduces the blood supply and dries up the nose. With repeated coke use, ulcers form, cartilage is exposed and the nasal septum can be perforated, requiring repairs by plastic surgery. (Savvy users rinse their noses with water after sniffing to wash away the irritants.)

To avoid the impurities of street coke and obtain a greater jolt, more users are resorting to freebasing. After dissolving a substantial quantity of coke in an alkaline (basic) solution, they boil the brew until a whitish lump, or freebase, is left. The lump can be purified further by washing it in a strong solvent. Then it is smoked, often in a water pipe. That way a highly concentrated dose is absorbed into the blood even faster via the lungs than through the nasal membranes.

A few users inject a solution of it directly into the bloodstream. "Shooting" is especially perilous. Not only can the high initial dose send the body into a frenzy, but just a little more than a gram of pure coke can be fatal. There is also a great risk

14.1 *continued* EXHIBIT 14.1

of deadly reactions from dirty syringes or contaminants in the coke. Dr. Charles Wetli, deputy chief medical examiner for Florida's drug-plagued Dade County, reports seeing cases where the needle was still in the dead victim's arm.

As lethal as shooting or freebasing may be, in proper hands cocaine can be medically useful. During the nineteenth century it was widely used as a local anesthetic because of its numbing properties. Since it constricts blood vessels and thus inhibits bleeding, it was particularly helpful during surgery on such sensitive, blood-rich parts of the body as the eye. It is still the anesthetic of choice for surgery on the nose, throat, larynx and trachea.

Unlike such downers as heroin or Quaaludes, cocaine is physically non-addictive, without strong withdrawal symptoms. Still, it can damage the liver, cause malnutrition and, especially among those with cardiac problems, increase the risk of heart attacks. Equally disturbing, says Siegel, "it is the most psychologically tenacious drug available." Coming down from a high may cause such deep gloom that the only remedy is more cocaine. Bigger doses often follow, and soon the urge may become a total obsession, with all its devastating consequences.

Source: Demarest, M. "Cocaine: Middle Class High," *Time* (6 July 1981). 

## DISCUSSION QUESTIONS

1. What do you think are some of the reasons why recreational use of cocaine is reaching epidemic proportions?

2. Differentiate between the psychological dependence common to cocaine users and the physical dependence that occurs with many other drugs.

## Marijuana

Long before the city of El Paso, Texas, passed the first law against it in 1914, **marijuana** had an extensive history as an herbal drug used for medicinal, religious, and recreational purposes.

The major psychological effects of marijuana at the most usual dosage levels are much the same as the effects of small doses of alcohol or the sedative-hypnotic prescription drugs.[46] These effects are relaxation, drowsiness, euphoria, lowering of inhibitions, and relief of mild anxiety. More severe anxiety, however, may be worsened by use of marijuana.[47] Unlike alcohol or the sedative-hypnotics, marijuana does not increase aggressiveness; in fact it inhibits aggressiveness.

One of the most common effects of marijuana is mirthfulness—a tendency to find things funny, often with uncontrolled laughter or giggling. Impairment of short-term memory and loss of train of thought are also common effects of marijuana. Perceptions of space and time may be distorted. Very much unlike alcohol or any other depressant, marijuana heightens sensitivity to external stimuli. Reaction time is slowed in first-time marijuana users but is speeded up in experienced users.[48] (See Exhibit 14.2.)

Other physical effects of marijuana are not very impressive. The primary effects are bloodshot eyes, dry throat, cough, and increased appetite and thirst. Heart rate is increased. Blood pressure seems to be lowered by marijuana use when the user is standing, but remains normal or increases when lying down.[49] This can result in dizziness or even faintness when a user goes from a lying to a standing position.

14.2 EXHIBIT 14.2

## Marijuana and Driving

The effects of marijuana on driver performance are important to us all. With sixteen million regular marijuana smokers and several million more occasional marijuana smokers in America, there are inevitably a good many drivers on the highways under the influence of marijuana. If their driving ability is seriously impaired, our safety is affected.

Early studies of this question compared the effects of marijuana on driver performance to the effects of alcohol on driver performance. Given such a comparison, marijuana was reported to present no hazard for driving. Marijuana clearly impairs driving ability to a much lesser degree than alcohol does. But, of course, we know that drinking drivers are a danger to us all; the real question was whether people drove significantly worse under the effects of marijuana than when not under the effects of any psychoactive drug.

The finding by Weil, Zinberg, and Nelsen (1968) that marijuana slowed reaction time in first-time users but speeded up reaction time in experienced users was also cited as evidence for lack of hazard. In fact, it was argued that by speeding up reaction time marijuana use might improve driving ability and safety, especially with regard to emergency braking.

Marijuana users, meanwhile, reported that they felt that marijuana impaired their ability to drive. Most frequently reported was a tendency to drive much too slowly. Marijuana users also reported that they had trouble deciding when it was safe to pass another car, pull away from a stop sign, or merge with traffic, and that they tended to be excessively cautious in doing so.

Klonoff (1974) tested the effects of high and low doses of marijuana and placebos (cigarettes looking, tasting, and smelling like marijuana but containing no THC) on driving performance on a closed course and in traffic. In the driving course the abilities to drive between cones, judge whether there was enough distance to drive between cones, and brake in an emergency were tested. Some drivers were unaffected, but the average performance without marijuana was better than the performances with either high or low doses of marijuana. In traffic the drivers were rated on the same test used to examine drivers for their driver's license. High doses of marijuana significantly impaired driving ability as measured by this test. Low doses did not.

It is true that marijuana is less hazardous to drivers than alcohol, but it is definitely a hazard. The situation is further complicated when drivers use both marijuana and alcohol.

Source: From *Drugs and the Whole Person,* by D. F. Duncan and R. S. Gold (New York: Macmillan, 1982). Reprinted by permission of the publisher.

### DISCUSSION QUESTIONS

1. Do you think that smoking marijuana and driving poses an important public-health problem?

2. What could be done to prevent the problems that arise from combining alcohol and marijuana consumption with driving?

**Table 14.3 Attitudes toward Marijuana**

**Trends in Attitudes Regarding Marijuana Laws (Entries are percentages)**

| *Q. There has been a great deal of public debate about whether marijuana use should be legal. Which of the following policies would you favor?* | Class of 1975 | Class of 1976 | Class of 1977 | Class of 1978 | Class of 1979 | Class of 1980 |
|---|---|---|---|---|---|---|
| Using marijuana should be entirely legal | 27.3 | 32.6 | 33.6 | 32.9 | 32.1 | 26.3 |
| It should be a minor violation like a parking ticket, but not a crime | 25.3 | 29.0 | 31.4 | 30.2 | 30.1 | 30.9 |
| It should be a crime | 30.5 | 25.4 | 21.7 | 22.2 | 24.0 | 26.4 |
| Don't know | 16.8 | 13.0 | 13.4 | 14.6 | 13.8 | 16.4 |
| N = | (2,617) | (3,264) | (3,622) | (3,721) | (3,278) | (3,211) |
| *Q. If it were legal for people to* USE *marijuana, should it also be legal to* SELL *marijuana?* | | | | | | |
| No | 27.8 | 23.0 | 22.5 | 21.8 | 22.9 | 25.0 |
| Yes, but only to adults | 37.1 | 49.8 | 52.1 | 53.6 | 53.2 | 51.8 |
| Yes, to anyone | 16.2 | 13.3 | 12.7 | 12.0 | 11.3 | 9.6 |
| Don't know | 18.9 | 13.9 | 12.7 | 12.6 | 12.6 | 13.6 |
| N = | (2,616) | (3,279) | (3,628) | (3,719) | (3,280) | (3,210) |
| *Q. If marijuana were legal to use and legally available, which of the following would you be most likely to do?* | | | | | | |
| Not use it, even if it were legal and available | 53.2 | 50.4 | 50.6 | 46.4 | 50.2 | 53.3 |
| Try it | 8.2 | 8.1 | 7.0 | 7.1 | 6.1 | 6.8 |
| Use it about as often as I do now | 22.7 | 24.7 | 26.8 | 30.9 | 29.1 | 27.3 |
| Use it more often than I do now | 6.0 | 7.1 | 7.4 | 6.3 | 6.0 | 4.2 |
| Use it less than I do now | 1.3 | 1.5 | 1.5 | 2.7 | 2.5 | 2.6 |
| Don't know | 8.5 | 8.1 | 6.6 | 6.7 | 6.1 | 5.9 |
| N = | (2,602) | (3,272) | (3,625) | (3,711) | (3,277) | (3,210) |

Source: Lloyd D. Johnston, Jerald G. Bachman, and Patrick O'Malley, *Highlights from Student Drug Use in America,* Department of Health and Human Services, Public Health Service, DHHS Publication No. (ADM) 81–1066 (Washington, D.C.: U.S. Government Printing Office, 1980).

Chronic effects of marijuana on the lungs and heart have been serious concerns in recent years. The best available evidence suggests that respiratory damage from smoking marijuana is roughly equal to that of smoking tobacco on a cigarette-for-cigarette basis.[50] The evidence regarding the cardiovascular system is less adequate but so far it does not indicate any damage due to marijuana use.[51] Reports of male breast enlargement and lowered testosterone levels have not been confirmed by subsequent studies.[52] CAT scans and psychological tests have failed to detect brain damage among marijuana users. Marijuana may increase susceptibility to respiratory infections and there is some evidence for a general impairment of immune response in marijuana users.[53]

Much attention was focused at one time on the idea that marijuana caused a loss of achievement motivation or of attachment to conventional goals. This was called amotivational syndrome.[54] Evidence accumulated since then seems to refute this theory fully.[55]

## LSD

**LSD,** a psychedelic drug, is a white, crystalline powder that dissolves readily in water. As a liquid or in large volumes it has a slightly bluish or purplish appearance. It is odorless and tasteless. The most potent drug known, the dosage of LSD must be measured in micrograms (millionths of a gram) rather than the milligram (thousandths of a gram) used to measure most drugs.[56] No other psychedelic has an effective dose less than 200 milligrams, but 20 micrograms of LSD will produce effects.

LSD was not the first psychedelic drug—psychedelics played a major role in the development of primitive religions early in human social evolution—but it has been the most important one for modern America.[57] Properly known as lysergic acid diethylamide, LSD was twenty-fifth in a series of lysergic-acid derivatives synthesized by Albert Hofmann in 1938; it came to be known by its laboratory abbreviation, LSD-25.[58] It was not until 1943 that Hofmann accidentally discovered the psychedelic effects of LSD-25.[59] Harvard psychologist Timothy Leary and San Francisco novelist Ken Kesey developed a large following in the 1960s by widely popularizing LSD.

The physical effects of LSD are not terribly impressive for such a notorious drug. It increases heart rate and produces a slight rise in blood pressure and temperature.[60] It increases the activity of the digestive tract and often produces feelings of nausea. Reflexes are speeded up and more easily triggered, muscular twitches or tremors commonly occur, and the pupils of the eyes become dilated. Moderate pain relief is afforded by LSD use. Perspiration, salivation, and tears are all increased.

The psychological effects are considerably more profound. LSD typically produces an exaggerated sense of well-being known as **euphoria.** Less commonly it may produce the exact opposite effect—an exaggerated sense of wrongness and uneasiness known as **dysphoria.** Although LSD usually reduces anxiety and tension, it may instead increase anxiety. LSD usually shortens attention span and results in a wandering mind. It appears in some cases, however, to increase the ability to concentrate.[61]

LSD increases introspection, lowers psychological defense mechanisms, and facilitates focusing on subjective experiences.[62] Aggressiveness is consistently reduced by LSD. Esthetic appreciation for art or music is usually enhanced by LSD. Users often believe that the drug has enhanced their creativity but objectively this does not seem to be so. Peak or mystical experiences in which the user feels a sense of oneness with nature or the universe are common experiences in LSD use.[63]

Contrary to popular belief, LSD only rarely produces **hallucinations**—perceptions for which there are no actual sensory stimuli.[64] What commonly do occur are illusions and closed-eye imagery. **Illusions** are distortions of actual stimuli—walls that seem to move, faces that grow distorted, lights that seem to prism into many colors or segment into splinters of light. **Closed-eye imagery** refers to seeing things with your eyes closed. LSD also may produce an effect known as synesthesia in which sensory messages seem to become crossed—sounds are seen, smells are heard, or colors are felt.[65]

LSD's potential for "bad trips" as well as "good trips" is obvious, given its potential for producing dysphoria as well as euphoria and for increasing as well as decreasing anxiety. Despite widespread media reports about LSD users having bad trips which result in "permanent insanity," there is no evidence that such things ever happened.[66] Borderline psychotics, however, may be pushed over the border into a full-blown psychosis by LSD use—whether a "bad trip" or a "good trip."[67] Flashbacks, in which some elements of an LSD experience occur again at a later time without further LSD use, occur to only a relatively small percentage of LSD users and usually last for less than a minute.[68]

## PCP

Once thought to have medicinal value as an anesthetic, **phencyclidine** (or **PCP**) proved to have side effects that made it unacceptable for medical use. Those side effects were delirium, dysphoria, and hallucinations. PCP did, however, come into widespread use as an animal tranquilizer, especially in fattening hogs for market.

In the 1970s PCP became a street drug when it began to be sold as **THC** (one of the major active ingredients in marijuana). Real THC was too expensive to produce and too difficult to store to be a successful street drug, so PCP became a common substitute. Eventually most street-drug users learned of the deception, but many had learned to like PCP and it continued to be sold as "angel dust," "dust," or "tea"—the latter coming from THC. Angel dust usually refers to a granular crystalline form of PCP that is usually sprinkled on marijuana or tobacco and then smoked. Tea usually refers to a fine powdered form of PCP that is usually snorted or sometimes injected.

PCP is a deliriant rather that a psychedelic drug. A typical dose (5 milligrams or less) causes a drunken state similar to that produced by alcohol or a sedative-hypnotic, along with a loss of sensitivity to light pain (such as a pinprick).[69] A dose of 5 to 10 milligrams causes delirium and hallucinations, loss of sensitivity to pain or temperature, and fever accompanied by shivering and possibly nausea and vomiting.[70] Larger doses can result in a sudden drop in blood pressure, coma, convulsions, or even death. Soon after taking PCP the user feels an intensification of experience, followed by vivid hallucinations and paranoia. In a later phase the user becomes extremely withdrawn and feels divorced from reality. The user can become so withdrawn as to experience a state of virtual nothingness.[71] Such a state of nothingness seems to be highly appealing to persons who find their ordinary reality extremely unpleasant.

Death due to PCP overdose is distinctly possible. PCP users may also suffer injury due to reduced sensitivity to pain and temperature, lack of coordination, and their own aggressive behavior.

## SOCIAL BARRIERS TO RESPONSIBLE DRUG USE

In the last few chapters we have shown that drugs of all kinds are a part of the fabric of our society; most people use drugs of some kind. Current research indicates that by the time someone reaches high-school age today, that person will have seen more than 17,000 hours of commercial-television programming. Much of that television programming is supported by commercials about psychoactive substances. We would like to turn now to some issues regarding the extent of the influence of drugs in our society today.

### Drugs and Sports

Both print and electronic media have recently reported that a very high percentage of professional athletes are drug users.[72] Athletes use psychoactive drugs recreationally. Reports also indicate extensive use of drugs as **ergogenic aids** (a substance that is felt to alter the performance capabilities of an athlete).[73] The Addiction Research Foundation of Toronto, Ontario, reports that there are no data available yet that accurately indicate the extent of psychoactive drug use among athletes. The Addiction Research Foundation has found the following information in published reports:

1. Forty percent of all major-league baseball players use amphetamines and barbiturates.
2. At least half of the National Football League players use amphetamines during their games.
3. Twenty-five percent of all Canadian Football League players use amphetamines during their games.
4. Seventeen percent of all players in an Italian soccer league were found to use amphetamines.
5. Sixty-eight percent of all coaches/trainers recommend vitamin supplements for their athletes.
6. One in ten women professional bodybuilders use **steroids** (hormones to increase body size and strength).
7. Ninety-nine percent of male professional bodybuilders use steroids.
8. Cocaine use in professional sports is estimated to be high, with 40 to 75 percent of the players in the National Basketball Association using it.
9. "Everyone" in cycling uses amphetamines or other ergogenic aids.
10. Over one-third of the U.S. track-and-field team used steroids in pre-1980 Olympic training.
11. All throwers or weight lifters have used steroids at some time.
12. Ten percent of both male and female high-school athletes use stimulants.[74]

These are levels of *reported* use, and do not come from empirically designed studies of such drug use. However, these reports are consistent with the kind of information we hear from coaches, players, and management.[75] (See figure 14.5.)

Reports of drug use (for performance improvement) by high-school and college athletes have also been a cause for concern for educators and health specialists. Particularly for young people who are not yet fully matured physically, use of drugs to enhance athletic abilities may result in long-term—even permanent—adverse effects.[76]

### Attitudes toward Drug Use

Lloyd Johnston and others have conducted longitudinal studies on drug use since 1975.[77] Their data indicate some changes over that period of time. Table 14.4 contains the results of a question regarding whether people feel that drug use should be prohibited by law. A review of the data in this table suggests that for almost all illicit drugs, respondents felt

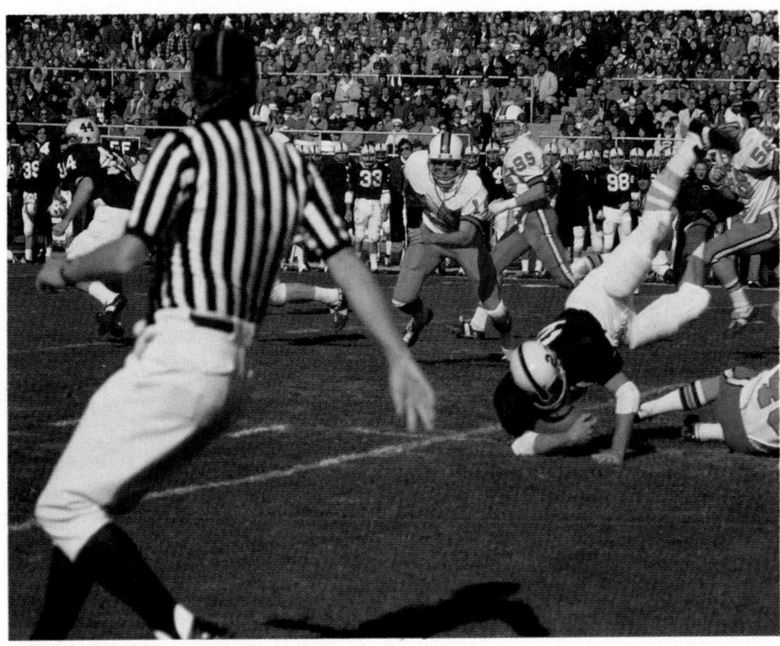

**Figure 14.5**
Drug use and misuse is common in both amateur and professional sports.

## Table 14.4 Attitudes toward Drug Use

### Trends in Attitudes Regarding Legality of Drug Use

| | Percent Saying "Yes"[a] | | | | | | |
|---|---|---|---|---|---|---|---|
| *Q. Do you think that people (who are eighteen or older) should be prohibited by law from doing each of the following?*[b] | Class of 1975 | Class of 1976 | Class of 1977 | Class of 1978 | Class of 1979 | Class of 1980 | 1979–1980 *change* |
| Smoke marijuana in private | 32.8 | 27.5 | 26.8 | 25.4 | 28.0 | 28.9 | *+0.9* |
| Smoke marijuana in public places | 63.1 | 59.1 | 58.7 | 59.5 | 61.8 | 66.1 | *+4.3 ss* |
| Take LSD in private | 67.2 | 65.1 | 63.3 | 62.7 | 62.4 | 65.8 | *+3.4 s* |
| Take LSD in public places | 85.8 | 81.9 | 79.3 | 80.7 | 81.5 | 82.8 | *+1.3* |
| Take heroin in private | 76.3 | 72.4 | 69.2 | 68.8 | 68.5 | 70.3 | *+1.8* |
| Take heroin in public places | 90.1 | 84.8 | 81.0 | 82.5 | 84.0 | 83.8 | *−0.2* |
| Take amphetamines or barbiturates in private | 57.2 | 53.5 | 52.8 | 52.2 | 53.4 | 54.1 | *+0.7* |
| Take amphetamines or barbiturates in public places | 79.6 | 76.1 | 73.7 | 75.8 | 77.3 | 76.1 | *−1.2* |
| Get drunk in private | 14.1 | 15.6 | 18.6 | 17.4 | 16.8 | 16.7 | *−0.1* |
| Get drunk in public places | 55.7 | 50.7 | 49.0 | 50.3 | 50.4 | 48.3 | *−2.1* |
| Smoke cigarettes in certain specified public places | NA | NA | 42.0 | 42.2 | 43.1 | 42.8 | *−0.3* |
| N = | (2,620) | (3,265) | (3,629) | (3,783) | (3,288) | (3,224) | |

Note: Level of significance of difference between the two most recents classes:
*s* = .05, *ss* = .01, *sss* = .001.
[a]Answer alternatives were: (1) No, (2) Not sure, and (3) Yes.
[b]The 1975 question asked about people who are *"twenty or older."*
Source: Lloyd D. Johnston, Jerald G. Bachman, and Patrick O'Malley, *Highlights from Student Drug Use in America.* Department of Health and Human Services, Public Health Service, DHHS Publication No. (ADM) 81-1066. (Washington, D.C.: U.S. Government Printing Office, 1980).

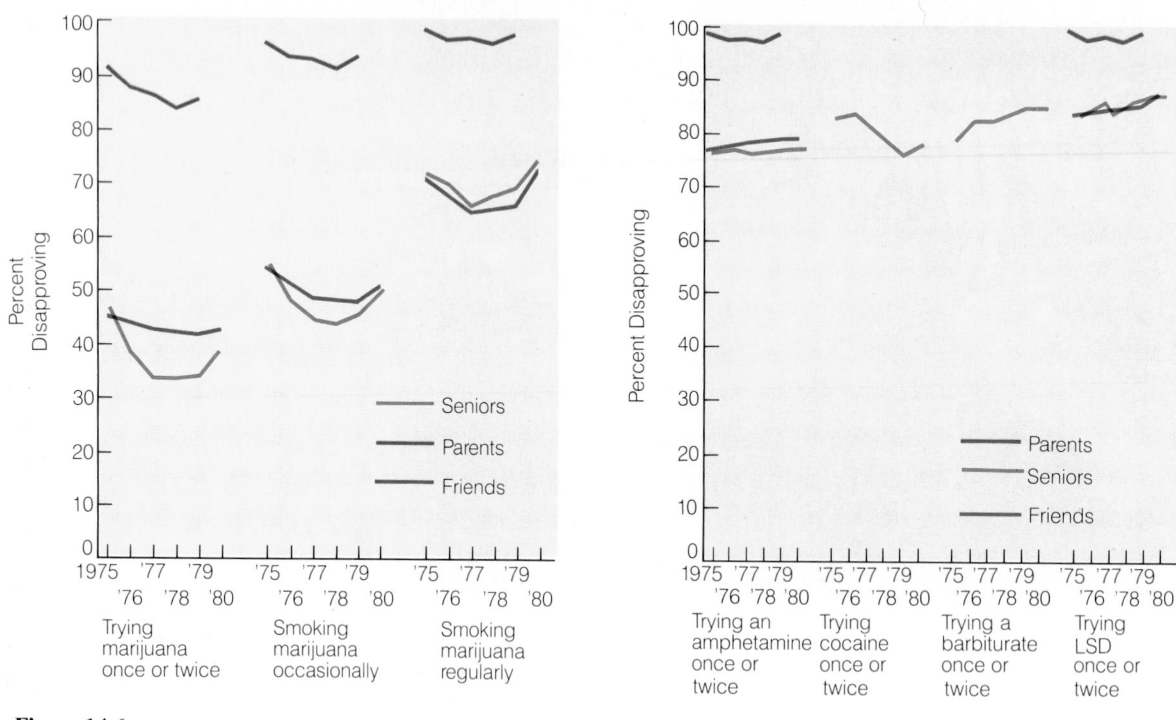


**Figure 14.6**
Trends in disapproval of drug use. *Source:* Johnston, Lloyd D., Jerald G. Bachman, and Patrick Y. O'Malley, *Highlights from Student Drug Use in America.* Department of Health and Human Services, Public Health Service, DHHS Publication No. (ADM) 81–1066. (Washington, D.C.: U.S. Government Printing Office, 1980).

such use should be prohibited. This was not the case, however, for the responses regarding drunkenness and cigarette smoking.

Figure 14.6 contains a graphic representation of trends in disapproval of illicit drug use. For all drugs asked about, there was an increase between 1979 and 1980 in the percentage of respondents disapproving of their use.

## WHERE DO WE GO FROM HERE?

All these data seem to produce some conflicting signals for young adults today. Everywhere we read about increases in the use of recreational and ergogenic aids by athletes. These athletes are often seen as important role models in our society. Many reports are also found regarding the use of psychoactive substances by other role models such as actors and actresses. Yet at the same time, data seems to indicate increasing disapproval regarding the use of drug substances. These conflicts make responsible decisions a difficult task for some. Lack of knowledge and disagreements regarding the facts about drug use also complicate the issue. We have included here a drug knowledge survey to use as a self-assessment device for your own levels of knowledge. (See Activity for Wellness 14.1.)

In general, the increasing use of recreational drugs during adolescence and young adulthood results in growing numbers of problems, particularly when these drugs are used as an escape valve from stress or the pressures of life. These drugs produce some negative physical and psychological effects; they also have a dependence-producing potential. But a drug user's inability to learn how to cope with reality is an even more substantial problem resulting from such escapism. There are times when the moderate use of socially approved recreational drugs is appropriate, just as there are times when self-administered OTC drugs or supervised use of prescription drugs can be appropriate. But unsupervised, unrestricted, and unrestrained use of any drug diminishes our potential for achieving wellness.

14.1 ACTIVITY FOR WELLNESS 14.1

# Are You a Drug Quiz Whiz?

Directions: Mark your choices, then check the answers on the following pages.

1. The most commonly abused drug in the United States is
   _____ marijuana
   _____ alcohol
   _____ cocaine
   _____ heroin
2. People who are dependent upon heroin keep taking it mostly to
   _____ experience pleasure
   _____ avoid withdrawal
   _____ escape reality
   _____ be accepted among friends
3. Which of these is *not* a narcotic?
   _____ heroin
   _____ marijuana
   _____ morphine
   _____ methadone
4. Which age group has the highest percentage of drug abusers?
   _____ 10–17
   _____ 18–25
   _____ 26–35
   _____ 36–60
   _____ 61 and over
5. Which drug does not cause physical dependence?
   _____ alcohol
   _____ morphine
   _____ peyote
   _____ secobarbital
   _____ codeine
6. Most drug users make their first contact with illicit drugs
   _____ through "pushers"
   _____ through their friends
   _____ accidentally
   _____ through the media
7. What is the most unpredictable drug on the street today?
   _____ PCP
   _____ heroin
   _____ LSD
   _____ alcohol
8. Which of the following is not a stimulant?
   _____ amphetamine
   _____ caffeine
   _____ methaqualone
   _____ methamphetamine
9. The majority of inhalant abusers are
   _____ men
   _____ children
   _____ women
   _____ the elderly
10. Which of the following poses the greatest health hazard to the most people in the United States?
    _____ cigarettes
    _____ heroin
    _____ codeine
    _____ LSD
    _____ caffeine
11. Which of the following poses the highest *immediate* risk to users?
    _____ marijuana
    _____ nicotine
    _____ LSD
    _____ inhalants
12. This drug was believed to be nonaddictive when it was developed in the 1800s as a substitute for morphine and codeine.
    _____ LSD
    _____ heroin
    _____ horseradish
    _____ PCP

14.1 *continued*

## ACTIVITY FOR WELLNESS

13. When does a person become hooked on heroin?
    _____ first time
    _____ after four or five times
    _____ 20 times or more
    _____ different for each person
14. What sobers up a drunk person?
    _____ a cold shower
    _____ black coffee
    _____ a traffic ticket
    _____ time
    _____ walking
15. Which of the following should *never* be mixed with alcohol?
    _____ amphetamines
    _____ sedatives
    _____ cocaine
    _____ cigarettes
16. Medical help for drug problems is available without legal penalties:
    _____ if the patient is under 21
    _____ under the protection of federal law
    _____ in certain states
17. Stopping drug abuse before it starts is called
    _____ prevention
    _____ withdrawal
    _____ tolerance
    _____ education
18. How long does marijuana stay in the body after smoking?
    _____ one day
    _____ 12 hours
    _____ up to a month
    _____ one hour
19. The use of drugs during pregnancy
    _____ should be limited to tobacco and alcohol
    _____ may be harmful to the unborn child
    _____ should cease at 26 weeks
20. What makes marijuana especially harmful today?
    _____ younger kids are using it
    _____ it is much stronger
    _____ it could affect physical and mental development
    _____ none of these
    _____ all of these

*Answers to Drug Quiz*

1. *Alcohol.* It is estimated that about 10 million people in the United States are dependent on alcohol. About two-thirds of all adults are occasional drinkers of either wine, beer, or some other alcoholic beverage. About half of all junior high-school students have tried some type of alcoholic drinks.

2. *Avoid withdrawal.* When heroin addicts are deprived suddenly of the drug, they develop physical withdrawal symptoms. These symptoms may include shaking, sweating, nausea, runny nose and eyes, muscle spasms, headaches and stomachaches. Sudden withdrawal from certain drugs can be dangerous. For instance, a person who has been using barbiturate sedatives for a long time should not attempt withdrawal without a physician's assistance.

3. *Marijuana.* Marijuana was legally declared a narcotic in the past but it is not now. The way the drug works on a person's mental and physical system differs from the effects of narcotics.

4. *18–25.* The findings from the 1979 National Survey on Drug Abuse showed that of the three major age groups surveyed (12–17, 18–25, and 26 and over) illicit drug abuse was more prevalent among young adults, ages 18–25.

5. *Peyote.* The active ingredient of the peyote cactus is mescaline, a hallucinogen. Physical dependence on this class of drugs has not been verified.

## ACTIVITY FOR WELLNESS 14.1

6. *Through their friends.* The pressure from friends to experiment with drugs can influence many people to try drugs, especially young people. Being accepted by friends is strong pressure. But showing friends that you care when they feel bad about themselves and their lives, and helping them solve problems can prevent them from becoming involved with drugs.

7. *Phencyclidine (PCP).* This illicit drug can produce unpredictable, erratic, and violent behavior in users. These actions can be directed at themselves or at others, and, in some cases, have led to serious injuries and death. Drownings, burns, falls from high places, and automobile accidents have also been reported. Since the drug is usually manufactured illegally, users cannot be certain of its purity.

8. *Methaqualone.* This is a nonbarbiturate sleep-inducing drug called a "lude" or "sopor" on the street. Abuse can lead to convulsions or coma.

9. *Children.* Inhalant abuse is rising among children between the ages of 12 and 17. These substances are readily available in household products, often found in aerosol sprays. Inexpensive and available aerosol products can cause irregular heartbeats, breathing problems, and sudden death.

10. *Cigarettes.* There are over 50 million cigarette smokers in the United States. It is estimated that 300,000 deaths each year are related to tobacco use. Some of the long-term effects of smoking are emphysema, chronic bronchitis, heart disease, and cancer of the lungs, mouth, larynx, and esophagus. Women who smoke during pregnancy run the risk of having babies that weigh less, or of losing their babies through stillbirth or death after birth. Therefore, the health risks associated with tobacco are extremely high.

11. *Inhalants.* These compounds are found among common household products. Sniffing these substances can result in immediate death. Irregular heartbeat and interference with breathing can cause suffocation. This can happen the first time or any time a person uses these substances.

12. *Heroin.* In 1898 when heroin was placed on the market, it was not believed to be habit forming. However, in a few more years, researchers found heroin more addictive than morphine or any other narcotic drug. This knowledge made it necessary for the government to begin passing laws to restrict the sale and use of heroin.

13. *Different for each person.* The time it takes for a person to become dependent on heroin varies. But repeated use will eventually cause physical dependence. Some people become hooked on heroin after using it a few times. Developing an addiction to any drug varies with the form and potency of the drug, the dosage, the frequency, the pattern of use, and the personality of the user.

14. *Time.* There are no shortcuts to sober a drunk person. Once alcohol is in the bloodstream, it takes time for the body to rid itself of the alcohol. This process, called metabolism, takes about 2 hours for each drink taken.

15. *Sedatives.* (Also known as tranquilizers and sleeping pills.) Most people do not realize that alcohol is a sedative drug. Combining sedatives with alcohol increases their effects. Judgment is impaired and lapses in memory can occur. In this confused state, users can unintentionally take larger or repeated amounts of these substances. This can result in comas and death. More Americans die from overdoses of barbiturates (another sedative) than from heroin addiction.

14.1 *continued* — ACTIVITY FOR WELLNESS — 14.1

16. *Under the protection of federal law.* Under federal law persons can seek help for drug problems. Federal law in most instances requires doctors, psychologists, and drug treatment centers to keep confidential any information received from drug patients, if the drug treatment program is federally assisted. However, it may be necessary for information to be given to other doctors to help in treating patients, or to insurance companies to help to provide benefits for patients. This can only be done with the patient's consent.

17. *Prevention.* Children are confronted with drugs and the pressure to use drugs. This occurs wherever they live. Young people are faced with alcohol and tobacco at a very young age. They should be taught how to say "no" when drugs are offered. The purpose of prevention is to provide young people healthy and attractive alternatives to drug abuse. This involves the whole community and includes helping young people to develop meaningful relationships with parents, teachers, and peers.

18. *Up to a month.* The major active ingredient in marijuana is tetrahydrocannabinol (THC). Scientists have discovered that THC accumulates in the fatty tissues of the cells and is eliminated slowly. It takes approximately 4 weeks for the body to rid itself of THC.

Source: National Institute on Drug Abuse, 1981.

19. *May be harmful to the unborn child.* Pregnant women should be extremely careful about taking any drug, even aspirin, without consulting a physician. Research has shown that heavy smoking and drinking can harm the fetus. Babies born of narcotic- and barbiturate-dependent mothers are often born drug dependent and must receive special care.

20. *All of these.* Recent studies of teenage marijuana use show that 59 percent of high school seniors have tried it. Eight percent of the 12- to 13-year-olds report that they have smoked marijuana at least once, and half of this group were current users. Of the 14- to 15-year-olds, 32 percent have tried it, and 17 percent still use it. Many children in the 12- to 17-age group report that they first tried marijuana while they were in grade school.

In 1975 marijuana street samples rarely exceeded 1 percent THC (tetrahydrocannabinol) content; in 1980 marijuana samples containing 5 percent were common. The amount of THC determines its psychoactive potential. The more potent marijuana increases the physical and mental effects, and the possibility of health problems to the user.

Research shows that marijuana effects can interfere with learning by impairing thinking, reading comprehension, and verbal and arithmetic skills. Young people need to learn how to make decisions, to handle success, and to cope with failures. Drug abuse can prevent them from growing up to become mature, responsible people.

## SUMMARY

1. This chapter reviewed the herbal, OTC, prescription, unrecognized, and illicit drugs. Each have the potential to be misused or abused.

2. A brief overview of each of the categories of drugs was provided.

3. Almost all of the categories of drugs contain substances which are psychoactive, and have either stimulatory, depressant, or mind-altering properties.

4. Perhaps the most widely used drug in our society is caffeine, an unrecognized drug.

5. Among the illicit drugs, cocaine is perhaps the most prominent today in terms of its levels of use and its abuse potential.

6. The use of drugs in sports has become an increasing problem, particularly in professional sports leagues.

7. Perhaps more than the importance of looking at the effects of any single drug, it is essential that we recognize the role of drugs in our society. Although drugs are readily available, and easy to get for most people, they can have lifesaving or life-threatening effects. We must learn to make reasonable decisions regarding their use.

### Recommended Readings

Blum, Richard H., & Associates, *Society and Drugs: Social and Cultural Observations* (San Francisco: Jossey-Boss, 1970).

Brecher, Edward M., and the Editors of *Consumer Reports, Licit and Illicit Drugs* (Boston: Little, Brown, 1972).

### References

1. R. S. Gold, D. F. Duncan, and M. S. Sutherland, (1975) "College Student Interests Go Further than Illicit Drugs," *Journal of Drug Education* 10, 79–88.

2. Varro E. Taylor, *The Honest Herbal: A Sensible Guide to the Use of Herbs and Related Remedies* (Philadelphia: George F. Stickley Co., 1981), 224.

3. William A. R. Thomson, *Herbs That Heal* (New York: Charles C. Scribner's Sons, 1976), 80.

4. Ray S. Oakley, *Drugs, Society and Human Behavior* (St. Louis: C. V. Mosby, 1974), 373.

5. Thomson, *Herbs That Heal,* 77.

6. Thomson, *Herbs That Heal,* 77.

7. Johnson Lightfoote, Joseph Blaire, and James R. Cohen. "Lead Intoxication in an Adult Caused by Chinese Herbal Medicine," *Journal of the American Medical Association,* 238, 14 (1977): 1,539.

8. David R. Zimmerman, *The Essential Guide to Nonprescription Drugs* (New York: Harper & Row, 1983), xvii.

9. Zimmerman, *The Essential Guide to Nonprescription Drugs,* xvii.

10. Zimmerman, *The Essential Guide to Nonprescription Drugs,* xviii.

11. Zimmerman, *The Essential Guide to Nonprescription Drugs,* xix.

12. American Society of Hospital Pharmacists, *Consumer Drugs Digest* (New York: Facts on File, Inc., 1982), 415.

13. Am. Soc. Of Hosp. Pharm., *Consumer Drugs Digest,* 414.

14. Am. Soc. Hosp. Pharm., *Consumer Drugs Digest,* 241.

15. Zimmerman, *The Essential Guide to Nonprescription Drugs,* 664.

16. Zimmerman, *The Essential Guide to Nonprescription Drugs,* 728.

17. H. I. Abelson and R. B. Atkinson, "Public Experience with Psychoactive Substances: A Nationwide Study among Adults and Youth: Part I, Main Findings," ERIC document, 1975.

18. Zimmerman, *The Essential Guide to Nonprescription Drugs,* 662.

19. Helen I. Green and Michael H. Levy, *Drug Misuse . . . Human Abuse* (New York: Marcel Dekker, Inc., 1976), 278.

20. Green and Levy, *Drug Misuse,* 388.

21. Green and Levy, *Drug Misuse,* 383.

22. Oakley, *Drugs, Society and Human Behavior,* 114.

23. Oakley, *Drugs, Society and Human Behavior,* 116.

24. Oakley, *Drugs, Society and Human Behavior,* 116.

25. Oakley, *Drugs, Society and Human Behavior,* 116.

26. Oakley, *Drugs, Society and Human Behavior,* 115.

27. Oakley, *Drugs, Society and Human Behavior,* 116.

28. Zimmerman, *The Essential Guide to Nonprescription Drugs,* 729.

29. Zimmerman, *The Essential Guide to Nonprescription Drugs,* 729.

30. Zimmerman, *The Essential Guide to Nonprescription Drugs,* 729.

31. Thomson, *Herbs That Heal,* 123–124.

32. Thomson, *Herbs That Heal,* 124.

33. Taylor, *The Honest Herbal,* 202.

34. Oakley, *Drugs, Society and Human Behavior,* 1974, 19.

35. Oakley, *Drugs, Society and Human Behavior,* 198.

36. Oakley, *Drugs, Society and Human Behavior,* 199.

37. Oakley, *Drugs, Society and Human Behavior,* 199.

38. Oakley, *Drugs, Society and Human Behavior,* 204.

39. Oakley, *Drugs, Society and Human Behavior,* 204.

40. Oakley, *Drugs, Society and Human Behavior,* 204.

41. Norman E. Zinberg, "Nonaddictive opiate use," in *Handbook on Drug Abuse*, eds. Robert L. Dupont, Avram Goldstein, and John O'Donnell (Washington, D.C.: U.S. Government Printing Office, 1979).

42. Oakley, *Drugs, Society and Human Behavior,* 204.

43. Oakley, *Drugs, Society and Human Behavior,* 204.

44. Oakley, *Drugs, Society and Human Behavior,* 161.

45. Richard G. Schlaadt and Peter T. Shannon, *Drugs of Choice: Current Perspectives on Drug Use* (Englewood Cliffs, N.J.: Prentice-Hall, 1982), 74.

46. Oakley, *Drugs, Society and Human Behavior,* 264.

47. Oakley, *Drugs, Society and Human Behavior,* 408.

48. Charles T. Tart, "Marijuana intoxication: Common experiences," *Nature,* 226 (1970): 704.

49. Oakley, *Drugs, Society and Human Behavior,* 261.

50. Institute of Medicine, *Marijuana and Health.* (Washington, D.C.: National Academy Press, 1982), 59.

51. Institute of Medicine, *Marijuana and Health,* 59.

52. Institute of Medicine, *Marijuana and Health,* 94.

53. Institute of Medicine, *Marijuana and Health,* 59.

54. Institute of Medicine, *Marijuana and Health,* 124.

55. Institute of Medicine, *Marijuana and Health,* 125.

56. Green and Levy, *Drug Misuse,* 226.

57. Oakley, *Drugs, Society and Human Behavior,* 213.

58. Green and Levy, *Drug Misuse,* 226.

59. Oakley, *Drugs, Society and Human Behavior,* 233.

60. Oakley Ray, *Drugs, Society and Human Behavior,* 1974, 357.

61. Duncan and Gold, *Drugs and the Whole Person,* 148.

62. Duncan and Gold, *Drugs and the Whole Person,* 148.

63. Oakley, *Drugs, Society and Human Behavior,* 365.

64. Duncan and Gold, *Drugs and the Whole Person,* 149.

65. Duncan and Gold, *Drugs and the Whole Person,* 149.

66. Duncan and Gold, *Drugs and the Whole Person,* 150.

67. Oakley, *Drugs, Society and Human Behavior,* 363.

68. Duncan and Gold, *Drugs and the Whole Person,* 151.

69. Sachindra N. Pradhan and Samarendra N. Dutta, *Drug Abuse: Clinical and Basic Aspects* (St. Louis: C. V. Mosby, 1977), 194.

70. Pradhan, *Drug Abuse,* 194.

71. Pradhan, *Drug Abuse,* 194.

72. Thomas Burks, "Drug Use By Athletes," in *Drug Abuse in the Modern World: Perspective for the Eighties,* eds. Gabriel G. Nahas and Henry Clay Frick II (New York: Pergamon Press, 1981), 112.

73. Burks, Drug Use By Athletes, 112.

74. Addiction Research Foundation, *Information Review: Drugs and Sports* (Toronto: Alcoholism and Drug Addiction Research Foundation of Ontario, 1981), 25.

75. Addiction Research Foundation, 1.

76. Addiction Research Foundation, 2.

77. Lloyd D. Johnston, Jerald G. Bachman, and Patrick O'Malley, *Highlights from Student Drug Use in America.* Department of Health and Human Services, Public Health Service, DHHS Publication No. (ADM) 81–1066. (Washington, D.C.: U.S. Government Printing Office, 1980).

CHAPTER FIFTEEN

# Noncommunicable Diseases: Threats to Wellness



Cardiovascular disease, cancer, diabetes, emphysema, and other noncommunicable diseases present significant threats to wellness. Your greatest probability of achieving wellness occurs by moderating the risk factors that contribute to the disease process, and by selecting a prudent life-style from among an array of alternatives. Individual involvement and self-responsibility are vital to pursuing the goal of high-level wellness.

This chapter addresses the important noncommunicable diseases that may be roadblocks to high-level wellness. We discuss the cause, development, treatment and prevention of, and adaptation to the leading noncommunicable diseases. We also suggest how one can minimize personal risk in order to maximize the opportunities for full and fruitful living. We begin by seeing how life-style choices affect the development of cardiovascular disease, the number-one killer of Americans.

# CARDIOVASCULAR DISEASE AND YOUR HEART

Cardiovascular disease is responsible for more than 50 percent of all deaths in the U.S.; many of these deaths are premature. It is responsible for almost three times as many deaths each year as cancer, the second leading killer. (See figure 15.1.) The economic costs are staggering, amounting to more than $50 billion a year in lost wages, lost productivity, and medical expenses. (See figure 15.2.) Beyond these costs are the intangible costs of losing a family member or friend who is in the prime of life. The most common forms of cardiovascular disease include:

- hardening of the arteries (arteriosclerosis)
- heart attack (myocardial infarction)
- chest pain (angina pectoris)
- irregular heartbeat (arrhythmia)
- congestive heart failure
- high blood pressure (hypertension)
- congenital heart defects
- rheumatic heart disease
- stroke (cerebrovascular accident)

Before we explore these disorders, a brief examination of normal heart function is in order.

## Normal Heart Function

The heart is a four-chambered muscular organ a little larger than one's fist, which continually pumps blood through the circulatory system. A heart contracts about 100,000 times per day, and moves in excess of 4,300 gallons of blood, thus performing an enormous quantity of work.

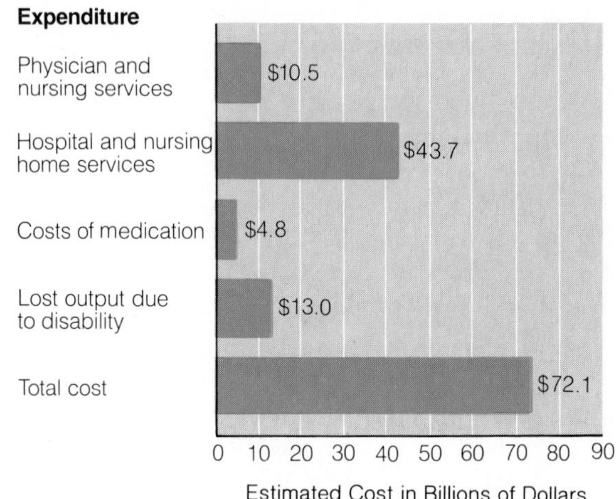


The costs illustrated in this chart are for physician and nursing services, hospital and nursing home facilities and medications, as well as the lost occupational output as a result of disability.

**Figure 15.2**
Estimated economic costs in billions of dollars of cardiovascular diseases by type of expenditure. *Source:* Reproduced with permission from *Heart Facts 1985.* © American Heart Association.

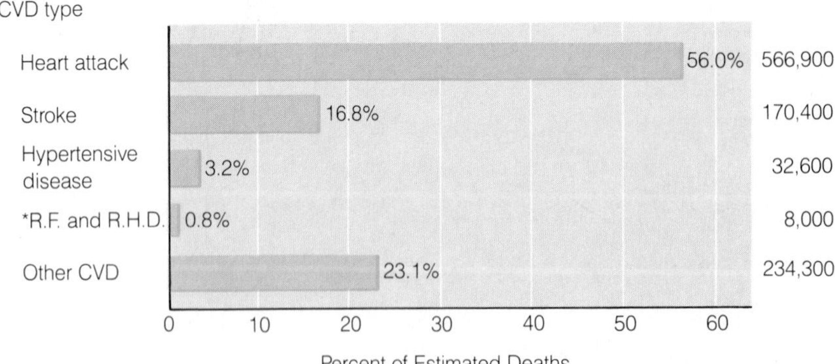


*Rheumatic fever and rheumatic heart disease

**Figure 15.1**
Estimated deaths due to cardiovascular diseases by major type of disorder. (United States: 1985 Estimate) *Source:* National Center for Health Statistics, U.S. Public Health Service, DHHS.

In human beings and other mammals, the heart is divided into a left and a right side. Each side contains an **atrium,** a chamber in which blood collects, and a **ventricle,** a chamber that contracts to force (i.e., pump) blood out of the heart. The right atrium receives **deoxygenated blood** concentrated with carbon dioxide from the body. This blood moves from the right atrium into the right ventricle, where it is pumped to the lungs to exchange its carbon dioxide for oxygen. Oxygen-rich blood moves from the lungs to the heart's left atrium, and subsequently moves into the left ventricle. The left ventricle is the largest and most muscular of the heart's chambers so its contractive force can be sufficient to pump blood throughout the body. (See figure 15.3.)

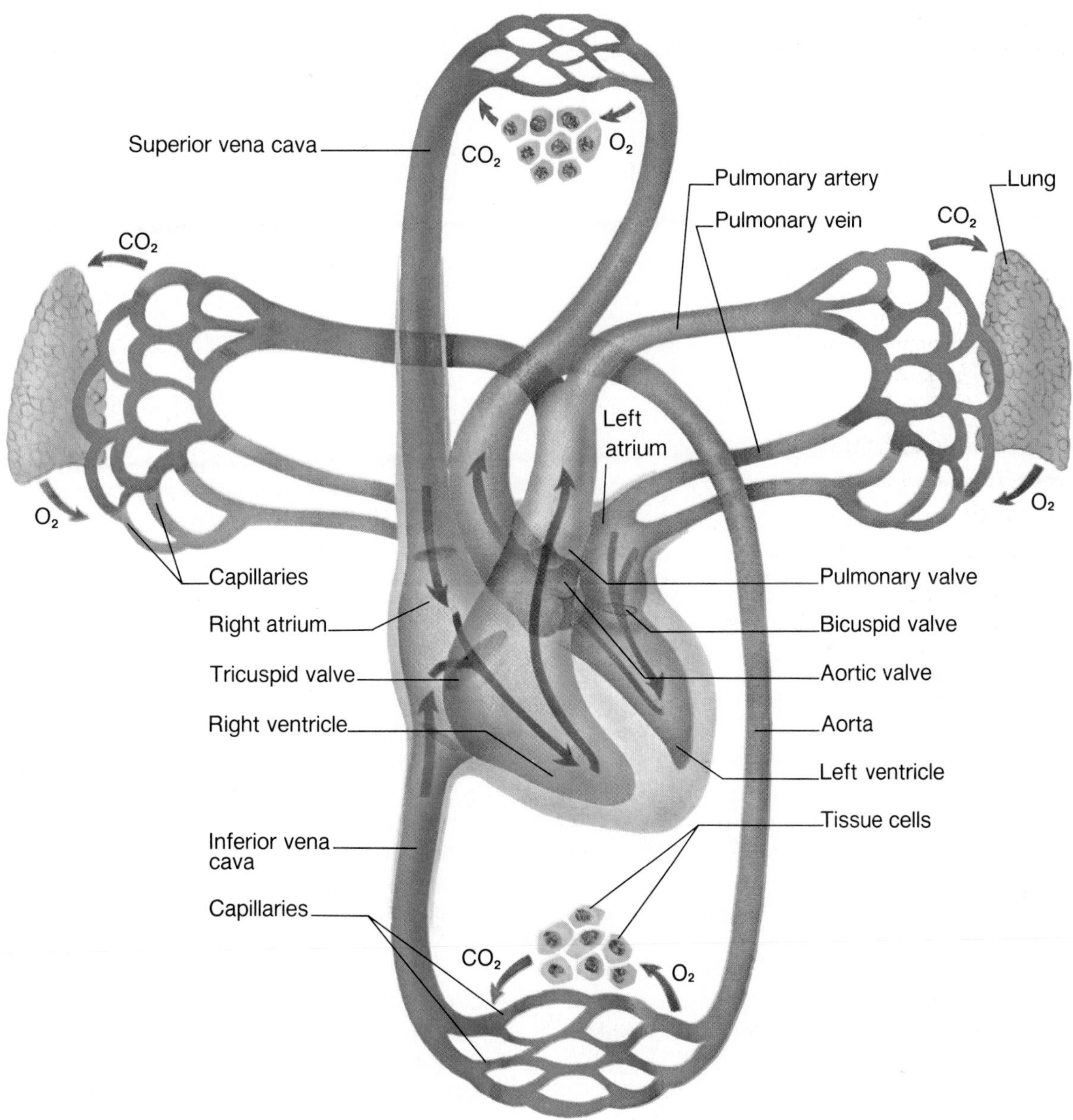


**Figure 15.3**
Your heart and how it works. *Source:* From Hole, John W., Jr., *Human Anatomy and Physiology,* 3d ed. © 1978, 1981, 1984 Wm. C. Brown Publishers, Dubuque, Iowa. All rights reserved. Reprinted by permission.

The circulation of blood begins in the heart and lungs, moving oxygen and nutrients through **arteries, arterioles,** and **capillaries** to provide nourishment for the cells of the body, then through *venules* and *veins* back to the heart to repeat the process. The heart, then, is a pump that "squeezes" blood through the body. The most vital part of the heart is the muscle itself, called the **myocardium.** Like all of the body's muscles, the myocardium must use oxygen and nutrients to do its work. The myocardium, however, is unable to use the blood in the chambers directly. Instead, oxygen and other nutrients are supplied by coronary arteries. These arteries originate at the base of the aorta, the largest artery of the body, through which blood is pumped as it leaves the left ventricle of the heart.

The pumping action or "beat" of the heart is regulated by a natural pacemaker consisting of specialized cells that generate electrical impulses. These minute electrical impulses coordinate ventricular contractions.

After each contraction of the left ventricle, blood flows into the heart because of the change in pressure. Valves between the atria and the ventricles open to permit blood flow. When the ventricle receives the electrical impulse to contract, the valves between both atria and ventricles are closed by the pressure, and the blood is forced out of the heart to the lungs from the right ventricle, and to the rest of the body from the left ventricle.

## Common Cardiovascular Diseases

The cardiovascular system then, consists of the heart, lungs, and a network of blood vessels that carry blood to the various parts of the body. Cardiovascular disease occurs when any of a number of events take place. Some of the things that can go wrong include a partial or complete block in the coronary arteries or elsewhere in the body, a loss in the contractive force of the heart muscle, a malfunction of the valves, or an alteration of the heart's electrical activity. Some cardiovascular diseases are more prevalent than others.

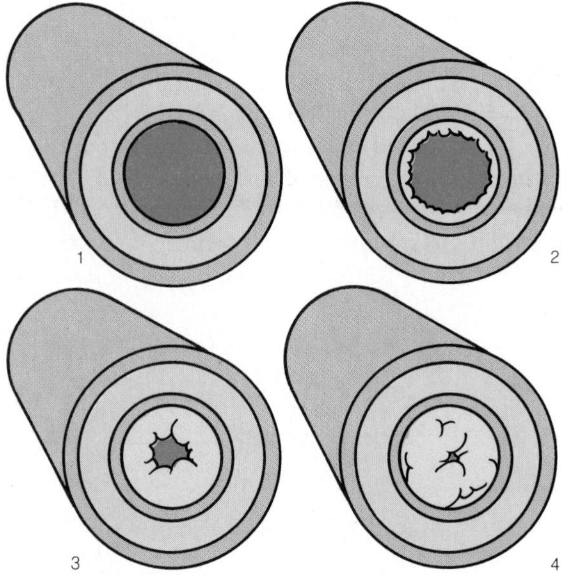


**Figure 15.4**
Progressive artherosclerotic buildup on artery walls.

**ARTERIOSCLEROSIS** **Arteriosclerosis,** commonly called "hardening of the arteries," includes several conditions that cause the walls of the arteries to thicken and lose their elasticity. The most frequently occurring form of arteriosclerosis is **atherosclerosis.** (See figure 15.4.)

Atherosclerosis is a lifelong process in which arterial walls become thickened by deposits of fat, minerals, and other cellular debris. As atherosclerosis progresses, arteries become less elastic, thereby prohibiting blood from moving smoothly, and making blood more susceptible to forming clots. When a clot blocks a coronary artery, the result is called a **coronary thrombosis,** one example of a heart attack. Similarly, a clot in an artery of the brain produces a **cerebral thrombosis,** a form of stroke.

**HIGH BLOOD PRESSURE** By definition, blood pressure is the force exerted against the walls of the arteries as the heart contracts and relaxes. The force is measured in millimeters of mercury (mm Hg), and a "typical" blood pressure is 120/80 (read 120 over 80). The "120" refers to the force exerted by the blood just as the heart contracts, and is called the **systolic** pressure. The "80" refers to the force exerted when the heart muscle is relaxed, and is called the **diastolic** pressure.

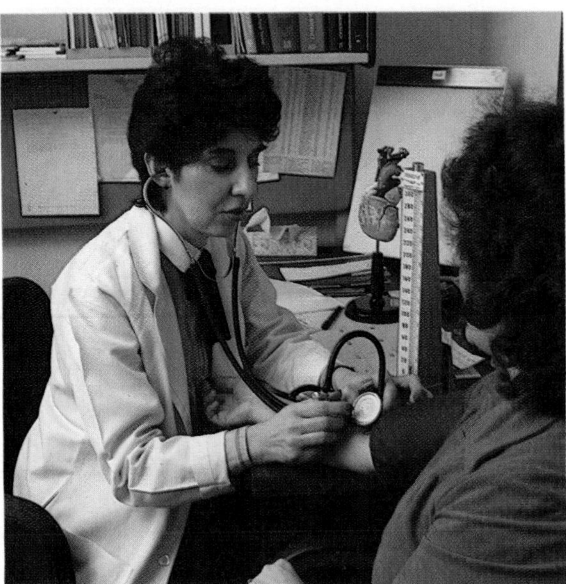

**Figure 15.5**
Several blood pressure readings are necessary before hypertension can be diagnosed.

When arteries are constricted, as in atherosclerosis, blood does not flow easily through them. As a result, the heart must pump harder to exert the same force to move the blood. This process increases blood pressure above normal levels. If this pressure elevation is maintained, the result is **hypertension,** or high blood pressure.

Hypertension and atherosclerosis are closely linked. As arteries narrow due to plaques, blood pressure increases. As blood pressure increases, arterial walls become increasingly damaged, leading to the development of still more plaques. Once underway, the process is difficult to modify.

How "high" is high blood pressure? Medical practitioners disagree about the answer. A person whose systolic pressure is consistently above 160 mm Hg or whose diastolic pressure is consistently above 95 mm Hg may have hypertension. The American College of Cardiology is more conservative in specifying its upper limit of "normal," suggesting that readings above 140/90 signal a problem.

One can never rely on a single blood pressure measurement to determine hypertension, as blood pressure can fluctuate widely. Stress, exercise, and certain drugs are common factors which may cause short term elevations in blood pressure. A health care professional will measure a person's blood pressure on at least 3 separate occasions before making a diagnosis of hypertension. (See figure 15.5.)

Several steps can be taken in combatting hypertension. One can avoid foods heavily concentrated with sodium. Weight loss in obese persons can also help regulate blood pressure. In addition, many medications are available that reduce blood pressure. Most physicians, however, attempt to control a person's hypertension through diet modifications before prescribing drugs. The most important advice for a hypertensive person is to follow a physician's recommendations. Too often, persons with hypertension either fail to realize it or fail to take decisive action to correct it.

Hypertension is sometimes called the "silent killer," because it has no major signs or symptoms. Many people never realize they have high blood pressure until extensive, life-threatening damage has occurred. Because of this, it can be useful to monitor your blood pressure regularly. The wide availability of home blood-pressure devices makes this a realistic secondary prevention practice. If you decide to do this, though, avoid purchasing cheap and unreliable equipment.

Unfortunately, the mechanisms in the development of hypertension are poorly understood. In fact, it is estimated that 90 percent of all cases of hypertension are of unknown origin.[1]

**HEART ATTACK** A heart attack is the result of any one of many cardiovascular disorders that affect the heart muscle. The most commonly encountered disorder giving rise to a heart attack is **coronary artery disease,** also known as **coronary heart disease.**

When the coronary arteries are unable to supply the heart with an adequate supply of blood, as in the advanced stages of atherosclerosis, the condition is known as coronary heart disease (CHD), and the person's health may be seriously threatened. A blood clot may form in a narrowed coronary artery, thus blocking the flow of blood to the heart muscle. When cells of the heart muscle are deprived of oxygen due to insufficient blood flow those cells die. This type of heart attack is called a **myocardial infarction.** If the blocked artery is a major blood supplier to the heart, the result may be sudden death or serious heart damage. This is the event that occurs when one is said to have suffered a "massive coronary."

The heart appears to be able to develop a limited back-up system for obtaining blood flow when an artery is blocked. This system is known as **collateral circulation.** Collaterals are tiny vascular channels that connect with major arteries that supply blood to particular organs or tissues. Normally, they carry little blood. If blood flow in a major artery becomes restricted, the small collaterals dilate and attempt to perform the work of the injured artery. How many collaterals the heart possesses and to what extent they can compensate for a major arterial block are questions that need further research.

The symptoms of a myocardial infarction or heart attack may vary, but generally include one or more of the following events. The most commonly experienced symptom is severe pain in the midchest area. Persons who have survived heart attacks describe the pain as "crushing" or "viselike," or compare it to an elephant sitting on their chest or to being wrapped tightly in a rope. The pain often radiates to other areas of the upper trunk, especially the neck, jaw, shoulder, and arms. A person may also experience dizziness, nausea, and even vomiting. The person may appear pale and cold, but have beads of perspiration on the forehead. Pulse may be weak, but rapid. The person may begin to go into shock.

A person who is with another individual experiencing severe chest pain, especially in combination with other symptoms, should seek prompt emergency care. Many persons die unnecessarily each year by delaying help because they fail to recognize symptoms. Everyone ought to know how to get in touch with the local emergency medical system. This means knowing the telephone number of the fire-rescue service, or having the number written in several prominent locations in one's home. In some areas, the emergency system can be contacted by dialing 911, a central dispatch number for all emergency situations. Persons with a heart condition should record emergency numbers when staying in hotels or other places away from home. Such knowledge may be valuable in a variety of unexpected emergency situations.

A heart attack may be so severe that heartbeat and breathing cease. This situation is termed a **cardiac arrest.** When this crisis arises, the well-prepared individual is in a position to perform a life restoring procedure known as **cardiopulmonary resuscitation** or CPR. CPR combines mouth-to-mouth resuscitation with closed heart massage to maintain breathing and circulation for the victim until help arrives. Physicians, nurses, and emergency medical and paramedical personnel have used CPR for many years. It is now being encouraged as a skill that all people should develop. It is a highly specialized skill, however, that requires both appropriate preparation and practice. It is *not* a procedure to be performed by an *unskilled* individual. Each member of a family that includes a heart patient ought to learn it. Persons interested in learning CPR can contact their local affiliates of the American Heart Association or the American National Red Cross. Many hospitals also offer citizen training and practice in CPR. (See figure 15.6.)

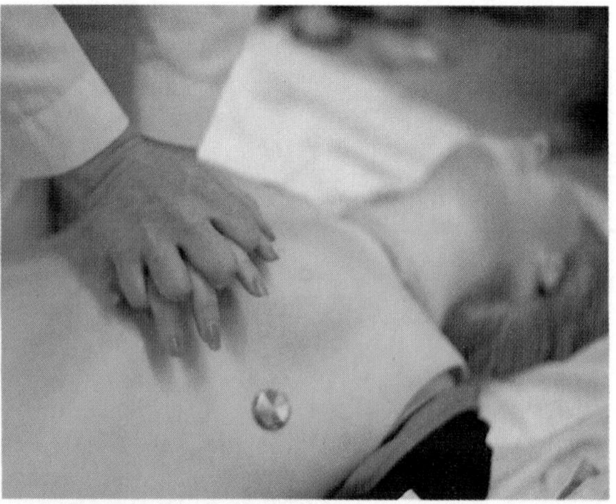

**Figure 15.6**
Cardiopulmonary resuscitation is a skill that all people can develop in specially designed CPR classes.

**ANGINA** Another consequence of CHD is chest pain known as **angina pectoris,** or simply, **angina.** Such pain results when restricted blood flow to the heart occurs. Angina may not be a constant source of discomfort for the CHD patient, but it can be a serious one during physical exertion, stress or emotional upset, or at other times when the blood-supply demands of the heart are increased. Angina's discomfort can be controlled in many CHD patients with a variety of drugs.

## Other Cardiovascular Disorders

So far, we have discussed the most common forms of cardiovascular disease. There are some other, less-common cardiovascular diseases that can also pose threats to one's well-being.

**ARRHYTHMIAS** Arrhythmia means an irregular heartbeat. Normal heartbeat is regulated by electrical impulses originating in specialized bundles of cardiac cells. This system can malfunction, however. In extreme cases of electrical misfiring, the heart experiences a life-threatening situation known as **fibrillation.** During fibrillation, the pumping action of the ventricles is so irregular and insufficient that adequate circulation cannot be maintained. As recently as the 1960s, half of sudden cardiac deaths had electrical causative factors.[2] Minor problems in the heart's electrical conduction system now can be controlled by drug therapy, or by implantation of a **pacemaker.** The pacemaker is a small, battery-operated unit that artificially produces the electrical impulses necessary to generate appropriate heart rhythm.

**CONGESTIVE HEART FAILURE** **Congestive heart failure** occurs when the heart muscle becomes damaged because of a heart attack, atherosclerosis, hypertension, rheumatic fever, or congenital heart defects. Damaged heart muscle lacks the contractive force to circulate blood properly. A failing heart may continue to work for years, but does so less efficiently than a healthy heart. As blood flow is retarded, blood returning to the heart "backs up," producing congestion or swelling in selective tissues. This swelling, called **edema,** tends to occur in the ankles and feet. Fluid may also accumulate in the lungs (pulmonary edema) resulting in shortness of breath and labored breathing. Congestive heart failure reduces the ability of the kidneys to excrete water and sodium. Water that is retained adds to the edema.

Treatment for congestive heart failure requires multiple approaches. Some of these include rest, dietary changes, modification of daily activities, and drug therapy.

**STROKE** A **stroke** results from damage to arteries supplying blood to the brain. Blockage of cerebral arteries can produce death of any brain cells usually nourished by these arteries. This cell death is a stroke. If many brain cells are destroyed, the result may be partial paralysis, speech impairment, other psychomotor dysfunction, or death. Minor strokes occur if blood flow to the brain is reduced. These small strokes present symptoms such as temporary dizziness, sensory loss, or confusion.

# CARDIOVASCULAR DISEASE: PERSONAL AND SOCIAL INFLUENCES

Clearly, the answer to the problem of cardiovascular disease is prevention before the problem occurs. Although we cannot control all the biological factors that contribute to cardiovascular disease, we can minimize many of the personal and social risks that encourage CHD.

## Risk Factors and Prudent Heart Living

Scientists can identify several life-style factors that promote development of cardiovascular disorders. Many people, however, have a difficult time following recommendations to decrease risk. Life-style options for risk reduction are presented in the following paragraphs.

**SMOKING** The more a person smokes, the greater is his or her likelihood of sustaining a heart attack or stroke. Risk is dose related. Thus, someone who smokes two packs of cigarettes per day is at greater risk than someone who smokes one pack of cigarettes per day. The death rate from heart attack is 200 percent higher for smokers than for nonsmokers. Smoking is the life-style factor that contributes most to cardiovascular disease. (See Exhibit 15.1.)

Most smokers find it difficult to quit smoking. Newspaper and magazine advertisements for cigarettes, as well as the constant availability of smoking paraphernalia and the presence of fellow smokers, can all undermine the best efforts. Chapter 13 provides many helpful suggestions for kicking the cigarette habit.

**HYPERTENSION** Hypertension enhances the development of atherosclerosis, aneurysms, and other disorders, and forces the heart to work harder. A hypertensive person should take medication as prescribed, eliminate excess sodium from the diet, and maintain optimal body weight. Annual blood-pressure monitoring is also helpful.

Changing eating habits, especially decreasing sodium consumption, is difficult for some people.

15.1 EXHIBIT 15.1

## Medical Costs of Smoking Equal Cost of Cigarettes, Study Says

The medical costs incurred by cigarette smokers as a result of their habit nearly equal the cost of their cigarettes, according to a recent study by the Minnesota health department.

The study estimated that the cost of treating smoking-related illnesses in Minnesota in 1983 surpassed $400 million—about 7.5 percent of the state's total health care bill.

The health department said that nearly 457 million packs of cigarettes were sold in Minnesota in 1983 at an average price per pack of 94 cents. The health care costs resulting from smoking translated to 89 cents per pack, the department said.

The department's calculations were based on "mortality comparisons," which use the proportion of smoking-attributable deaths to provide an estimate of the lifetime smoking-attributable illness rates.

The study estimated the direct costs of smoking-related illnesses, including hospital charges, physician fees, costs for prescription drugs, and fees for ancillary health services.

Not included were the health costs for former smokers, and costs associated with lost productivity and income. "It is apparent that the overall economic benefit of non-smoking to Minnesota will greatly exceed the gross income from the sale of cigarettes," the health department said.

Minnesota has been a leader in anti-smoking campaigns. The state was one of the first to require that all public places have designated no-smoking areas.

The health department broke down the medical costs of each cigarette pack to include:

- 12 cents for treating smoking-related cancer.
- 22 cents for heart and circulatory problems.
- 30 cents for emphysema and other respiratory problems.
- 23 cents for other illnesses such as ulcers.
- 1.5 cents for injuries in fires caused by smoking.

Source: © 1984 *American Medical News.* Reprinted with permission.

### DISCUSSION QUESTIONS

1. Who should be responsible for the high cost of treating smoking-related illnesses?

2. Would it be feasible and ethical to pass these costs on to the smoker by placing an additional tax on cigarettes, the proceeds of such a tax being directed toward the cost of health care?

Fortunately, there are many flavorful seasonings which can be substituted for salt and which do not seem to increase blood pressure. Chapter 4 presents these options in greater detail.

**DIETARY FAT** It is estimated that 40 to 45 percent of the caloric intake of Americans is in the form of fat; this is 10 to 20 percent more than recommended. Studies indicate that the incidence of cardiovascular disease is lower in populations consuming less saturated fat. Saturated-fat consumption contributes to elevated levels of cholesterol and triglyceride. It is also a factor in obesity. Obesity does not directly affect the heart itself. Excess weight increases blood pressure and inflates blood sugar and cholesterol levels. A person whose cholesterol level exceeds 250 milligrams has three times the risk of premature heart attack as a person whose cholesterol is in the desired range.

With moderate dietary changes, desirable cholesterol and trigylceride levels often can be maintained.

Many Americans are now discovering that low fat and predominantly vegetarian meals are both less costly than traditional meals, and deliciously refreshing! Chapter 4 presents information on how to implement tasty dietary changes which will help reduce your risk of coronary artery disease. (See Exhibit 15.2.)

15.2 EXHIBIT 15.2

## Heart Attack and Cholesterol

A ten-year government study has finally proved the connection. The good news: diet and drugs can help.

It seems harmless enough, a bit like liquid soap, as it courses through the bloodstream to the body's tissues. As much as 80 percent of it is manufactured naturally, exclusive of diet—most of it churned out by the liver at the rate of about 1,000 milligrams a day. And it is essential to human life. Without it, the body could not make hormones, or vitamin D, or bile acids, or the sheath that insulates nerve fibers.

Cholesterol is the name of this vital substance, known chemically as a steroid alcohol. But for all its benefits, cholesterol has emerged as America's public health enemy number one. It is the principal component of plaque, the fatty, yellowish deposit inside the arteries.

Despite strong warnings over the years from the American Heart Association to limit cholesterol intake to no more than 300 milligrams a day (a medium-sized egg yolk contains about 275), the average American adult consumes between 400 and 700 (see the table at the end of this Exhibit for a list of cholesterol-laden foods and some low-cholesterol alternatives).

Such gustatory abandon will be but a fond memory if Americans heed the results of a new government-sponsored study, which was conducted at twelve medical centers in the United States and Canada. Its message, delivered in a succinct, 39-page report in mid-January 1984, was painfully clear: lowering cholesterol reduces heart attacks and heart attack deaths, period. Just as significant, the study found that every one percent drop in the cholesterol level in the bloodstream means a two per cent decrease in the likelihood of a heart attack. Moreover, lowering cholesterol with a combination of diet and drugs can cut the risk of heart disease by as much as 50 percent in people with high cholesterol levels.

Exercise and avoiding cigarettes can also help. Although the study did not address the point, scientists know that when people exercise regularly and do not smoke, their blood levels of "good" fats—the so-called high-density lipoproteins (HDLs)—increase. HDLs, which contain less cholesterol than the more dangerous low-density lipoproteins (LDLs), may actually protect against atherosclerosis.

The notion that cholesterol makes unhealthy hearts is not new. Scientists have long known that a typical American diet raises cholesterol levels.

## 15.2 *continued* EXHIBIT

They know, too, that societies with low-fat, low-cholesterol diets, such as the Japanese, have fewer deaths from coronary artery disease. In the laboratory, the evidence is graphic: animals fed an American-style diet eventually develop plaque in their arteries.

Strong as the connection seemed, it was still not enough to tag cholesterol definitively as the culprit. Critics argued that although studies demonstrated that diet could increase cholesterol levels in the blood, none had shown any conclusive association between cholesterol and heart disease. Some of the same studies dismissed any possible danger from saturated fats—which occur in such foods as fatty meat, whole milk dairy products, and lard—even though they raise cholesterol levels. The new government report put an end to such wishful thinking. Says Dr. Basil Rifkind of the National Institutes of Health, co-director of the new study, "It is now indisputable" that lowering cholesterol pays off handsomely.

The study that prompted such a point-blank conclusion was carefully planned. Recruiting of the subjects began in 1973 with the screening of some 400,000 men between the ages of 35 and 59 whose blood cholesterol levels were above 265 milligrams per 100 milliliters (the average is around 210 to 220 milligrams). Although at the outset none of the men showed evidence of heart disease—that is, they had no history or symptoms of angina or heart attack—they were considered at high risk because of their high cholesterol levels. All the men—women, who are less susceptible to heart disease, were not included in the sample—were put on a low-cholesterol diet. Half were also treated with cholestyramine, a potent drug introduced in 1965 that lowers cholesterol; they took it two to four times a day in powdered form, mixed with water or orange juice. The other half of the group got a placebo powder that had no effect on cholesterol levels.

The outcome confirmed two hypotheses: first, that blood cholesterol could be lowered dramatically by diet, and even more so by a combination of diet and drugs; second, that lowering cholesterol reduces the risk of heart attacks. Even those who only changed their diet reduced their cholesterol levels by about four percent; among those who also took the drug, cholesterol dropped an average of twelve and a half percent. Still more important was the effect the lowered cholesterol levels had on the risk of heart disease. Over the ten years, those on both diets and drugs had 24 percent fewer fatal heart attacks than those on diets alone, and 19 percent fewer non-fatal heart attacks than the diet-only subjects. When the cholesterol level was reduced 25 percent, the incidence of heart disease fell an impressive 50 percent. The group taking cholestyramine also came out ahead on another score: 20 percent fewer attacks of angina and 21 percent fewer coronary bypass operations to detour blood around blocked arteries.

While the study did not say that Americans as a whole should follow the example of the high-risk men in the study by cutting their cholesterol intake, other scientists have been quick to make the inference. Says Dr. Antonio Gotto, president of the American Heart Association, "We believe that we can extrapolate from all this, that it does not just apply to middle-aged men with high cholesterol. It applies to other age groups, and to women as well."

Gotto also pressed for periodic monitoring: cholesterol levels should be checked at age 20 or 21, and every five years thereafter. For those with normal cholesterol levels, Gotto had some advice: "It depends on the circumstances and the person's age. If you're thirty-five years old, lower it, because it may go up later. If you're seventy-five, I don't recommend a change."

To keep cholesterol at a healthy level, the recommendations are straightforward: cut down on saturated fats and high-cholesterol foods, and substitute more fish and poultry; use skim milk; eat only two or three eggs a week; limit shrimp and organ meats, like liver, to one or two portions a month; cook with liquid polyunsaturated vegetable oils and margarine; avoid saturated vegetable fats like coconut oil.

By following such recommendations, the average person can lower his blood cholesterol from 10 to 15 percent, thereby substantially reducing his chances of heart disease. If that does not work for those with high cholesterol levels, then a cholesterol-lowering drug may be prescribed. Cholestyramine is expensive—about $150 a month per person for the doses used in the trial—and many of the others have unpleasant side effects. There is no argument, though, about the value of lowering cholesterol. Says Gotto, "If everyone goes

## EXHIBIT 15.2

along, by the year 2000 we will be talking about things other than atherosclerosis. I think we will have it conquered by then."

### CULINARY CULPRITS AND SAFE SUBSTITUTES

Nearly everyone knows that beef, eggs, and butter are high in cholesterol, but so are such less likely suspects as beef liver and shrimp. To get a more accurate gauge of the damage foods can do to blood cholesterol levels, you must also consider the amount of saturated fats they contain. A sampler of foods to eat sparingly, and others to substitute:

| *Culprits* | *Cholesterol (in milligrams)* | *Saturated Fat (in grams)* | *Substitutes* | *Cholesterol (in milligrams)* | *Saturated Fat (in grams)* |
|---|---|---|---|---|---|
| pork brains (3 oz.) | 2,169 | 1.8 | green or yellow vegetable or fruit | 0 | trace |
| beef kidney (3 oz.) | 683 | 3.8 | peanut butter (1 tbsp.) | 0 | 1.5 |
| beef liver (3 oz.) | 372 | 2.5 | angel food cake (3 oz. slice) | 0 | 1.96 |
| one egg | 275 | 1.7 | stick or tub margarine (1 tbsp.) | 0 | 2.1 |
| shrimp (3 oz.) | 128 | .2 | skim milk (1 cup) | 4 | 0.3 |
| Roquefort cheese (3 oz.) | 78 | 16.5 | parmesan cheese (1 tbsp.) | 4 | 1.0 |
| beef hot dog (30 percent fat, 3 oz.) | 75 | 9.9 | cheese pizza (3 oz. slice) | 6 | .8 |
| prime ribs of beef (3 oz.) | 66.5 | 5.3 | buttermilk (1 cup) | 9 | 1.3 |
| ice cream (10 percent fat, 1 cup) | 59 | 8.9 | uncreamed cottage cheese (1 cup) | 10 | .4 |
| lobster (3 oz.) | 46.5 | .075 | ice milk, soft (1 cup) | 13 | 2.9 |
| doughnut (3 oz.) | 36 | 4.0 | yogurt (1 cup) | 14 | 2.3 |
| whole milk (1 cup) | 33 | 5.1 | lean fish (3 oz.) | 43 | .08 |
| butter (1 tbsp.) | 31 | 7.1 | turkey, white meat (3 oz.) | 59 | .9 |
| creamed cottage cheese (1 cup) | 31 | 6.0 | chicken, white meat (3 oz.) | 72 | 1.1 |
| french fries (3 oz.) | 20 | 6.0 | lean beef (3 oz.) | 73 | 3.7 |
| milk chocolate bar (3 oz.) | 18 | 16.3 | lean veal (3 oz.) | 85 | 1.6 |
| | | | lean lamb (3 oz.) | 85 | 2.7 |

Source: John Langone. © *Discover Magazine* 3/85, Time, Inc.

## DISCUSSION QUESTIONS

1. Are you aware of the amount of cholesterol consumed in your daily diet? Do you know your current blood cholesterol level?

2. Do you agree with the major conclusions of this study? You may want to review the critical thinking approaches to reviewing research reports which was presented in chapter 1.

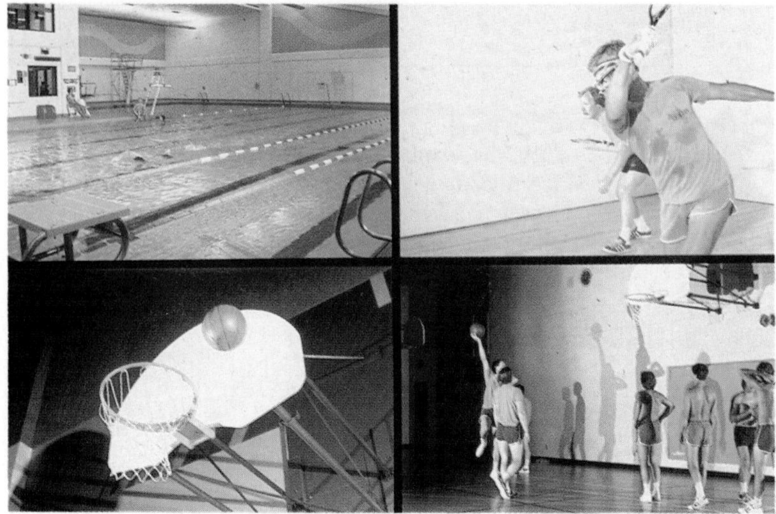

**Figure 15.7**
More and more businesses are providing their workers and executives with exercise facilities similar to those of Sentry Insurance Company of Stevens Point, Wisconsin.

**STRESS** It is generally accepted that cardiovascular disease is related to a behavior pattern referred to as the "Type-A" personality. The Type-A person is highly competitive, ambitious, and feels a profound sense of urgency to complete tasks once they are started.[3] Most Type-A people are male, perhaps because competitiveness and achievement orientation are more a part of the rearing process of males. Type A's, regardless of gender, subject themselves to high levels of stress. The best physiologic evidence suggests that persons designated as Type A's exhibit higher cholesterol levels and faster clotting times than their more relaxed Type-B counterparts, thereby increasing their risk of heart attack.

Authorities agree that the first step in combatting stress is recognizing its origins. Type-A people need to build relaxation into their daily routines. For the working person, this may mean breaks from work that involve more than just coffee or lunch. Many people identify moderate exercise as a source of stress reduction and fit it into their daily routines. Our society often makes it difficult to relax or exercise daily. Some large corporations, however, now recognize the importance of facilitating stress reduction programs for executives and other employees. Sentry Insurance Company of Stevens Point, Wisconsin, for example, offers organized recreational activities for employees and has on-site facilities that include basketball courts and a gymnasium with weight equipment. The company also provides a "quiet room" for employees. Employees need to speak up and request such opportunities for controlling stress. More information about stress management can be found in chapter 3. (See figure 15.7.)

**LACK OF EXERCISE** Although lack of exercise has not clearly been established as an independent risk factor for cardiovascular disease, it may play a role. A low activity level, when combined with overeating, predisposes one to obesity which *is* linked to cardiovascular disease. Regular aerobic exercise will strengthen the heart muscle, causing it to pump more highly oxygenated blood with each beat.

Exercise may aid efforts to control cigarette smoking, hypertension, lipid abnormalities, diabetes, obesity, and emotional stress. Evidence suggests that regular, moderate or vigorous occupational or leisure-time physical activity may protect against coronary heart disease and may improve the likelihood of survival from a heart attack.[4]

Chapter 6 provides valuable information about starting an aerobic exercise program which will best meet your needs and interest. The possible role of exercise in cardiovascular disease prevention is explored in Exhibit 15.3.

## A Last Word about Cardiovascular Disease

As we have seen, several life-style factors are implicated in the development of America's number-one killer, cardiovascular disease. These factors can be modified to reduce risk. Your risk profile is provided in Activity for Wellness 15.1.

15.3 EXHIBIT 15.3

## Aerobic Advice in Post-Fixx Era

Jim Fixx's death raises the question, is aerobic exercise truly protective against heart attacks? The American Heart Association (AHA) says yes, and the majority of cardiologists interviewed concurred. In its statement on exercise, the association declares that "physical training alters lipid and carbohydrate metabolism and may result in a blood lipid and lipoprotein profile consistent with a decreased risk of atherosclerotic vascular disease."

"Exercise is surely effective in improving longevity and functional capacity," said Dr. Selvester, chairman of the AHA's subcommittee on exercise and cardiac rehabilitation. "Our committee will not back away from promoting exercise because of Fixx's death, but we do emphasize the role of other risk factors such as cigarette smoking, hypertension, and obesity.

Dr. Cooper strongly advocated continued fitness programs and has signed a lucrative book contract to promote safe running, called *Avoiding the Jim Fixx Syndrome*. The death of Fixx, he noted, probably will not cause people who already jog to stop. Instead, "it will affect those who were thinking of jogging but are frightened by Mr. Fixx's death into thinking it's not the thing to do after all." Dr. Cooper cited a report in *JAMA* (252:487–490, 1984) by his colleague Dr. Steven N. Blair that showed a "good relationship between levels of fitness and protection from hypertension." And, in the same issue, a study of 16,936 Harvard alumni who entered the university from 1916 to 1950 found that even modest exercise—expending 2,000 or more calories per week in walking, climbing stairs, or playing sports—"reduced substantially" the risk of cardiovascular disease (*JAMA* 252:491–495, 1984). Of 640 men who died of cardiovascular disease, the adjusted death rates of sedentary persons were almost twice as high as in the group who expended 2,000 or more calories a week.

Dr. Cooper also quoted Gallup poll figures indicating a 12 percent increase over the past two years in the number of adults exercising regularly, with a "corresponding improvement in heart disease. We're now enjoying the best cardiovascular statistics we've ever had in this country," he said, "so if exercise and jogging are potentially dangerous to the heart, why aren't the streets full of dead joggers?"

Despite Dr. Cooper's enthusiasm, Dr. Paul D. Thompson, assistant professor of medicine, Brown University Program in Medicine, cited studies of runners who do drop dead in their tracks, suggesting that "excellent physical condition is no guarantee against sudden cardiac death during exercise." In his own most recent study of 81 exercise deaths, to be published in *Medicine and Science in Sports and Exercise,* Dr. Thompson found that "the absolute risk of dropping dead while jogging is very low—we calculated one death in 7,620 joggers per year for six years."

"Exercise is no panacea," he said, "and mine are not the first studies to point out the risk involved. A study of how soldiers die that was done in the '40s found a 10 times greater chance of dying while marching than while in bed. So I don't know why people get so upset when I say this about exercise, unless they cherish the mistaken notion that jogging is a guarantee against dropping dead from heart trouble."

Dr. Friedewald believes that "the chronic benefits—weight loss, cessation of smoking, dietary and life-style changes, lowering of blood pressure, and increase in HDL cholesterol—must certainly outweigh the small, but real, acute risk," of running.

Source: Reprinted courtesy *Medical Tribune*.

### DISCUSSION QUESTIONS

1. Do you believe Dr. Cooper and others who claim that, while exercise is not a guarantee against heart attacks, aerobic exercise does decrease the probability of their occurrence?

2. Did you use the critical thinking approach to reviewing research in reaching your conclusion? If not, you may want to review chapter 1.

15.1

ACTIVITY FOR

# WELLNESS

## Men

Find the column for your age group. Everyone starts with a score of 10 points. Work down the page *adding* points to your score or *subtracting* points from your score.

**54 or Younger**

Starting Score 10

**YOUR RISKO SCORE**

1. Weight
   *Locate your weight category in the table on the right.* If you are in . . .

| | | |
|---|---|---|
| ☐ | weight category A | Subtract 2 |
| ☐ | weight category B | Subtract 1 |
| ☐ | weight category C | Add 1 |
| ☐ | weight category D | Add 2 |
| | **Equals** | ☐ |

2. Systolic blood pressure
   *Use the "first" or "higher" number from your most recent blood-pressure measurement. If you do not know your blood pressure, estimate it by using the letter for your weight category.* If your blood pressure is . . .

| | | |
|---|---|---|
| A | 119 or less | Subtract 1 |
| B | between 120 and 139 | Add 0 |
| C | between 140 and 159 | Add 0 |
| D | 160 or greater | Add 1 |
| | **Equals** | ☐ |

3. Blood cholesterol level
   *Use the number from your most recent blood cholesterol test. If you do not know your blood cholesterol, estimate it by using the letter for your weight category.* If your blood cholesterol is . . .

| | | |
|---|---|---|
| A | 199 or less | Subtract 2 |
| B | between 200 and 224 | Subtract 1 |
| C | between 225 and 249 | Add 0 |
| D | 250 or higher | Add 1 |
| | **Equals** | ☐ |

4. Cigarette smoking
   If you . . .
   
   *(If you smoke a pipe, but not cigarettes, use the same score adjustment as those cigarette smokers who smoke less than a pack a day.)*

| | | |
|---|---|---|
| ☐ | do not smoke | Subtract 1 |
| ☐ | smoke less than a pack a day | Add 0 |
| ☐ | smoke a pack a day | Add 1 |
| ☐ | smoke more than a pack a day | Add 2 |
| | **Final Score Equals** | ☐ |

ACTIVITY FOR
# WELLNESS
15.1

**55 or Older**
Starting Score [10]

Subtract 2
Add 0
Add 1
Add 3

**Equals** [ ]

Subtract 5
Subtract 2
Add 1
Add 4

**Equals** [ ]

Subtract 1
Subtract 1
Add 0
Add 0

**Equals** [ ]

Subtract 2
Subtract 1
Add 0
Add 3

**Final Score Equals** [ ]

**Weight Table for Men**

Look for your height (without shoes) in the far left column and then read across to find the category into which your weight (in indoor clothing) would fall.

Because both blood pressure and blood cholesterol are related to weight, an estimate of these risk factors for each weight category is printed at the bottom of the table.

| Your Height FT IN | Weight Category (lbs.) A | B | C | D |
|---|---|---|---|---|
| 5 1 | up to 123 | 124–148 | 149–173 | 174 plus |
| 5 2 | up to 126 | 127–152 | 153–178 | 179 plus |
| 5 3 | up to 129 | 130–156 | 157–182 | 183 plus |
| 5 4 | up to 132 | 133–160 | 161–186 | 187 plus |
| 5 5 | up to 135 | 136–163 | 164–190 | 191 plus |
| 5 6 | up to 139 | 140–168 | 169–196 | 197 plus |
| 5 7 | up to 144 | 145–174 | 175–203 | 204 plus |
| 5 8 | up to 148 | 149–179 | 180–209 | 210 plus |
| 5 9 | up to 152 | 153–184 | 185–214 | 215 plus |
| 5 10 | up to 157 | 158–190 | 191–221 | 222 plus |
| 5 11 | up to 161 | 162–194 | 195–227 | 228 plus |
| 6 0 | up to 165 | 166–199 | 200–232 | 233 plus |
| 6 1 | up to 170 | 171–205 | 206–239 | 240 plus |
| 6 2 | up to 175 | 176–211 | 212–246 | 247 plus |
| 6 3 | up to 180 | 181–217 | 218–253 | 254 plus |
| 6 4 | up to 185 | 186–223 | 224–260 | 261 plus |
| 6 5 | up to 190 | 191–229 | 230–267 | 268 plus |
| 6 6 | up to 195 | 196–235 | 236–274 | 275 plus |
| | 119 or less | 120 to 139 | 140 to 159 | 160 or more |
| | 199 or less | 200 to 224 | 225 to 249 | 250 or more |

Estimate of Systolic Blood Pressure

Estimate of Blood Cholesterol

15.1 *continued*

ACTIVITY FOR
# WELLNESS

## Women

Find the column for your age group. Everyone starts with a score of 10 points. Work down the page *adding* points to your score or *subtracting* points from your score.

**54 or Younger**

**YOUR RISKO SCORE** Starting Score 10

1. Weight
   *Locate your weight category in the table on the right.* If you are in . . .

| | | |
|---|---|---|
| ☐ | weight category A | Subtract 2 |
| ☐ | weight category B | Subtract 1 |
| ☐ | weight category C | Add 1 |
| ☐ | weight category D | Add 2 |

**Equals** ☐

2. Systolic blood pressure
   *Use the "first" or "higher" number from your most recent blood-pressure measurement. If you do not know your blood pressure, estimate it by using the letter for your weight category.* If your blood pressure is . . .

| | | |
|---|---|---|
| A | 119 or less | Subtract 2 |
| B | between 120 and 139 | Subtract 1 |
| C | between 140 and 159 | Add 0 |
| D | 160 or greater | Add 1 |

**Equals** ☐

3. Blood cholesterol level
   *Use the number from your most recent blood cholesterol test. If you do not know your blood cholesterol, estimate it by using the letter for your weight category.* If your blood cholesterol is . . .

| | | |
|---|---|---|
| A | 199 or less | Subtract 1 |
| B | between 200 and 224 | Add 0 |
| C | between 225 and 249 | Add 0 |
| D | 250 or higher | Add 1 |

**Equals** ☐

4. Cigarette smoking
   If you . . .

| | | |
|---|---|---|
| ☐ | do not smoke | Subtract 1 |
| ☐ | smoke less than a pack a day | Add 0 |
| ☐ | smoke a pack a day | Add 1 |
| ☐ | smoke more than a pack a day | Add 2 |

**Equals** ☐

5. Estrogen use
   *Birth-control pills and hormone drugs contain estrogen. A few examples are: *Premarin *Ogan *Menstranol *Provera *Evex *Menest *Estinyl *Meurium*

- Have you ever taken estrogen for five or more years in a row?
- Are you age 35 years or older and are now taking estrogen?

| | |
|---|---|
| No to both questions | Add 0 |
| Yes to one or both questions | Add 1 |

**Final Score Equals** ☐

ACTIVITY FOR
# WELLNESS
15.1

**55 or Older**
Starting Score [10]

Subtract 2
Subtract 1
Add 0
Add 1

**Equals** [ ]

Subtract 3
Add 0
Add 3
Add 6

**Equals** [ ]

Subtract 3
Subtract 1
Add 1
Add 3

**Equals** [ ]

Subtract 2
Subtract 1
Add 1
Add 4

**Equals** [ ]

Add 0
Add 3

**Final Score Equals** [ ]

**Weight Table for Women**
Look for your height (without shoes) in the far left column and then read across to find the category into which your weight (in indoor clothing) would fall.

Because both blood pressure and blood cholesterol are related to weight, an estimate of these risk factors for each weight category is printed at the bottom of the table.

| Your Height FT IN | Weight Category (lbs.) | | | |
|---|---|---|---|---|
| | A | B | C | D |
| 4 8 | up to 101 | 102–122 | 123–143 | 144 plus |
| 4 9 | up to 103 | 104–125 | 126–146 | 147 plus |
| 4 10 | up to 106 | 107–128 | 129–150 | 151 plus |
| 4 11 | up to 109 | 110–132 | 133–154 | 155 plus |
| 5 0 | up to 112 | 113–136 | 137–158 | 159 plus |
| 5 1 | up to 115 | 116–139 | 140–162 | 163 plus |
| 5 2 | up to 119 | 120–144 | 145–168 | 169 plus |
| 5 3 | up to 122 | 123–148 | 149–172 | 173 plus |
| 5 4 | up to 127 | 128–154 | 155–179 | 180 plus |
| 5 5 | up to 131 | 132–158 | 159–185 | 186 plus |
| 5 6 | up to 135 | 136–163 | 164–190 | 191 plus |
| 5 7 | up to 139 | 140–168 | 169–196 | 197 plus |
| 5 8 | up to 143 | 144–173 | 174–202 | 203 plus |
| 5 9 | up to 147 | 148–178 | 179–207 | 208 plus |
| 5 10 | up to 151 | 152–182 | 183–213 | 214 plus |
| 5 11 | up to 155 | 156–187 | 188–218 | 219 plus |
| 6 0 | up to 159 | 160–191 | 192–224 | 225 plus |
| 6 1 | up to 163 | 164–196 | 197–229 | 230 plus |
| | 119 or less | 120 to 139 | 140 to 159 | 160 or more |
| | 199 or less | 200 to 224 | 225 to 249 | 250 or more |

Estimate of Systolic Blood Pressure
Estimate of Blood Cholesterol

15.1 *continued*

ACTIVITY FOR WELLNESS

## What Your Score Means

**0–4**

You have one of the lowest risks of heart disease for your age and sex.

**5–9**

You have a low-to-moderate risk of heart disease for your age and sex but there is some room for improvement.

**10–14**

You have a moderate-to-high risk of heart disease for your age and sex, with considerable room for improvement on some factors.

**15–19**

You have a high risk of developing heart disease for your age and sex with a great deal of room for improvement on all factors.

**20 & over**

You have a very high risk of developing heart disease for your age and sex and should take immediate action on all risk factors.

***Warning***

- If you have diabetes, gout, or a family history of heart disease, your actual risk will be greater than indicated by this appraisal.
- If you do not know your current blood-pressure or blood-cholesterol level, you should visit your physician or health center to have them measured. Then figure your score again for a more accurate determination of your risk.
- If you are overweight, have high blood pressure or high blood cholesterol, or smoke cigarettes, your long-term risk of heart disease is increased even if your risk in the next several years is low.

**HOW TO REDUCE YOUR RISK**

- Try to quit smoking permanently. There are many programs available.
- Have your blood pressure checked regularly, preferably every twelve months after age forty. If your blood pressure is high, see your physician. Remember blood-pressure medicine is only effective if taken regularly.

**Table 15.1 Risk-Factor Reduction for Health Promotion**

- Reduce saturated fats and cholesterol in your diet, and substitute heart-healthy foods.
- Monitor caloric intake and maintain an optimal body weight.
- Learn how to monitor your blood pressure at regular intervals, and have it checked by a physician at least annually.
- Be a nonsmoker, or else become a nonsmoker.
- Reduce stress where possible.
- Develop a pattern of exercise that is heart healthy and enjoyable to you.
- Have medical checkups as recommended by your physician for early detection of diabetes, hypertension, and other factors that contribute to the risk of cardiovascular disease.

## ACTIVITY FOR WELLNESS 15.1

- Consider your daily exercise (or lack of it). A half hour of brisk walking, swimming, or other enjoyable activity should not be difficult to fit into your day.
- Give some serious thought to your diet. If you are overweight, or eat a lot of foods high in saturated fat or cholesterol (whole milk, cheese, eggs, butter, fatty foods, fried foods) then make changes in your diet. Look for the American Heart Association Cookbook at your local bookstore.
- Visit or write your local Heart Association for further information and copies of free pamphlets on many related subjects including:
  - Reducing your risk of heart attack.
  - Controlling blood pressure.
  - Eating to keep your heart healthy.
  - How to stop smoking.
  - Exercising for good health.

**SOME WORDS OF CAUTION**

- If you have diabetes, gout, or a family history of heart disease, your real risk of developing heart disease will be greater than indicated by your RISKO score. If your score is high and you have one or more of these additional problems, you should give particular attention to reducing your risk.
- If you are a woman under forty-five years or a man under thirty-five years of age, your RISKO score represents an upper limit on your real risk of developing heart disease. In this case your real risk is probably lower than indicated by your score.
- If you are a woman whose use of estrogen has contributed to a high RISKO score, you may want to consult your physician. Do not automatically discontinue your prescription.
- Using your weight category to estimate your systolic blood pressure or your blood cholesterol level makes your RISKO score less accurate.
  - Your score will tend to overestimate your risk if your actual values on these two important factors are average for someone of your height and weight.
  - Your score will underestimate your risk if your actual blood-pressure or cholesterol level is above average for someone of your height or weight.

Source: Reproduced with permission. American Heart Association.

There is no guarantee that cardiovascular disease can be prevented, but making positive modifications in your risk profile provides the best chance for attaining higher levels of wellness. For the person who already has a cardiovascular disorder, risk-factor modification reduces the sense of helplessness and hopelessness that interfere with personal growth, an orientation toward the future, and optimal wellness. (See table 15.1.)

## CANCER: NUMBER-TWO KILLER IN AMERICA

Cancer, which is probably as old as the oldest forms of life, is not a single disease. Rather, it is a collection of diseases that share certain traits. Scientists identify more than 100 different types of cancer in humans.[5] All are diseases arising from an individual cell.

**Table 15.2 A Comparison of Benign and Malignant Tumors**

| Trait | Benign Tumor | Malignant Tumor |
|---|---|---|
| Method of growth | Grows by expansion, displacing normal tissue | Invades, destroys, or incorporates adjacent structures |
| Metastasis | Does not metastasize | Most metastasize and develop distant colonies |
| Rate of growth | Usually slow; may be self-limiting | Grows slowly or rapidly |
| Architecture | Encapsulated | Not encapsulated |
| Potential for harm | Most without lethal potential, but may grow to the point of compressing other cells or adjacent organs | Almost always has a lethal potential by killing the host by destroying essential cells; must be removed or destroyed |

In all living things known to get cancer, the disease process begins when something goes wrong within the cell's replication mechanism. Instead of an orderly and controlled pattern of growth and replacement, the abnormal cell follows a disorderly pattern of irregular and uncontrolled growth. How an error is introduced into the cell is poorly understood. Errors may result from many factors. Chemicals from the environment, solar radiation, X rays or other radiation, foods, and food additives are all implicated to some extent in cancer causation. Some cancers may be caused by certain viruses. In addition, there simply may be random breakdowns in the cell giving rise to viable but abnormal new cells.

Few abnormal cells survive long enough to do much harm. They are seldom as virulent as normal, healthy cells. They may simply die or be eliminated by the body's immune system. But in the person with cancer, at least one abnormal cell survives and begins to engage in processes that may lead to the destruction of the host.

Some abnormal cells produce a lump or swelling called a **tumor** or **neoplasm.** Rarely do these swellings become a threat. The lump you get after bumping your head is, after all, only an accumulation of fluid and other cellular material underneath the skin. Even a tumor resulting from abnormal cell growth is usually not cancerous. Most lumps or tumors are classified as **benign,** and do not pose an immediate threat. **Malignant** tumors are cancerous though, and almost always are life threatening.

These two types of tumors differ in many ways. Benign tumors are almost always enclosed in a fibrous sheath or capsule. The cells that comprise benign tumors have the same physical characteristics of the normal surrounding tissue. Benign tumors grow by expansion only, and seldom penetrate surrounding areas. They do not spread to distant parts of the body. Warts and moles are familiar benign tumors.

Malignant tumors do not confine themselves to the site of the body in which they arise. With rare exception, malignant tumors are not encapsulated and do not resemble surrounding cells. They fail to respond to normal growth-control mechanisms. They invade surrounding tissues, and often spread to distant parts of the body, a process known as **metastasis.**

Though not cancerous, benign tumors can be dangerous. A benign tumor inside the skull may give rise to a fatal stroke if it inhibits blood from reaching the brain. Benign tumors as large as basketballs have been surgically removed from people after causing a deficiency in blood flow to vital organs, producing pain and interfering with digestion and other bodily functions.

While malignant tumors can produce the same kind of results, their principal threat arises from their ability to metastasize. Metastasis begins when a cell or cell mass breaks away from its primary site, and is carried by the blood or lymph fluid elsewhere in the body. If even one cancerous cell exists, it has the potential of developing into billions of destructive cells. (See table 15.2.)

There are four major types of cancer, named according to the tissue from which they arise. **Carcinomas** are cancers of epithelial tissue such as the skin or the mucous membranes that line organs. **Sarcomas** are cancers originating in connective or supporting tissues such as bone, cartilage, fibrous tissue, and muscle. **Leukemias** are cancers of the blood-forming parts of the body, primarily the bone marrow and the spleen. *Lymphomas* arise in the lymphatic system.

**Table 15.3 Carcinogens and Occupations**

| Occupation | Suspected Carcinogen | Type of Cancer |
|---|---|---|
| Automobile mechanic | Petroleum products | Larynx, lung, nasal passages, scrotum, skin |
| Carpenter | Wood dusts | Nasal passages, sinus cavity |
| Dyer | Benzene and other aromatics | Bladder, leukemia |
| Farmer | Ultraviolet rays of the sun | Skin |
| Miner | Arsenic, asbestos, coal, iron oxide, uranium | (Liver, lung, skin); (lung); (bladder, larynx, lung, scrotum, skin); (larynx, lung); (bone, lung, skin) |
| Painter | Benzene | Leukemia |
| Rubber worker | Vinyl chloride | Liver |
| Textile worker | Cadmium | Kidney, lung, prostate |

# PERSONAL AND SOCIAL ISSUES IN CANCER CAUSATION

There will be approximately 870,000 new cases of cancer diagnosed and some 450,000 cancer deaths recorded in the U.S. this year.[6] Cancer is the second leading cause of death in the U.S., and has been called "the most feared of all diseases."[7] One person in four develops cancer.

While the mechanism that sparks abnormal cell development in human beings is not completely understood, some conditions are so frequently associated with cancer development that they are identified as predisposing factors. Montague Lane divides them into three categories: occupational factors, medical factors, and social factors.[8] To this list can be added a fourth category: biological factors.

## Occupational Factors

A number of agents found in occupational settings may be related to specific types of cancer. In their extensive review of avoidable cancer risks, Richard Doll and Richard Peto[9] estimate that at least 4 percent of all cancer deaths result from occupational exposures. Some of the agents encountered in various occupations are summarized in table 15.3.

Asbestos, one of the known occupational carcinogens, has recently received attention. Because of its flame- and friction-retardant properties, asbestos is used in the automotive industry (brake linings), shipbuilding industry, and construction industry (insulation). It probably poses its greatest health threat, however, to workers involved in asbestos mining and milling. The tiny asbestos fibers lodge in the lung, producing a condition known as **chronic obstructive lung disease.** This condition may be a precursor to an otherwise-rare form of lung cancer. Since asbestos has been used traditionally in the walls and ceilings of schools and other buildings, millions of people inadvertently may have received years of exposure to fibers. Other products now are substituted for asbestos where possible in construction projects. Because of the efforts of health personnel, scientists, labor-union personnel, and legislators, employers are now required by law to inform employees of known or suspected carcinogens in the work setting, and to take precautionary measures to minimize risk.

## Medical Factors

Medical exposure to carcinogens results from such things as radiation, hormonal drugs, chemotherapeutic agents, and immunosuppressive drugs. As many as 2,000 fatal cases of cancer are estimated to result annually from radiation exposure.[10]

Exactly how much radiation exposure is safe is unknown. Several factors, though, are considered crucial. Radiation is known to have a cumulative effect. Small doses spread over years are not as harmful, however, as a single large dose. For years, the calibration of X-ray equipment was inadequate.

Doses were sometimes greater than intended. Radiation was also scattered rather than directed at a particular target site. With improvement in both diagnostic and therapeutic radiation techniques, it is probable that radiation-induced cancer will diminish as a problem.

Another celebrated example of cancer arising from medical exposure involves the substance diethylstilbestrol or DES. DES was prescribed from the 1940s through the 1960s to women who experienced complications like bleeding or diabetes during pregnancy, or who were believed to be at risk of a miscarriage.[11] Several million pregnant women were treated with DES.

In 1971, scientists found a link between DES and a cancer of the female reproductive organs. The cancer did not affect the women who actually took the drug; instead, it affected their daughters. DES and DES-type drugs are no longer prescribed for pregnant women. They do continue to be used for a number of other medical problems, however. For instance, DES-type drugs are useful in treating some of the undesirable symptoms of menopause, and certain kinds of cancer of the breast and prostate. DES is also used as a "morning-after" birth-control pill in cases of rape and incest.

## Social Factors

Without much doubt, the largest percentage of fatal cancers result from social exposures, especially to tobacco and alcohol. In fact, Lane estimates that 30 percent of all cancer deaths are attributable to the use of tobacco and alcohol.[12] About 70 percent of these deaths are from lung cancer.

The Surgeon General's 1979 report, *Smoking and Health,* identifies several trends in the smoking activity of Americans. There appears to be an overall decline in the number of adults who smoke, particularly among males. However, an increasing number of smokers are smoking more heavily. Mortality and morbidity rates are lower for smokers of low-tar and nicotine cigarettes, the consumption of which now represents 40 percent of all cigarette sales. The gains made by changing to low-tar and nicotine brands may be negated, however, if smokers inhale more deeply or smoke more cigarettes to achieve the effect of higher tar and nicotine cigarettes.

While there is no evidence that alcohol is carcinogenic in itself, it does appear to act with other factors to cause cancers in the digestive tract. Because of its link to cirrhosis of the liver, alcohol may be at least indirectly responsible for the development of cancer of the liver as well.

There has recently been an increasing interest in the role of diet in both cancer causation and prevention. Dietary practices are closely related to tradition and culture, and certain cancers are linked to specific behaviors involving food preparation and consumption. In Japan, fish lovers enjoy such delicacies as salmon, salmon eggs, or codfish eggs, all heavily salted and seasoned. These large quantities of salt in the diet have been associated with inflated rates of stomach cancer that exist worldwide, wherever salted fish is a staple.

Certain food additives are linked to some cancers. Most additives, though, serve useful purposes. Some provide protection from spoilage; some mask an otherwise unappetizing color; others enhance flavor. A wise consumer must weigh these benefits against the potential risks. The great American hot dog, for instance, contains **sodium nitrite,** which adds color and acts as a preservative. Sodium nitrite is converted, when ingested, into suspected carcinogenic substances known as **nitrosamines.** However, the untreated hot dog is pale gray, instead of the familiar red and must be both fresh and carefully prepared to avoid growth of the bacteria that produce deadly botulism.

Other food additives have been associated with cancer. Artificial sweeteners, for example, have been the subject of much controversy. The first artificial sweeteners to come under suspicion and scrutiny were the **cyclamates.** Introduced in the 1950s and popularized in diet soft drinks during the 1960s, cyclamates were linked to bladder tumors. Because these substances had produced such tumors in laboratory rats, cyclamates were removed from the market in the U.S. in 1969. Cyclamates remain available in Canada today, and subsequent tests revealed that the initial conclusions about their carcinogenicity may have been incorrect.[13]

Another popular artificial sweetener, **saccharin,** came under attack in 1977. Canadian studies involving both humans and laboratory animals provided evidence that saccharin intake substantially increased one's risk of bladder cancer. The Canadian government banned the use of saccharin following publication of these studies.[14] When the U.S.

**Figure 15.8**
Efforts by the FDA to ban products containing saccharin resulted in great protest.

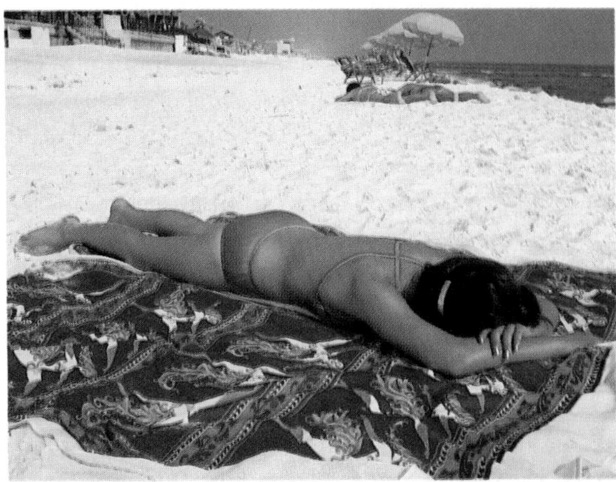

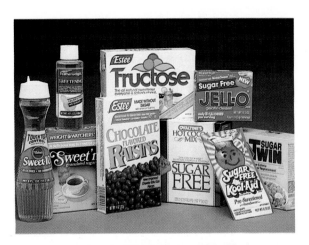

**Figure 15.9**
Sunbathers are susceptible to skin cancer from the sun's ultraviolet rays.

Food and Drug Administration announced its intent to carry out a similar ban, there was a loud protest from consumers. People raced to their grocers to buy up popular substances containing saccharin. Today, products containing saccharin are labeled with warning messages like those found on cigarette packages. Ironically, saccharin remains available in the U.S. today, but not in Canada, just the opposite of cyclamates. (See figure 15.8.)

Irish physician Denis Burkitt noted that cancer of the colon was second only to lung cancer as a cause of cancer death in Western Europe and North America, but was virtually nonexistent in East Africa and some other parts of the world. Africans, he observed, ate about three times the amount of fiber (e.g., fruits, vegetables, whole grain cereals) consumed by westerners, who process most of the fiber out of their food. Burkitt reasoned that fiber's ability to absorb liquids and its general indigestibility made it pass rapidly through the digestive tract, presumably removing carcinogenic substances in the process before they could do damage.[15]

Some investigators feel that it is the western diet of red meat and animal fats that is responsible for the high incidence of colon cancer. In many western countries, fats from beef, pork, lamb, fried foods, and cheese and other milk products account for 40 percent or more of the caloric intake. By contrast, in Japan, other Asian countries, and the East African countries studied by Burkitt where colon cancer is rare, fats constitute only 10 to 12 percent of the caloric intake.

The pursuit of the golden tan is yet another socio-cultural behavior that can have grave consequences. A tan provides various subtle messages in North America and elsewhere in the world. To some people, it represents affluence, indicating that the possessor can afford the Florida vacation, the Caribbean cruise, or the exotic "good life" described in travel brochures. To other people, a bronzed appearance is symbolic of health, of a rugged exterior, or of being in touch with nature. To still others, a tan is sensual or symbolic of sexual prowess. (See figure 15.9.)

For whatever reason a tan is pursued, sun worshipers are susceptible to the most common of all malignancies to attack humankind—skin cancer from the sun's ultraviolet rays. There are several varieties of skin cancer. They form on or near the surface of exposed areas of skin. Fortunately, skin cancers grow slowly, usually remain localized, and seldom metastasize. These qualities make them treatable, usually on an outpatient basis.

More dangerous is a skin cancer known as **melanoma.** Melanomas are cancers of the cells that produce **melanin,** the pigment that gives skin its color. Melanomas are life threatening if they metastasize. Although they are more likely to occur on exposed areas of the body, they may also occur on covered areas. A change in the appearance of a mole may signal the development of melanoma, and should promptly be examined by a physician.

Other socio-cultural factors seemingly related to cancer incidence include having multiple sex partners (cancer of the cervix), being obese (cancers of the uterus and gallbladder), being beyond age 30 during one's first pregnancy (breast cancer), and never having borne children (ovarian cancer). Not all of these relationships can be explained readily. However, even if cause-and-effect relationships are eventually confirmed, it is unlikely that significant life-style changes would result without accompanying and profound cultural changes.

### Biological Factors

Heredity does not appear to be a major predisposing factor in human cancer. Although some forms of cancer seem to "run in a family," such as breast cancer in mother, daughter, and sister, heredity does not explain most cancers. Obscuring the role of heredity is the fact that family members frequently observe similar life-styles, eat the same foods, and have nearly identical environmental exposures for much of their lives. They may therefore have similar carcinogenic exposure risk but no unique hereditary predisposition.

As cells and tissues grow older, they are less able to repair themselves, and may be more susceptible to abnormal activity. By the age of twenty-five, risk begins to increase, with more cancers showing up in women until about age fifty-five, when cancer starts to occur more often in men. Some authorities believe that if other diseases, such as those of the cardiovascular system, did not claim so many lives prematurely, cancer would ultimately cause nearly everyone's death.

Gender appears to be a factor in the development of some cancers. While breast cancer can indeed occur in men, it is nearly 132 times more common in women.[16] The role of gender is a difficult one to assess because of the intervention of life-style variables. For instance, thirty years ago, when cigarette smoking was a male-dominated behavior, lung cancer was virtually unknown in females. Today, more women than ever are smoking cigarettes, and lung cancer has become the leading cause of cancer deaths for both men and women. This link between changing life-styles and the resultant growth in lung cancer among women dispels some earlier views about the relation between gender and susceptibility to cancer.[17]

Research with human viruses has given rise to many suspected carcinogens. The herpes virus, which causes cold sores, fever blisters, and the sexually transmitted disease that bears its name, may be one culprit. It has been implicated as a factor in some cases of cervical cancer.[18]

## CANCER INCIDENCE AND MORTALITY

As previously mentioned, approximately 870,000 new cases of cancer are diagnosed per year, and 450,000 people die of their cancers.[19] While cancer can strike at virtually any part of the body, it most commonly develops at the sites indicated in figure 15.10. The most important cancers include lung cancer, colon and rectum cancer, breast cancer, uterine cancer, and testicular cancer.

### Lung Cancer

Lung cancer is the leading cause of cancer death among both men and women. It is estimated that as many as three-fourths of lung cancers would not occur if people did not smoke cigarettes. Lung cancer metastasizes easily and is one of the most virulent and difficult of all cancers to treat. It is seldom diagnosed in its early stages. Even with the most radical of therapeutic procedures, the five-year survival rate among lung cancer patients is less than 10 percent. Moreover, the survival rate with respect to lung cancer has not changed markedly in the past forty years, and no significant change in this rate is on the horizon.

### Colon and Rectum Cancer

Cancers of these two sites are sometimes referred to as the "cancers no one talks about."[20] As mentioned previously, dietary habits related to fat and fiber intake may be responsible, in part, for the relatively high U.S. incidence of these cancers.

Because colo-rectal cancer tends to metastasize slowly, early detection can often result in complete cure through surgery and follow-up therapy. Delayed diagnosis, however, makes treatment more difficult. Changes in bowel habits and stool consistency,

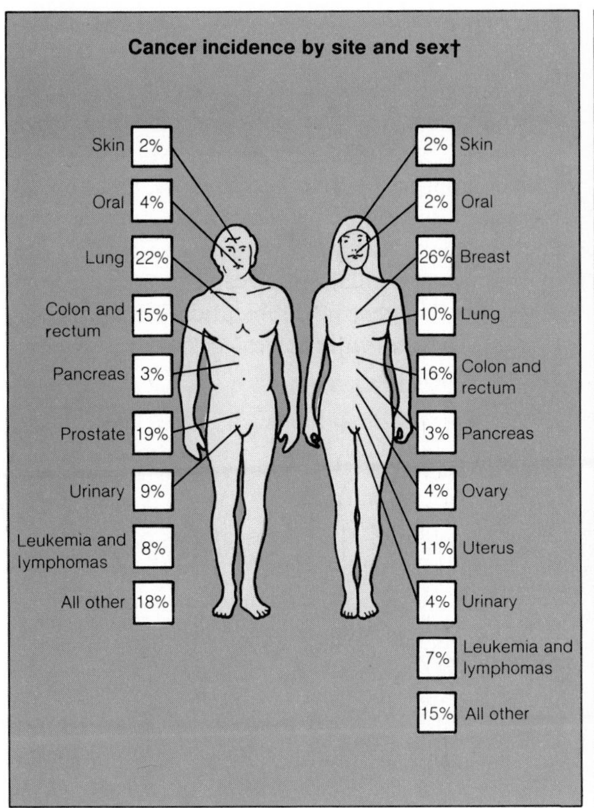


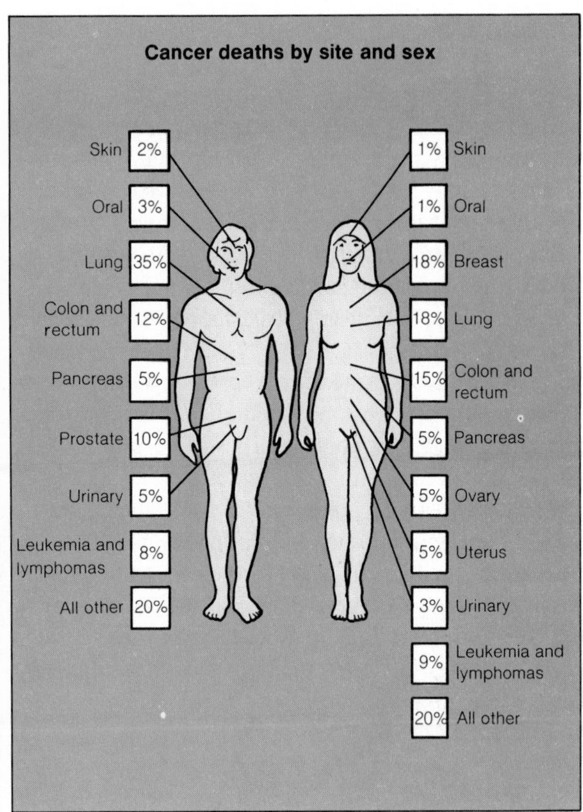


†Excluding non-melanoma skin cancer and carcinoma in situ

**Figure 15.10**
Cancer incidence and deaths by site and sex—1985 estimates. *Source:* Reprinted by permission of the American Cancer Society.

or rectal bleeding not attributable to hemorrhoids is cause for a medical checkup. As with other cancers, survival rate is dependent upon the actual site and stage of development.

## Breast Cancer

Cancer of the breast is the number-two cancer killer of women. Early detection of breast cancer is essential for successful treatment. With early detection and treatment, breast cancer can show a five-year survival rate as high as 87 percent. Delayed diagnosis can reduce the options for treatment and the probability of long-term survival to less than 50 percent. Under the age of thirty-five, the risk of breast cancer is minimal. Risk increases with age; about 75 percent of breast cancer patients are over the age of fifty. Women with a personal history of breast cancer are at high risk, as are women who have a history of breast cancer in their family (grandmother, mother, or sister).[21] Women with breast lumps or thickenings, nipple discharges, or other abnormalities may also be at greater risk.

Besides a lump, thickening, swelling, puckering, or dimpling of the breast, any persistent skin irritation of the breast or nipple can signify breast cancer. Changes in the shape or appearance of the nipples or areolae should be reported to a physician, as should unusual pain or breast tenderness. Breast self-examination (BSE) should be practiced on a monthly basis as a means of early detection. A physician or nurse practitioner can usually teach the BSE procedure in a few moments, and provide important performance feedback to the woman. Pamphlets that outline the steps of BSE are widely available as well. Women should ask their physicians for these pamphlets, or inquire about them through local affiliates of the American Cancer Society (ACS).

### Uterine Cancer

Most uterine cancers arise in the cervix, the "neck" of the uterus that descends to the posterior end of the vagina, or in the lining of the uterus. For both of these sites, early symptoms include unusual bleeding or discharge. At its earliest stage a tumor can be confined to a single area, allowing for a relatively uncomplicated surgical removal. The lack of early detection and prompt treatment permits metastasis to occur.

The Pap test, named for its creator, George N. Papanicolaou, is an examination of cells taken from the cervix to detect abnormalities. The procedure takes minutes to administer, creates only minor discomfort, and can be performed in a physician's office. If the test reveals any abnormality, additional diagnostic techniques may be necessary. While highly effective in detecting cervical cancer, the Pap test is less effective in detecting cancer of the uterine lining. Other diagnostic techniques are available, however.

### Testicular Cancer

Although testicular cancer represents only 1 percent of all cancers in the male, it is the most frequently occurring type of solid tumor seen in late adolescence and early adulthood.[22] Unfortunately, many adolescent males are unaware of this potentially dangerous type of cancer. Because of the seriousness of testicular cancer and the importance of early detection to allow for effective treatment, testicular self-examination (TSE) is now being promoted.[23]

## CANCER TREATMENT

At the turn of the century there was no proven treatment for cancer. Recent information indicates that about one-half of all patients in the U.S. who have cancer can be cured.[24] Four particular treatments are presently used, separately and in combination, depending on the stage of the disease at the time of diagnosis, and the aggressiveness of the individual cancer. These treatments include surgery, radiotherapy, chemotherapy, and immunotherapy. A fifth treatment, psychotherapy, is as yet unproven.

### Surgery

The development of successful cancer surgery was dependent on the development of modern medical technology, including blood transfusions, antibiotics, improved surgical techniques, and new anesthetics. Surgery is now the most common weapon against cancer. If tumors are confined to their sites of origin, surgery alone often can accomplish a complete cure. Surgery in combination with additional therapy can frequently achieve positive results, even after metastasis.

### Radiotherapy

About one-half of all cancer patients receive radiation treatment, either alone or combined with surgery or chemotherapy. Radiotherapy is based on the fact that X rays stop cell growth, and do so somewhat selectively. That is, X rays are more effective in destroying abnormal cells than in destroying healthy cells.

Surgery and radiotherapy share some similar limitations. Both are local forms of treatment, and therefore do not impact on tumor cells that have been shed into the blood. Both forms of treatment, by necessity, must do some damage to healthy tissue. Radiotherapy, while a useful tool, has drawbacks that require considerable research and continued technologic improvement.

### Chemotherapy

More than fifty different cancer drugs are now used in the U.S. Chemotherapy, or drug therapy, has a major advantage over surgery and radiotherapy in that it is useful for treatment of diffuse tumors, such as leukemias, and malignancies that have metastasized. Chemotherapy has produced astounding results for some forms of cancer.

A case in point is Hodgkin's disease. Precision X-ray treatments combined with chemotherapy have increased five-year survival rates to 70 percent for advanced disease patients, and 90 percent for patients whose disease is detected early. Significant improvements in survival have also been accomplished for cancers at several other sites.

Cancer chemotherapy has many side effects. Some side effects, such as nausea and vomiting, may be immediate and of short duration but intense.

Though time passes and the patient begins to feel better, the prospect of another treatment day and the return of the unpleasantness must be faced. Side effects such as hair loss, weight loss, and fatigue are both less immediate and more cumulative in nature. Their presence, however, may be damaging to the patient's self-image and act as a constant reminder of the disease.

Many experimental drugs are presently undergoing clinical study to determine their effectiveness and safety. For the time being, existing drugs are saving many lives of cancer patients who only a few years ago would have been without hope.

### Immunotherapy

Immunotherapy, the newest approach to cancer management, is based upon a search for ways to stimulate the body's defenses to fight cancer cells. The goal is to accomplish the type of immune system mobilization that occurs when the body fights off chicken pox, an infected cut, or the common cold.

A problem is that since cancerous cells come from within the body, the body does not recognize them as hostile or alien. Thus, the immune system is not stimulated. Another problem relates to the fact that cancer is a collection of diseases rather than a single disease. There is, therefore, little chance of a single "immunization" being able to build up the body's resistance to all forms of cancer. Promising results are now coming from the world's laboratories, though.

Scientists recently became excited over an antiviral protein produced in the body, called **interferon,** which helps to combat colds, influenza, and possibly cancer as well. However, theories that attempt to explain interferon's actual role in cancer management still greatly outnumber facts. In addition, interferon is expensive to produce and retrieve in pure form. While early experiments hint that interferon may be useful in cancer management, it is likely to be many years before sufficient research evidence substantiates these claims.

## CANCER QUACKERY

Cancer quackery is a multi-million-dollar industry in the U.S. alone each year. When cancer strikes, many people do foolish, irresponsible, or dangerous things. One of the things they do is turn to "quacks." These practitioners offer the cancer patient friendly attentiveness, hope, or "secret" cures. The person with cancer may be desperate, so the practitioner who can make these offers has appeal. Quacks may be professionally educated physicians. However, many times they have no degree and no medical education whatsoever. (See Exhibit 15.4.)

15.4 EXHIBIT 15.4

### Investigators Testify: Billions Wasted Annually on Dangerous 'Cures'

When 7-year-old Chuckie Peters was diagnosed as having leukemia, Paulette Peters did what most mothers would do—she panicked. She helplessly watched the devastating effects of spinal taps, bone marrow aspirations, biopsies, chemotherapy, and radiation therapy.

Seeking a way to sustain her son's strength, Paulette turned to Robert Baldwin, MD, a retired Texas physician. He urged a diet of vitamins, herbs, and fresh fruits and vegetables, and referred her to the American International Hospital in Zion, Ill.

Physicians there said Chuckie should be pulled off chemotherapeutic drugs before he suffered "injurious side effects" or "irreversible damage." Special vitamin A injections would boost his immune system, they advised.

Not long after undergoing such treatment, Chuckie began experiencing waves of nausea and itching of his skin. Suddenly sensitive to light, he asked that his bedroom be darkened. His right arm was seized by spasms and jerked when he tried to eat. Each day brought more pain.

15.4 *continued* EXHIBIT 15.4

The diagnosis: vitamin A toxicity. Emergency hospitalization revealed severe cranial swelling and bone inflammation. "Three years of chemotherapy never produced the pain he experienced during 3½ months of vitamin A therapy," his mother said. Two months after discharge, he was confined to a wheelchair, unable to attend school.

Chuckie still is alive—having survived both the treatment and the disease.

Edith Schneider will not be so lucky. Her physicians gave her a 95 percent chance of recovery from breast cancer if she underwent a mastectomy. Fearful of surgery, however, Mrs. Schneider went to New York City's Institute of Applied Biology, where Emanuel Revici, MD, gave her injections of selenium to "burn the cancer out of her body." The tumor, once the size of a marble, now resembles a baseball. The diagnosis: terminal.

Thousands of patients have been harmed by such "quack" cures, according to an investigation recently completed by a subcommittee of the House Select Committee on Aging.

The elderly are its most frequent victims. Older people—because they are trusting, unfamiliar with modern remedies, and most frequently in need of medical help—are quick to welcome strangers who take an interest in their health, the congressional investigators discovered.

Roughly $10 billion each year is wasted on these bogus "cures," the investigation found. Americans spend an average of $44 a year per person on unproven therapies, compared with 25 cents on senility research, 35 cents on arthritis research, and $4.40 on cancer research. "This money could be routed into a search for legitimate cures," said Val J. Halamandaris, who initiated the congressional inquiry.

More than 75 percent of these so-called cures are dangerous or potentially dangerous. Fewer than 5 percent offer any benefits; of these, the benefits are cosmetic and expensive.

Purveyors of such "cures" are inventive—quick to capture the desperate imagination. Cancer victims are offered such "cures" as ground-up diamonds, a tonic made from warts of horses, or serums drawn from human urine and feces.

Such cures, although comical, have dangerous consequences. "By the time many of these people realize they have been deceived, it may be too late to prevent serious consequences. Patients often aggravate existing conditions, or even die needlessly, because they utilize an unproven or useless treatment," Harrison L. Rogers Jr., MD, speaker of the American Medical Association House of Delegates, told members of the subcommittee.

"It's a new dimension of murder," said Helene Brown of the American Cancer Society (ACS). "Survival rates [with accepted treatment] approach 90 percent for breast cancer, 82 percent for cervical cancer, and 77 percent for colon-rectal cancer. These quack "cures" deny patients life-saving treatment," she added.



## DISCUSSION QUESTIONS

1. Do you agree with Helene Brown of the American Cancer Society when she states "Cancer quackery is a new dimension of murder"?

2. What do you think can and should be done to deal with the problem of disease-cure quackery?

Responsible physicians do not offer secret cures or make guarantees about treatment interventions. Quack treatments can be especially dangerous to the patient who has early-stage cancer. Trying useless gadgets or therapeutically worthless drugs is costly and wastes valuable time. Quacks may have no conscience about telling patients that they have cancer when in fact they do not. After a series of worthless, but expensive "treatments," the patient is declared "cured." The practitioner takes the credit, which opens the door for the testimonial and exploitation of more people. Quacks cannot be recognized by their appearance alone. They are smart, friendly, and impressively attired. They provide warmth, act concerned, and give reassurance to patients who are filled with anxiety.

## CANCER PREVENTION AND EARLY DETECTION

The technology needed to prevent cancer or detect it early (when therapy is most beneficial) is evolving. As a result of new knowledge, the American Cancer Society provides the recommendations for prevention and early detection contained in this section. Important cancer risk factors are summarized in table 15.4.

As previously mentioned, certain dietary factors have been statistically associated with both the cause of some cancers and the prevention of others.

**Table 15.4 Summary of Cancer's Risk Factors**

**Colo-rectal**
- History of rectal polyps
- Rectal polyps run in family
- History of ulcerative colitis
- Blood in stool
- Over age forty

**Lung**
- Heavy cigarette smoker over age fifty
- Started smoking before age fifteen
- Smoker working with/near asbestos

**Uterine—Endometrial**
- Unusual bleeding or discharge
- Late menopause (after age fifty-five)
- Diabetes, high blood pressure, and overweight
- Over age fifty

**Uterine—Cervical**
- Unusual bleeding or discharge
- Frequent sex in early teens or with many partners
- Low socioeconomic background
- Poor care during or following pregnancy

**Breast**
- Lump or nipple discharge
- History of breast cancer
- Close relative with history of breast cancer
- Over age thirty-five; especially over age fifty
- Never had children; first child after age thirty

**Skin**
- Excessive exposure to sun
- Fair complexion
- Work with coal tar, pitch, or creosote

**Oral**
- Heavy smoker and drinker
- Poor oral hygiene

**Ovary**
- History of ovarian cancer among close relatives
- Over age fifty
- Never had children

**Prostate**
- Over age sixty
- Difficulty in urinating

**Stomach**
- History of stomach cancer among close relatives
- Diet heavy in smoked, pickled, or salted foods

In February 1984, the American Cancer Society, in a joint statement with the National Cancer Institute and the National Academy of Sciences, made the following seven recommendations with respect to diet and cancer:

1. Avoid obesity. A twelve-year ACS study of more than a million Americans showed that overweight persons were at greater risk of cancer, especially if 40 percent or more overweight.
2. Eat less fat. Persons who eat less fat have significantly lower rates of cancer of the breast, colon, and prostate.
3. Eat more high-fiber foods. This recommendation remains controversial, but even if the lack of fiber in the diet is not an independent risk factor in the development of colon and other cancers, the addition of more fiber is a wholesome substitute for fatty and high-calorie foods.
4. Include adequate supplies of vitamins A and C in the diet. This statement is not the same as saying "have an excessive amount." High levels of vitamin A are toxic, but at recommended daily levels they may introduce protective factors.
5. Eat "cruciferous" vegetables such as cabbage, broccoli, brussels sprouts, kohlrabi, and cauliflower. There is evidence that these vegetables are protective against some chemically induced cancers.
6. Consume alcoholic beverages in moderation. Heavy alcohol consumption is linked to cancers of the oral cavity, larynx, esophagus, and liver.
7. Minimize intake of salt-cured, smoked, and nitrite-cured foods. There is evidence that foods prepared by these processes, when eaten in excess, contribute to cancers of the stomach and esophagus.

Lung cancer and nonmelanoma skin cancer are the best examples of malignancies largely preventable through prudent life-style choice. Since lung cancer is related to cigarette smoking, the best prevention against it is never to start smoking, to quit or reduce smoking if you already smoke, or to change to a lower-tar brand. Smoking-cessation programs have helped many smokers overcome dependency on cigarettes. Some of these programs are discussed in chapter 13.

If you must pursue the golden tan, or if prolonged exposure to the sun is unavoidable, you can still minimize the risks. Special caution should be exercised when in the mountains, where thin air transmits more of the sun's ultraviolet rays, or near water, where they are multiplied. When you are in the sun, be cautious:

1. Wear light clothing and a hat to protect exposed areas.
2. Use lotions that block the sun's rays and apply them often, especially after swimming. Sunscreen products are those that contain para-aminobenzoic acid (PABA) or related ingredients. They are graded from 2 to 15, with the higher numbers providing greater screening protection.
3. Avoid using baby, mineral, olive, or vegetable oils during exposure. Although these products may moisturize the skin, they also enhance the burning power of the sun.
4. Avoid exposure during the midday hours when the sun's rays are particularly damaging. During the summer months, these hours are approximately 10:00 A.M. to 2:00 P.M.
5. Be aware of hazy or partially overcast days. Ultraviolet radiation can penetrate haze or clouds.

Methods for early detection of many cancers are described in table 15.5. Most of these procedures require a visit to a physician's office. One test that can be self-administered by women is monthly breast self-examination (BSE). (See Activity for Wellness 15.2.) Although a woman's risk of breast cancer remains low until she is in her forties, BSE is encouraged among women in their twenties and thirties, as well as among older women. (See Activity for Wellness 15.3.) BSE allows the woman to become familiar with the feel and texture of normal breast tissue. Unfamiliar lumps or changes can then be identified more easily.

An early-detection test for testicular cancer in men can also be self-administered. The procedure for testicular self-examination (TSE) is easy to perform. (See Activity for Wellness 15.4.)

15.2 ACTIVITY FOR WELLNESS 15.2

# Breast Self-Examination

1. In the shower:

Examine your breasts during bath or shower; hands glide easier over wet skin. Fingers flat, move gently over every part of each breast. Use the right hand to examine the left breast, left hand for the right breast. Check for any lump, hard knot, or thickening.

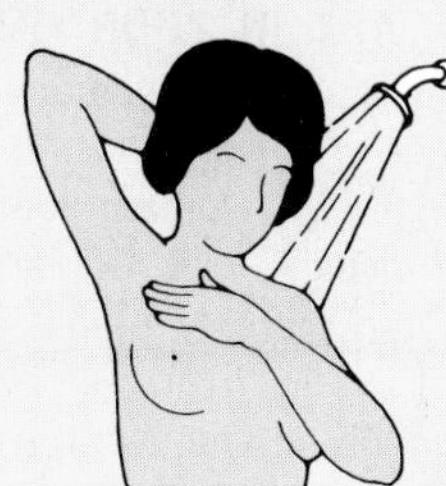

2. Before a mirror:

Inspect your breasts with arms at your sides. Next, raise your arms high overhead. Look for any changes in the contour of each breast: a swelling, dimpling of skin, or changes in the nipple.

Then rest palms on hips and press down firmly to flex your chest muscles. Left and right breast will not exactly match; few women's breasts do.

Regular inspection shows what is normal for you and will give you confidence in your examination.

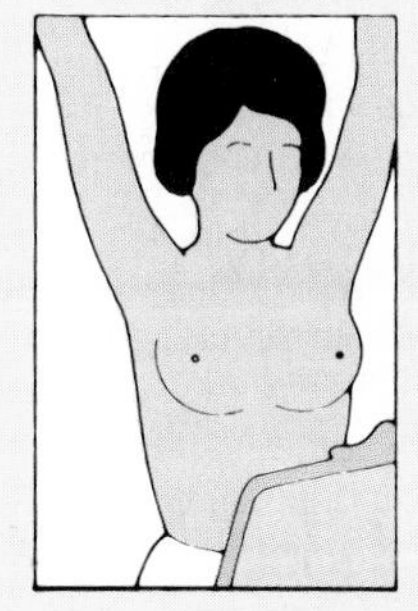

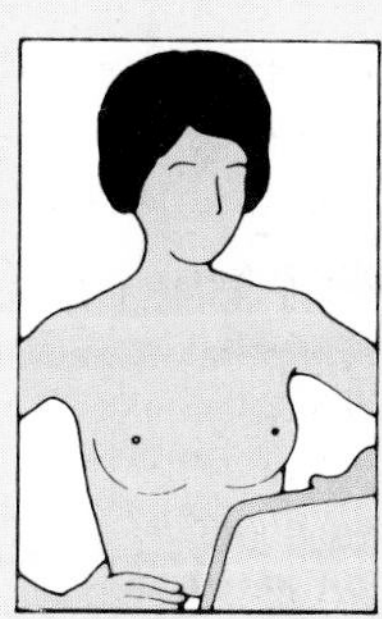

3. Lying down:

To examine your right breast, put a pillow or folded towel under your right shoulder. Place right hand behind your head—this distributes breast tissue more evenly on the chest. With left hand, fingers flat, press gently in small circular motions around an imaginary clock face. Begin at outermost top of your right breast for 12 o'clock, then move to 1 o'clock, and so on around the circle back to 12. A ridge of firm tissue in the lower curve of each breast is normal. Then move in an inch, toward the nipple, keep circling to examine *every part of your breast,* including nipple. This requires at least three more circles. Now slowly repeat procedure on your left breast with a pillow under your left shoulder and left hand behind head. Notice how your breast structure feels.

Finally, squeeze the nipple of each breast gently between thumb and index finger. Any discharge, clear or bloody, should be reported to your doctor immediately.

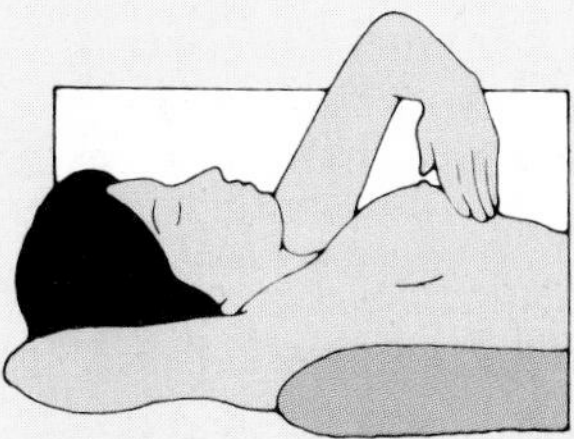

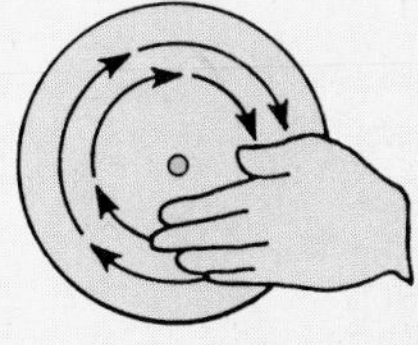

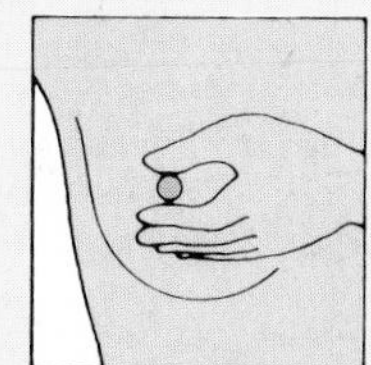

Source: Reprinted by permission of the American Cancer Society.

15.3 ACTIVITY FOR WELLNESS 15.3

# Assessing Your Risk of Breast Cancer

**THE ODDS ARE IN YOUR FAVOR . . .**
Fourteen of every fifteen women will never get breast cancer.

However, every woman needs to guard against the disease with regular physical examinations and monthly breast self-examination (BSE). Certain "risk factors" need your careful attention so you can have the advantage of early detection. When breast cancer is found early, before it has spread, the chances of cure are very high.

No woman can predict for sure whether she will or won't get breast cancer. But there is a way you can estimate your own risk, by entering the number that applies to you in each group below and adding the numbers.

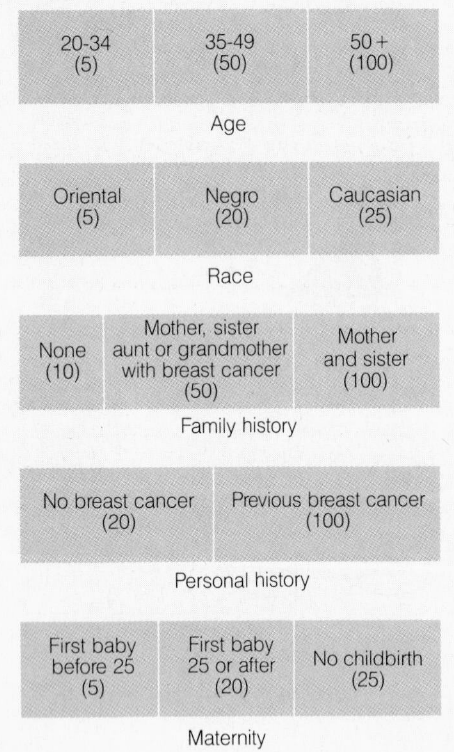

| 20-34 (5) | 35-49 (50) | 50+ (100) |
|---|---|---|

Age

| Oriental (5) | Negro (20) | Caucasian (25) |
|---|---|---|

Race

| None (10) | Mother, sister aunt or grandmother with breast cancer (50) | Mother and sister (100) |
|---|---|---|

Family history

| No breast cancer (20) | Previous breast cancer (100) |
|---|---|

Personal history

| First baby before 25 (5) | First baby 25 or after (20) | No childbirth (25) |
|---|---|---|

Maternity

**WHAT YOUR SCORE MEANS TO YOU**
*Women 225 and higher* on the scale should practice monthly breast self-examination (BSE) and have physical examination of the breast every six months, with breast X ray (mammography) annually or as the doctor may advise.

*Women between 100 and 220* on the scale should practice monthly BSE and have physical examination of the breast as part of an annual checkup. Periodic breast X ray, especially when there is a personal or family history of breast cancer, should be included as the doctor may advise. Many physicians feel an initial breast X ray for all women age 40 and over is valuable in the study of breast changes that may occur later.

*Women below 100* on the scale should practice monthly BSE and have physical examination of the breast as part of an annual checkup.

Other screening techniques being developed may also help identify women who should receive more complete testing; these can be discussed with your doctor during your annual checkup.

*All changes* . . . lumps, nipple discharge, unusual sensation or other breast change should always receive prompt, expert medical examination. No matter where you are on this scale!

Source: Reprinted by permission of the American Cancer Society.

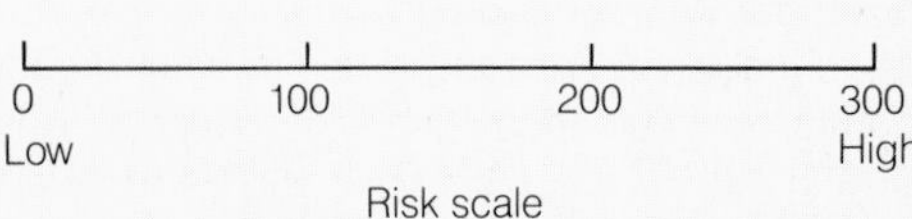

15.4 ACTIVITY FOR WELLNESS 15.4

## Testicular Self-Examination

1. Examine each testis separately with your fingers.
2. Your index finger, middle fingers, and thumb should be positioned as shown in the sketch.
3. Your testis should be gently rolled between your thumb and fingers; feel for small lumps or other abnormalities.
4. This examination ought to be conducted on a monthly basis; the best time is after a shower or hot bath when the scrotum is relaxed, and your testes are easily felt.
5. If you identify an abnormality, bring it to the attention of your physician.

Source: American Cancer Society.

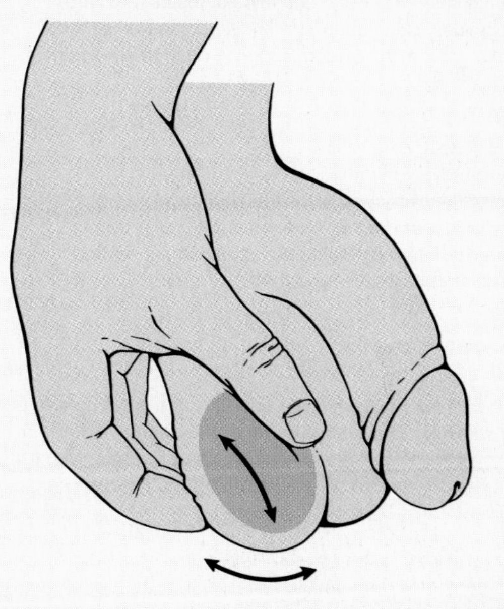

**Table 15.5 Guidelines for the Early Detection of Cancer in People without Symptoms. Talk with your doctor. Ask how these guidelines relate to you.**

**Age Twenty to Forty**

*Cancer-related Checkup Every Three Years*

Should include the procedures listed below plus health counseling (such as tips on quitting cigarettes) and examinations for cancers of the thyroid, testes, prostate, mouth, ovaries, skin and lymph nodes. Some people are at higher risk for certain cancers and may need to have tests more frequently.

*Breast*

- Exam by doctor every three years
- Self-exam every month
- One baseline breast X ray between ages thirty-five and forty. Higher risk for breast cancer: personal or family history of breast cancer, never had children, first child after age thirty.

*Uterus*

- Pelvic exam every three years

*Cervix*

- Pap test—after two initial negative tests one year apart—at least every three years, includes women under twenty if sexually active. Higher risk for cervical cancer: early age at first intercourse, multiple sex partners.

Source: © 1980, American Cancer Society, Inc.

**Table 15.5** *Continued*

**Age Forty and Over**

*Cancer-related Checkup Every Year*

Should include the procedures listed below plus health counseling (such as tips on quitting cigarettes) and examinations for cancers of the thyroid, testes, prostate, mouth, ovaries, skin, and lymph nodes. Some people are at higher risk for certain cancers and may need to have tests more frequently.

*Breast*

- Exam by doctor every year
- Self-exam every month
- Breast X ray every year after age fifty (between ages forty to fifty, ask your doctor). Higher risk for breast cancer: personal or family history of breast cancer, never had children, first child after age thirty.

*Uterus*

- Pelvic exam every year

*Cervix*

- Pap test—after two initial negative tests one year apart—at least every three years. Higher risk for cervical cancer: early age at first intercourse, multiple sex partners.

*Endometrium*

- Endometrial tissue sample at menopause if at risk. Higher risk for endometrial cancer: infertility, obesity, failure of ovulation, abnormal uterine bleeding, estrogen therapy.

*Colon and Rectum*

- Digital rectal exam every year
- Guaiac slide test every year after age fifty
- Procto exam—after two initial negative tests one year apart—every three to five years after fifty. Higher risk for colorectal cancer: personal or family history of colon or rectal cancer, personal or family history of polyps in the colon or rectum, ulcerative colitis.

Remember, these guidelines are not rules and only apply to people without symptoms. If you have any of the seven Warning Signals see your doctor or go to your clinic without delay.

Source: Reprinted by permission of the American Cancer Society.

**Table 15.6** **Cancer's Seven Warning Signals**

Change in bowel or bladder habits
A sore that does not heal
Unusual bleeding or discharge
Thickening or lump in breast or elsewhere
Indigestion or difficulty in swallowing
Obvious change in wart or mole
Nagging cough or hoarseness

If YOU have a warning signal, see your doctor!

Source: Reprinted by permission of the American Cancer Society.

Become acquainted with cancer's seven warning signals. (See table 15.6.) Although these signs of cancer are not comprehensive, they do provide a clue to the most common cancers. It is important to remember what Lane advises: "The importance of 'warning signals' is not solely early detection and treatment of cancer, but determination that the signal may not be due to cancer."[25]

## OTHER NONCOMMUNICABLE DISEASE THREATS

In addition to cardiovascular disease and cancer, there are a number of other noncommunicable diseases that threaten a person in quest of high-level wellness. Some of these diseases include diabetes, emphysema, and chronic bronchitis.

### Diabetes

Diabetes is a disease of the pancreas in which the body cannot make use of sugars and other carbohydrates in a normal way. The sixth leading cause of death in the U.S., diabetes is also a contributing cause of death due to other conditions, such as cardiovascular disease.

Normally, complex carbohydrates, when consumed, are broken down into a simple sugar called **glucose. Insulin,** a hormone produced by the pancreas, then acts on the glucose to facilitate its use by the body for energy. The diabetic either does not

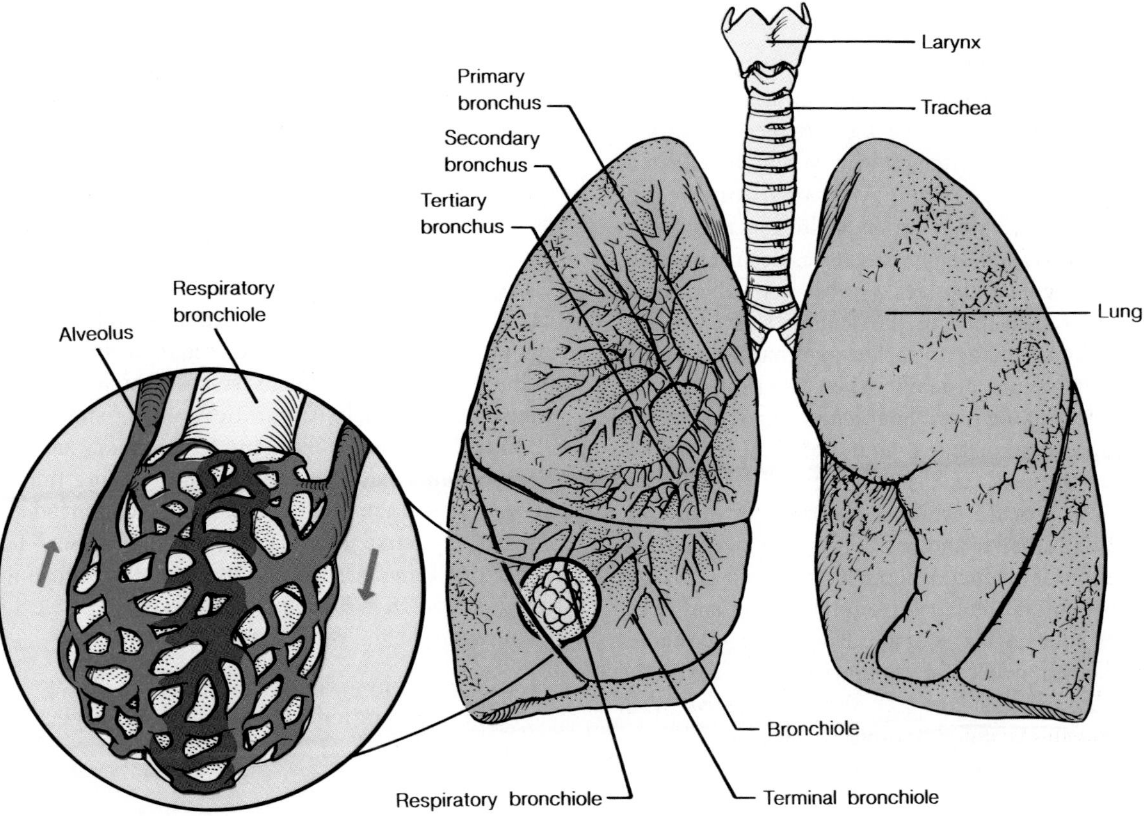


**Figure 15.11**
The bronchial tree consists of the passageways that connect the trachea and the alveoli. *Source:* From Hole, John W., Jr., ***Human Anatomy and Physiology,*** 3d ed. © 1978, 1981, 1984 Wm. C. Brown Publishers, Dubuque, Iowa. All rights reserved. Reprinted by permission.

produce sufficient insulin, or is unable to mobilize the insulin. Thus, excess glucose accumulates in the blood and may appear in the urine.

There are an estimated ten million diabetics in the U.S. Perhaps four million are unaware of their disease. It is a serious disease in itself, but even more so because of the complications which can arise. High levels of glucose in the blood can have many harmful effects. Diabetes leads to damaged or narrowed coronary arteries. It precipitates hemorrhages in the capillaries of the retina of the eye, a condition that now ranks as the leading cause of blindness in the U.S. Diabetes contributes to kidney failure, when the body's waste-and-disposal system is no longer able to maintain the body's delicate chemical balance. Furthermore, diabetes gives rise to peripheral vascular disease, in which the extremites of the body do not receive an adequate supply of blood and thus lead to tissue death. In some cases, amputation of the affected body part may be necessary.

Symptoms of diabetes include frequent urination and thirst, extreme hunger, rapid weight loss, blurred vision or a sudden change in visual acuity, easy tiring, drowsiness, or general weakness after completion of relatively simple physical tasks. If these symptoms recur or persist, consult your physician.

Simple, relatively painless tests can detect the presence of diabetes. A physician may prescribe some combination of the following therapies for diabetes: diet modification, structured exercise, insulin injections as needed, and oral medication. Diabetes cannot currently be cured, but it can be managed, especially with early detection.

## Emphysema

Emphysema is presently an incurable, destructive disease. It mainly strikes males between the ages of fifty and seventy, although women may be affected. A high percentage of emphysema patients are cigarette smokers. Air pollution is also associated with the incidence of emphysema. It has been suggested, too, that people who lack a substance called **alpha one antitrypsin** may be particularly susceptible to emphysema, and at an earlier age than normal.

Emphysema develops when the **bronchi,** passageways leading from the trachea (windpipe) to the lungs, become irritated and obstructed. Air becomes "trapped" in the lung beyond the obstruction. The bronchi are like the branches of a tree, branching smaller and smaller until they terminate in clusters of air spaces in the lung, known as **alveoli.** Oxygen enters the blood from the alveoli and is exchanged for carbon dioxide. Emphysema damages the alveolar walls; the capillaries which carry the blood for gas exchange may also be damaged. With less oxygen exchange possible, the person with emphysema experiences shortness of breath, making even simple physical tasks difficult. Even breathing is laborious for people who have advanced emphysema. Since emphysema also interferes with blood flow through the lung, the heart works harder in an effort to compensate. Under such strain, the heart may enlarge, leading to congestive heart failure.

The exact cause of emphysema is unknown, but the strong evidence of a relationship among cigarette smoking, air pollution, and emphysema suggests the wisdom of avoiding these agents.

If emphysema is diagnosed early, progressive disease may be halted. Breathing retraining, light exercises, and careful effort to minimize respiratory congestion can help people with emphysema to make the best use of their breathing capacity and lead ordinary lives.

## Chronic Bronchitis

Bronchitis is an inflammation of the lining of the bronchi. Accompanying this inflammation, typically, is an impaired air flow. Acute bronchitis, with its characteristic coughing and spitting, is often associated with the common cold or with influenza. Chronic bronchitis includes all the symptoms of the acute state, except that they are almost always present.

Bronchitis is caused by the irritation brought on by disease or infection, and contact with air pollutants. A major pollutant is cigarette smoke. The person with chronic bronchitis experiences occasional acute episodes. If the source of the acute bronchitis is bacterial infection, antibiotic therapy can provide relief. However, permanent relief of the symptoms of chronic bronchitis requires elimination of the sources of irritation to the nose, throat, mouth, sinuses, and bronchi. Cigarette smoking should be eliminated, as should exposure to secondary smoke. If a person is exposed to dust and irritating fumes at work, a change of employment is recommended. That is, of course, more easily said than done. The American Lung Association provides the following suggestions for persons particularly susceptible to frequent bronchial infections:

1. See your physician at the beginning of any cold or respiratory infection. Do not neglect even a slight cold.
2. Do not smoke.
3. Follow a nutritious diet and avoid obesity.
4. Participate in mild, but daily exercise, taking care not to tire yourself.
5. Ask your physician about being immunized against pneumococcal pneumonia and influenza.
6. Avoid exposure to colds and influenza at home or in public.[26]

# SUMMARY

1. Cardiovascular disease is the number-one cause of death in the U.S.

2. Cardiovascular disease is really several diseases that affect the heart and the circulatory system.

3. The major risk factors in cardiovascular disease include gender, age, race, cigarette smoking, hypertension, high cholesterol, and diabetes. Obesity, lack of exercise, and stress may be additional risk factors.

4. Arteriosclerosis, also known as hardening of the arteries, includes several conditions that cause the walls of the arteries to lose their elasticity. Atherosclerosis is the most common form of arteriosclerosis.

5. Hypertension is diagnosed when a systolic reading above 140 mm Hg or a diastolic reading above 90 mm Hg is obtained on a regular basis.

6. Heart attack is a nonspecific term that describes the result of any one of many cardiovascular disorders that affects the heart muscle. A heart attack occurs when part of the heart muscle is deprived of oxygen.

7. A person who experiences severe chest pain and other symptoms of a heart attack should seek prompt medical attention.

8. A stroke is a form of cardiovascular disease that affects the arteries that supply blood to the brain. A stroke occurs when part of the brain is deprived of oxygen.

9. While many high-technology procedures are available to diagnose and treat cardiovascular disease, the most economic solution to the control of this problem is through prevention.

10. Cancer ranks second to cardiovascular disease as a killer of Americans.

11. Cancer is a collection of diseases that share the trait of abnormal cell growth.

12. Benign tumors are not cancerous and pose no immediate threat to health in most cases. Malignant tumors are cancerous and are usually life threatening if not diagnosed and treated early in the disease process.

13. The causes of cancer can be grouped by occupational factors, medical factors, social factors, and biological factors.

14. Many cancers are preventable. Lung cancer could virtually be eliminated if people did not smoke cigarettes. Some skin cancers could be eliminated if people took greater precautions to avoid excessive exposure to the sun.

15. Cancers may be treated by surgery, radiotherapy, chemotherapy, or immunotherapy. Combinations of these therapies are also used.

16. Cancer quackery is a multi-million-dollar operation. People fall prey to "quacks" because of fear and desperation.

17. Not all cancers have early self-detection procedures that can be performed in the privacy of one's home. However, women can do breast self-examination (BSE), and men can perform testicular self-examination (TSE).

18. Diabetes, a major disease in and of itself, is also a principal risk factor in the development of cardiovascular disease.

19. Emphysema and chronic bronchitis are potentially serious respiratory ailments. Changes in life-style, however, can allow for a close-to-normal life.

## Recommended Readings

American Cancer Society. *Cancer Facts & Figures.* New York: 1985.

American Heart Association. *Heartbook: A Guide to Prevention and Treatment of Cardiovascular Diseases.* New York: Elsevier-Dutton, 1980.

Beattie, Edward J., Jr., and Cowan, Stuart D. *Toward the Conquest of Cancer.* New York: Crown Publishers, 1980.

Duncan, T. G. *The Diabetes Fact Book.* New York: Charles Scribner's Sons, 1982.

## References

1. American Heart Association, "Heart Facts," Dallas, Tex.: 1983.

2. Robert I. Levy, *Heart Attacks* (Washington, D.C.: U.S. Department of Health and Human Services. NIH Publication no. 81–1803, 1981).

3. Meyer Friedman and R. H. Rosenman, *Type A Behavior and Your Heart* (New York: Fawcett Books, 1978).

4. American Heart Association's Subcommittee on Exercise/Cardiac Rehabilitation, *Statement on Exercise* (Dallas, Tex.: American Heart Association, 1981).

5. P. Rubin and R. F. Bakemeier, *Clinical Oncology for Medical Students and Physicians* (New York: American Cancer Society, 1978).

6. *Cancer Facts and Figures* (New York: American Cancer Society, 1984).

7. Ruth D. Abrams, "The Patient With Cancer—His Changing Pattern of Communication," *New England Journal of Medicine* 288 (1966): 317–22.

8. Montague Lane, "Cancer Prevention: An Oncologist's Prespective," *Health Values: Achieving High Level Wellness* 6.3 (1982): 12–18.

9. Richard Doll and Richard Peto, "The Causes of Cancer: Quantitative Estimates of Avoidable Risks of Cancer in the United States Today," *Journal of the National Cancer Institute* 66 (1981): 1193–1308.

10. Doll and Peto, "The Causes of Cancer," 1193–1308.

11. National Institutes of Health, *Questions and Answers about DES Exposure before Birth* (Washington, D.C.: U.S. Department of Health, Education and Welfare. NIH Publication no. 77–1118, 1977).

12. Lane, "Cancer Prevention."

13. *Fighting Cancer* (Alexandria, Va.: Time-Life Books, 1981).

14. *Fighting Cancer.*

15. Denis P. Burkitt, "Epidemiology of Cancer of the Colon and Rectum," *Cancer* 28 (1970): 3.

16. *American Cancer Society Statistics* (New York: 1985).

17. *American Cancer Society Statistics.*

18. James H. Nelson, Jr., Henry E. Averette, and Ralph M. Richart, "Dysplasia, Carcinoma in Situ, and Early Invasive Cervical Carcinoma," *C.A.—A Cancer Journal for Clinicians* (1985): 306–27.

19. *Cancer Facts and Figures.*

20. *American Cancer Society Statisics.*

21. *Facts on Breast Cancer,* American Cancer Society.

22. Nasser Javadpour, "Germ Cell Tumor of the Testis," *CA—A Cancer Journal for Clinicians* 30 (1980): 242–55.

23. Phillip J. Marty and Robert J. McDermott, "Teaching about Testicular Cancer and Testicular Self-Examination," *Journal of School Health* 53 (1983): 351–56.

24. Vincent T. DeVita, *Cancer Treatment* (Washington, D.C.: U.S. Department of Health and Human Services. NIH Publication no. 80–1807, 1980).

25. Lane, "Cancer Prevention."

26. American Lung Association, *Chronic Bronchitis* (New York: American Lung Association, 1978).

CHAPTER SIXTEEN

# Sexually Transmitted Diseases: Threats to Wellness from the STDs



Unlike the cardiovascular diseases, cancer, and the other disease threats to wellness discussed in chapter 15, the sexually transmitted diseases, or STDs, are communicable. It is this property of communicability that makes the STDs of critical importance. Formerly called venereal diseases (VD), after Venus, the Greek goddess of love, these disorders have been around for a long time. Some of these problems are even described in the Bible: "When any man has a discharge from his penis, the discharge is unclean, whether the penis runs with it or is stopped up by it. Any bed on which he sits or lies is unclean." [Book of Leviticus]

These diseases were also known to such early physicians and scholars as Hippocrates of Cos and Claudius Galen. Most historians agree that Christopher Columbus' crew brought smallpox and other communicable diseases to the inhabitants of the New World. A lesson seldom taught in history books, however, is that the New World natives passed along syphilis and other STDs to the Spaniards whom Columbus commanded. Columbus himself was stricken with syphilis, and, along with his men, may have been responsible for introducing some types of venereal disease to Europe.

The term STD now stands for all the disorders that are transmitted through sexual contact of some kind—sexual intercourse primarily, but other forms of intimacy and sex play as well, including kissing. (See Activity for Wellness 16.1.) The control of STDs is probably a bigger problem today than at any previous time. There are numerous factors that have led to the growth of the problem.

16.1 ACTIVITY FOR WELLNESS 16.1

## Do You Know Your STD IQ?

Below are some True-False questions about STDs. They are representative of some, but not all of the important concepts contained in this chapter. By the time you have finished reading this chapter, you should be able to answer all of them correctly. Develop your own "key" to this test as you read.

_____ 1. It is possible to contract some STDs through kissing.

_____ 2. It is always easy for a person to tell if he or she has an STD.

_____ 3. STDs must always be reported to public-health authorities.

_____ 4. Most STDs are now being controlled effectively thanks to the availability of preventive vaccines.

_____ 5. Once its symptoms disappear, an STD cannot be contagious.

_____ 6. Once a person has a particular STD and is treated, he or she can never be infected with that STD again.

_____ 7. Next to the common cold, gonorrhea may be the most prevalent communicable disease in the U.S. today.

_____ 8. Untreated gonorrhea or syphilis may result in irreversible complications.

_____ 9. Condoms can be instrumental in minimizing one's personal risk of contracting many STD's.

_____ 10. Genital herpes is an incurable STD whose prevalence is rising.

_____ 11. Differential diagnosis for some STDs can be difficult since the symptoms of one STD can mimic those of another.

_____ 12. Persons treated for an STD are required by law to report the names of their sexual contacts.

## PERSONAL AND SOCIAL ISSUES RELATED TO STD CONTROL

Part of the reason why STDs pose a problem of such great magnitude stems from the fact that treatment of the infected individual solves only half the STD problem. Adequate treatment of sex partners through **contact investigation** is also necessary, although both laborious and expensive. There is even some disagreement as to who has the responsibility for contact investigation. Is it the patient? the physician? public health officials? Moreover, diagnosis of some STDs is occasionally difficult because most physicians do not screen for them on a routine basis, and some individuals, particularly women, may be infected but not notice any symptoms. The lack of early symptoms in women is characteristic of more than one of the STDs.

Also contributing to the proliferation of STDs is the fact that exact diagnosis of some STDs is extremely difficult without the availability of laboratory transfer facilities. This is especially true of such

By sexually active, we don't mean simply having a lot of sex. Instead we are using the term to mean having sex with different people.

In general, the fact of life is that sooner or later, sexually active people will either be exposed to an STD, or get one.

By STD, of course, we mean sexually transmitted disease—that group of infections spread from person to person by sexual contact. The term STD includes syphilis, gonorrhea, nongonococcal urethritis, genital herpes, trichomoniasis and more than ten other diseases, all of which are sexually transmissible.

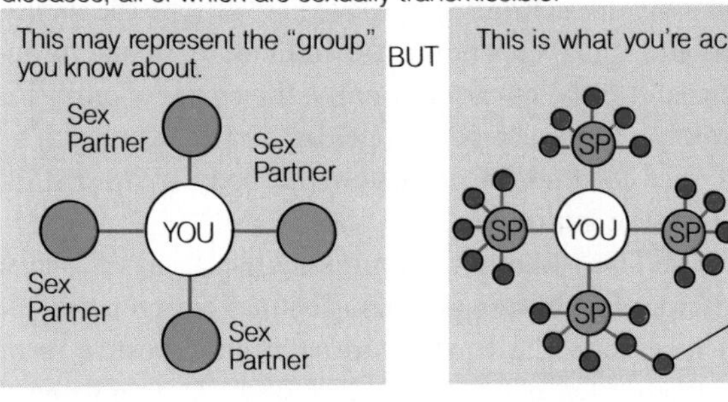

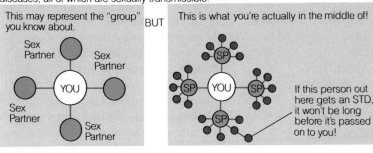

**Figure 16.1**
STD's: a fact of life for the sexually active. *Source:* Figure and text courtesy of American Social Health Association.

STDs as gonorrhea, nonspecific urethritis, and nonspecific vaginitis, all of which have similar symptoms early in their development. Laboratories are expensive to build, staff, and supply, and therefore, are luxuries not found in all communities. Samples often must be sent great distances for accurate diagnoses, resulting in delays of several days.

Adding to this problem is the fact that some physicians fail to report cases of STDs to public-health agencies. Not all STDs require reporting, but certain ones do. Support for physician training in the areas of STD diagnosis, treatment, and reporting may not be as strong as in many other areas of medical education.

Perhaps the most prevalent myth about STDs is that once symptoms disappear or treatment occurs, reinfection cannot take place. In fact, there are no vaccines and no acquired immunities for the STDs. People can be infected over and over, and the reservoir for such disorders can be maintained indefinitely. Reinfection often occurs in the individual who is careless or reckless about his or her sexual activity.

Due to the easing of sexual mores, there may also be greater opportunity than ever before for the transmission and spread of STDs. Improved fertility-control measures may enhance the frequency of sexual participation, or the number of sexual partners, thus increasing the chances of infection. Fertility-control measures such as birth-control pills may actually promote the proliferation of a natural yeast organism of the vaginal flora, **Candida albicans.** The Pill creates an environment in some women that permits periodic growth of this yeast, leading to irritation of the genital area and other symptoms. Although the woman may not have contracted the organism by sexual activity, she can certainly transmit it to her partner by that means. Thus, the "technology" of birth control has been somewhat of a mixed blessing. At the same time, use of the condom, the only birth control option that provides a measure of protection against some of the STDs, has been on the decline. A recent survey of college students shows that the condom is not perceived as a desirable fertility-control measure.[1]

There is an expectation among adolescents and many young adults that sexual participation is part of "growing up." There is a strong perception of peer pressure to participate in sexual activity. There has been a clear shift in recent years toward earlier sexual participation, and participation with more partners.[2] This trend has been especially significant among females.[3] The result is an enhanced STD risk. (See figure 16.1.)

Finally, the present STD incidence can be attributed in part to public apathy about the subject. In some communities, the subject of STDs cannot be raised in conversation, talked about in a public forum such as a newspaper, or taught to pupils in schools. The result is often widespread ignorance and personal vulnerability. There is a tendency to ignore threats to wellness until they reach crisis proportions. With some of the STDs, such a crisis may have already occurred.

# THE INFECTIOUS DISEASE CYCLE AND STDs

Each communicable disease has a unique cycle of progression that may aid in transmission and spread. The STDs are no exception. All STDs have cycles that share some common traits.

The first trait or condition in a disease cycle is the presence of disease causing organisms. Such organisms are called "germs," as everyone knows, or more precisely, **pathogens.** Pathogenic organisms, then, are disease causing, and each kind of pathogen is usually responsible for a specific disease or set of symptoms. Pathogens may be viruses, bacteria, fungi, spirochetes, protozoa, tiny wormlike creatures, insects, and other plant and animal organisms. What they have in common is that they are all small, often invisible to the naked eye.

A **reservoir** where pathogenic organisms can thrive and reproduce until they can infect people is a second condition that needs to be present to facilitate disease transmission. Some common reservoirs are animals (including people), soil, air, water, food, and inanimate objects. Some pathogens, such as those that cause STDs require special environments. For most STD-producing species, the warm, moist mucous membranes of the oral, genital, or anal regions of the body provide the receptive reservoir.

Pathogens require a **place of exit** from their reservoir to get to another person. For instance, germs from the common cold exit through the mouth and nose in the form of droplets when the infected person sneezes. Most STD-causing organisms, however, leave the body by means of the genitals, though they may also leave by way of the mouth, anus, or, in some cases, open sores or wounds in the skin.

Communicable diseases have to have a **mode of transmission** from reservoir to person or from person to person. A mode of transmission is the means by which germs leave one person and enter another. Sexual intercourse and other intimate physical contact are the usual mechanisms for transmitting the STDs, hence the name.

Pathogens require a **portal of entry,** or place where they can get into the body. For the more familiar communicable diseases (such as the common cold, influenza, chicken pox) this place is the nose or the mouth. The portal of entry for the STDs is usually the genitals, though it may also be the mouth or the anus depending on individual sexual practices. Rarely, but occasionally, the portal of entry for some STDs may be an opening in the skin, such as a sore located on a part of the body quite distant from the genitals.

STDs, like all communicable diseases, have various **incubation periods.** The incubation period of a disease is the time lapse between exposure to or introduction of the pathogen, and the actual onset of symptoms. Incubation periods are disease specific, which is another way of saying that they vary from disease to disease.

A disease may have a stage in which it is more easily transmitted than during other stages. This time is called its **period of communicability.** For example, a cold is most easily transmitted during its early stages. Genital herpes, an STD that appears to be growing in incidence, is most easily transmitted during an outbreak in the infected individual; at other times, the risk of transmission may be relatively low. Syphilis, another important STD, may be easily transmitted during its primary or secondary stages, but rarely transmitted at other times. Some STDs, however, are readily communicable virtually all of the time. (See figure 16.2.)

Pathogens may never make a person sick unless that person is what is called a **susceptible host.** That is, exposure to infection does not automatically result in disease. The body's arsenal of natural defenses includes the immune system, whose principal functions are the detection of and protection against disease. Good overall health that results from proper nutrition, rest, and exercise may help to fight potential disease-causing invaders. However, for many STDs, good health may not be adequate protection. Additional preventative steps to minimize personal risk for the sexually active are necessary. These steps are identified at the end of chapter 16.

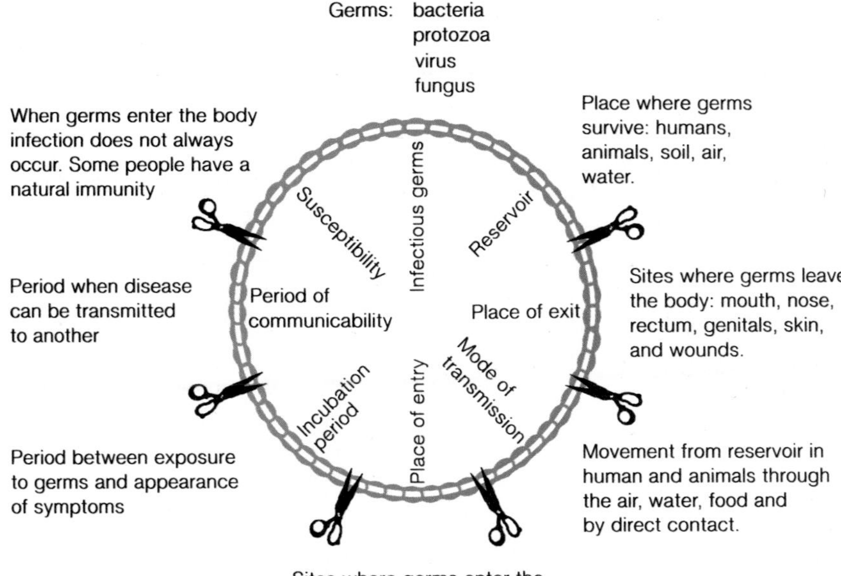
Scissors indicate points at which chain of infection can be interrupted.
Germs: bacteria
protozoa
virus
fungus
Place where germs survive: humans, animals, soil, air, water.
When germs enter the body infection does not always occur. Some people have a natural immunity
Susceptibility
Infectious germs
Reservoir
Period when disease can be transmitted to another
Period of communicability
Place of exit
Sites where germs leave the body: mouth, nose, rectum, genitals, skin, and wounds.
Incubation period
Place of entry
Mode of transmission
Period between exposure to germs and appearance of symptoms
Movement from reservoir in human and animals through the air, water, food and by direct contact.
Sites where germs enter the body: mouth, nose, rectum, genitals, skin or wounds.

**Figure 16.2**
Infectious disease cycle. *Source:* Reprinted by permission of the American Council on Healthful Living, 439 Main Street, Orange, N.J. 07050.

# THE COMMON STDs

Although authorities now recognize more than twenty disorders as being transmitted primarily by sexual means, there are a few STDs that are most likely to be problematic for sexually active persons, especially for persons who have casual or multiple sexual partners.[4] Many of these STDs may already be familiar to you. The more familiar STDs discussed in this section are gonorrhea, syphilis, genital herpes, candidiasis, nonspecific urethritis, nonspecific vaginitis, trichomoniasis, pediculosis, scabies, and urinary-tract infections.

## Gonorrhea

Many people are surprised when they learn that gonorrhea is one of the most frequently encountered communicable diseases in the U.S. Known by such street names as "clap," "drip," "dose," "strain," "gleet," and "jack," gonorrhea is caused by a bacterium named **Neisseria gonorrhoeae** which is common all over the world today. There is evidence to suggest that gonorrhea is increasing in incidence,[5] and despite the more than one million cases each year in the U.S. alone, it is probably underreported.

Susceptibility to gonorrhea is considered to be general—that is, there appear to be no factors that predispose one to acquiring gonorrhea, other than being sexually active. Human beings are the only known reservoirs for N. gonorrhoeae. There is no way to acquire immunity to the disease, either by vaccine or by actually contracting gonorrhea.

Gonorrhea is transmitted via direct contact with the secretions of mucous membranes such as those of the urethra, cervix, vagina, anus, eyes, and throat. The contact involved in transmitting gonorrhea is almost always sexual in nature. However, an infant may acquire a gonorrhea infection of the eyes during passage through the birth canal of an infected mother. Because of this risk, the eyes of newborn infants are routinely treated with a 1 percent silver-nitrate solution moments after birth to eliminate the possibility of infection developing.

It is possible that one's contaminated fingers can also transfer infection from one region of the body to another. However, nonsexual infection (such as from touching inanimate objects) is highly unlikely because N. gonorrhoeae dies rapidly when denied the warmth and moisture of mucous membranes.

Symptoms of infection usually appear within two to ten days after exposure, but may take up to thirty days in some cases. These symptoms can vary for males and females.

In males, gonorrhea usually strikes first at the urethra, the tubelike structure that extends from the bladder to the tip of the penis. Urine is eliminated through the urethra and semen passes through it during sexual intercourse. Males are most likely to experience a burning sensation during urination due to the irritation of the urethra's mucosal lining. Many males may also notice an abnormal discharge from the penis. The penis itself may be red or swollen at the tip. Urination may become more frequent, or become difficult. In between 5 and 20 percent of males who have gonorrhea, no symptoms are immediately evident.

In the female, gonorrhea seems to strike selectively at the cervix (the entrance of the uterus), but it also can appear elsewhere. As many as 80 percent of the females with gonorrhea have no immediate signs or symptoms to signal that something is wrong. In women with symptoms, there may be a foul smelling vaginal discharge. Since vaginal discharges are not uncommon, women should be alert to any change in the color, odor, or other appearance of discharges. If gonorrhea has affected the urethra, a woman may experience a burning sensation upon urination.

Gonorrhea can also infect the anal region, the oral cavity, and the eyes. Symptoms for males and females are identical. Gonorrhea that has affected the anus produces severe burning or itching. There may be a mucous discharge or blood and pus present in the stool. A throat infection acquired through oral-genital contact is likely to be only mild; it could easily be mistaken for a cold or other ailment. Eye involvement usually produces acute **conjuctivitis,** often severe, and accompanied by pain and discharge.

The period of communicability for gonorrhea is uncertain, but probably lasts as long as discharges continue. This may be anywhere from three to six months. It is possible for gonorrhea to be transmitted even after clinical symptoms of the disease have subsided.[6]

Diagnosis of gonorrhea is complicated by other STDs, nonspecific urethritis and vaginitis in particular, which are caused by a host of pathogens and which mimic many of gonorrhea's symptoms. Precise diagnosis, therefore, requires cultures of discharge specimens. Repeated cervical cultures in females may be necessary to detect any residual infection.

Under most circumstances gonorrhea is easily treated. Penicillin, given in two intramuscular injections, is the treatment of choice.[7] It is now clear, however, that larger and larger doses of penicillin may be necessary to kill some resistant strains. Moreover, there are some strains that can even render the penicillin useless.[8] While many antibiotics are effective against N. gonorrhoeae, some health personnel fear that the day may come when existing antibiotics will be unable to cure an infected person.[9]

Untreated gonorrhea may result in irreversible complications. In the male, infection may spread throughout the urinary and reproductive tracts. The channels through which sperm must pass may constrict or become blocked completely, thus decreasing fertility. In females, similar results may produce **pelvic inflammatory disease (PID).** PID can constrict the fallopian tubes, or even cause a complete blockage. If blockage is complete, sterility results. If it is partial, there is an increased risk of a tubal (ectopic) pregnancy, a medical emergency that can cause rupture, hemorrhage, or even death. Untreated gonorrhea in either sex may produce gonococcal arthritis in major joints, and a generalized infection which irreversibly damages the brain, heart, liver, and other key organs.

To minimize their risk of contracting gonorrhea, sexually active people who have casual or multiple partners should use condoms during sexual episodes. This is their most reliable form of protection. The sexually active individual should also be

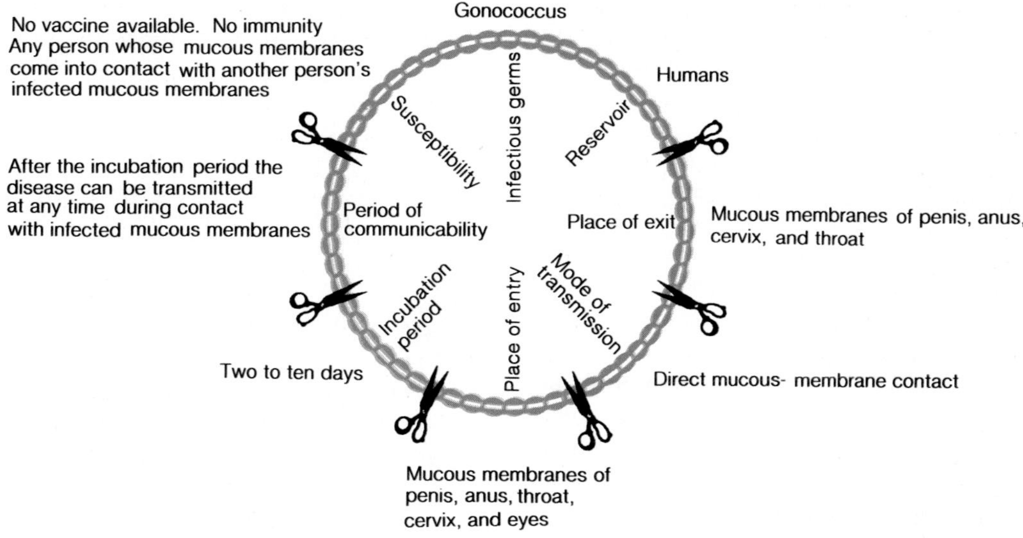


**Figure 16.3**
Gonorrhea infectious disease cycle.
*Source:* Reprinted by permission of the American Council on Healthful Living, 439 Main Street, Orange, N.J. 07050.

selective about sexual partners and stay alert to obvious signs and symptoms of disease. (See figure 16.3.)

## Syphilis

Nicknamed "syph," "pox," or "bad blood," syphilis is perhaps the best known of all the STDs. Once confined to certain parts of the world, syphilis now occurs universally. Its causative agent, **Treponema pallidum,** belongs to a group of organisms that resemble bacteria, called **spirochetes.** Humans provide the only known reservoir for T. pallidum. As with gonorrhea, there is no vaccine or other acquired immunity for syphilis. Although the potential for exposure to T. pallidum can be found throughout the world, only about 10 percent of exposures result in infection.[10]

Syphilis is transmitted by direct contact with infectious sores, (called **chancres**), syphilitic skin rashes, or mucous patches on the tongue and mouth during kissing, necking, petting, or sexual intercourse. The disease may also be transmitted from a pregnant woman to a fetus after the sixteenth week of pregnancy.[11] (Such transmission occurs when spirochetes in the mother's blood enter the circulatory system of the fetus.) Syphilis is not generally transmitted by inanimate objects such as drinking glasses or toilet seats, as spirochetes die rapidly when away from warmth and moisture. The incubation period for syphilis is from ten to ninety days, with twenty-one days being common. The blood test that is used in the diagnosis of this STD is likely to be negative during the incubation period.[12]

Syphilis may proceed through several stages or phases. In its **primary stage,** this STD is characterized by the appearance of a chancre at the primary site of infection. A chancre resembles a blister, pimple, or raised open sore. It is infectious and contains a large number of spirochetes. Despite their appearance, chancres are often painless, and may be hidden in the mouth, throat, vagina, cervix, or anus, making detection difficult. Chancres are said to be self-limiting.[13] That is, they heal themselves in from two to six weeks. After healing, however, a population of infectious spirochetes is left behind. Occasionally, primary syphilis may also be accompanied by swollen glands near the site of primary infection. (See figure 16.4.)

The primary stage ends with the disappearance of the chancre. The **secondary stage** then begins. Secondary stage symptoms may occur from six weeks to six months after the primary infection "disappears." These new symptoms usually include the presence of a rash or raised lesions anywhere on the skin surface. The rash is neither painful nor itchy, but it is infectious. In addition, patches of white in the mouth, nose, or rectum may appear. These mucous patches can also transmit disease. Additional symptoms at this stage may include patchy hair loss, mild fever and body aches, swollen glands, and some flulike symptoms. Secondary symptoms disappear in two to six weeks, but may recur for up to two years.

If still untreated, syphilis enters what is called the **latent stage.** At this point, symptoms are absent and the person is probably no longer infectious to others. The exception is the pregnant woman who is still able to transmit disease to the unborn. The length of the latent stage is variable, but can last at least five years, and perhaps as many as twenty years or more.[14] Some cases of syphilis remain dormant for an indefinite length of time. Others, however, evolve into the final stage or set of symptoms.

**Tertiary** or **late-stage syphilis** usually occurs between five and twenty years following initial infection. This condition leads to permanent disabilities, even death. Neurosyphilis, in which the brain and the spinal cord are affected, produces paralysis (tabes dorsalis), insanity (paresis), and blindness. Cardiovascular syphilis includes major damage to the heart and the aorta, possibly resulting in death. A condition called late benign syphilis is characterized by the appearance of large destructive lesions virtually at any internal or external site. (See figure 16.5.)

Congenital syphilis can result from the infection of the unborn child. Spirochetes travel readily across the placenta from the woman to the fetus.

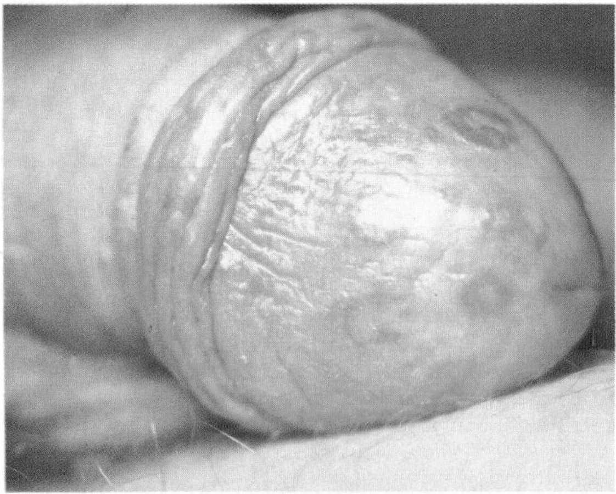

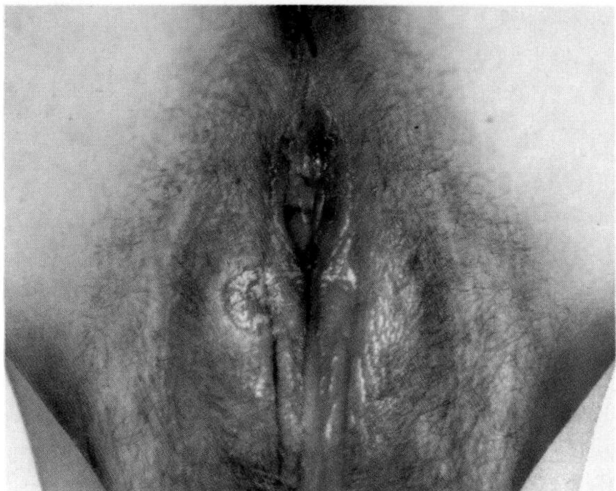

**Figure 16.4**
Infectious sores, called chancres, characterize the primary stage of syphilis and often appear on the genitalia.

Prior to the sixteenth week of pregnancy the fetus is protected by a membrane known as Langhan's layer, but this membrane is temporary. Infection of the unborn can produce stillbirth, mild to severe damage of many body systems, or destruction not apparent until many years after birth.[15]

The period of communicability for syphilis is variable. It is clearly infectious in its primary and secondary stages. Active spirochetes are rendered harmless in twenty-four to forty-eight hours by adequate treatment with long acting penicillin. For penicillin-sensitive individuals, antibiotics such as erythromycin or tetracycline are also effective. Infected individuals need to be followed closely after

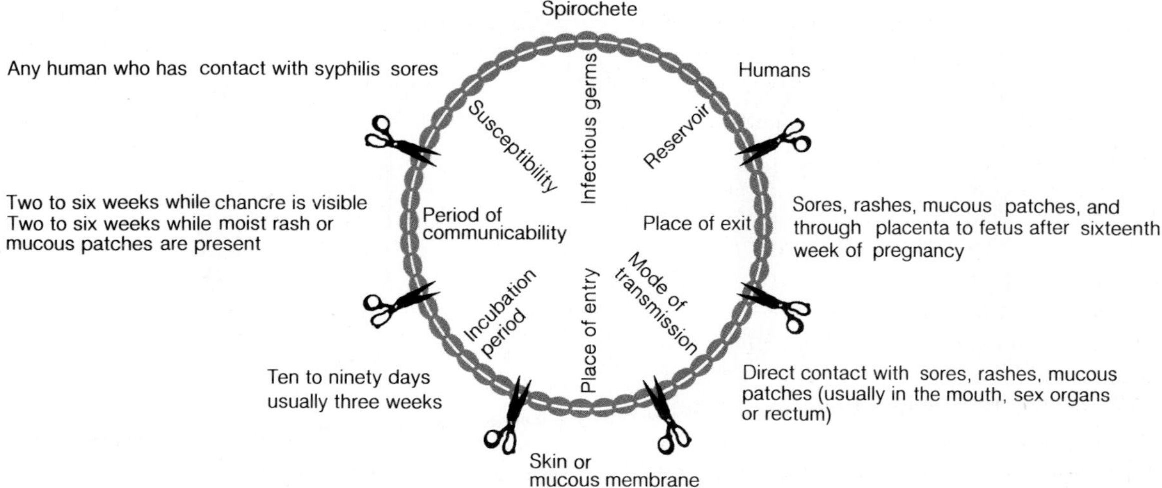


**Figure 16.5**
Syphilis infectious disease cycle.
*Source:* Reprinted by permission of the American Council on Healthful Living, 439 Main Street, Orange, N.J. 07050.

treatment, and repeated blood tests need to be performed to assure the complete absence of disease.

People hoping to avoid syphilis must avoid contact with syphilitic lesions. The use of the condom during sexual intercourse can assist in this, but a condom will not protect other exposed surfaces that may come into contact with lesions. Sexually active people who have multiple sex partners may be wise to undergo periodic screening for syphilis and other STDs. Early prenatal tests for this STD and periodic testing during pregnancy can assure that both mother and infant are free of disease. Most states continue to require blood tests for syphilis for people who are to be married. While this is one of the few good control measures for syphilis, many states are undertaking initiatives to repeal the requirement for the premarital-blood-test, charging that it is not a cost-effective strategy. (See figure 16.6.)

## Genital Herpes

Most people are familiar with **herpes simplex virus type I.** It is the cause of cold sores that occasionally affect many children and some adults. Cold sores generally appear on or around the mouth, and their symptoms are usually mild. Genital herpes, produced by **herpes simplex virus type II (HSV-II),** presents a different story. The sores caused by HSV-II form on the genitals and are transmitted during sexual intercourse. An infected pregnant woman may also pass on the virus to her infant during childbirth. The result for the newborn infant can be blindness, severe mental retardation, neurological damage, or even death.

Genital herpes is rapidly gaining considerable attention as an STD. One reason is that thousands of new cases are being identified each year. Another reason for the recent concern is the lack of any known cure. The fact that herpes is a virus makes antibiotic drugs useless in treating the symptoms and eliminating infection from the body. In most instances, the herpes sores—the blisters and crusts they later form on the genitals—heal and disappear on their own in a few days or weeks. The virus itself, however, stays in a dormant stage; the absence of symptoms does not necessarily mean the absence of active virus. Herpes may reassert itself from time to time, causing the sores to reappear. The sores are usually visible and painful in both sexes. However, signs of

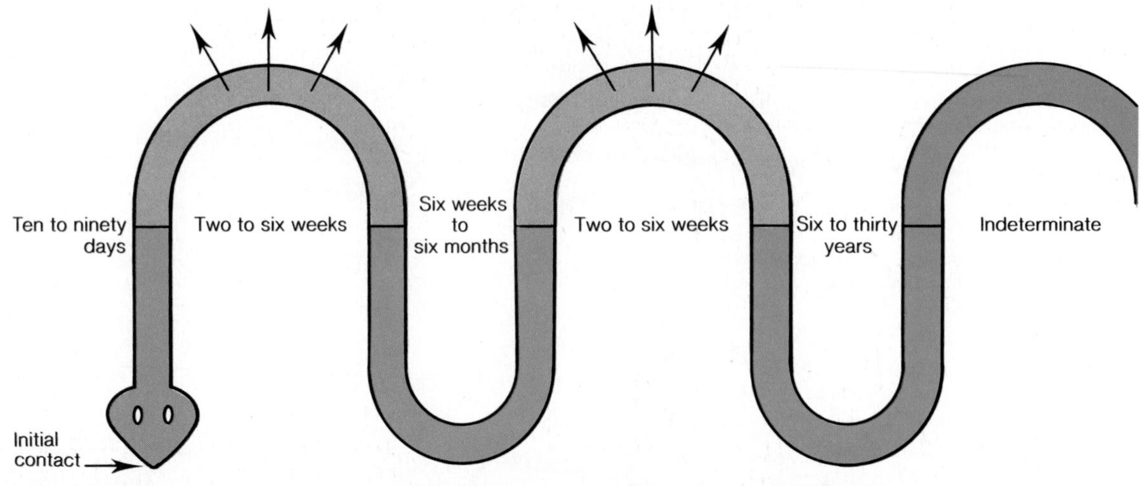


| Incubation stage | Primary stage | Latent stage | Secondary stage | Latent stage | Tertiary stage |
|---|---|---|---|---|---|
| Noninfectious | Infectious | Noninfectious | Infectious | Noninfectious | Noninfectious |
| No symptoms | Primary chancre<br>Swollen glands | No symptoms | Rashes, mucous patches, hair loss, swollen glands, sore throat | No symptoms | Permanent damage to any organ of the body |
| Not detectable in blood tests | Detectable in blood tests | Detectable in blood tests | Detectable in blood tests | Detectable in blood tests | Detectable in blood tests |
| Period after germs enter the body until first sign appears | | | Symptoms may reoccur during two-year period | | |

During pregnancy, infection can be transferred to the unborn child at any time following the incubation stage

**Figure 16.6**
Stages of syphilis (snake chart).
*Source:* Reprinted by permission of the American Council on Healthful Living, 439 Main Street, Orange, N.J. 07050.

herpes in women can be internal and painless. Therefore, as with some of the other STDs, it is possible for women to be unaware of the virus's presence. (See figure 16.7.)

What triggers recurrences of herpes is not well understood. Lowered resistance, other infections, chafing or irritation of the affected area, emotional upset, and even certain foods are factors implicated to some extent.[16] In women, the onset of menstruation may occasionally produce a flare-up of this STD.

Though herpes has an effect on all of its victims, it need not "paralyze" them emotionally. If a few sensible points are observed, and some life-style alterations made, life can continue to be lived fully and enjoyably. First, herpes victims are advised to be even more conscientious about controlling the stressors that may aggravate the dormant HSV-II organism. Stress-management programs and routine relaxation, valuable assets for anyone's level of wellness, are particularly helpful for the person with herpes. During recurrence, sexual contact ought to be avoided. Even at other times, if procreation is not an objective, it is advised that a condom be used during intercourse to provide protection for one's partner. The person who eats a well-balanced diet, receives adequate rest, and practices the routines identified above should experience only minimal life disruptions resulting from herpes.

The woman who has herpes needs to take a couple of additional precautions. There is a statistical association between HSV-II infection and the development of cancer of the cervix. Thus, a woman with herpes may be advised to have Pap tests slightly more often than other women her age. She should also be more conscientious about noticing any unusual vaginal bleeding. One's physician is probably best able to determine the optimal frequency for periodic examinations.

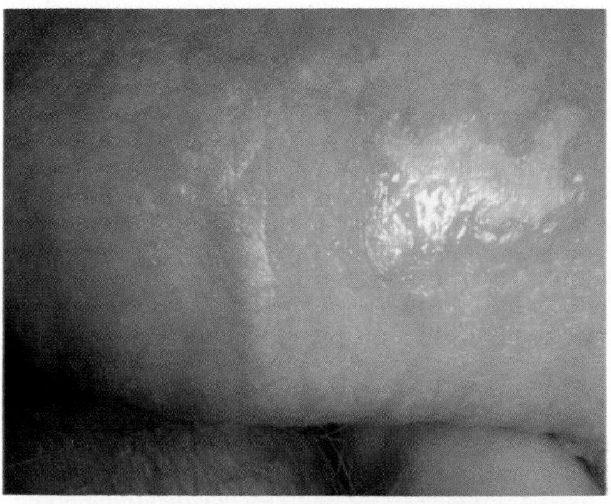

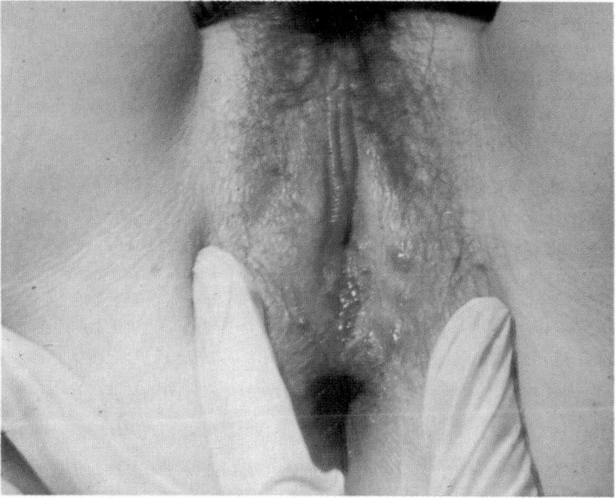

**Figure 16.7**
Blisters on the male and female genitals are a symptom of herpes.

Because of the danger of infecting the newborn infant, women who know they have herpes need to share this information with their physicians. Caesarean deliveries are generally advised when herpes is actively present.

Although no cure for genital herpes has been identified, some progress toward the relief of symptoms has occurred. Most traditional medical remedies are ointments applied topically to the affected areas. Most promising among these remedies is **acyclovir,** an antiviral drug, which has demonstrated remarkable effects in recently infected individuals who received it. It has not, however, proven effective for persons experiencing a recurrent episode of herpes.

## Candidiasis (Monilia)

This STD, also known as monilia vulvovaginitis or just monilia, is a common yeast-fungus infection caused by **Candida albicans.** It produces clinical symptoms more frequently in women than in men. Unlike most of the other STDs discussed so far, candidiasis may be acquired by other than sexual means. In fact, Candida albicans is probably a normal part of the human flora, such as that which resides inside of the vagina. If this is so, why does it flare up? Why is candidiasis labeled an STD?

Acute episodes of candidiasis seem to occur when certain other predisposing factors are present. It is known to be more common in people with diabetes, individuals with certain immune deficiencies, women taking birth control pills, and patients under broad-spectrum-antibiotic therapy.[17] Such circumstances may alter the normal acidity of the vagina, thus promoting an outbreak of the yeast organisms. Acute infections are accompanied by intense itching at the infected site, along with redness and perhaps swelling. In women, candidiasis may also produce vaginal discharges of a white, curdlike quality.

Complications from candidiasis are more aggravating than they are medically serious. The principal complication is recurrence, resulting when the infection is passed back and forth (Ping-Pong style) between partners. Consequently, when flare-ups occur, both partners are often treated. The most common and reliable treatment is topical application of nystatin for both partners, along with vaginal suppositories for the female.[18] Some women achieve relief from mild cases by douching with a solution of water and vinegar. The yeast organisms do not do well in acidic environments. Because candidiasis is so common, especially in women, some physicians may prescribe topical nystatin over the telephone without examination or microscopic evidence. If your physician does this, you might consider changing doctors. However, if nystatin is used, special notice should be made of the progress of symptoms. If they persist beyond a week, examination by a physician is recommended. Acute episodes of candidiasis can generally be avoided or minimized by using condoms during intercourse, wearing clothes that are not tight fitting (to reduce perspiration), and keeping the genital area dry.

## Nonspecific Urethritis

**Nonspecific urethritis** (NSU), also called **non-gonococcal urethritis** (NGU), is apparently very common and increasing in incidence. In the United States, cases of NSU caused by the intracellular parasite **Chlamydia** outnumber those of gonorrhea by a factor of 2- to 10-fold.[19]

NSU involves an inflammation of the urethra, though no symptoms may be readily evident. If symptoms are present, they may resemble those of gonorrhea. NSU is said to be nonspecific because it appears to have a host of causative agents, including Chlamydia trachomatis, organisms known as T-mycoplasmas, and unidentified bacteria and protozoans. Chlamydia currently accounts for approximately 50% of NSU cases.[20] Transmission of NSU, however, is probable during sexual intercourse, and transfer from mother to infant at birth is also possible. Infected newborns may experience conjuctivitis, pneumonia, and infections of the middle ear from these agents.

Differentiation of NSU from gonorrhea requires cultures of smears or discharges examined in laboratory settings. The very organisms that are implicated in NSU may actually be present in healthy, asymptomatic individuals, too. The treatment of choice for NSU is tetracycline. Both partners should be treated in order to avoid the so-called Ping-Pong effect. Untreated acute NSU can produce multiple complications including inflammations of the prostate, epididymis, and rectum in the male, and inflammations of the vagina, cervix, and rectum in the female. The most severe complication of NSU in females is PID. It is estimated that between 20 and 35 percent of PID cases are the result of Chlamydial infection.[21] PID is a serious complication, as it often leads to infertility. NSU can be controlled by using condoms during sexual intercourse, washing the genitals with soap and water before and after intercourse, and contacting sex partners when applicable.

## Nonspecific Vaginitis

Nonspecific vaginitis (NSV) is probably caused by the bacterium **Gardnerella vaginalis,** also known as **Haemophilus vaginalis,** whenever other organisms identified in the cause of NSV cannot be implicated. Symptoms of NSV are almost always restricted to females, though a male may experience itchy, burning symptoms of disease in his penis, similar to the vaginal symptoms that females report.

Symptoms in the female include a foul-smelling vaginal discharge, vaginal itching, and burning upon urination. However, the complete absence of symptoms is not uncommon. Treatment is accomplished with oral metronidazole and transfer is prevented by the use of condoms.

## Trichomoniasis

This STD is caused by the presence of **Trichomonas vaginalis,** a protozoan, which may exist without symptoms, in the vaginal flora of 50 percent of the females in the U.S. between the ages of sixteen and twenty-five. Susceptibility to "trich" is general, though clinical disease is usually restricted to females. Though the organisms can be acquired during sexual intercourse, they may also be picked up by nonsexual means from freshly soiled bedclothes, towels, and other items.

The female with trichomoniasis is most likely to notice acute disease during or shortly after menstruation. Symptoms may include a foul-smelling discharge, localized itching, redness, and burning during urination. Or, there may be no symptoms. Treatment of choice is oral metronidazole, usually given to both partners, since "trich" is another of the so-called "Ping-Pong" STDs. Males seldom experience any demonstrable symptoms. Females who suspect trichomoniasis should not douche before an examination, as this could make diagnosis difficult.

## Pediculosis and Scabies

These two disorders are more accurately labeled infestations than infections. Both are caused by parasites, pediculosis by the crab louse, and scabies by the itch mite. These organisms may be found anywhere on the body, but show a selective preference for the pubic hair. They lay their eggs at the base of the hair, just underneath the skin. The presence of these "bugs," "wee beasties," "creepy crawlers," or "crotch critters," as they are called, is highly irritating. Crabs and mites can produce an agonizing itch after their eggs hatch. Transfer of these organisms can occur from person to person in a variety of ways. Direct body contact, particularly during physical intimacy, is a common mode. Contact with personal items such as clothes and bedsheets can often accomplish transfer. Other means are also possible.

Complications are rare, though secondary infections can result from breaks in the skin due to intense itching and irritation. Tight clothing and perspiration can aggravate the condition further. Treatment is provided by application of medicated shampoos. Reinfestation is prevented by good personal hygiene and careful laundering and ironing of clothes and bedding items.

### Urinary-Tract Infections (UTIs)

UTIs are often classified as bladder infections or cystitis, and occur when pathogenic organisms enter the urethra and migrate to the bladder. A host of bacteria and other organisms may produce a UTI. Intestinal bacteria can produce infection when they are present in fecal matter that comes into contact with the urethra. This might occur when wiping the anal area following a bowel movement. Contact between the hands and the urethra or between the urethra and inanimate objects may also lead to infections. Women, perhaps because of their shorter urethras, are much more susceptible to UTIs than men. UTIs may be chronic in some women. Pathogens can sometimes be "flushed" from the system by having the individual drink large quantities of water (eight to ten glasses per day). Some physicians recommend the consumption of liquid high in acidity, such as cranberry juice, to lower the risk of UTIs. However, Myron Brin[22] suggests that 1.5 to 4 liters of cranberry juice is required on a daily basis to have even a slight effect on the urine's acidity. Cranberry juice in that quantity may exceed the body's tolerance, and it is high in calories as well. If you should have persistent symptoms of a UTI, be sure to consult a physician.

## LESS COMMON STDs

There are many other STDs that can be serious threats to wellness. Most of these STDs have long and strange-sounding names, such as chancroid, condyloma, Granuloma inguinale, and Lymphogranuloma venereum.

### Chancroid

This STD is caused by the bacterium **Hemophilus ducreyi,** and is rare or absent in most temperate climates (such as the kind found in most parts of the U.S.). Chancroid is more common in tropical or subtropical regions. As the name of this disease implies, it produces chancrelike sores that can cause it to be confused with primary stage syphilis. Infection usually requires contact with these sores, which most often occur in the genital or anal areas of the body. Diagnosis to distinguish chancroid from syphilis requires a biopsy or culture of affected regions. Extensive destruction of surrounding tissue can occur if chancroid is not properly treated, but this disease fortunately responds well to sulfanoamide and other antibiotics.

### Condyloma

Condyloma acuminata or **"venereal warts"** are caused by a DNA virus of the papova virus group. Although this disease occurs worldwide, it is only known to occur in sexually active individuals, and primarily by direct contact. These warts are benign tumors, varying in size and shape, but generally clustering in the genital and anal areas. Occasionally they are hidden from view. Taking several weeks or months following exposure to appear, these unsightly growths can transmit infection as long as they are present. Fortunately, condyloma seldom results in complications, and can be treated by surgical removal or topical application of medication. As with some other of the STDs, condyloma can pose a threat to the newborn infant.

### Granuloma Inguinale

Because of association with tropical and subtropical environments, this STD is not commonly seen in the U.S. A bacterium with a real tongue twister of a name, Calymmatobacterium granulomatis, is responsible for this disease. Granuloma is more common in men than women, and occurrence is possibly associated with male homosexual activity. This STD produces painless sores or blisters on or near the sex organs, but the blisters can ulcerate and spread infection throughout the genital and anal regions. If untreated, tissue destruction can occur in

16.1 EXHIBIT

# AIDS: A New and Dreaded STD

Q: What is AIDS?

A: AIDS stands for "acquired immune-deficiency syndrome." It is a disorder, first documented in 1981, in which the body's immune system is impaired to varying degrees of severity. "Acquired" refers to the fact that AIDS is not inherited and is not explained by an underlying illness. "Immune deficiency" is the common trait that persons with confirmed cases of AIDS demonstrate. This trait refers to the body's inability to defend itself against a host of what are called "opportunistic diseases." These diseases include certain infections and otherwise-rare tumors. "Syndrome" refers to the variety of specific diseases that can occur. People with AIDS, therefore, are predisposed to have diseases that immunologically healthy individuals would not normally encounter. Two of the diseases often associated with AIDS include an unusual cancer known as Kaposi's sarcoma and a severe infection, *Pneumocystis carinii* pneumonia.

Q: How does the healthy immune system work?

A: The main line of defense in the body is comprised of a group of cells known as *lymphocytes*. Lymphocytes are concentrated in the body at strategic sites, called lymph nodes. In healthy persons, specialized lymphocytes, called T-cells, act as "attack cells" to foreign substances that are detected in the body, and attempt to render them harmless. In the AIDS victim, the effectiveness of the T-cells becomes lessened, allowing disease processes to develop.

Q: What causes AIDS?

A: The exact cause of AIDS is not known. Most of the research up to this point indicates that AIDS is a result of a virus. The leading culprit is believed to be *human T-cell lymphotropic virus variant III* (HTLV-III). Other agents, including cytomegalovirus, Epstein-Barr virus, and herpes simplex virus have also been implicated as possible causes.[1] HTLV-III and other agents frequently have been isolated in blood samples of persons with AIDS. A test to screen blood for AIDS virus antibodies is now available.

Q: How many cases of AIDS are there?

A: According to the Centers for Disease Control in Atlanta, Georgia, through November of 1984 there had been 6,993 patients meeting the surveillance definition for AIDS.[2] About 48 percent of patients were known to have died, but the suspicion was that case mortality could eventually reach 100 percent. Approximately 86 percent of the adult and 82 percent of the pediatric cases of AIDS had been reported since January 1983. Among adult patients, 59 percent were white, 25 percent were black, 14 percent were Hispanic, and 2 percent were of other or unknown ethnicity. About 75 percent of the adult victims of AIDS were reported to be residents of New York, California, Florida, or New Jersey.[3]

Q: Who gets AIDS?

A: About 96 percent of the confirmed AIDS cases have been in persons belonging to one of four distinct groups: 1) homosexual and bisexual men (73 percent); 2) intravenous drug users (17 percent); 3) Haitians (4 percent); and 4) people with hemophilia (a disorder where the blood does not clot normally) and recipients of blood transfusions (2 percent). A fear has arisen that some asymptomatic individuals in the early stages of AIDS may have donated blood that can transmit the disorder when the blood is used for transfusion.[4] Others who are at greatest risk are sexual partners of persons who have AIDS, and infants of mothers who have AIDS.[5]

Q: How communicable is AIDS?

A: The occurrence of AIDS in the affected groups is consistent with the hypothesis that AIDS results from an agent transmitted sexually or, less commonly, through exposure to contaminated needles or blood. According to the Centers for Disease Control,[6] person-to-person transmission through ordinary social or occupational contact has not been shown. Also, there is no evidence of airborne or foodborne transmission. The incubation period for AIDS is estimated to be from six to thirty-six months, or longer.[7]

Q: What are the early-warning signs of AIDS?

A: The early-warning signs of AIDS are vague, and could indicate many unrelated diseases. These

## EXHIBIT 16.1

symptoms include: fever, night sweats, persistent cough, chronic fatigue, loss of appetite, diarrhea, enlarged lymph nodes, yeast infections, and weight loss. The first indication of an AIDS-related problem may be when a person presents with these symptoms and a series of infections that signal a declining immune response. Each of these symptoms can occur as part of many disease processes not caused by or associated with AIDS. However, people with prolonged or persistent symptoms should consult a physician.

Q: How is AIDS treated?
A: There is currently no specific protocol for treating victims of AIDS. Effective remedies do exist for certain of the opportunistic infections, like *Pneumocystis carinii* pneumonia, however. To date, no effective remedy for restoring the normal function of the immune system has been identified.

Q: What preventive measures can minimize the occurrence of AIDS?
A: The United States Public Health Service[8] recommends that occurrence can be minimized with these measures: 1) avoid intimate sexual contact that involves the exchange of body secretions with persons known to have AIDS, persons suspected of having AIDS, persons in the high-risk groups, and persons who are sexual partners of members of the high-risk groups; 2) members of high-risk groups and their sexual partners should refrain from donating blood; 3) individuals using intravenous drugs should not share needles and syringes; and 4) physicians should order blood transfusions only when medically necessary. For individuals in high-risk groups, certain other practices may help to reduce one's personal risk. These practices include avoiding unnecessary stress, maintaining good nutrition, getting adequate rest and exercise, and minimizing use of toxic substances such as tobacco, alcohol, and recreational drugs that suppress immune response.

Q: Who has the most up-to-date information on AIDS?
A: Because of increased public concern about AIDS, some cities have established telephone hot lines to address questions about the disorder.[9] The National Gay Task Force operates a toll-free long-distance crisis line at 1-800-221-7044, and a local New York City number at 212-807-6016. The United States Public Health Service also operates a hot line from 8:30 A.M. to 5:30 P.M. on weekdays (1-800-342-AIDS) at which referrals can be made, if necessary. Finally, the Center for Disease Control—AIDS Activity has a telephone service available by dialing 1-404-329-3162. Some state health departments also offer telephone services for people with questions about AIDS. Telephone numbers can be obtained from local directories in most instances.

[1]Centers for Disease Control, "Update on Acquired Immunodeficiency Syndrome (AIDS)—United States," *Morbidity and Mortality Weekly Report* 31 (1982): 507–14.
[2]Centers for Disease Control, "Acquired Immunodeficiency Syndrome (AIDS) Update—United States," *Morbidity and Mortality Weekly Report* 33 (1984): 661–64.
[3]Centers for Disease Control, "Acquired Immunodeficiency Syndrome Update (AIDS) Update—United States," (1984): 661–64.
[4]J. W. Curran, D. N. Lawrence, H. Jaffe, et al., "Acquired Immune Deficiency Syndrome (AIDS) Associated with Transfusions," *New England Journal of Medicine* 310 (1984): 69–75.
[5]Gwendolyn B. Scott, Billy E. Buck, Joni G. Leterman, et al., "Acquired Immunodeficiency Syndrome in Infants," *New England Journal of Medicine* 310 (1984): 76–81.
[6]"Update on Acquired Immunodeficiency Syndrome (AIDS)—United States" (1984).
[7]"Update on Acquired Immunodeficiency Syndrome (AIDS)—United States" (1984).
[8]*AIDS Information Bulletin,* Public Health Service (Washington, D.C.: U.S. Department of Health and Human Services, 18 July 1983).
[9]Carol B. Persons and Roxie L. Tabor, "AIDS Precautions," *Journal of Practical Nursing* 33–32 (September 1983): 51–53.

## DISCUSSION QUESTIONS

1. Are the present steps being used to control the spread of AIDS adequate? What additional steps would you approve of?
2. Should people who are sexually active and members of groups at risk for AIDS have free access to early detection blood-screening tests?

these areas. Diagnosis almost always requires laboratory assistance, and infection of partners is possible as long as sores are present. Antibiotic therapy with tetracycline or erythromycin has generally been successful. This disease has been associated with subsequent cancer of the penis.[23]

## Lymphogranuloma Venereum

Lymphogranuloma venereum (**LGV**), is caused by **Chlamydia trachomatis,** an organism sharing traits of both bacteria and viruses. This STD is more common than formerly believed. Though found worldwide, it is particularly prevalent in tropical and subtropical environments.[24]

Transmission doubtlessly results from direct contact with lesions during sexual intercourse. These sores usually appear on the genitals and resemble pimples. LGV is more common in homosexuals and persons having multiple sex partners. Complications from LGV are rare, though inflammation of the urethra, cervix, and rectum are possible. PID is an occasional complication that can result in sterility if left unchecked. Tetracycline provides reliable therapy for this STD.

# WHAT TO DO AND WHERE TO GO FOR HELP

The symptoms of STDs vary, though some STDs show symptoms that are remarkably similar to one another. A summary of the STD signs and symptoms is presented in Tables 16.1 and 16.2.

Anyone who has one or more symptoms that arouse suspicion of an STD should seek medical help. Consultation with a physician may also be advisable if one suspects that exposure to an infected person has occurred, whether or not signs of infection have appeared. Although the family physician is an appropriate person to contact, many people are reluctant to consult someone they know because of guilt or embarrassment. Other physicians can certainly be considered. Many communities have clinics exclusively for people with STDs. College campus health services can usually direct people to an appropriate source for STD tests.

**Table 16.1 Symptoms of STDs in Females**

1. Burning during urination.
2. Pain, itching, soreness, or redness on or around the vaginal or rectal areas.
3. Sores, pimples, warts or other unusual lesions on or near the genital area.
4. Any unusual or abnormal discharge from the vagina.

**Table 16.2 Symptoms of STDs in Males**

1. Burning during urination.
2. Any abnormal drip or discharge from the penis.
3. Any unusual or abnormal coloring in the urine.
4. Obvious presence of blood in the urine.
5. Sores, pimples, warts or other unusual lesions on or near the genital area.
6. Soreness or redness on the penis or anus.

Remember that not all physicians or clinics provide STD diagnostic and treatment services. If you are making an appointment to be examined for a suspected STD, be sure to ask if such services are available. Health centers and hospitals provide services with variable costs. Investigate these services and costs, and also look into the availability of free or low-cost clinics.

What is likely to happen during a trip to a clinic for an STD examination? In the waiting room you are likely to be instructed to "take a number." This ensures that names are not used in public and each person's confidentiality is protected.

You will be requested to complete forms that ask for information about your purpose for coming in and your medical history. By law, all information that is provided must be held in strict confidence.

Regardless of the exact STD symptoms, each patient is likely to be given a specific test for syphilis and possibly for gonorrhea as well. These tests are precautionary and routine. In the syphilis test, a blood sample is drawn from the arm. If any sores are present, fluid samples may be taken for examination.

If test results indicate the presence of one or more STDs, medications may be prescribed immediately. With women whose symptoms are vague or even absent, a complete pelvic examination may be

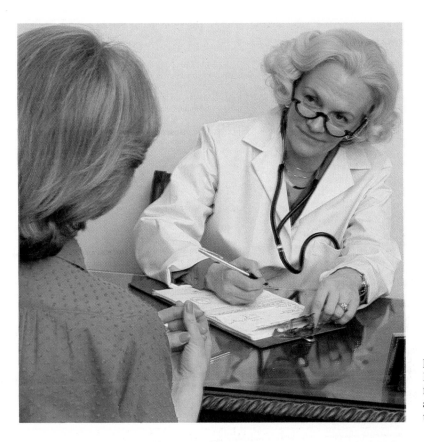

**Figure 16.8**
Health counselors provide guidance for individuals suffering from STD's and help them control the spread of their disease.

required. Some tests take several days to a week for interpretation. If such tests are performed, the patient is usually asked to avoid any sexual contact until results are available and a diagnosis is made.

Next, you are likely to talk to a health counselor. This person may be a physician, nurse, health educator, or other specially designated member of the health-care team. Part of the counseling process includes discussion of how you can help sexual partners. You may be requested to name sexual contacts. Withholding this information will not be doing your partners a favor, though you are under no legal obligation to identify your sexual contacts. Providing the names of contacts will assist, however, in case control of STDs. If you are too embarrassed or uneasy about informing a partner, designated personnel from the clinic are likely to be available for such purposes. The counseling process concludes with a discussion of ways to prevent contracting STDs and usually a request to return to the clinic at least once for a follow-up examination. This return trip is to assure complete cure; it is a vital part of disease control. You can usually rely on clinic personnel to be sensitive to your needs. (See figure 16.8.)

## MINIMIZING THE RISK OF STDs

The best way of dealing with STDs is to prevent their occurrence in the first place. Most of the recommended precautions are simple enough for everyone to follow. These suggestions are summarized in table 16.3.

Do not forget that with many STDs, it is what you cannot see that can hurt you. When symptoms do appear, have them checked out. If you are sexually active with more than one partner, periodic routine STD checkups may be a responsible precautionary measure on behalf of partners, as well as advisable for personal peace of mind. Embarrassment and guilt should not be barriers to informing a partner if you have an STD. Wouldn't you want to be informed if a partner just had an STD diagnosed? Having an STD is not likely to be looked upon as the highlight of your life, but it need not be the end of the world, either.

**Table 16.3 Personal Prevention Methods**

| | |
|---|---|
| Abstinence | Not engaging in any intimate body contact is an effective way of preventing VD. |
| Limited partners | If two partners limit their contact to each other, chances of acquiring a venereal disease are minimal. |
| Selectivity | If a partner is having contact with others who may be infected, a disease may be transmitted through that partner. |
| Soap and water | Cleansing all areas of contact immediately before and after any type of contact will wash away some of the germs. Douching is not recommended as it may force germs into the uterus. |
| Observation | Examine partner discreetly for rashes, sores, blisters or discharges. Avoid contact with those areas of possible infection. |
| Urination | Urinating after contact may wash away the germs in the urethra. |
| Prophylactic | A condom used before and during any intimate contact is one of the most effective venereal-disease-preventive measures. |
| Foams and jellies | Effectiveness is uncertain. |
| Periodic VD Checkups | Special examinations to detect VD will reveal unidentified infections. They should be done once or twice each year to detect hidden infections or more often when there is a reason to be suspicious. |
| Treatment of Partners | All sex contacts should be treated simultaneously to prevent reinfection. |

Although no single preventative method is 100 percent effective, when used properly and in combination with other preventative measures, they can provide adequate protection against VD.

Source: Reprinted by permission of the American Council on Healthful Living, 329 Main Street, Orange, N.J. 07050.

## SUMMARY

1. Unlike many disease threats to wellness, the STDs are communicable in nature.

2. The existence of STDs has been known since the beginning of civilization.

3. Numerous cultural, behavioral, and other factors act as barriers to adequate STD control. Appropriate contact investigation is a particularly vital STD control measure that often is not practiced.

4. Like most infectious diseases, the STDs go through the infectious-disease cycle.

5. Some STDs are more common than others. These include gonorrhea, syphilis, genital herpes, candidiasis, NSU, NSV, trichomoniasis, pediculosis, scabies, and a variety of UTIs.

6. Less-common but potentially dangerous STDs include chancroid, condyloma, granuloma inguinale, lymphogranuloma venereum, and acquired immune deficiency syndrome (AIDS). AIDS is the newest of the STDs and one of the most dangerous.

7. Some STDs are treated easily and effectively, but for others, there is no cure. Some STDs, such as herpes, may recur in the infected person. The absence of STD symptoms does not always mean the absence of disease.

8. For people who have an STD, there is help available through many channels. The best STD protection, however, is reliable prevention.

## Recommended Readings


1. Barlow, D. *Sexually Transmitted Diseases: The Facts*. New York: Oxford University Press, 1979.

2. Corsaro, M. and Korzeniowsky, C. *STD: A Commonsense Guide*. New York: St. Martin's Press, 1980.

3. Kassler, J. *Gay Men's Health: A Guide to the AIDS Syndrome*. New York: Harper & Row, 1983.

4. Neumann, H. H. *Dr. Neumann's Guide to the New Sexually Transmitted Diseases: Symptoms, Treatment, Prevention*. Washington, D.C.: Acropolis Books, 1983.

5. Wickett, W. H. *Herpes: Cause and Control*. New York: Pinnacle Books, 1982.


## References


1. Robert J. McDermott and Robert S. Gold, "Gender Differences in Perception of Contraception Alternatives by Never-Married College Students," paper presented at the 100th Annual Meeting of the American Alliance for Health, Physical Education, Recreation and Dance, Atlanta, Ga., 1985.

2. Karl King, Jack O. Balswick, and Ira E. Robinson, "The Continuing Premarital Sexual Revolution among College Females," *Journal of Marriage and Family* 39 (1977): 455–59; and Bo Lewin, "The Adolescent Boy and Girl: First and Other Early Experiences with Intercourse from a Representative Sample of Swedish School Adolescents," Archives of Sexual Behavior, 11 1982: 417–28.

3. King et al., "The Continuing Premarital Sexual Revolution among College Females"; and James F. Keller, S. S. Elliott, and E. Gunberg, "Premarital Sexual Intercourse among Single College Students: A Discriminant Analysis," *Sex Roles* (1982): 21–32.

4. Abram S. Benenson, ed., *Control of Communicable Diseases in Man*. Washington, D.C.: American Public Health Association, 1975, 315.

5. Benenson, *Control of Communicable Diseases in Man*, 315.

6. Benenson, *Control of Communicable Diseases in Man*, 315.

7. William M. McCormack, "Treatment of Gonorrhea—Is Penicillin Passe?" *New England Journal of Medicine* 296 (1977): 934–36.

8. McCormack, "Treatment of Gonorrhea," 934–36; and William M. McCormack, "Penicillinase-producing Neisseria Gonorrhoeae—A Retrospective," *New England Journal of Medicine* (1982): 438–39.

9. McCormack, "Penicillinase-producing Neisseria Gonorrhoeae," 438–39; and H. H. Handsfield et al., "Epidemiology of Penicillinase-Producing Neisseria Gonorrhoeae Infections," *New England Journal of Medicine* 306 (1982): 950–54.

10. Benenson, *Control of Communicable Diseases in Man*, 315.

11. Benenson, *Control of Communicable Diseases in Man*, 315.

12. Benenson, *Control of Communicable Diseases in Man*, 315.

13. Benenson, *Control of Communicable Diseases in Man*, 316.

14. Benenson, *Control of Communicable Diseases in Man*, 315.

15. Benenson, *Control of Communicable Diseases in Man*, 315.

16. Benenson, *Control of Communicable Diseases in Man*, 315.

17. Benenson, *Control of Communicable Diseases in Man*, 60.

18. Benenson, *Control of Communicable Diseases in Man*, 61.

19. Robert B. Jones, "Chlamydia: The Most Common Sexually Transmitted Pathogen," *Medical Aspects of Human Sexuality* 18. 2 (1984): 236–61.

20. Robert B. Jones, and K. H. Fife, "Update on Sexually Transmitted Diseases," *Medical Times* (April 1982).

21. Jones, "Chlamydia."

22. Myron Brin, "Drug-Vitamin Interrelationships," *Nutrition and the M.D.*, (November 1976): 1.

23. Benenson, *Control of Communicable Diseases in Man*, 138.

24. Benenson, *Control of Communicable Diseases in Man*, 315.

# UNIT FOUR

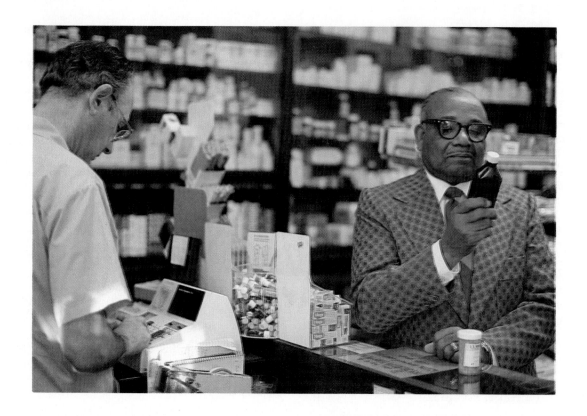

# Self-Responsibility: Enhancing Positive Life Habits

In unit 3, we concentrated on minimizing negative life habits as one essential part of a wellness life-style. You also need to enhance positive life habits in order to achieve high-level wellness. Chapters 17 through 20 will introduce you to some important wellness skills and habits that will be useful to you now, and later as you adapt to aging.

One prescription for wellness is to become a better consumer. We live in a consumer society and it is important to be aware of your own behavior as a consumer. As a consumer, you need to make decisions regarding health-related products and services ranging from beauty aids and eyeglasses to funerals and exercise equipment. Taking responsibility for your own wellness involves learning consumer skills such as assertiveness, budgeting, and comparison shopping.

Consumer skills are also important when you make decisions about health-care providers. In the U.S., there are many different kinds of health-care providers, including physicians, dentists, nurses, physician assistants, and providers of alternative kinds of care. Health care is provided on three levels—primary, secondary, and tertiary—and in different kinds of facilities, from hospitals to offices. There are also various ways to finance health care, including private health insurance and prepaid health-insurance plans. Unit 4 will give you a background for utilizing this array of health-care services wisely.

Taking responsibility for your own personal wellness inevitably leads to concerns about the larger environment. Unit 4 will present the four laws of ecology and show how they relate to daily life aboard "spaceship Earth." Our consuming way of life has profound implications for our own future and that of generations to come. Unit 4 shows some ways we can contribute to making our environment more healthy.

As we age, a wellness life-style becomes even more important. Unit 4 discusses some of the myths about aging. There are several different theories about how and why biological aging occurs. People age emotionally and socially as well. Unit 4 presents several different theories about both the biological and the sociological patterns of aging. We must adapt to aging if we are to maintain a wellness life-style.

CHAPTER SEVENTEEN

# Better Consumerism: Rx for Wellness



Each of us must make decisions that affect wellness. Deciding whether or not to purchase health-related goods and services, for example, requires us to be informed consumers. Poorly informed consumers may purchase goods and services on blind faith or "gut feelings" alone, a practice that can be detrimental to both one's health and pocketbook. Wise consumers ask questions, perform background research, and identify people and agencies to whom they can take their complaints.

The purposes of this chapter are to explore some of the determinants of consumer behavior, to examine essential consumer skills, to identify a host of fraudulent practices in the health marketplace, to indicate what to look for when purchasing some specific items, and to inform you about consumer-protection laws and agencies that can be mobilized if you are victimized by manufacturers and service providers. In the words of Esther Peterson, Director of the U.S. Office of Consumer Affairs during the Carter administration:

> Consumers do have many resources available to assist them, but often they just don't know how to find them. Many of the problems and frustrations consumers face stem from a lack of knowledge about where to go for help. . . . Today, we must be educated consumers. We cannot afford to make purchases without information about all the alternatives. Before handing over our hard-earned dollars, we should all learn as much as we can about the choices available to us. When buying a product or service, we are all well advised to remember the old saying "an ounce of prevention is worth a pound of cure."[1]

## PSYCHOLOGICAL AND SOCIOLOGICAL FOUNDATIONS OF CONSUMER BEHAVIOR

Thomas Robertson[2] identifies two reasons why people purchase services or products. First, a purchase may satisfy a "want" characteristic, a perceived need, or a tangible desire for an item. Second, a purchase may serve a "social-symbolic" function, such as raising an individual's self-esteem, sense of importance, or psychological-comfort level.

Successful marketing specialists appeal to basic psychological forces. Advertisers identify the most appropriate medium for delivering a product message. Audience perception is achieved in a variety of ways. One way is through **media bombardment.** In this strategy, a product becomes familiar by mere repetition. Bombardment results in consumers internalizing product messages like "Weekends were made for Michelob," "Get the Signal," "Coke is it," and "No more medicine breath." Vignettes from life that are humorous and sometimes even a little aggravating help get the advertiser's message internalized by breaking through our perceptual barriers. Marketing experts know that success has been achieved because consumers hum and whistle the jingles to their commercials while driving, showering, or performing household chores.

**Subliminal advertising** also appeals to basic drives and needs as a way to sell products. Subliminal techniques are aimed at the subconscious mind and often focus on sexual motivations. Wilson Bryan Key[3] has examined a variety of subliminal messages in product advertising. He claims that advertisers sell products by embedding words like "sex" on product labels or in product ads. Magazine ads for liquor show ice cubes in glasses that feature nude human figures embracing. Also according to Key, advertising may depict people whose hands are placed provocatively to suggest that a sexual act is about to occur or has recently been completed. The language of such pictorials also may be suggestive of sex. Not all subliminal selling, though, is based on sexual innuendo. Producers of suntanning products have achieved selling success in recent years by appealing to consumers' olfactory senses. The addition of fragrances such as coconut that suggest tropical paradises subliminally appeal to people's desires to seek the "good life" of the islands.

Marketing specialists attempt to understand the relationship between consumer attitudes and eventual behaviors. Successful marketing reaffirms existing positive feelings about a product, changes negative attitudes to more favorable ones, or creates new attitudes. Traditional marketing strategies typically include creating a need for a product that results in demand for that product, and then directing advertising in a way that reaffirms the demand. Americans have been persuaded to pursue white teeth, fresh breath, smooth skin, and comfortable underarms, and to fight unending battles with dandruff and split ends. Reinforcing the marketer's campaign is the next-door neighbor who has accepted the advertising message. People don't want to deviate too far from the norm, and if friends confirm the message of the television or magazine ad, most people will brush with Brand X toothpaste, shampoo with Brand Y protein enhancer, and rub on, roll on, or spray on Brand Z twenty-four-hour underarm-odor protector.

Peer pressure, the need for group membership, and a tendency toward conformity help to explain much consumer behavior. Group pressure can help determine one's health beliefs, especially where trends or fads are concerned.

Yet another influence on consumer behavior is the advertising technique of **appealing to authority.** In this scenario, a well-known actor, athlete, or other performer poses as an authority to make a pitch for a particular product. Because they elicit respect from consumers, such personalities can entice would-be shoppers into purchasing an item. Thus, such notables as Martha Raye can propel sales of denture products, Lorne Greene, Art Linkletter, Michael Landon, and Ed McMahon can promote life-insurance with success, and Robert Young can alter the coffee-drinking habits of millions of Americans.

## SELECTING HEALTH-RELATED PRODUCTS

Consumers spend a large sum of money on health-related products each year. These products include skin and beauty aids, drugs, and health devices, and should be selected wisely. This may mean challenging some of your own long-held beliefs. (See Activity for Wellness 17.1.) In the following pages, hints for the wise selection and purchase of some of

17.1 ACTIVITY FOR WELLNESS 17.1

## Why Do I Buy Certain Products?

Consider the brief list of products below. If you can, record the main reason you bought a particular brand during your last purchase. Is there a rationale behind the particular brands that you select? Are you getting most of the incentive for your purchases from TV or other advertising media? Are product claims upheld? As you read through chapter 17, decide if you are making wise decisions before spending money.

| ITEM | BRAND | REASON FOR BUYING THAT PARTICULAR BRAND |
|---|---|---|
| Deodorant or antiperspirant | | |
| Toothpaste | | |
| Mouthwash | | |
| Shampoo | | |
| Hair conditioner | | |
| Tanning product | | |
| Pain reliever | | |
| Cold medication | | |

these products are presented. It is possible that many readers will have some long-held beliefs challenged here. If that is so, this chapter will have performed a useful function.

### Skin and Beauty Aids

Skin and beauty aids are **cosmetics** and as such must be considered chemicals as well. They are regulated by the **Food and Drug Administration (FDA)** under the Food, Drug and Cosmetic Act, and include any products that cleanse, beautify, enhance attractiveness, or modify appearance. The most popular cosmetics are soaps, toothpastes, shampoos, mouthwashes, powders, and hand or body lotions. These products comprise 22 percent of annual cosmetic sales, exceeding eight million dollars in expenditures each year.

The majority of cosmetic preparations are safe for general use when instructions are followed carefully. This is largely due to the fact that over-the-counter (**OTC**) cosmetics contain mostly inert ingredients. The Food, Drug and Cosmetic Act does not require testing of products for safety prior to marketing. Moreover, manufacturers need not report problems with cosmetic products, nor must they report product formulas. In certain instances some people may have a hypersensitivity to a given product such as a particular brand of soap. As a consumer aid, the FDA has made it mandatory since 1977 for manufacturers to list all ingredients that comprise 1 percent or more of their product. This enables the consumer to identify potential sources of allergy or irritation. Some manufacturers label their products as **"hypoallergenic."** The FDA permits a product to be so labeled, however, only if testing demonstrates

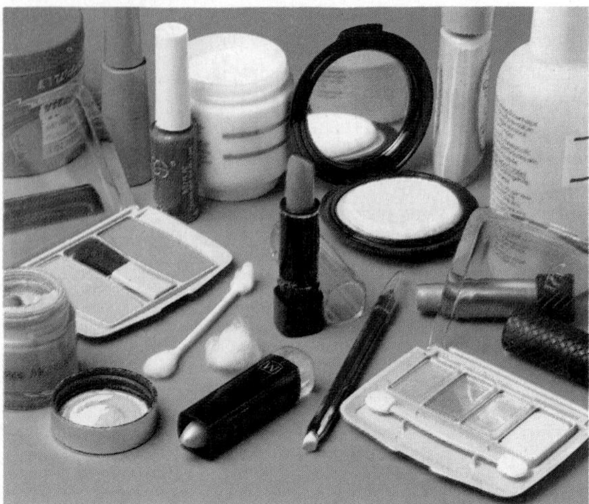

**Figure 17.1**
While the FDA does not require testing of cosmetic products, it does require the submission of test results to support specific product claims.

**Table 17.1. Sun Protection Factor (SPF) Designations**

| | |
|---|---|
| 2 to 4 | Offers limited protection and allows tanning. Recommended for persons who tan readily and rarely burn. |
| 4 to 6 | Offers moderate protection from the sun's burning rays. Recommended for persons who burn minimally and generally tan. |
| 6 to 8 | Offers extra sun protection. Recommended for persons who prefer to tan gradually or who burn moderately easy. |
| 8 to 15 | Offers near maximum protection and allows virtually no tanning. Recommended for persons who seldom develop tans, but who burn readily. |

that it produces significantly fewer allergic reactions in individuals than do other similar preparations. Thus, although the FDA does not require testing for safety, it does require the submission of test results to support particular product claims. (See figure 17.1.)

Soaps are used primarily for their cleansing properties. Occasionally, soaps that contain moisturizing agents are desirable for some individuals. These agents usually are lanolin, glycerin, or vegetable oils of various kinds. Such soap additives are generally effective in promoting moisture retention. Many products are advertised as containing "special" organic or natural ingredients. A number of ingredients such as avocado, estrogen, turtle oil, milk, honey, and vitamin E have been advocated as additives to restore beauty, retard aging and wrinkling, and perform a wide range of miracles.[4] There is no clinical evidence to support these claims.

Little by little the FDA is asking manufacturers to submit test results that support these assertions. The FDA is hampered by two things: (1) this government agency probably has too much responsibility for its typical budget allotment, and (2) some manufacturer's "claims" are more implied than they are real. Most people have little need for special high-priced soaps or facial-wash preparations. The best skin-cleansing care comes from washing rather than scrubbing, and from using mild soaps and warm water, rather than medicated soaps and hot water.[5]

Bathing often in the winter and exposing the skin to sun and wind in the summer promote drying or flaking of the skin. Moisturizers may minimize this process. Another important skin-care product with real value is the sunscreen lotion. Although more and more tanning products contain a **sun-protection factor (SPF),** not all do. A common SPF is para-aminobenzoic acid (**PABA**). PABA and similar ingredients help protect skin from burning, drying, wrinkling, and developing cancer. Sunscreen products are assigned different ratings from two to fifteen according to the degree of protection offered. These designations are clearly marked on most sunscreen preparations, and are summarized in table 17.1. Although sunscreens offer some protection from the sun's effects, they are not substitutes for reason and common sense about moderating sun exposure.

Shampoos are cosmetic products that can mislead poorly informed consumers. Shampoos are much like soaps, except that their cleansing agent is a detergent that leaves hair clean and shiny. Regular soaps applied to hair leave the hair dull and filmy unless very soft water has been used. In addition to detergents, most shampoos contain lathering agents, fragrances, and several miscellaneous compounds such as lemon juice, eggs, proteins, milk, herbs, and vitamins. Most of the miscellaneous ingredients have little or nothing to do with the ultimate outcome of a shampoo.[6]

Many shampoo products are advertised as pH-balanced or as nonalkaline. While marketers have led the public to believe that this factor makes the shampoo less irritable to the scalp, skin and eyes, the editors of *Consumer Reports* indicate that pH differences among shampoos are too insignificant to be of any practical importance.[7]

Some manufacturers add protein to their shampoo formulas, claiming that protein-enriched products repair broken hairs and split ends. It is unlikely, though, that protein-enriched formulas serve the repair process any better than the nonenriched formulas of other shampoos.[8] The added expense, therefore, may not be justified.

Hair products are frequently marketed on the basis of their fragrance. Lemon is quite popular, as are apple and strawberry. Fragrances are said to provide the "freshness of spring," an obvious attempt to appeal to the olfactory senses. Other than masking some less appealing odors, fragrance adds nothing to the product but cost.

Finally, some makers of shampoos have special formulas for dry hair and oily hair. There is nothing wrong with this practice, but curiously enough, *Consumer Reports* indicates that persons with oily hair often prefer dry-hair preparations and vice versa.[9]

In general, shampoo performance results from how it is applied and rinsed, and how the hair is dried and combed after washing. For best results shampoo should be applied only once. Directions to shampoo and rinse twice are probably of no practical value except to the manufacturer who is able to sell more of the product. Gently massage the shampoo through your scalp and spread around the lather. Then rinse thoroughly and gently towel dry. Following shampooing, comb your hair with a wide-toothed comb. Using a narrow-toothed comb or brush is likely to snag or break wet hair. Remember that although some products perhaps provide a little extra glisten or shine to your hair, the results seldom justify their higher price tags.[10]

Two types of personal-care products that receive attention in all advertising media are deodorants and antiperspirants. Almost all of us have been convinced by media messages that wet underarms or offensive underarm odor will lose us that important date, job, or client.

What exactly happens when we perspire and to what extent can it be controlled? Perspiration is a normal body product that assists in maintaining skin-surface moisture and regulating body temperature. Perspiration itself does not smell bad, but takes on an unpleasant odor when it reacts with skin-surface bacteria. There are two common approaches to dealing with this "problem": (1) masking odor with antibacterial soaps, deodorant soaps, or other preparations; and (2) reducing sweat buildup with antiperspirant preparations.

**Deodorizing products** contain substances such as alcohol that inhibit bacterial metabolism. Some products also contain vitamin E, which serves as an antioxidant to retard the degradation of perspiration's components. Products containing vitamin E are suspected, however, of causing skin allergies in people who have a particular sensitivity. **Antiperspirants** work by contracting the skin and inhibiting perspiration flow. The effectiveness of antiperspirants is in the 20 to 33 percent range; roll-on products are the most dependable.[11]

Recent years have seen the proliferation of genital deodorants, vaginal sprays, and "intimate hygiene" preparations, such as douches. With rare exception, genital deodorants have been designated for women and have been the cause of much unnecessary anxiety and self-consciousness. According to Margaret Morrison, "No evidence has been submitted to the FDA, and the FDA has found no substantial evidence that feminine sprays have any hygienic or therapeutic advantage. And for the purposes of cleanliness, soap and water are more effective than perfumed sprays."[12]

Although of little hygienic value, some of these products are actually the cause of irritations. One is well advised to avoid them. A woman who does experience unpleasant genital odor can follow several recommended courses of action. First, odor can be controlled by washing the genital area carefully with soap and water daily. Mild antibacterial soaps may be of some value unless the woman is allergic to them. Second, clothing plays an important role in the amount of genital perspiration. Pantyhose and tight-fitting slacks limit absorption and evaporation processes. Similarly, nylon panties or briefs inhibit evaporation. Cotton underwear, because of its better absorbancy, should always be worn with pantyhose.

Such practices reduce both unpleasant odors and susceptibility to genital infections. The use of commercially prepared douches may contribute to an infection in the first place by changing the natural acid balance of the vagina, thus causing the odor.

Part of society's obsession with offensive odors, created in part by the advertising media, is reflected in the annual expenditures on mouthwashes to sanitize, odorize, purify, or otherwise sweeten the breath. Common causes of bad breath include poor oral hygiene, gum disease, smoking, and the consumption of alcohol, garlic, coffee, or onions. Chronic bad breath (**halitosis**) may be a symptom of serious oral infection, diabetes, or other disorders.

People who buy mouthwashes for other than their breath-freshening effects often do so to clean their teeth, kill germs, or treat colds and sore throats. In fact, mouthwashes perform none of these functions effectively.[13]

Mouthwashes can freshen the breath momentarily but they cannot get at the source of the odor if it is from bacteria and decaying food particles embedded in the gums. Mouthwashes are no more effective than water in cleaning the teeth, but certainly more costly.[14] Some are able to kill surface germs on contact, but germs soon return, so any effect is temporary. Some mouthwash manufacturers claim their product can result in a person having fewer or milder colds if used daily. A case in point is the Warner-Lambert Company that made such an assertion for years in TV advertising about its product, Listerine. The company was taken to court for misleading and fraudulent advertising and forced by the **Federal Trade Commission (FTC)** to pay a penalty as well as to remove any references to Listerine having cold-preventive properties. Moreover, because it was believed that the effects of years of misleading advertising could not be eliminated simply by dropping the claim, the FTC required Warner-Lambert to announce during its commercials that Listerine was ineffective against colds.[15] Mouthwashes are relatively expensive preparations that provide little more than temporary relief of the symptoms of bad breath, but do nothing toward eliminating their causes.

Toothpastes assist in the removal of food particles, plaque, and stains from the teeth. Table 17.2 summarizes the seven principal components of commercial dentifrice preparations.[16] In addition to these ingredients, many toothpastes now contain fluoride, an anticaries agent. Not all dentifrices have fluoride and it should never be assumed that a given product does unless it is marked on the label.

**Table 17.2. Ingredients of Commercial Dentifrices**

| | |
|---|---|
| Binding agents | To prevent separation of the product into its solid and liquid parts. |
| Detergent agents | To enhance sudsing properties. |
| Abrasives | To remove debris from the surface of teeth. |
| Flavoring agents | To enhance taste and freshen breath temporarily. |
| Humectants | To help the toothpaste retain moisture when it is exposed to the air. |
| Water, oils, and preservatives | To retard spoilage and maintain moisture. |
| Antienzyme agents | To enhance whitening and stain removal capabilities. |

Some toothpastes are said to "whiten teeth" and "brighten smiles." Often these products contain highly abrasive substances that are not good for teeth; they should be avoided. An often-forgotten fact is that teeth are naturally off-white in color.[17]

Some people have "sensitive" teeth that ache when they come into contact with things that are extremely hot, cold, or sweet. Special toothpastes have been designed for this problem. However, the American Dental Association's Council on Dental Therapeutics does not endorse the claims of these preparations.[18] People may develop "sensitive" teeth from frequent brushing or scrubbing with a hard-bristled toothbrush, resulting in actual exposure of a nerve. This problem can be prevented or minimized by brushing thoroughly, but less vigorously with a soft-bristled toothbrush.

## Eyeglasses and Contact Lenses

Proper evaluation of the eyes is performed by either an ophthalmologist (M.D.) or an optometrist (O.D.). These examinations typically last thirty to forty-five minutes and are likely to cost between thirty-five and seventy-five dollars.

If an examination reveals the need for glasses, the examiner will prepare a prescription. It is not unusual for ophthalmologists or optometrists to be associated with dispensing opticians in the same office or building. While this arrangement is a time-saving convenience for consumers, it may not necessarily be the most economical one. Prices for frames, lenses, and fittings vary. Most frames cost between twenty-five and seventy-five dollars, while lenses are an additional twenty-five to fifty dollars. A person who desires high fashion frames may pay over one hundred dollars. Tinted lenses, plastic lenses, or photosensitive lenses cost more. Each type of lens has both advantages and disadvantages. These factors can be explained by the examiner. Fitting is usually done at no cost if it is performed at the place of purchase. Sales people are sometimes available to help consumers select frames and lenses that complement facial features and colorings.

Contact lenses have become an enormously popular alternative to eyeglasses in recent years. These lenses are small and thin, and fit directly over the eyeball. Presently, there are three widely available types of contact lenses. Hard lenses are rigid and may be either clear or tinted; they fit over about two-thirds of the cornea. Soft lenses are more flexible and absorb water more readily. The eye adapts more easily to soft than hard lenses, but soft are more expensive. They cover the entire cornea when fitted properly, and can be worn for longer periods of time. Gas-permeable contact lenses are similar to hard lenses, though somewhat less rigid. They allow better flow of oxygen and other gases to the eye surface and therefore tend to cause fewer problems for the wearer than hard contacts.

All contact lenses need to be fitted by an ophthalmologist or optometrist. Lenses may vary in price from one hundred to four hundred dollars and average around one hundred fifty dollars. Prices have come down markedly in recent years and will probably continue to do so. Contact lenses have a life expectancy of from two to four years, which is not quite as long as regular eyeglasses. However, most people who can wear contact lenses comfortably report that they see better and with less distortion than with eyeglasses. An optometrist or ophthalmologist can best advise you on how to care for your lenses to prolong their life and to promote comfortable wear.

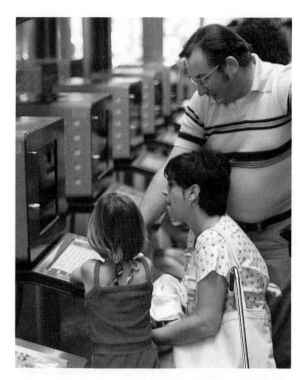

**Figure 17.2**
Blood-pressure kits and coin-operated blood-pressure machines often provide dubious readings and can't replace professional quality equipment.

## Self-Diagnosis Equipment

Consumers today are accepting more personal responsibility for selected health matters. Among the most popular self-care skills are blood-pressure screening and early-pregnancy testing (**EPT**). Manufacturers have responded by offering accessories to the public to assist the development of these skills. (See figure 17.2.) In principle, there is nothing wrong with the notion of saving on physician fees and avoiding possible delays in clinic waiting rooms. However, not all of the equipment and devices available are of sufficient caliber to provide accurate self-assessments.[19]

Blood-pressure kits include a **sphygmomanometer** to assess blood pressure, and a **stethoscope** for listening to arterial sounds. Three types of kits are marketed. They are described in table 17.3. The mercury-type is the most expensive, but also the most

**Table 17.3. Commercially Available Blood Pressure Kits**

| | |
|---|---|
| Mercury type: | Includes stethoscope and sphygmomanometer. As pressure in the cuff is increased, the column of mercury rises. As pressure in the cuff decreases, the height of the column of mercury decreases. |
| Aneroid type: | Does not contain mercury. A needle moves on a pressure-sensitive dial to indicate blood pressure reading. |
| Electronic aneroid type: | Requires no stethoscope. Contains a microphone under the blood pressure cuff that records the arterial sounds instead. |

accurate.[20] Unfortunately, it is clumsy and heavy, making it difficult to transport. The aneroid (non-mercury) variety is light and mobile, but requires recalibration at regular intervals. A kit of the aneroid type costs approximately twenty-five dollars, but inferior-quality devices may sell for less. The electronic-aneroid type eliminates the need for a stethoscope and for interpreting arterial sounds. However, *Consumer Reports* found its output to be of unsatisfactory quality. The quality of blood-pressure kits is generally so low that they make unnecessary purchases except when advised by a physician.[21] If you must screen your blood pressure often, it might be advisable to invest in professional-quality equipment.

Consider one last note on blood-pressure screening. It is fashionable these days for stores, shopping malls, and even libraries and airports to offer coin-operated blood pressure machines. While depositing fifty cents in a machine may be a way to pass the time or give you and a friend something to talk about, such equipment provides dubious readings.[22]

Early-pregnancy tests, or EPTs, have also become popular recently, especially through ads in women's magazines. (See figure 17.3.) Their operation is relatively simple. A few drops of a woman's urine are added to a test tube provided in the kit. The test tube already contains chemicals that react with the urine if pregnancy has actually occurred.

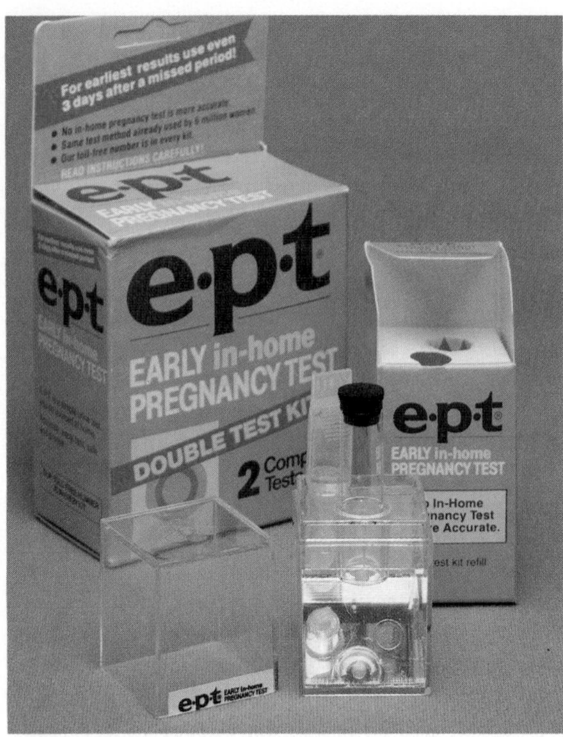


**Figure 17.3**
Early pregnancy tests (EPTs) have become popular recently, although their results are not always reliable.

The reactive substance found in the urine of pregnant women is a hormone known as **human chorionic gonadotropin** (HCG). (EPT kits sell for ten dollars or more and are available in most drug stores.)

There is a certain ill-conceived logic about the use of EPTs. Although the tests themselves are sensitive, their results are not always reliable. In fact, the test tends to produce some false-negative results. A person who gets false-negative results may do one of two things. She might delay seeking prenatal care since she remains unaware of her pregnancy. In the interim, she may encounter substances that could later pose a problem for her or the fetus, such as oral contraceptives or other drugs. A false-negative test might also direct her to repeat the test, and therefore, incur added costs without any assurance that the second result is more credible than the first.

A positive pregnancy indication produces a similar predicament. It probably will lead to a visit to the physician, who will repeat the test and have it interpreted by professionals. Thus, the EPT result will be confirmed or refuted, making the original test an unnecessary expense. If you suspect you are pregnant, contact an appropriate medical professional who can schedule a test, if necessary.

## Other Health-Related Devices

There are a variety of other health-related devices. Depending on their quality and validity, they can either aid or hinder your search for wellness.

**SUNLAMPS** One product found in many health clubs, and in drugstores for home purchase, is the sunlamp. These lamps contain mercury gases and give off ultraviolet (UV) radiation when electricity is passed through them. The radiation from sunlamps is similar to that given off by the sun, only intensified. If you are not properly protected, you can receive severe burns from a sunlamp. The hazards of UV radiation have been described in chapter 15. Use of sunlamps (or the tanning booths available in many sports clubs and "health" spas) may accelerate skin aging as well as promote the development of skin cancer. Although it is best to avoid these products, if you must use them, observe these precautions:

1. Avoid the bare-mercury-type sunlamp.
2. Use sunlamps that have timers.
3. Observe product recommendations regarding safe distance from the lamp during its use.
4. Protect your eyes during all exposures with goggles or dark glasses.
5. Avoid washing or bathing right before exposure to the sunlamp's radiation. Cleansing the oils from your skin may result in an intensified response.

**EXERCISE EQUIPMENT** Buying exercise equipment also requires information and common sense. People invest in exercise equipment ranging from barbells and exercycles to jogging suits and wrist sweat bands. There are many high quality products made and sold by reputable firms, but there are also costly products created by phony "experts" that do little if any good.

The benefit that results from exercise depends on the nature of the exercise itself. Weight lifting builds muscle and strength, but has minimal cardiovascular benefits. Aerobic exercises like running, swimming, or bicycling can have significant cardiovascular effects, and tone muscles as well. Being able to move large volumes of oxygen throughout the body to perform a variety of tasks is more useful than to have bulging muscles and little ability to oxygenate them.[23] Thus, identifying your objective for exercising determines to a large extent the type of accessories, if any, you will purchase.

Carefully assess ads that promote a product said to be "a total exercise program all by itself." No single product can do that. Employ similar skepticism when an ad suggests that you "can see real changes in only moments a day." A recent ad featured "a way to lose weight and trim waistlines without exercise." The ad advocated wearing a tight-fitting synthetic rubber suit (resembling a diver's wet suit) during the course of normal daily activities. The suit sells for about forty-nine dollars and works by dehydrating the body. The person literally sweats away up to fifteen pounds a day, a dangerous system of weight loss. The weight is quickly gained back as you replace the lost water. This deal and others like it often come with money-back guarantees that appear to enhance the legitimacy of the product prior to purchase. Many consumers, though, are too embarrassed to ask for their money back once they have been "taken."

**MAIL ORDER GIMMICKS** Many health products and devices are sold by mail order and are advertised in popular magazines. Consumers frequently and falsely assume that reputable magazines screen out all fraudulent advertisers. The products typically promoted include sex aids (pleasure enhancers, vibrators, penis enlargers and erection aids) and beauty aids (bust enlargers, spot reducers, and hair removers/growers). Numerous devices and "secrets" are advocated for breast enlargement. Among the most popular have been gravity devices, water-massage devices, and elastic stretch devices. None of them work, and, so far as anyone knows, no process or device can permanently increase the amount of breast tissue. Exercising the chest muscles can improve appearance somewhat as can better posture, but neither alters breast size. Any health-related device or gimmick that is available exclusively through mail order ought to be considered prone to failure.

# MORE ABOUT FRAUD AND THE CONSUMER

We have discussed various schemes that attempt to lure the unsuspecting consumer into buying an item not needed or purchasing an item at a higher price than necessary. There are other, common fraudulent schemes.

A frequently practiced scheme is the **"bait-and-switch"** tactic. It begins when a retailer advertises a product at an unusually low price to lure customers into the store. Upon arrival, customers learn that the advertised merchandise is "sold out" or that it is of inferior quality. A salesperson may try to persuade the customer to purchase a brand that is of "higher quality" but also higher priced. Retailers concerned about their reputation are not likely to engage in this practice; instead they offer customers "rain checks" to be used when the particular item is restocked. Potential danger exists with this practice too. Once lured to the retail outlet, you may purchase other items simply because you have made the trip and do not want to waste it. After receiving the raincheck, you may return to purchase the original item, but again make additional purchases. The retailer gains in either case.

Another technique employed is the **"brand-loyalty"** approach. The retailer or advertiser convinces people that a brand name is the trademark of quality. Well-known products for such items as antacids and pain relievers are usually more expensive but seldom of better quality than more obscure brands or generic products. The key is to read the product label and examine the so-called active ingredients. Be wary of an ad that proclaims: "Buy the name you have come to rely on" or "Accept no substitute." Although the product may be perfectly acceptable, the price tag may be unnecessarily inflated.

Another favorite strategy for attracting customers is product **"misrepresentation."** Almost everyone has seen a TV commercial that begins: "Nine out of ten doctors recommend . . . Brand X for the relief of the headache and congestion of cold and flu." Before rushing out to the corner drugstore, consider such questions as: Which doctors were asked? How were they selected? Were they paid to respond? Obviously, this information is not shared in the commercial. Another common misrepresentation begins: "Studies from a major university reveal . . . Brand Y provides help for hemorrhoidal sufferers." What studies? Which university? Under what conditions and with which research methods? One begins to see how subtle and repetitious media messages can work their way into our repertoire of buying habits.

"Bait-and-switch" and "misrepresentation" tactics are sometimes combined to bring in potential customers. Recently a national retail outlet store advertised the availability of hard contact lenses in their optics department for forty-nine dollars. People flocked to the optics department, accepting the merchandiser's bait. Once there, consumers discovered that there were additional charges for examination, fitting, follow-up, and storage cases. Total cost: One hundred sixty-nine dollars or about the same as the standard retail cost. Even though the "bargain" price was misrepresented, many customers had, nevertheless, entered a stage of "psychological readiness" to complete the purchase. Sales clerks then went on to argue the advantages of soft contacts (the switch), available for only forty dollars more.

The wise consumer needs to ask questions, and to be on guard for deception, manipulation, misrepresentation, and even complete fraud. Some measure of protection can be attained by identifying reputable retailers who have a long history of service, and who provide written guarantees. (See figure 17.4.)

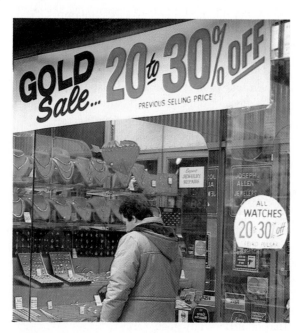


**Figure 17.4**
Special sales trigger a "psychological readiness" to buy among many consumers.

# THE FUNERAL INDUSTRY AND THE CONSUMER

At the time of the death of a close relative, we are placed in a position of vulnerability as consumers. When selecting funeral services, family members of the deceased can be financially victimized because of their emotional state. This is not an indictment of funeral directors. Reputable funeral directors conscientiously uphold professional ethics and standards. However, consumers are often unaware of their options until they must plan a funeral on short notice. To assist consumers, the FTC has sponsored legislation to regulate the funeral industry. The FTC-sponsored legislation requires that funeral directors submit itemized bills to consumers and provide unit costs upon request, including over the telephone. The idea was to get away from "package deals" where the consumer had no idea how much the casket was versus the vault versus the funeral director's services for embalming, cosmetics, vehicles, etc.

## Choosing a Funeral Director

Just as it is wise to select a physician and dentist prior to needing their services, it is wise to identify a funeral director before a crisis arises. Selection considerations are summarized in table 17.4. The best way to evaluate services is to visit funeral establishments and see how services are carried out. Many proprietors of funeral homes view themselves as public servants and are available to talk to people who want the "mystery" of the industry clarified for them.

## Range of Services Provided

The death of a loved one usually requires a consultation with a funeral director. The director handles a variety of tasks, such as:

1. Obtaining personal information about the deceased.
2. Determining the time, place, and type of funeral service.
3. Casket selection, perhaps even if cremation is to be performed.
4. Burial-vault selection, if desired, unless cremation is to be performed.
5. Cemetery arrangements.
6. Floral arrangements.
7. Preparation of death notice for local newspaper.

You may wish to discuss other details with the funeral director, but these items are the ones most frequently discussed.

**Table 17.4. Criteria by which Persons Select a Funeral Director**

| |
|---|
| Personal acquaintance with the funeral director. |
| Funeral director's reputation; previous use of services and satisfaction. |
| Counseling and guidance ability of the funeral director. |
| Funeral director's sensitivity to the stress on the family. |
| Funeral director's willingness to discuss prices in straightforward terms in person or over the telephone. |
| Religious affiliation (if any) of the funeral home. |
| Convenience of the funeral home's location. |
| Recommendation by others. |
| Funeral director's knowledge of community resources for the bereaved family. |

## Pricing

In the past, many funeral directors have offered families funeral "packages" that included costs in the purchase price of the casket. The package may have included unnecessary or undesired services. The 1984 FTC legislation discourages such packages and promotes itemized price lists that allow consumers to see exactly what they are buying. Funeral directors themselves are split over the merit of this legislation. There is evidence that itemized price lists might lower the cost of a funeral, as well as evidence to the contrary. The price of funeral goods and services is affected by many factors, such as:

1. **Newspaper notices.** Many newspapers will print a simple death notice at no cost. A formal obituary, however, does involve costs. It may be written by a family member or the funeral director, and will cost more if handled by the director.
2. **Flowers.** Floral arrangements are customary but not required. They may be ordered by either a family member, a florist, or the funeral director, and prices vary.
3. **Cemetery fees.** The charge for opening and closing a grave ranges from 50 to 250 dollars depending on location in the U.S. Purchasing a cemetery lot is a substantial additional cost.
4. **Embalming.** Most states do not require this practice unless the deceased died of a highly contagious disease. However, if there is to be a funeral-home visitation with showing of the body, embalming is almost always advised.
5. **Minimum service charge.** Most funeral homes charge for such services as pickup and delivery of the body, filing a death notice, and other services, such as paying an honorarium to a clergyman.
6. **Use of facilities.** Visitations are optional, but if a visitation is held, there is a fee for use, setup, and arrangement of the funeral parlor or chapel.
7. **Hearse.** The fee charged for use of the hearse may vary according to how far the body of the deceased is transported for burial or cremation. A flat fee may be charged for local service.
8. **Limousine.** A fee is charged to transport family members from the funeral home to the church or cemetery. This service is optional.
9. **Casket.** A casket is required for burial, but not for cremation. If a visitation is to be held before cremation, a rented casket may be required. Caskets vary in cost from about two hundred to eight thousand dollars depending on material and workmanship. Caskets are categorized as sealers and nonsealers. The sealer casket, which contains a rubber gasket that makes it air- and water-tight, thus slowing down the decomposition process, is higher priced, but it is seldom necessary to buy one. Some funeral directors may try to suggest one as a "final gesture of love for the deceased." Try to ignore such suggestions unless having a sealed casket is of great importance to you. Caskets made primarily from wood or other nonmetallic materials seldom have a sealing mechanism.
10. **Alternative containers.** Most places that perform cremations require the body to be in a container. This container does not have to be a casket. It is made of wood, pressed board, or even cardboard. Cremation containers can frequently be purchased from the funeral director for under fifty dollars.
11. **Burial garments.** Most families provide burial clothes for the deceased. If the family has no appropriate clothes, funeral directors can supply them at cost. If there is no visitation or if the body is to be cremated, the deceased may simply be covered by a sheet or other wrapping.

12. **Burial vault.** State laws do not require the use of grave liners or burial vaults. They are also not required if the body is to be interred in a mausoleum. However, many cemeteries do require vaults for burial to avoid the collapse of the grave and to reduce maintenance. Check local requirements before making a decision. Vaults, like caskets, vary in price. Depending on the materials used, they can cost from four hundred to five thousand dollars.

Each family will arrange a funeral according to its own needs and preferences, making it as simple or as elaborate as desired. There are some good concepts to keep in mind when planning a funeral. Remember that funerals are for the living. A person who has died cannot know of or appreciate any posthumous funeral arrangements. Life goes on for those left behind, and choosing an extravagant funeral can involve an unnecessary and stressful economic burden. When in doubt, choose a funeral that is consistent with the deceased's former life-style and financial means.

## Planning Your Own Funeral

We seldom think seriously about our own funeral; most of us deny or reject the notion of personal mortality. Anyone who has made funeral arrangements, however, knows of the difficult decisions involved. By planning your own funeral, you can spare your survivors such decisions. They may already be deeply burdened with feelings of loss, sorrow, and grief.

It is frequently difficult to obtain all the necessary information required for death certificates. You can assist your survivors by preparing a document that contains your full name, social security number, city and state of official residence, date and place of birth, U.S. armed forces serial number if applicable, occupation, father's name and date and place of birth, and mother's maiden name and date and place of birth.

It is also of enormous practical value to identify the locations of important papers and documents, such as your will, cemetery deeds, insurance policies, bank accounts, real-estate deeds, birth and marriage certificates, stocks and bonds, negotiable papers, mortgages, contractual agreements, promissory notes, trust-fund information, and any other pertinent materials.

Finally, prepare general directions for the kind of funeral you prefer. Specify the funeral home, clergyman, type of funeral, pallbearers, music, readings, flowers, special requests, type of casket, type of vault, type of burial, name of cemetery, and cemetery plot numbers (if you have purchased a plot). This information seems excessive, but it has tremendous practical value.

You can provide your survivors with guidance on one final aspect of dying. Innovations in medical technology now make it possible for machines to provide limited heartbeat and breathing actions for the person unable to perform these functions. Such advances pose certain dilemmas for physicians, lawyers, patients, and members of a patient's family. If your body is hopelessly ill or if your brain is irreparably damaged, should you be kept alive by artificial means? If so, for how long? Family members often must make such agonizing decisions.

The "living will" is the result of attempts to deal with these issues. The **"living will"** document is available from Concern for Dying, an educational and service council that promotes death with dignity and patient involvement in decisions that affect the future quality of life.[24] The living will has increasing validity as a legal document in at least eleven states. Its legal validity aside, it can provide guidance for physicians, family members, and others who may find themselves in a situation where a life versus death decision has to be made. (See figure 17.5.)

## LIVING WILL DECLARATION

**To My Family, Doctors, and All Those Concerned with My Care**

I, ______________________________, being of sound mind, make this statement as a directive to be followed if for any reason I become unable to participate in decisions regarding my medical care.

I direct that life-sustaining procedures should be withheld or withdrawn if I have an illness, disease or injury, or experience extreme mental deterioration, such that there is no reasonable expectation of recovering or regaining a meaningful quality of life.

These life-sustaining procedures that may be withheld or withdrawn include, but are not limited to:

SURGERY ANTIBIOTICS CARDIAC RESUSCITATION
RESPIRATORY SUPPORT ARTIFICIALLY ADMINISTERED FEEDING AND FLUIDS

I further direct that treatment be limited to comfort measures only, even if they shorten my life.

*You may delete any provision above by drawing a line through it and adding your initials.*

Other personal instructions:

These directions express my legal right to refuse treatment. Therefore, I expect my family, doctors, and all those concerned with my care to regard themselves as legally and morally bound to act in accord with my wishes, and in so doing to be free from any liability for having followed my directions.

Signed ______________________________ Date __________

Witness ______________________________ Witness ______________________________

### PROXY DESIGNATION CLAUSE

*If you wish, you may use this section to designate someone to make treatment decisions if you are unable to do so. Your Living Will Declaration will be in effect even if you have not designated a proxy.*

I authorize the following person to implement my Living Will Declaration by accepting, refusing and/or making decisions about treatment and hospitalization:

Name ______________________________

Address ______________________________

If the person I have named above is unable to act on my behalf, I authorize the following person to do so:

Name ______________________________

Address ______________________________

I have discussed my wishes with these persons and trust their judgment on my behalf.

Signed ______________________________ Date __________

Witness ______________________________ Witness ______________________________

**Figure 17.5**
Sample of the "living will." *Source:* Courtesy of the Society for the Right to Die, 250 West 57th Street, N.Y., N.Y. 10107.

## PERSONAL AND SOCIAL ISSUES FOR THE CONSUMER

Great technological advances are occurring in science and medicine. Consumers, nevertheless, remain vulnerable to quackery because of their lack of adequate knowledge, and feelings of hopelessness, helplessness, or despair. Quackery is a lucrative business for its practitioners, accounting for five billion dollars or more in annual income.[25] Most susceptible to the quack's persuasion are people who are incurably ill, who face surgery, who experience chronic and unending pain, and who have difficulty in adjusting to the prospects of growing older.

For the incurably ill patient, the will to live may be an important determinant in the eventual outcome of an illness. Those with the spirit to survive sometimes reach out for any sign of hope that is offered. Often such hope is provided by quacks. The dilemma of the incurably ill patient is a difficult one to comprehend for all but those who have been confronted with a similar situation. The patient must almost hope for a miracle, yet accept the best that medical science has to offer, recognize its limitations, and avoid the temptations of quackery.

Surgery is usually a frightening prospect. Even minor surgical procedures can require anesthesia, hospitalization, and other obtrusive procedures. Some people fear postoperative pain or are dismayed by the reality of the two million or so unnecessary surgical procedures that are performed each year.[26] Unless prospective surgical patients receive reassurance both from physicians and family members, they may have severe reservations about proceeding with an operation. If such social support is lacking, the appeal of an alternative practitioner who promises healing without surgery is inviting.

Other people, who are confronted with neither terminal illness nor surgery, are also susceptible to the hucksters of the health marketplace. These are the chronic pain sufferers whose desperate search for relief opens the door to quackery. Few ailments, for example, cause the physical anguish and mental frustration brought about by arthritis. Arthritis quackery is estimated to be a three-hundred-million to seven-hundred-fifty-million-dollar-a-year business.[27] Quacks have exploited this situation by offering such items as "magical" copper bracelets, mineral waters, condensed seawater, and a multitude of other gimmicks and concoctions of no curative value.

The inability to cope with the inexorable process of aging causes still other people to consider quackery. Quacks target both the elderly and the middle aged, offering help for wrinkles, balding, declining interest in sex, or decreasing vigor through cosmetics, diets, drugs, exercises, and other equipment and paraphernalia.

Quackery has survived centuries of exposure and is likely to be around as long as there are vulnerable individuals. Perhaps being aware of times you are most likely to be susceptible to quackery's inviting promises and schemes can direct you toward more beneficial practices.

## CONSUMER SKILLS AND SELF-RESPONSIBILITY

We have examined many techniques used by advertisers, retailers, quack practitioners, and others to persuade and influence consumer behavior. There are some skills that good consumers can develop to defend themselves in the health marketplace, or, where appropriate and necessary, to fight back. Corry delineates five important skills, including assertiveness, bargaining and bidding, budgeting, comparison shopping, and data collection.[28]

### Assertiveness

**Assertiveness** sometimes has a negative connotation; it is equated with being exploitative, aggressive, or unnecessarily obnoxious. Being assertive means to stand up for your rights, to be a self-advocate. Unfortunately, many of us are taught not to challenge health practitioners. But engaging in constructive confrontation, where appropriate, not only gives the consumer a more positive self-image, but may benefit the other party as well.[29] Learning to be assertive, like learning to play the French horn, requires practice. Some people fear the prospect of being assertive. As Corry states: "If this prospect terrifies you, keep in mind that through practice and role playing, your fear will pass."[30]

17.1 EXHIBIT

# Bee Pollen As a Health Food

It seems there's always someone willing to consider unlikely substances as capable of curing an illness or promoting better health. In the case of bee pollen, the philosophy seems to be that what's good for bees will be better for humans.

Bee pollen is flower pollen gathered by the common honeybee and carried to the hive on the bee's legs as tiny pods formed by mixing the pollen with nectar. The pollen is used as food by the bees.

But some bees don't get their food because humans have intervened to claim the supply for themselves. Humans get into the act by placing devices in the hive that strip the bee of her pollen before she can deliver. The purloined pollen is collected in trays, processed into several forms, and marketed as an extraordinarily nutritious food, often accompanied by claims of therapeutic qualities.

The idea of what's good for the bee is good for the beekeeper needs examination. Following are some of the principal claims made for bee pollen, along with scientific evidence and other facts associated with those claims.

*Claim:* Pollen is a "giant germ killer in which bacteria cannot exist."

The most authoritative scientific study of the biology, biochemistry and management of pollen (*Pollen,* by R. G. Stanley and H. F. Linskens) shows that pollen, when exposed to air, is rapidly attacked by bacteria, yeast and other fungi. Therefore, consumers should use the same precautions when storing pollen as with any other perishable food product.

*Claim:* Pollen is nature's most perfect food.

There is no one perfect food, only those that are better for various forms of life. The perfect food for the sea cucumber is organic debris sucked up from the ooze at the ocean's bottom. To larva of the silphid beetle, decaying meat is a perfect food. For the hookworm, there's nothing better than blood. According to studies by the National Academy of Sciences, the best dog food differs from the best cat food which differs from the best guinea pig food, and all of them differ from the ideal human diet. Thus, because pollen may be the best food for bees (or at least the best they can lay their hind legs on), there is no basis for a conclusion that it is the best, or anywhere near the best, food for human beings.

*Claim:* Pollen retards aging, as witness the longevity of natives of the mountains of Russian Georgia who owe it all to their pollen-rich diet.

According to a study of the eating habits of elderly persons in the Caucasus region of Soviet Georgia, "Sixty percent ate a mixed diet of milk, vegetables, meats, and fruits. Seventy percent of the calories were of vegetable origin and the remainder from meat and dairy products. Seventy to 90 grams of protein were included in the diets. Milk was a main source of protein." Although honey (which does contain some pollen) was sometimes included in the breakfast menu, along with cheese, bread and tea, the scientists conducting the study made no mention whatever of bee pollen, even though they were looking for some dietary clue that might explain why these people live so long. One centenarian's recipe might be less than attractive to those men who believe bee pollen wards off old age. Gabriel Chapnian, estimated to be 117, gave his prescription for longevity as: "Active physical work, and a moderate interest in alcohol and the ladies."

*Claim:* Pollen is the richest source of protein known to science.

The major constituent of pollen is carbohydrate, not protein. And the protein quality of pollen varies, depending on the plant from which it comes. As pointed out by Dr. Hachiro Shimanuki, director of the Bee Laboratory at the U.S. Department of Agriculture Research Center in Beltsville, Md., the protein content varies, ranging from 5 to 28 percent. A study by the United Nations Food and Agriculture Organization shows that many foods contain more protein than even the bee pollen with the highest protein content. For example, soybean cake contains 46 percent protein; raw soybeans, 38 percent; dry pumpkin seed, 29 percent; brewer's yeast, 39 percent. For comparison, round steak is about 20 percent protein.

The gross amount of protein does not give the full picture, however. Some protein sources contain all the essential amino acids in the proper balance needed by humans, but others do not. Thus, dry gelatin, which is about 86 percent protein, has a low biological value because it is very low in some essential amino acids. Most bee pollen does contain all the essential amino acids, but the amounts

EXHIBIT 17.1

of individual acids will also vary with the climatic and nutritional conditions of the plants on which the pollen matures.

Biological value means the amount of protein actually digested and transformed into food value. Tests on rats by several researchers have produced information on weight gain related to protein intake of various kinds. This ratio—called the "protein efficiency ratio"—ranges from a high of 3.80 for eggs and 3.55 for fish to a low of −1.25 for gelatin. Legumes (beans and peas) are good protein sources, having protein efficiency ratios of about 1.5. No tests of this kind have ever been carried out for bee pollen. Indeed, we do not really know what percentage of ingested bee pollen, if any, is actually capable of being absorbed by the human digestive system. It should be noted, however, that the amounts usually contained in a capsule of bee pollen provide an insignificant amount of protein.

It should also be pointed out that even if bee pollens were rich in biologically available protein, there are far less expensive protein sources, including filet mignon.

*Claim:* Bee pollen relieves allergies, asthma and hay fever.

There are no scientific studies to support this claim. On the contrary, scientists believe that bee pollen is especially hazardous for persons with allergies, asthma or hay fever. Dr. M. D. Levin, director of the Carl Hayden Bee Research Center in Tucson, Ariz., warns pollen users ". . . to be aware of its potential to trigger an allergic reaction."

This view is supported by cases in scientific studies. In one instance, 15 minutes after a 46-year-old man with a history of seasonal allergy took bee pollen he developed anaphylactic shock and required emergency treatment.

Dr. Steven Cohen, an allergy specialist conducting research on stinging insects and bee pollen at the Milwaukee County Medical Complex, tested two women who experienced acute allergic reactions after eating small quantities of bee pollen. He stated that bee pollen can be deadly to persons with allergies. "Some people are sensitive enough that oral exposure to it will cause a significant reaction," he said. An entomologist with the Mississippi Cooperative Extension Service, Dr. James Jarratt, also pointed out that, "If you were not aware of a specific allergy, one that you didn't notice due to the low levels of the allergen you encounter in day-to-day behavior, you might ingest a pretty good-sized slug of it in bee pollen and have an allergic reaction." This is fair warning for the 10 to 20 percent of the U.S. population that suffers from some form of allergy.

*Claim:* Various athletes state that bee pollen has improved their performance.

Assuming the person making such a statement is not doing it for a fee, such claims, called testimonials, are based on personal belief, not evidence of effectiveness. Medical history (as well as the history of food fads) is crammed with instances of people claiming various types of benefit from useless, and sometimes even harmful, substances, primarily from the plant world.

During a high point of the quack patent medicines era, just before the 1906 Food and Drugs Act, magazines and newspapers were full of testimonials about the curative powers of "medicines" that were little more than alcohol and colored water. Such ads, then and now, capitalize on an oddity of human nature: People are often (temporarily) helped, not by the food or drug being touted, but by a profound belief it will help. The renowned physician Sir William Osler had this in mind when he advised physicians ". . . to treat as many patients as possible with a new drug while it still has the power to heal." Some testimonials are sincere expressions of erroneous belief, and the still mysterious translation of hope magnified by belief into benefit, but others are fraudulent. And some are purchased. Noting how people lend their names to preposterous claims, one cynical newspaper editor said, "If your brains won't get you into the papers, sign a 'patent medicine' testimonial. Maybe your kidneys will."

*Claim:* Scientific tests prove that bee pollen enhances athletic performance.

In a 1975 test sponsored by the National Association of Athletic Trainers, the Louisiana State University swimming team participated in a six-month experiment in which half the team took 10 pollen tablets a day, one-quarter received 10 placebo tablets (externally identical to the pollen tablet but devoid of pollen), and the other quarter

17.1 *continued* EXHIBIT 17.1

received five pollen and five placebo tablets. There was no measurable difference in performance among the three groups.

The test later was repeated with 30 swimmers and 30 high school cross-country runners. As one of the researchers, Dr. John Wells of LSU, said, the bee pollen was "absolutely not a significant aid in metabolism, workout training or performance."

*Claim:* Bee pollen can alleviate a virtual encyclopedia of ailments, including sexual malfunction and tendencies toward suicide. (One promotional pamphlet listed 80 separate afflictions, from "growing pains" to cancer, which it claimed bee pollen had treated successfully.)

There is no valid scientific evidence for any therapeutic benefit from bee pollen. In view of what's known about bee pollen, compared with what's claimed, the conclusion of the authoritative Stanley-Linskens study is worth repeating. "While pollen, or its equivalent, may be irreplaceable in the bee diet," the study said, "we fail to see a correlation with suggested benefits to man. . . ."

What is the position of the Food and Drug Administration regarding bee pollen? Under the law, since the pollen has not been shown to be harmful other than to those suffering from an allergy, bee pollen may be marketed as a food, provided no nutrition or therapeutic claims are made or implied regarding it.

Thus, if the labeling (including pamphlets or advertising associated directly with the product) does not suggest that it is intended for use other than as food, bee pollen marketed as a food need meet only the same general labeling requirements as other foods, and be prepared, packed and held in a sanitary manner.

Although FDA has legal authority to require that new food additives pass certain tests before being allowed on the market, it cannot demand the same proof of foodstuffs, such as bee pollen. This is not the case with drugs.

If those selling bee pollen, or anything else, claim it can cure or alleviate any illness or produce some therapeutic benefit, the law says the product is a drug and must meet rigid scientific requirements for both safety and effectiveness. The exact language of the law is strict and precise. To gain approval as a new drug, a product must support its claims by "adequate and well controlled investigations, including clinical investigations, by experts qualified by scientific training and experience to evaluate the effectiveness of the drug involved, on the basis of which it could be fairly and responsibly concluded by such experts that the drug will have the effect it purports or is represented to have under the conditions of use prescribed, recommended or suggested in the labeling or proposed labeling."

Obviously, some bee pollen distributors have been making drug claims. In a recent instance, FDA asked that all shipments of a particular product and its promotional literature be immediately recalled by the manufacturer. The firm responsible swiftly complied, possibly aware that FDA can take other steps. These include seizure, injunction, and criminal prosecution where the law is violated regarding sale of an unapproved drug or a product classified as a drug due to therapeutic claims made for it.

Source: Larkin, Tim, "Bee Pollen as a Health Food," *FDA Consumer* (April 1984), 21–22.

## DISCUSSION QUESTIONS

1. What groups of people might be most vulnerable to the health food "quackery" of bee pollen?

2. Why would manufacturers of bee pollen want to avoid making curative claims about their product?

### Bargaining and Bidding

These are strategies used to pay the lowest reasonable price possible when making a purchase. In some settings, such as at automobile dealerships, bargaining has long been a common and expected practice. A car has a retail price known as the sticker price. A customer makes an offer at something less than the sticker price. The salesperson makes a counteroffer at something between the customer's bid and the sticker price. The familiar process of haggling begins. Perhaps the customer has received an offer from another dealer, that is, has engaged in comparison shopping. At some point, the buyer and the seller agree on a compromise price.

Such practice has not been common in the health marketplace. It may be that the purchase of practitioner services could become similar to the purchase of a car someday. If that seems improbable, then clearly the prospect of bargaining for a means of paying off practitioners' fees over time is not.

### Budgeting

This is a practice which can save you much anguish and prevent overspending. When you decide to purchase an item or service, establish an upper spending limit. Adhere to it. Such a practice discourages being lured into the bait-and-switch trap.

### Comparison Shopping

Comparison shopping can often be a fruitful source of savings. One of the realities of the health marketplace is that stiff competition exists. The purchase price of both prescription and non-prescription drugs can be moderated by calling different pharmacies. A month's supply of a particular oral contraceptive may be $12.95 at the clinic pharmacy, but only $8.95 at a pharmacy a block away. Make phone calls—lots of them.

Although it is rarely done, there is no practical reason why the cost of many practitioner services cannot be given over the telephone. Though cost is not the only criterion to be considered when selecting a service provider, think about the merit of paying twenty-seven dollars for preventive dental services with Dr. Smith compared to forty-eight dollars for equivalent services from Dr. Jones.

### Data Collection

This may be the most tedious and laborious part of being a good consumer. Most of us do not take the time or expend the energy necessary to make the best purchase for our money. It is easier to gamble and keep our fingers crossed. Often we do not get "burned" gambling, so we are tempted to gamble again. When we finally get a bad product and feel "stung," we act as if the toilet backed up into our living room and we did not have any control over it. The merchandiser knows of this flaw in consumers' characters and exploits it. At the moment we are ready to buy, our only "data" may be what we remember from that TV commercial or magazine ad.

What can we do to reduce the chances of being victimized? Any consumer who can read can become a self-advocate. A number of informative and worthwhile publications are widely available. These publications include such periodicals as *Consumer Reports, Changing Times,* and *FDA Consumer.* When in a physician's office, a wise consumer should seek information, especially if handed a prescription. Pharmacists are also good sources for information about medications. You can develop the necessary assertiveness to find out what information you need and how to find it.

## HELP FOR THE CONSUMER

As a consumer, you may sometimes feel compelled to complain about the performance of a product or the outcome of a service. Before making a complaint, it is wise to be sure that it is justified. If you failed to follow directions or improperly handled the product, your complaint may not be legitimate. But if you are sure your complaint is justified, be sure you stay coolheaded and diligently follow up on the complaint. There are several private and governmental agencies to assist consumers.

## Private Organizations

Professional associations like the **American Medical Association** and the **American Dental Association** are instrumental in the war on quackery. These organizations are represented at local levels by state or county affiliates. These groups are usually listed in the telephone book, and can address questions about adherence of practitioners to professional and ethical standards. Professional organizations representing other groups such as optometrists and funeral directors exist, and also may have local affiliates.

The local **Better Business Bureau** is not an enforcement agency and does not give legal advice, but it can direct consumers to the most appropriate source of help for their complaint or problem. The Better Business Bureau may be able to provide you with information concerning an establishment's reputation before you spend your money there. It can be a valuable community resource in overseeing consumer satisfaction, arranging for appropriate adjustments when necessary, and acting as an intermediary when a consumer's complaint seems unwarranted.

There are many other private organizations available to aid a troubled consumer. Such organizations are often listed in the telephone book. You can also seek help at the public library, in the local newspaper, or sometimes, by contacting radio and television stations. If all else fails, a comprehensive list of consumer organizations in your state can be obtained from Division of Consumer Organizations, U.S. Office of Consumer Affairs, Washington, D.C. 20201.

## Governmental Agencies

Help for the consumer is at hand from three major federal agencies: the Food and Drug Administration (FDA), the Federal Trade Commission, (FTC), and the United States Postal Service (USPS).

The **FDA** is an agency of the U.S. Department of Health and Human Services responsible for consumer protection in the areas of falsely represented or worthless drugs, medical devices, and cosmetics. It also protects consumers against food contaminants. The safety and effectiveness of new drugs are regulated by the FDA. Complaints can be addressed to: Director, Consumer Communications, FDA, 5600 Fishers Lane, Rockville, Md. 20857.

The **FTC** provides consumer safeguards against deceptive claims in advertisements. It addresses claims concerning OTC drug products and cosmetics, medical devices, hearing aids, contact lenses, dental appliances, so-called hair restorers and bust developers, and funeral services. Fraud must be evident before the FTC can take legal action. Unfortunately, it may take years before some claims can be completely settled by the FTC. Complaints can be filed by writing: Office of the Secretary, Federal Trade Commission, Washington, D.C. 20580.

The **USPS** attempts to protect the public from fraud and quackery conducted through the U.S. mail. Conviction of people operating fraudulent businesses or selling worthless products through the mail requires only the proof of product misrepresentation. If you receive falsely promoted, misrepresented, or unwanted products in the mail, contact your local postmaster or write: Consumer Advocate, U.S. Postal Service, Washington, D.C. 20260.

## Writing a Complaint Letter

Resolving a consumer problem to your satisfaction does not always require the help of a consumer advocacy or regulatory agency. Most complaints are settled to everyone's satisfaction through direct communication between parties. Learn to be a self-advocate.

To prepare a letter of complaint, first find out if the company has a local office. If there is no local listing, consult a reference available at most public libraries entitled *Standard & Poor's Register of Corporations, Directors and Executives*. This reference lists the names and addresses of more than 37,000 American businesses.

Type your letter, if possible, and include your name, address, and home and business telephone numbers. Be brief and to the point. Letters that are longer than one page and contain an extensive case history are undesirable. Pertinent facts such as date of transaction, item involved, and the store name should be included. You should state your proposal for a fair and just settlement. Attach documentation to support your claim (sales receipts, cancelled checks, etc.) Send photocopies of the documentation rather than originals. It is seldom justified in a first letter to be sarcastic, threatening, or insulting, no matter how tempting it may be. The person reading your letter doubtlessly had nothing to do with creating your complaint, but may be instrumental in settling it. Finally, keep a copy for your records. A sample letter that can be adapted for a variety of situations is shown in figure 17.6.

Your address
Your city, state, zip

Date

Appropriate person
Company name
Street address
City, state, zip

Dear Appropriate person:

Recently I purchased a (name of product with serial or model number or service performed). I made this purchase at (location, date, and other pertinent details of the purchase transaction).

Unfortunately, your product (or service) has not performed in a satisfactory manner (or the service was not adequate) because ______________

______________________________________________

______________________________________________

______________________________________________

Therefore, to solve this problem, I am requesting that you (state the specific action you want taken). I have enclosed copies (copies—NOT ORIGINALS) of my records of this transaction (receipts, guarantees, warranties, cancelled checks, contracts, model or serial numbers, and any other pertinent documents).

I am looking forward to hearing from you and learning how this problem is to be resolved. I shall wait three weeks before seeking third-party assistance. I may be contacted at the above address, or by telephone at (place your home and business numbers here).

Sincerely,

Your name

______________________________________________

**Figure 17.6**
Sample of a complaint letter written by a consumer.

## A LAST WORD ABOUT CONSUMERISM

The health marketplace may be perceived by the uninformed consumer as a "jungle." Everyone is likely to have bad experiences from time to time. However, the number of complaints and problems, as well as their eventual outcomes, are often within the consumer's control. By being a self-advocate, you can protect both yourself and others from being victimized. A great many problems can be avoided by arming yourself with what it takes to be an informed consumer.

## SUMMARY

1. Everyone must make decisions about the purchase of health-related goods and services.

2. People purchase goods and services to satisfy perceived needs and the desire for self-esteem.

3. Peer pressure, the need to belong, perceptions about group norms, and belief in authority are important forces in determining product purchases by consumers.

4. Wise selection and use of health-related products require that a consumer possess both knowledge and common sense.

5. Marketing of health products includes appealing to basic psychological desires of people through such strategies as media bombardment and subliminal advertising.

6. A variety of deceptive or fraudulent sales techniques can mislead unsuspecting and poorly informed consumers. Some common schemes include bait and switch, brand loyalty, and product misrepresentation.

7. Considerable sums of money are spent by consumers on such things as skin and beauty aids, eyeglasses and contact lenses, self-diagnosis equipment, and other health-related devices. Shopping around to price items, purchasing only what is needed, and observing caution about fraudulent practices are practices that can assist consumers in getting the most for their money.

8. Vulnerability to quackery and other fraudulent practices can sometimes be predicted and prevented. People most at risk include the incurably ill, those facing surgery, chronic pain sufferers, and those who deal unrealistically with the prospects of advancing age.

9. Certain consumer skills can be learned and practiced to minimize the probability of being defrauded. These skills include assertiveness, bargaining and bidding, budgeting, comparison shopping, and data collection.

10. Funeral services provide a special challenge to the consumer. It is important for consumers to know how to select a funeral director, to understand the range of services provided by funeral directors, and to recognize how pricing is performed. It is of practical importance that you do some advance planning for your own death in order to assist your survivors in the task of making funeral arrangements.

11. Consumers have many resources available to assist them. In the private sector, organizations like the American Medical Association (AMA) and the American Dental Association (ADA) can be helpful. The Better Business Bureau can be of great assistance in mediating consumer complaints, though it has no enforcement authority. It can also provide information to consumers prior to both service utilization and product purchase. Federal government agencies such as the Food and Drug Administration (FDA), the Federal Trade Commission (FTC), and the U.S. Postal Service (USPS) attempt to protect the public from fraud and quackery.

12. Everyone should know how to write a letter of complaint when necessary, and to direct it to the most appropriate person.

13. Learn to be a self-advocate.

## Recommended Readings

Editors of Consumer Reports Books. *The Medicine Show,* 5th ed. Mount Vernon, N.Y.: Consumers Union, 1980.

Kaufman, Joel et al. *Over the Counter Pills that Don't Work.* New York: Pantheon Books, 1983.

Key, Wilson Bryan. *Subliminal Seduction.* Englewood Cliffs, N.J.: Prentice-Hall, 1973.

Mechanic, David, ed. *Handbook of Health, Health Care, and the Health Professions.* New York: Free Press, 1983.

Pinckney, C., and Pinckney, E. R. *The Patient's Guide to Medical Tests.* New York: Facts on File, 1982.

## References

1. *Consumer's Resource Handbook* (Pueblo, Colo.: Consumer Information Center, 1979).

2. Thomas S. Robertson, *Consumer Behavior* (Glenview, Ill.: Scott, Foresman and Co., 1970).

3. Wilson Bryan Key, *Subliminal Seduction* (Englewood Cliffs, N.J.: Prentice-Hall, 1973).

4. J. W. Smith and S. S. Baker, *Doctor, Make Me Beautiful* (New York: David McKay, 1973).

5. H. J. Cornacchia and S. Barrett, *Consumer Health* (St. Louis: C. V. Mosby, 1980).

6. "Shampoos," *Changing Times* 33 (April 1979): 19–20.

7. Editors of Consumer Reports, "Shampoo," *Consumer Reports* 41 (1976): 617–21.

8. Editors of Consumer Reports, "Shampoo," 617–21.

9. Editors of Consumer Reports, "Shampoo," 617–21.

10. Editors of Consumer Reports, "Shampoo," 617–21.

11. A. Hecht, "Aerosol Antiperspirants under a Cloud," *FDA Consumer* 13 (November 1978): 10–11.

12. Margaret Morrison, "The Great Feminine Spray Explosion," *FDA Consumer* (October 1973): 16–17.

13. Editors of Consumer Reports Books, *The Medicine Show,* 5th ed. (Mount Vernon, N.Y.: Consumers Union, 1980).

14. James M. Corry, *Consumer Health: Facts, Skills, and Decisions* (Belmont, Calif.: Wadsworth, 1983), 225.

15. Corry, *Consumer Health: Facts, Skills, and Decisions,* 224–25.

16. G. B. Griffenhagen and L. L. Hawkins, eds., *Handbook of Nonprescription Drugs* (Washington, D.C.: American Pharmaceutical Association, 1973).

17. Cornacchia and Barrett, *Consumer Health,* 45.

18. Cornacchia and Barrett, *Consumer Health,* 46.

19. J. F. Greene, "Coin-Operated Blood Pressure Machines," *FDA Consumer* 12 (October 1978): 11–13.

20. Editors of Consumer Reports, "Blood Pressure Kits," *Consumer Reports* 44: (March 1979): 142–46.

21. Editors of Consumer Reports, "Blood Pressure Kits," 142–46.

22. J. F. Greene, "Coin-Operated Blood Pressure Machines," *FDA Consumer* 12 (October 1978): 11–13.

23. Corry, *Consumer Health: Facts, Skills, and Decisions,* 225.

24. Concern for Dying, 250 West 57th Street, New York, N.Y. 10107.

25. Corry, *Consumer Health: Facts, Skills, and Decisions,* 15.

26. Corry, *Consumer Health: Facts, Skills, and Decisions,* 119.

27. Corry, *Consumer Health: Facts, Skills, and Decisions,* 119.

28. Corry, *Consumer Health: Facts, Skills, and Decisions,* 47.

29. Corry, *Consumer Health: Facts, Skills, and Decisions,* 47.

30. Corry, *Consumer Health: Facts, Skills, and Decisions,* 47.

CHAPTER EIGHTEEN

# Health-Care Consumerism: Selecting Care Wisely



It might be hypothesized that in no other area of human health and wellness is there a greater premium placed on knowledge, assertiveness, and foresight than in our dealings with the health-care delivery system. Astronomical levels of growth and sophistication of medical technology, as well as significant advancements in the training of health-care professionals, speak strongly to the capacity of modern science and medicine effectively to diagnose, treat, and rehabilitate consumers for most known diseases. These advancements are not free from higher health-care costs. In order not only to deal with these rising costs, but also to make sound health-care decisions, consumers need to possess at least a general understanding of the health-care delivery system and how it works.

Most Americans grow up possessing a multitude of beliefs and attitudes about health, health care, health professionals, and health institutions and organizations. The nature and extent of the beliefs held present no particular problem, unless within these belief structures we have a majority of inaccurate notions that may cause us to make some faulty health-care consumer decisions.

Occasional poor decision making on the part of consumers cannot be entirely eliminated by increased understanding of the health-care system, but the probability of repeated or significant errors may be reduced.

This chapter will introduce you to the major components of the U.S. health-care system. Health-care practitioners, resources, and services will be highlighted, as well as various means of financing health care. It is hoped that as we, the consumers of health services, products, and information, assume a more assertive and intelligent posture relative to our well-being, we can begin to exert a greater influence on the direction and future emphasis of health care delivery in this country.

# HEALTH-CARE PERSONNEL

The delivery of health care in the U.S. is accomplished through the interaction of a variety of professionals, institutions, and agencies. The most visible element of the system might be those persons who directly provide care. Physicians, dentists, nurses, and other allied health personnel comprise this element of the health-care system.

## Physicians

Within the medical profession, there are two approaches to the practice of medicine that we would define as being orthodox. The two are known specifically as allopathy and osteopathy.

### ALLOPATHY

**Allopathy** is the term that is applied to persons graduating from schools of medicine where the doctor of medicine (M.D.) is awarded. The M.D. degree is awarded to an individual following successful completion of four years of schooling at an institution that is accredited by the American Medical Association and the Association of American Medical Colleges. Most states require that graduates of medical schools complete at least one year of hospital internship following graduation. Medical-school graduates must also pass either state or national board examinations before they are eligible to be licensed by a state board of medical examiners. People completing this series of events are referred to as **General Practitioners (G.P.)**. For individuals wishing to specialize in a particular field of medicine, an additional amount of schooling and internship activity is required. Additionally, students must pass specialty group examinations. Terms such as "board certified," "boarded," and "diplomate" are used to refer to individuals who have successfully completed this process. Some physician specialists do not complete the entire process of becoming board certified. Consumers can determine if a physician is board certified by checking *The Directory of Medical Specialists,* a national publication containing biographical information on practicing physician specialists. A listing of the various medical specialties can be found in table 18.1.

### OSTEOPATHY

Osteopathy, as a form of medical practice, has been in existence for quite a long time. The founder of osteopathy was Andrew Taylor Still, M.D., who expressed the basic principle and theory in 1874. He went on to organize the first school of osteopathy in Kirksville, Missouri, in 1894. **Osteopathy** is a system of medical practice that emphasizes integrity of the muscular and skeletal systems working in harmony. Over the years, osteopathic medicine has evolved to the point where some states (California, Michigan) allow persons who have been awarded the degree of osteopathy (D.O.) to use the M.D. designation if so desired.

The training of an osteopathic physician involves four years of medical training following at least three years of preprofessional undergraduate college education. A one-year hospital internship is also required of people graduating from an accredited school of osteopathic medicine. Osteopaths may also choose to specialize in a number of medical fields. Specializing requires additional study and testing following the one-year internship.[1] Osteopathic medicine is recognized as a form of legitimate medical practice in all fifty states.

### CHOOSING AND RATING A PHYSICIAN

Some of the most important and useful skills we can possess as health-care consumers come into play when selecting a physician. We not only need to seek out the names of physicians who might be willing to take on new patients, but also apply information gathered concerning this individual as an extension of the selection process. Initially, we need to identify the names of potential physicians. The following are examples of sources which may be useful in compiling such a list:

1. telephone book (yellow pages)
2. referrals from a former physician
3. friends and relatives
4. the American Medical Association, state or local medical societies

**Table 18.1 Selected Medical Specialties and Subspecialties**

*Allergy:* A subspecialty of internal medicine that concerns the diagnosis and treatment of allergic reactions.

*Anesthesiology:* Administration of drugs to block pain or induce unconsciousness during surgery, diagnostic procedures, or childbirth.

*Cardiology:* A subspecialty of internal medicine that concerns the diagnosis and treatment of disorders of the heart and blood vessels.

*Child Psychiatry:* A subspecialty of psychiatry that concerns nervous and emotional problems of children.

*Colon and Rectal Surgery (Proctology):* Diagnosis and treatment of disorders of the lower digestive tract.

*Dermatology:* Diagnosis and treatment of skin disorders.

*Family Practice:* Provides general medical care to patients and their families.

*Gastroenterology:* A subspecialty of internal medicine that concerns the diagnosis and treatment of disorders of the gastrointestinal tract.

*Internal Medicine:* Diagnosis and nonsurgical treatment of internal organs and organ systems of the body.

*Neurology:* Diagnosis and nonsurgical treatment of disorders of the brain, spinal cord, and nerves.

*Neurosurgery:* Diagnosis and surgical treatment of nervous system disorders.

*Nuclear Medicine:* Use of radioactive substances for the diagnosis and treatment of disease.

*Obstetrics and Gynecology:* Care of women during pregnancy, childbirth and the postnatal period, and/or diagnosis and treatment of disorders of the female reproductive system.

*Occupational Medicine:* Deals with the diagnosis, treatment, and prevention of diseases associated with health risks at the workplace. It is a subspecialty of preventive medicine.

*Oncology:* Diagnosis and treatment of neoplastic growths or tumors.

*Ophthalmology:* Medical and surgical care of the eye, including the prescribing of corrective lenses.

*Orthopedics:* Treatment of diseases, fractures, and deformities of the bones and joints, and diseases of the muscles.

*Otolaryngology:* Diagnosis and treatment of ear, nose, and throat disorders.

*Pathology:* Examination of body organs, tissues, body fluids, and excrement to detect disease.

*Pediatrics:* The medical care of children through adolescence.

*Physiatry:* The treatment and rehabilitation of physical handicaps.

*Plastic Surgery:* The correction or repair of body or facial structures through surgery.

*Preventive Medicine:* Disease prevention through health habits, immunization, and environmental control.

*Psychiatry:* Diagnosis and treatment of mental and emotional disorders.

*Public Health:* A subspecialty of internal medicine concerned with the promotion of the general health of the community.

*Pulmonary Medicine:* A subspecialty of internal medicine, concerned with diseases of the lungs.

*Radiology:* The use of radiation to diagnose and treat disease.

*Urology:* Diagnosis and treatment of disorders of the urinary tract in both males and females, and the genital organs in the male.

Source: From Price, J. H., N. Galli and S. Slenker, *Consumer Health: Contemporary Issues and Choices.* 

Once a list of potential physician candidates has been assembled, we can then attempt to rate these persons by acquiring additional information. Activity for Wellness 18.1 will assist you in locating a physician you will feel comfortable with.

By gathering information on potential physicians, you increase the probability that the person you select as either your primary-care or specialty physician will meet your expectations for high-quality health care. Assuming a passive role in such an important consumer area may result in later dissatisfaction and disappointment.

## Other Health-Care Practitioners

Physicians and osteopaths, by virtue of their medical licensing, can perform a full, unlimited range of legitimate medical procedures. Other types of health-care providers are limited in what they can perform. Some of the more common of these practitioners are dentists, podiatrists, nurse practitioners, optometrists, clinical psychologists, and physician assistants.

18.1 ACTIVITY FOR WELLNESS 18.1

# Issues to Consider in Selecting a Physician

Use this checklist to rate potential physicians. How many of these criteria do your potential (or current) physicians meet?

*On the Telephone*

[ ] Is the physician willing to consult with you on the telephone?
[ ] Do you feel that your questions are answered without you being rushed?
[ ] Is the receptionist willing to share information on the physician's credentials, hospital affiliation, and fee schedule?
[ ] Does the receptionist allow you sufficient time for interaction?

*In the waiting area*

[ ] Is the atmosphere friendly and reassuring?
[ ] Are you informed ahead of time if there is likely to be a delay?
[ ] Are you provided privacy in responding to questions of a personal nature?
[ ] Are there too many people waiting to see the physician?
[ ] Are there educational materials available in the waiting area?
[ ] Office accepts insurance, or does it require you to pay and wait to be reimbursed?

*During your examination*

[ ] Is a detailed medical history taken?
[ ] Does the physician explain the purpose of the exam and any tests given?
[ ] Does the physician use medical jargon?
[ ] Are your questions welcomed and answered in a helpful manner?
[ ] Is there a willingness to talk about matters such as medical training, hospital affiliation, and fees?

*When discussing diagnosis and treatment*

[ ] Does your doctor explain your diagnosis and treatment alternatives?
[ ] Does he encourage you to ask questions?
[ ] Does your doctor explain why a particular drug is prescribed? Does he give you directions on how to take it properly?
[ ] Does the physician support your obtaining a second opinion if surgery is recommended? Does he use surgery only as a last resort?
[ ] Does the physician suggest referrals when a specialist seems appropriate?

Source: From Price, J. H., N. Galli and S. Slenker, *Consumer Health: Contemporary Issues and Choices.* 

**DENTISTS** The **Doctor of Dental Surgery (D.D.S.)** and the **Doctor of Medical Dentistry (D.M.D.)** are concerned with the diagnosis and treatment of diseases and conditions of the teeth, gums, and associated oral structures. Most dentists are general practitioners. However, some dentists specialize in areas such as children's dentistry, treatment of poorly positioned teeth, treatment of tissues supporting the teeth, and treatment of diseases of the inner portion of the tooth.[2]

**PODIATRISTS** **Podiatrists** are medical specialists who deal with disorders of the foot. The podiatrist may use surgery, drugs, manipulative therapy, braces, and the like to diagnose and treat foot problems. Podiatrists possess the degree of either Doctor of Podiatric Medicine (D.P.M.) or the Doctor of Podiatry (D.P.).

**NURSE PRACTITIONERS** **Nurse practitioners** are professional nurses (R.N.s) who have graduated from specific specialty programs and as a result can engage in a variety of expanded health-care services. Nurse-practitioner programs are increasing rapidly, with the most notable ones being in the areas of pediatrics, family health, and obstetrics and gynecology. Nurse practitioners typically work under the direction of an allopathic or osteopathic physician.

**OPTOMETRISTS** An **optometrist** is a professionally prepared person who diagnoses visual problems and improves vision. The work of optometrists primarily involves prescription of glasses and contact lenses.

**CLINICAL PSYCHOLOGISTS** **Clinical Psychologists** concern themselves with the nonmedical aspects of human behavior and mental health. Clinical psychologists usually possess an academic doctorate (Ph.D.) in psychology and often specialize in a particular client population or a setting such as schools or worksites.

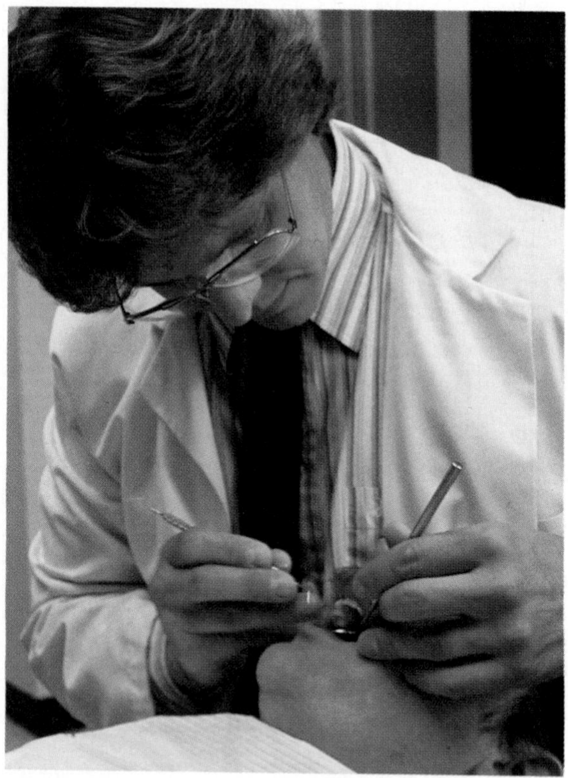

**Figure 18.1**
Dentists are crucial members of the health-care team.

**PHYSICIAN ASSISTANTS** **Physician Assistants (P.A.s)** are usually educated in two-year programs sponsored by medical schools, universities, or technical colleges. They perform routine medical procedures on patients under the supervision and legal obligation of a physician.

## Alternative Health Practitioners

In contrast to the orthodox full and limited practitioners discussed, a wide variety of alternative systems of healing and healers exist. These alternative approaches to medicine are considered somewhat questionable in that the techniques and methodologies have not been subjected to the rigors of scientific testing and evidence. Although these theories and approaches may work for some people with certain ailments, the likelihood that they can cure a wide

18.2 ACTIVITY FOR WELLNESS 18.2

# Deciphering Doctor Talk

Hypoglycemia may sound like a difficult word, but its meaning should be apparent to persons with a knowledge of medical terminology. The word parts, all derived from ancient Greek, are *hypo,* meaning under, or deficient; *glyco,* referring to sugar; and *emia,* referring to blood. When put together, the word hypoglycemia means an abnormally low level of sugar in the blood.

Thousands of medical words can be constructed in the same manner. To the famed Greek physician Hippocrates, who lived from 460 to 377 B.C., goes the credit for contributing to modern medical language most of these mix-and-match prefixes, suffixes and root words.

The Romans adopted Greek medicine and most of the terminology used by Greek physicians by the third century B.C., although they often gave the words Latin spelling. The use of Latin and Greek in medical terminology received new currency during the Renaissance when these languages became the medium of intellectual inquiry, providing a ready source of medical words for physicians of the times. Translations of Arabic medical texts also contributed new terms.

Modern medical terminology thus consists largely of Greek words and roots that have been Latinized. (Only a few purely Latin words have survived, and these are associated primarily with anatomy.) According to *Dorland's Illustrated Medical Dictionary,* 75 percent of the scientific words commonly used can be traced to these ancient languages. Other words are of more modern origin and come to us from French or German.

Some medical terms are based on a single root. For instance, "muscle" comes from the Latin "musculus"—a little mouse—describing the way certain muscles move under the skin. Coccyx, a small bone at the base of the spine, gets its name from the fact that it looks like the bill of the cuckoo, or *kokkyx,* in Greek.

Most medical words combine two or more words or word elements to form a new word. Because ancient Greek and Latin are "dead" languages, the meanings of these elements have not changed over the centuries. Thus, medical terms formed from them are logical and precise. The combinations have become a kind of condensed language that doctors the world over can understand.

Although it is true that doctors of old wrote their prescriptions in Latin to keep the patient from knowing what was in them, modern medical personnel don't use medical terminology to confuse the patient. It's just more convenient to use these universally accepted terms. For example, it's easier to say "arthritis" than "inflammation of the joints."

Here's a sampling of the bits and pieces that make up some familiar medical language.

**PREFIXES**

a, an = without, not
ad = near
anti = against
end(o) = within
ep(i) = on, upon, over
hyper = above, over, excessive
hypo = below, under, deficient
inter = between
intra = within
macro = large
micro = small
peri = around
pre = before, in front of
poly = many

**COMBINING FORMS***

angio, angi = blood or lymph vessel
arterio = artery
arthro = joint
brady = slow
cardio = heart

*Combining form = root word + a vowel

18.2 *continued*

ACTIVITY FOR WELLNESS

**COMBINING FORMS***

chole, cholo = bile
colo = colon
cysto, cystido = sac, cyst, bladder
dys = difficult, painful, abnormal
glyco = sugar
hema, hemo, hemato = blood
hepato = liver
hystero = uterus
leuco, leuko = white
lipo = fat
meno = menses
nephro = kidney
osteo = bone
pneumato, pneuma = air, gas
rhino = nose
sclero = hard
tachy = swift, rapid
veno = vein

*Combining form = root word + a vowel

**SUFFIXES**

algia = pain
cyte = cell
ectomy = excision of
emia = blood
itis = inflammation of
megaly = very large
oma = tumor, swelling
osis = disease, morbid process
ostomy = artificial opening
otomy, tomy = incision into
pathy = disease of
pnea = breathing
rhage, rhagia = bleeding, bursting forth
rhea = flow
uria = urine

By combining root words with prefixes and suffixes, words such as the following are formed:

arteriosclerosis = hardening of the arteries
bradycardia = slowness of the heartbeat
colostomy = surgical creation of an opening between the colon and the surface of the body
dyspnea = difficult or painful breathing
glycosuria = presence of sugar in the urine
hemorrhage = escape of blood from the vessels; bleeding
hepatitis = inflammation of the liver
hepatomegaly = enlargement of the liver
hyperlipemia = excessive fat in the blood
hysterectomy = removal of the uterus
intravenous = within a vein or veins
leucocyte = white blood cell
lipoma = a fatty tumor
macrocyst = a large cyst
neuralgia = severe sharp pain along the course of a nerve
periangioma = a tumor which surrounds a blood vessel
rhinitis = inflammation of the nasal passages

spectrum of health problems, as professed, is remote. The number of alternative health practices preclude detailed and comprehensive coverage in this chapter. A few of the more common alternative health practices are chiropractic, naturopathy, homeopathy, and acupuncture.

**CHIROPRACTIC** The **chiropractic** approach to healing is generally characterized as being both nonmedical and nonsurgical. It is a form of therapy whose theory states that health is contingent upon the structural integrity of the spinal column. Diagnosis is usually made by X ray of the full torso. Then through manipulation of the vertebrae by the chiropractor, changes in the health status of the patient are expected to occur. Chiropractors are trained in chiropractic colleges, wherein it takes four years

## ACTIVITY FOR WELLNESS 18.2

For a blockbuster of a medical word there is "hepatocholangiocystoduodenostomy," which any student who has done the required homework knows means "the establishment of drainage of bile ducts into the duodenum through the gallbladder."

There are thousands of other words in the medical lexicon. Listed below are a few that a patient might well hear when talking to the doctor, or read in medical articles. Some are not exclusive to medicine:

arrhythmia = an irregularity in the rhythm of the heartbeat
biopsy = removal of a small piece of tissue for examination under the microscope
cardiac arrest = sudden stopping of heart function
cardiovascular = pertaining to the heart and blood vessels
caries = gradual decay and disintegration of bone or tooth
comatose = in or of a coma, an abnormal deep stupor occurring in illness
contraindication = any condition that renders some line of treatment improper or undesirable
data = things known or assumed; information
diuretic = an agent or drug that increases the secretion of urine
edema = local or generalized condition in which the body tissues contain an excessive amount of fluid; swelling
efficacy = power to produce effects or intended results; effectiveness
etiology = the cause(s) or origin of a disease
ingestion = the act of taking food, medicine, etc., into the body by mouth
myocardial infarction = death of tissue in the heart muscle, usually following an interruption of the blood supply to the heart
pathogenic = productive of disease
prognosis = the forecast as to the probable outcome of a disease
psychogenic = a symptom having an emotional or psychologic origin, as opposed to an organic one
renal = pertaining to the kidney
serum = the clear portion of any animal fluid, separated from its more solid elements
stenosis = constriction or narrowing of a passage or opening
subcutaneous = beneath the skin

Consumers who turn to sources such as *The Merck Manual* or the *Physicians' Desk Reference* for health information may need a medical dictionary close by. But once the Greek and Latin roots are mastered, they should be able to solo without lexicographic assistance.

Source: *FDA Consumer* 18.4 (1984): 7–9. U.S. Food and Drug Administration, Office of Legislation and Information, Rockville, Md.

to earn the D.C. degree. Additionally, chiropractors must pass state licensing examinations in order to practice chiropractic.

Within the chiropractic profession there are two types of healers.[3] One group, known as the "straights," rely solely on manual manipulation as the therapeutic modality. The other, "mixers," rely on a wide variety of techniques such as "colonic flushes" (enemas administered by a machine),[4] heat, moisture, and ice in the treatment of their patients' problems.

Orthodox medical practitioners have expressed concern with the chiropractic profession's potential misuse of X rays and dangerous adjustments involving pressure on the spine.[5] To date, neither the straights nor the mixers have been able to gain any type of hospital privileges in institutions accredited by the Joint Commission on Accreditation of Hospitals.

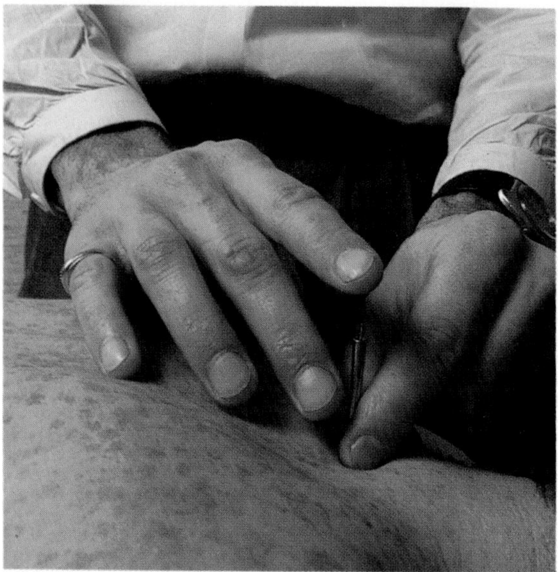

**Figure 18.2**
Acupuncture is an ancient Chinese healing art.

**NATUROPATHY** Individuals adhering to **naturopathy** rely on natural elements to restore health to the afflicted. Sunlight, water, electricity, gravity, heat, and herbs are examples of the prescriptions offered for health care.[6] Naturopaths believe that as we get our bodies out of balance with nature we encounter ill health.

**HOMEOPATHY** **Homeopaths** believe that people who are ill need to be treated with substances and therapies that in a normally healthy person would cause those symptoms. The notion of treating like with like is basic to their profession.[7] This theory is in direct opposition to allopathic practitioners who generally treat diseases with opposites.

**ACUPUNCTURE** **Acupuncture** is the ancient Chinese healing art whereby fine needles of varying length are inserted at specific points on the body known as loci. The insertion of the needles is an attempt to restore a balance to the Yin (cold, dark, female, and body interior) and Yang (hot, light, male, and body exterior). As needles are inserted by the acupuncturist and left for a determined period of time, the balance of Yin and Yang is restored and some good health supposedly regained.[8]

# HEALTH-CARE RESOURCES AND FACILITIES

A second major component of the health-care delivery system are the many health-care resources and facilities which exist to provide care to patients. Usually there is a correlation between the levels of care that are required and the place where that care is received.

## Levels of Care

**PRIMARY CARE** **Primary care** is provided to individuals requiring routine health checkups, or those experiencing illness for the first time. Outside of a serious medical emergency, this level of care is typically provided in a practitioner's private office or in an outpatient type of clinic.

**SECONDARY CARE** **Secondary care** is usually delivered by physicians who are specialists within a particular area of medicine, upon referral from a patient's primary-care physician. This level of care is provided either in the private office or clinic of the attending physician, or in a hospital where more extensive care can be delivered.

**TERTIARY CARE** **Tertiary care,** the highest level of care, is typically delivered in a hospital. This care is almost always supplied by highly technologically oriented professionals and resources. (See figure 18.3.)

## Places of Care

As we discuss the levels of care we generally refer to specific places where such care may be delivered.

**PRIVATE PRACTITIONER'S OFFICES** Depending on whether the practitioner is considered a primary-care practitioner or a specialist, the types of care will vary in extensiveness. In either case, the care is generally defined as ambulatory or outpatient.

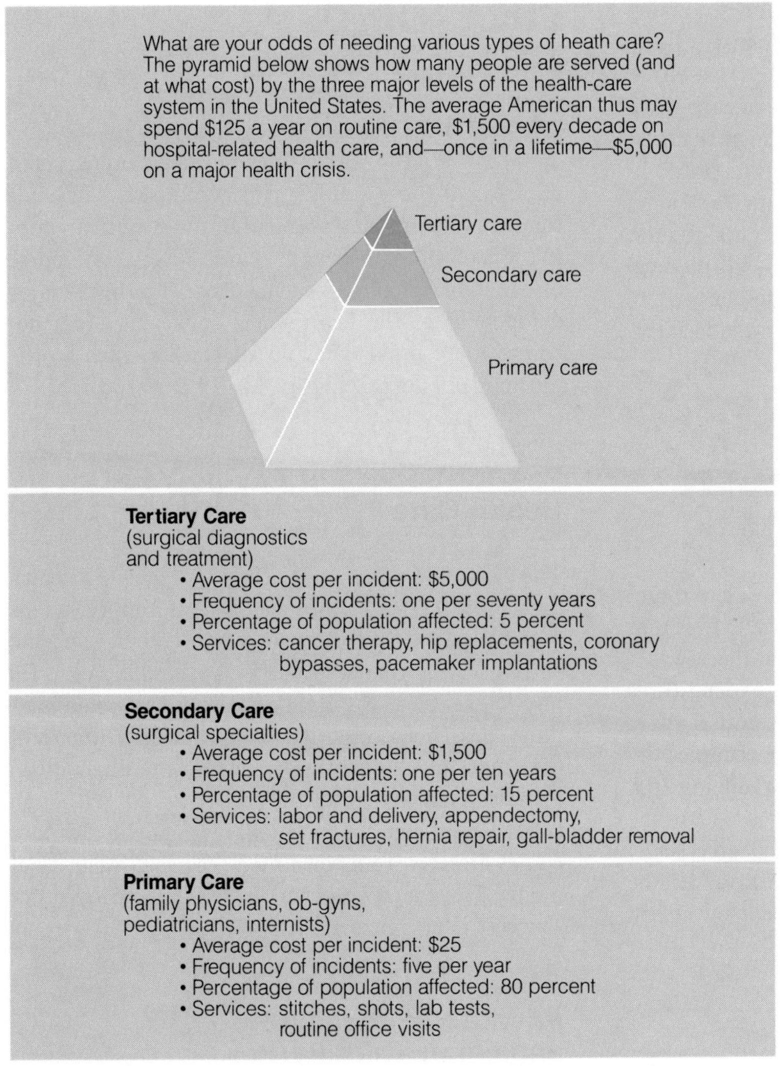

What are your odds of needing various types of heath care? The pyramid below shows how many people are served (and at what cost) by the three major levels of the health-care system in the United States. The average American thus may spend $125 a year on routine care, $1,500 every decade on hospital-related health care, and—once in a lifetime—$5,000 on a major health crisis.
Tertiary care
Secondary care
Primary care
Tertiary Care
(surgical diagnostics and treatment)
• Average cost per incident: $5,000
• Frequency of incidents: one per seventy years
• Percentage of population affected: 5 percent
• Services: cancer therapy, hip replacements, coronary bypasses, pacemaker implantations
Secondary Care
(surgical specialties)
• Average cost per incident: $1,500
• Frequency of incidents: one per ten years
• Percentage of population affected: 15 percent
• Services: labor and delivery, appendectomy, set fractures, hernia repair, gall-bladder removal
Primary Care
(family physicians, ob-gyns, pediatricians, internists)
• Average cost per incident: $25
• Frequency of incidents: five per year
• Percentage of population affected: 80 percent
• Services: stitches, shots, lab tests, routine office visits


**Figure 18.3**
The health-care system. *Source:* Copyright © 1981 by Keith W. Sehnert. Reprinted from *The Family Doctor's Health Tips,* with permission of Meadowbrook, Inc.

**HEALTH CLINICS** Clinics can be categorized as either private or public. Public-health clinics may offer the same range of outpatient, ambulatory care services as a private clinic, but differ in that public-health clinics are supported by either federal, state, or local tax funds.

**HOSPITALS** A wide variety of institutions are called hospitals. These institutions provide the most extensive level of care, which is usually performed on an in-patient basis. Any institution that attempts to qualify as a hospital is urged to submit to an accreditation process which is conducted by the Joint Commission on the Accreditation of Hospitals (JCAH). Such an accreditation process will not guarantee that errors in diagnosing or treating an illness cannot occur. Accreditation insures that the institution meets standards for providing care and conducting business that should translate into the probability that a high standard of care is likely to be conducted there. The Joint Commission is composed of the American College of Surgeons, the American College of Physicians, the American Hospital Association, and the American Medical Association.

Most hospitals are classified as short-term or acute care which means patients are there fewer than thirty days. Hospitals are also classified by the type of treatment rendered (clinical) or by the type of management or ownership.

**NURSING HOMES** In many instances, nursing homes are referred to as long-term care institutions. Nursing homes are typically classified as either skilled-nursing facilities or intermediate-care institutions. In a **skilled-nursing facility** the patients or residents require daily medical attention by a licensed physician and professional nurses. In an **intermediate-care institution** the residents require assistance but not necessarily professional medical attention. Tender loving care might be one way to describe the care to be rendered to persons in intermediate-care facilities.

## THE COST OF HEALTH CARE IN THE U.S.

The area that has recently seen the most rapid and sustained level of economic growth in the U.S. is that of health-care spending. In 1983 alone there was a 10.3 percent increase in health-care expenditures over the previous year. In terms of the actual share of the gross national product (GNP) occupied by health care spending, it accounts for a whopping 10.8 percent, or $355 billion. This is an increase from the 9.8 percent share occupied in 1981.[9] (See table 18.2.) By the year 1990, the average American will be spending an estimated $3,000 each year on health care.[10]

**Table 18.2 The Cost of Health Care in the U.S.**

| | Health-care expenditures | |
|---|---|---|
| *Year* | *In billions of dollars* | *As a % of GNP* |
| 1965 | $ 41.7 | 6.0% |
| 1967 | 51.3 | 6.4 |
| 1969 | 65.6 | 7.0 |
| 1971 | 83.3 | 7.7 |
| 1973 | 103.2 | 7.8 |
| 1975 | 132.7 | 8.6 |
| 1977 | 169.2 | 8.8 |
| 1979 | 215.0 | 8.9 |
| 1981 | 286.6 | 9.8 |
| 1983 | 355.0 | 10.8 |

Source: Data from Health Care Financing Administration.

## FINANCING HEALTH CARE

The cost of health care is extremely high with no apparent relief in sight. With dramatic increases in all areas of the system, it is becoming very difficult for a rapidly growing segment of the American population to afford necessary care. With this picture of economic gloom as a backdrop, the third major component of the health-care delivery system becomes more important and visible: specifically, the mechanisms for paying for health care received.

### Fee-for-Service or Pay-as-You-Go Health Care

The vast majority of Americans are receiving health care on a fee-for-service basis. This simply means that we pay either the provider or facility for the actual service rendered. As we witness increases in physicians' fees, hospital costs, drug costs, and auxiliary health services, it becomes readily apparent that most of us desperately need some mechanism to assist us in paying for the care required. Although twenty-eight cents of each dollar spent on health care comes directly from consumers, the vast majority of money (seventy-two cents) is reimbursed by other sources. (See figure 18.4.)

### Private Health Insurers and Other Third Parties

It is estimated that in excess of 80 percent of our nation's population is covered by some form of private health insurance. These insurance plans are generically referred to as standard indemnity plans. Blue Cross/Blue Shield is an example of such a plan. The insurance usually is written to cover one or more elements of costs incurred. The two costs that are most commonly covered are hospital-cost insurance and medical insurance, which is designed to cover mainly physician-related expenses. Additional forms of private health insurance may be secured, such as major medical (catastrophic), disability, and miscellaneous (which might cover things such as a prosthesis, blood, or specialized allied health care).

**Where the nation's health dollar came from**

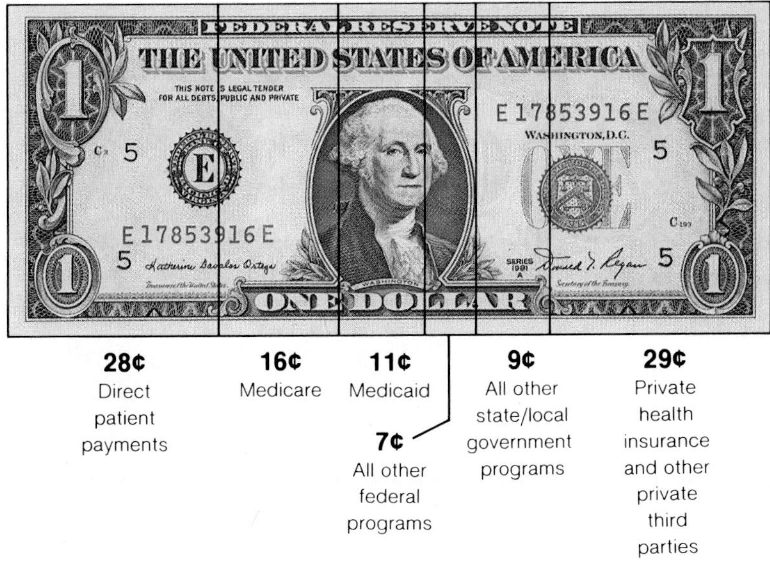


**Where it went**

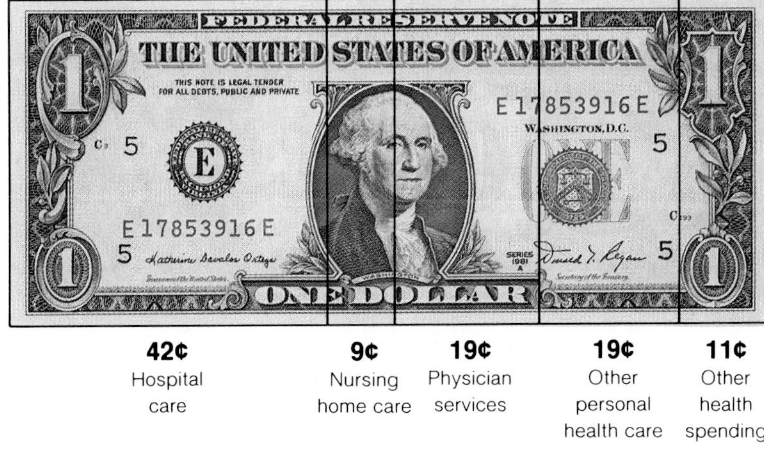


**Figure 18.4**
The origins and destinations of the nation's health-care dollar.

## Prepaid Health Insurance Plans

The concept of prepaid health insurance plans or **health-maintenance organizations (HMOs)** has been around for quite some time. The Ross-Loos plan, begun in the 1920s in California, is perhaps the first example of such a program. Health-maintenance organizations provide comprehensive health care to voluntarily enrolled subscribers for a fixed, prepaid fee. In the U.S. today, there are more than 230 such programs enrolling over ten million people.[11]

**TYPES OF HMOs** The three major types of HMOs are group, staff, or individual-practice HMOs.[12] Contractual arrangements differ from one plan to the next, which may cause them to have a slight variation in structure.

1. **Group Models**—In a group HMO, the HMO (administrative arm) contracts with an independent group of physicians to perform necessary services on persons enrolled in the HMO. Members of the HMO select their physician from among those in the physician group. The physicians are paid according to the number of patients they provide care for.

2. **Staff Model**—In a staff HMO, the HMO actually employs the physicians and typically pays them on a salaried basis. The HMO often builds and owns the facilities where the care is offered. Most university health centers are staff HMOs.
3. **Individual-Practice Association (IPA)**—In an individual-practice HMO, the HMO contracts with either individual private practicing physicians, or with a legal entity known as an individual practice association to which privately practicing physicians belong, for an agreed-upon fee schedule. In this form of HMO, physicians typically work out of their own offices.

Health-maintenance organizations have received strong support for development, including passage of the federal HMO Act of 1973. Economic times have reduced the monetary support of the federal government in the development of the programs. The philosophical base of support has remained strong, however, because HMOs represent a form of competition in the health-care marketplace.

A unique feature of HMOs is the reimbursement philosophy which stresses more care rendered on an outpatient, ambulatory basis than on an inpatient basis. Most private health-insurance companies will not reimburse for a number of procedures unless they are done in a hospital setting. Even casual observers of the system can quickly see that outpatient care should be less costly. Additionally, a well member is an asset to an HMO, as the fewer services required by a member the greater the monetary savings for the HMO. Most HMOs, therefore, are motivated to enhance levels of wellness by providing health-maintenance services such as prenatal care, physical fitness, and nutritional counseling.

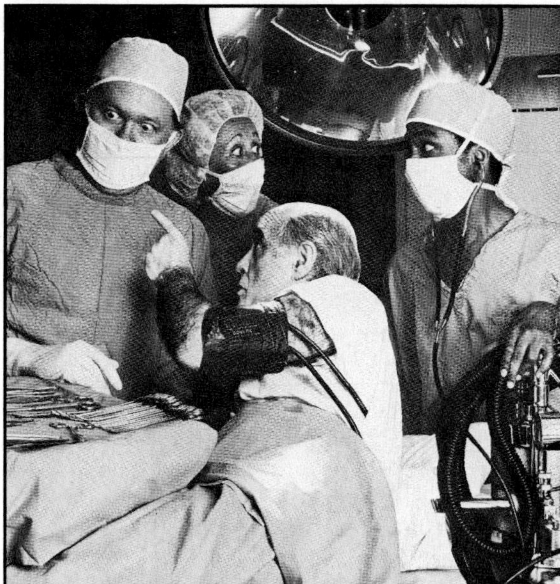

**"$1500 for everything... and that's my final offer!"**

How absurd it sounds—a consumer of medical care who's actually concerned about the price!

But while he may be greeted with amazement by the hospital staff, it isn't really *he* who's amazing—it's the rest of us, who've been buying health care as if money grew on trees.

**Figure 18.5**
HMOs stress economic health care through their reimbursement philosophy.

## Federal Financing of Health Care

Many people might want to debate what the federal government's role should be concerning matters of health care for the public. Specifically, should government, at any level, sponsor agencies for actually providing health care, or should it pay for care rendered? Presently, outside of special programs for military personnel and their dependents, the government sponsors two programs—medicare and medicaid.

**MEDICARE** **Medicare** is a social program that assists in the payment of health expenses for persons sixty-five years and older who are entitled to Social Security benefits.[13] The Medicare program consists of two parts. Medicare Plan A provides coverage for hospital-related expenses and is available to all eligible parties. Medicare Plan B is a form of optional medical insurance that pays for provider-related expenses. Even with Medicare coverage, a large number of the elderly carry additional private insurance to cover areas that may be exempted by Medicare.

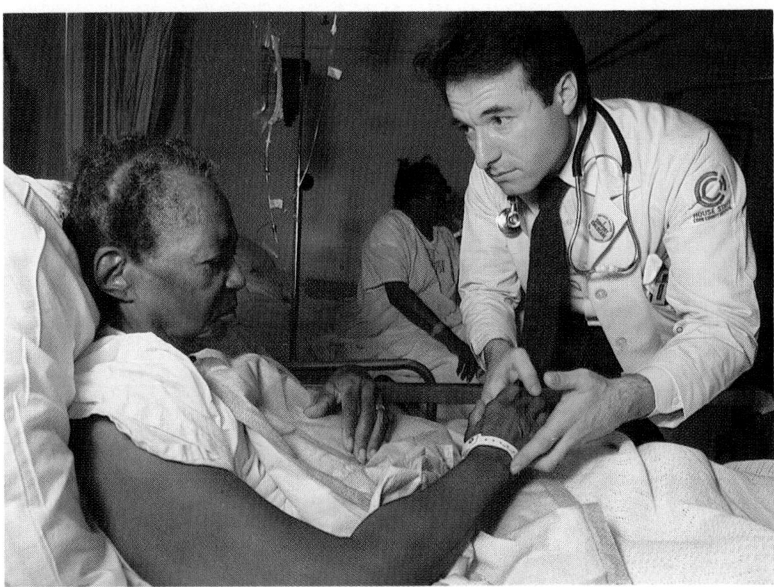

**Figure 18.6**
Medicare and Medicaid programs are an important source of health-care financing for the elderly.

**MEDICAID** **Medicaid** is the government-sponsored program of health insurance that was established to assist the socioeconomically disadvantaged, people determined to be in need of such assistance due to a health disability (such as blindness), and the aged poor.[14] This particular program, which covers basic health costs such as hospital expenses, physician's expenses, nursing home expenses, and some others, is shared economically with the federal government by the fifty state governments.

**PEER REVIEW ORGANIZATIONS (PROs)** As more and more federal and state dollars are being used to support both the Medicare and Medicaid programs, there becomes a growing need to establish some agency to monitor costs. Professional Standards Review Organizations (PSROs) came into being when Congress amended, in 1972, the Social Security Act. Physicians in each state were encouraged to organize PSROs and monitor the necessity, appropriateness, and quality of health-care services provided to Medicare beneficiaries and Medicaid recipients. This program did not develop without understandable resistance from many groups. Over the years PSROs were criticized as being expensive without demonstrating substantial cost savings or increases in the quality of care.[15] Based on such criticism, the federal government decided to phase out PSROs and replace them with **PROs (Peer Review Organizations).**[16] This action, as a part of the Tax Equity and Fiscal Responsibility Act of 1982, has also received its share of criticism. The major concern appears to involve the emphasis on cost control at the expense of quality care for the consumer.

## National Health Insurance

Even though there is presently no form of nationalized health insurance in the U.S. it seems prudent to mention the possibility of its emergence in the future. National health insurance, an idea first introduced in the U.S. by President Harry Truman, would provide health insurance to all U.S. citizens regardless of ability to pay.[17] Many politicians have spoken strongly about the need for some type of national insurance. Senator Edward Kennedy has been perhaps the most well-known proponent of a national health-insurance program. As more and more is learned about such a program, consumer input will certainly become extremely important. National health-insurance programs in Britain and Canada demonstrate that such a program, even on a limited scale, will be very costly and almost certainly cause our costs of health care to continue to rise rapidly.

# PERSONAL AND SOCIAL INFLUENCES ON HEALTH CARE

Some problems related to the delivery of health care in our society are perhaps beyond the influence of the average consumer and may actually act as barriers to the efficient and effective delivery of health care. Additionally, all of us possess personal beliefs and values that influence our use of the health-care system.

## Availability of Services

One of the most-cited barriers to health-care delivery is the availability of services. This barrier may now be less of a problem in light of recent studies indicating a potential surplus of physicians, which should translate into more available care. A study conducted by the Rand Corporation and Tufts University School of Medicine has found that few towns with 2,500 or more people are without ready access to a general physician.[18] The proportion of physicians in family practice and other primary-care fields, however, has not grown with the overall physician supply, and many areas remain underserved. In addition, many elderly and socioeconomically disadvantaged people have no means of getting to a health provider in their area.

## The Cost of Health Care

A second barrier to health care might be simply the cost of care. As health-care costs skyrocket, fewer people are able to afford necessary care. Not only are many consumers unable to pay directly for care rendered, they are also unable to afford any type of needed health-insurance coverage.

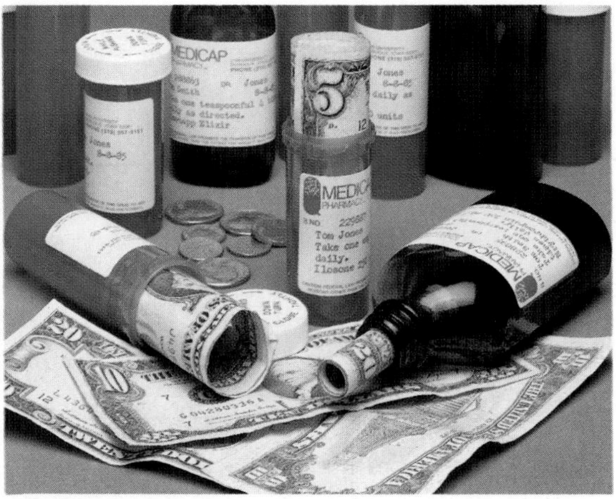

**Figure 18.7**
The high cost of health care is a barrier for many Americans.

## Disorganization of the Health-Care System

The health-care delivery system is an extremely large, complex social structure. Within this structure there appears to be a significant lack of organization which translates into a very fragmented system. Consumers usually need to travel among a variety of providers and institutions to receive necessary care. This situation creates a very costly and undesirable environment for the delivery of medical care.

The health-insurance industry itself contributes to the less than desirable situation through its shortsighted reimbursement policies. In most instances, insurance companies refuse payment for outpatient preventive health services. Providers are therefore not only encouraged but almost required to institutionalize patients so that they can be guaranteed reimbursement and patients can receive necessary care. This policy definitely translates into more costly health care.

## Personal Attitudes and Beliefs

Many of the conditions and situations that contribute to the high cost of health care are out of the control of the consuming population. However, many consumer attitudes and beliefs may, in fact, contribute a great deal to our current dilemma. Donald

M. Vickery, M.D., in his text *Life Plan for Your Health,* discusses ten myths of medicine that support such a contention.[19]

Vickery's Ten Myths of Medicine*

1. *Health depends most on good medical care,* and
2. *Your doctor manages your health.* For many people, the notion of self-responsibility and control of their own well-being is non-existent. In reality, we can have a good deal of control over our health. What we choose to do or not do as a component of our behavioral pattern perhaps dictates more than any other element the quality of life we will experience.
3. *Doctors, and only doctors, can tell whether you are healthy.* Health is a very difficult concept to define. In the absence of severe health problem symptoms, we are usually the best judge of our well-being. Only as we understand, to a greater degree, the impact behavioral factors such as excessive drinking, smoking, eating, stress, etc., have on our well-being, can we begin to modify our lifestyles in an attempt to improve our health.
4. *It is vital to see the doctor as soon as a problem develops so that the disease may be treated early.* It has been estimated that seventy-five percent of those persons visiting a physician are suffering from a condition that is self-limited and will be cured by the body itself. By taking appropriate care of ourselves and resisting the impulse to immediately see a physician, we might actually save dollars and rejoice in the ability of our bodies to control our health.
5. *Good doctors can almost always make the diagnosis right away.* The ability of a doctor to make an immediate diagnosis may not be as important as the ability to consider the wide range of health infirmities that may exist. The key to good health care might be in the overall management planning for a patient and their problems.
6. *A regular complete checkup is important to staying healthy.* Certain types of checkups, such as blood pressure screenings, breast examinations and Pap smears, may be warranted on a regular basis. The notion of having a yearly total physical checkup does not seem warranted unless an individual's personal or family history suggests it. (See tables 18.3 and 18.4.)
7. *Medicine has a cure for almost every disease.* This represents the most incredible myth and is not true. As was previously mentioned, most diseases will be cured by bodily processes with medicine treating effectively a portion of the others.
8. *Doctors are responsible for the rise in medical costs.* This statement is partially true. Physicians currently receive approximately 19 cents out of each health care dollar spent. The overwhelming majority of money is spent for care rendered in the hospital (42 cents).[20]
9. *Competent medical care involves little risk.* All medical care involves some element of risk. As consumers, we need to realize this and take this into account when evaluating the overall competence of the medical practitioner and the procedure performed. Medicine is more a form of art than an absolute science.
10. *Medical and surgical procedures must be tested and approved before they are used on the public.* Only drugs and medical devices would fall into this category.[21] Licensed physicians may perform any operation, X-ray procedure, or other treatment they deem appropriate.[22]

In summarizing these ten myths and the other barriers to health care we discussed, we could say that, to a large extent, the attitudes, beliefs, and feelings we possess about health care, in conjunction with our knowledge of the system and individual lifestyles, directly affect the cost of care rendered. To the extent that we can assume a greater level of responsibility for our own well-being, we may be able to exert some influence over the cost and nature of health-care services provided. (See Activity for Wellness 18.3.)

*Excerpted from Donald M. Vickery, *Lifeplan for Your Health.* © 1978 Addison-Wesley, Reading, Mass. Reprinted with permission.

## Table 18.3 Important Health Examinations and Procedures

| Period of Life | Physical Examination | Laboratory Test or Procedure |
|---|---|---|
| First week | Complete physical examination, including head size and hip examination to detect dislocation | PKU and $T_4$ blood tests to detect phenylketonuria and hypothyroidism (potential causes of mental retardation) |
| First year | Checkups every three months, including growth, development, and head size | At age nine months, hemoglobin test to detect anemia |
| Childhood | Checkups every year<br>Dental examination at age two or three and every six to twelve months thereafter<br>At age four, hearing and eyesight check, including examination to detect crossed eyes | At age four, tine test to detect tuberculosis, and urinalysis |
| Puberty | Assessment of sexual development<br>Check of spine to detect scoliosis (abnormal curvature)<br>Examination of male scrotum and female breast at age sixteen to eighteen and annually thereafter | Complete blood count, urinalysis |
| Age twenty-one + | Annual female pelvic examination with Pap smear<br>Complete physical examination, including rectal examination, every five years<br>Blood pressure check once a year during other visits | At age twenty-one, computerized blood chemistry screen to establish baseline for later comparison |
| Age forty + | Physical examination every three to five years<br>Rectal examination every two years<br>Sigmoidoscopy every five years<br>Tonometry (eye pressure check) every two years | Complete blood count, urinalysis, and ECG with each physical examination<br>Check for occult blood in feces every year |
| Age fifty + | Physical examination every two to three years, including pedal pulses and neck murmurs<br>Sigmoidoscopy every two to three years<br>Tonometry every two years | Complete blood count, urinalysis, and ECG with every physical examination<br>Check for occult blood in feces every year |
| Age sixty + | Annual physical examination<br>Sigmoidoscopy every two years<br>Tonometry every two years | Complete blood count and urinalysis with every physical examination<br>ECG every two to three years<br>Check for occult blood in feces every year |

Source: From Cornacchia, Harold J., and Barrett, Stephen, *Consumer Health: A Guide to Intelligent Decisions,* 3d ed. St. Louis, 1985. Times Mirror/Mosby College Publishing.

## Table 18.4 Recommended Timing of Vaccinations

| | | Two months | Four months | Six months | Fifteen months | Eighteen months | Four to six years | Every ten years |
|---|---|---|---|---|---|---|---|---|
| | Oral polio | ✓ | ✓ | * | | ✓ | ✓ | |
| Usually given as a single combination vaccine | Diphtheria | ✓ | ✓ | ✓ | | ✓ | ✓ | ✓ |
| | Tetanus | ✓ | ✓ | ✓ | | ✓ | ✓ | ✓ |
| | Pertussis | ✓ | ✓ | ✓ | | ✓ | ✓ | |
| Usually given as a single combination vaccine | Measles | | | | ✓ | | | |
| | Mumps | | | | ✓ | | | |
| | Rubella | | | | ✓ | | | |

*Some doctors give an additional dose of the oral polio vaccine at age six months.

Source: From Barton, Leslie L., "Immunization 1983," *Drug Therapy* 13.8 (1983): 197. Reprinted by permission of Biomedical Information Corporation, New York.

18.3 ACTIVITY FOR WELLNESS 18.3

# Twelve Ways to Cut Health-Care Costs

How many of these cost-saving behaviors do you already do? Begin today to be a conscientious consumer of health-care services.

[ ] 1. When you receive medical service, don't be reluctant to ask the doctor for a discount if you pay on the spot. This saves some billing costs.

[ ] 2. Select a doctor to be "your doctor." Set up a relationship with the physician. Ask questions about costs. Ask for referrals if needed. Don't try to do your own "shopping" for specialists—often an expensive undertaking.

[ ] 3. Use the telephone. Most doctors don't charge for telephone advice. Describe your symptoms as completely as possible.

[ ] 4. When it's not an emergency, go to the doctor's office, not the hospital's E.R., which will cost two or three times more than an office call.

[ ] 5. If you are going to a hospital for surgery, inquire about "pre-admission testing." Such service provides for having the necessary lab tests done before you are admitted. Every day cut off the stay can save a bundle.

[ ] 6. Ask if your surgery can be done on a one-day, come-and-go basis. If not, find out the earliest date you can get out of the hospital.

[ ] 7. While in the hospital you have the right to ask the doctor why a certain test or procedure is being done—and what it costs.

[ ] 8. Join a blood donor program *before* you need blood.

[ ] 9. Don't pester your doctor to give you a prescription. Many drugs such as antibiotics and tranquilizers are overprescribed because patients feel they need one. If you do need one, ask for a proven, reliable generic form (rather than a brand name); it may be 50 percent less expensive.

[ ] 10. Keep good records about drug and medical expenses so you can file for credit on your income tax.

[ ] 11. Take a medical self-care course. You should be able to cut $100 to $200 a year from your medical bills when you can handle routine ailments and common injuries yourself.

[ ] 12. Don't hesitate to request a second opinion if you're faced with a serious health problem. The added expense may only confirm some unpleasant news, but it could lead to alternative treatments or shed light on a confusing situation.

18.1 EXHIBIT

# The Life-and-Death Choices Created by Medical Technology

When Representative Ron Wyden (D-Ore.) was told that 30 percent of the coronary bypass operations performed in the U.S. were probably unnecessary, the congressman demanded an explanation for this flagrant abuse of the operation. "Do you want me to decide whether you should have one?" retorted Dr. John Marshall, director of the National Center for Health Services Research, who was testifying before a congressional subcommittee on health care.

Making such life-and-death decisions about the use of costly medical technology is something that few policymakers—and even fewer doctors—would be willing to do. Yet the question of who will receive medical care and who will not is cropping up with disturbing frequency. And it is a question that medical experts believe will soon demand an answer as advanced technology pushes up the cost of health care. "We are nearing the day when we will have to confront the rationing of very high-tech, very costly procedures," predicts Dr. Paul M. Ellwood, Jr., president of InterStudy, a health care research firm in Excelsior, Minn.

**ARTIFICIAL ORGANS.** For three decades, the U.S. has pumped billions of dollars into medical research. And that effort has created a cornucopia of new technology that is revolutionizing medical care. "The hope and goal of that enormous investment was that out of this would grow diagnostic and therapeutic discoveries that would be useful—and we're getting what we paid for," says Dr. William B. Schwartz, a professor of medicine at Tufts University.

In just the last decade, coronary bypasses, hip replacement surgery, and kidney dialysis have become commonplace. The CAT scan made a quantum jump in diagnosis, and the pace is still accelerating. Magnetic resonance imaging is extending the physician's ability to see inside the body, and laser light is replacing the surgeon's scalpel. The success rate of heart and lung transplants has improved dramatically. On the horizon are artificial hearts and other organs and powerful new drugs based on the body's immune system.

But the problem is how to pay for these advances. The bills for some procedures are already staggering. Costs for 70,000 U.S. kidney dialysis patients come to $2 billion a year. Intensive care for some 200,000 seriously premature or ill infants ran to $2 billion in 1983, as did some 100,000 coronary bypass operations. Even though many new technologies reduce costs by allowing doctors to perform procedures in their offices that once required hospitalization, studies estimate that new technology is responsible for more than half of the annual increases in the cost of a day in the hospital.

Technology now being developed promises to push costs up even more. An estimated $200 million has already been spent on developing artificial hearts, but that amount is sure to be dwarfed by the cost of using them. A study conducted by the congressional Office of Technology Assessment estimates that 33,000 people each year would require heart replacements. The annual bill for the operation and ongoing care would approach $3 billion.

Critics of such big-ticket research projects argue that the costly technology will be used, whether or not it produces significant benefits. The OTA report on the artificial heart, for example, points out that it can be expected to add only six months to the lives of the recipients.

Others complain that costly intensive-care units—which are the fastest-growing facilities in U.S. hospitals—are being used more often to prolong life in comatose, hopelessly ill patients than they are to save those whose health can be restored. "We spend an inordinate amount sustaining people in the last months of their lives. And in many cases, we're not appreciably improving health," notes Alan Greenspan, president of Townsend-Greenspan & Co. in New York.

**BITTER PILL.** Reconciling the need to protect public health with impossibly huge costs is now "the No. 1 issue of medical ethics," says Daniel J. Callahan, director of the Hastings Center, a think tank that wrestles with ethical issues in medicine. Callahan and others are convinced that the only direction the U.S. can take is to limit the availability of medical treatment.

## EXHIBIT 18.1

"The only way to cut costs will be to deny benefits to some people or deny benefits for some diseases," says Tufts's Schwartz, who conducted a study of the problem for the Brookings Institution. That, in fact, is just the way it is done in Britain, where the health care system clearly discriminates against the poor and the old by stringently rationing some procedures. Two-thirds of British patients with kidney failure are denied dialysis, for example, while virtually all patients in the U.S. are treated.

Such a system would be a bitter pill for the U.S. to swallow. More than 85 percent of the public is covered by health insurance and is accustomed to receiving costly treatment without question. Suggestions that medical technology should be withheld from certain patients have been greeted with howls of outrage in the past. Colorado Governor Richard D. Lamm's comment !ast April that the terminally ill elderly "have a duty to die" met resounding protest. And in the 1960s, a Seattle committee that was unabashedly selecting the first patients for dialysis on the basis of their "value to society" caused such a furor that Congress covered all kidney patients under medicare.

Still, there are indications that the medical free-for-all may be ending. Medical-Plan administrators are trying to limit the use of high technology as a way of cutting costs. Increasingly they are taking the decision out of the hands of the employee and his doctor.

**PLAYING GOD.** Honeywell Inc., for example, recently became one of the first companies to approve heart-lung and liver transplants for its employees, but it reviews requests on a case-by-case basis. Approval for the surgery is made by the company's medical director, who then manages the case with the patient's physicians. Other companies are considering putting a greater share of the cost burden on the patient. "We pay for transplants now, but should it be unlimited?" asks Richard G. Wardrop, general manager of compensation and benefits at Aluminum Co. of America.

The difficult questions are only beginning to be addressed. At issue is not who should be spared a prolonged death by pulling the plug from high-tech life support devices, but literally who should be allowed to live. And ultimately, the question revolves around how much a life is worth. For example, should a baby born two months prematurely be maintained in intensive care at a cost of more than $200,000 until it can survive on its own? Should medical insurers pay for test tube fertilization that will allow childless couples to conceive? Or should coronary bypasses and other major operations be limited to those younger than fifty years?

So far, no one is standing in line for a chance to play God. Doctors argue that they are obligated to take whatever steps are necessary to save lives and that decisions about the accessibility of health care must be made by policymakers. "Medicine does not want to make these ethical and moral decisions," declares Dr. Allan B. Weingold, chief of George Washington University's Obstetrics & Gynecology Dept. Meanwhile, policymakers are arguing that doctors must decide what is reasonable care and take steps to limit the use of costly technology themselves. The decision, says Marshall of the National Center for Health Services Research, rests "not on bureaucrats but on the physicians."

Nevertheless, both groups are convinced the U.S. must make some agonizing choices. If it continues on its present course of doing everything that might help a patient, it will have to learn to live with an ongoing escalation in health care costs. On the other hand, cutting costs will mean limiting the use of medical technology. Either way, deciding where to draw the line promises to be a painful process.

Source: Reprinted from the October 15, 1984 issue of *Business Week* by special permission. © 1984 by McGraw-Hill, Inc.

## DISCUSSION QUESTIONS

1. Do you believe that very costly, high-tech medical procedures should be rationed in order to control the cost of health care? If so, what criteria should be used in the rationing process?

2. Who do you think should be involved in the decision-making (or policy-making) process regarding the rationing of health-care technology and services?

# SUMMARY

1. Consumers need to accept a greater level of responsibility for their well-being and their utilization of the health-care system.

2. Careful selection of health-care professionals is a skill of great importance for enhancing consumer satisfaction with health care. Understanding differences between the various health-care specialties and subspecialties is crucial to the appropriate selection of health professionals.

3. The consumer should be aware of levels of care and their various costs.

4. Health-care spending has continued to skyrocket, accounting for as high as 10 percent of the U.S. gross national product (GNP) in recent years.

5. The cost of health care remains an important barrier to the average consumer. Other important health-care barriers include the availability of services, the organization of the health-care system itself, and mythical beliefs held by consumers about the health-care system.

6. Consumer knowledge of health-care financing alternatives must be heightened in an effort to aid in cost-control measures.

### Recommended Readings

Corry, James M. *Consumer Health: Facts, Skills and Decisions.* Belmont, Calif.: Wadsworth Publishing, 1983.

Price, James A., Galli, Nicholas, and Slenker, Suzanne. *Consumer Health: Contemporary Issues and Choices.* Dubuque, Iowa: Wm. C. Brown Publishers, 1985.

Sehnert, Keith W. *The Family Doctor's Health Tips.* Deephaven, Minn.: Meadowbrook Press, 1981.

Vickery, Donald M., and Fries, James F. *Take Care of Yourself: A Consumer's Guide to Medical Care.* Reading, Mass.: Addison-Wesley Publishing, 1976.

### References

1. Harold J. Cornacchia and Stephen Barrett, *Consumer Health: A Guide to Intelligent Decisions* (St. Louis, Mo.: C.V. Mosby Company, 1980), p. 24.

2. James H. Price, Nicholas Galli, and Suzanne Slenker, *Consumer Health: Contemporary Issues and Choices* (Dubuque, Iowa: Wm. C. Brown Publishers, 1985).

3. Cornacchia and Barrett, *Consumer Health,* 79.

4. James M. Corry, *Consumer Health: Facts, Skills and Decisions* (Belmont, Calif.: Wadsworth Publishing, 1983), 90.

5. Corry, *Consumer Health,* 89.

6. Corry, *Consumer Health,* 91; Cornacchia, *Consumer Health,* 80.

7. Corry, *Consumer Health,* 82.

8. Cornacchia, *Consumer Health,* 76.

9. Robert M. Gibson, and Daniel R. Waldo, "National Health Expenditures, 1981," *Health Care Financing Review* 4.1 (1982): 1–35; "Health Spending Increase in 1983 at 10-Year Low," *Hospitals* (16 November 1984): 32.

10. Mark S. Freeland, and Carol Ellen Schendler, "National Health Expenditure Growth in the 1980's: An Aging Population, New Technologies, and Increasing Competition," *Health Care Financing Review* 4.3 (1983): 1.

11. HMO Fact Sheet OHHS, PHS, Office of Health Maintenance Organizations, Rockville, Md., July 1983.

12. P. D. Lairson, "Why Informed Consumers are Choosing HMOs," *Patient Care* 16.18 (1982): 67–80.

13. U.S. Department of Health and Human Services, *A Brief Explanation of Medicare* (Washington, D.C.: U.S. Government Printing Office, July 1983), 2–14.

14. Cornacchia, *Consumer Health,* 260.

15. Corry, *Consumer Health,* 332.

16. Judith Frabotta, "Fed's New PROs Dismay Peer Review's Fans and Foes," *Medical World News* 23.25 (1982): 58–60, 65–66, 75–78.

17. National Issues Forum, *The Soaring Cost of Health Care* (Dayton, Ohio: Domestic Policy Association, 1984), 21.

18. "More Physicians Opt for Rural Life," *Physicians' Washington Report* 5.3 (1982): 4.

19. Donald M. Vickery, *Life Plan for Your Health* (Reading, Mass: Addison-Wesley, 1978).

20. "National Spending for Health Care," *Geriatric Consultant* 2.5 (1984): 24.

21. Arthur H. Hayes, "How the FDA Regulates Medical Devices," *Journal of Cardiovascular Medicine* 8.5 (1983): 597–600.

22. Corry, *Consumer Health,* 82.

CHAPTER NINETEEN

# Ecology: Establishing a Healthy Environment



Environmental sensitivity is an important dimension of both health and wellness. We face many personal life-style choices involving "spaces" in which we live, work, and play.

The media daily expose us to examples of the environmental crisis. Carbon dioxide levels in the air we breathe are excessively high and may cause dangerous climate changes in the coming years; the ozone layer is in serious danger of being destroyed, thereby increasing our exposure to harmful radiation from the sun; we are rapidly running out of places to dump our garbage. These seemingly endless crises overwhelm many people, often leading to the attitude that "there is nothing I can do about any of this." This attitude paves the way for three traps of personal inaction: (1) blind technological optimism—a belief that technology and science will "save" us; (2) gloom-and-doom pessimism—a belief that there is no hope; and (3) apathy—a lack of caring due to a fatalistic outlook.[1]

There is another attitude you can take toward the environment, however. You can accept the challenge of creating a personal life-style that is both fulfilling and ecologically sound. Environmental sensitivity of this sort will affect your personal "space," providing valuable support for your wellness life-style. Additionally, it will affect the larger environment, fostering higher levels of wellness for your community.

Once you understand the basic concepts of ecology, you will have the information and skills necessary for the development of a personal life-style that is ecologically sound. We cannot afford to wait for governments, industry, or technology to solve our environmental dilemma. As environmentalist John Lobell puts it, "When each one of us takes greater responsibility for our lives, our families, our communities, and the ecological health of the planet, we will see a better world."[2]

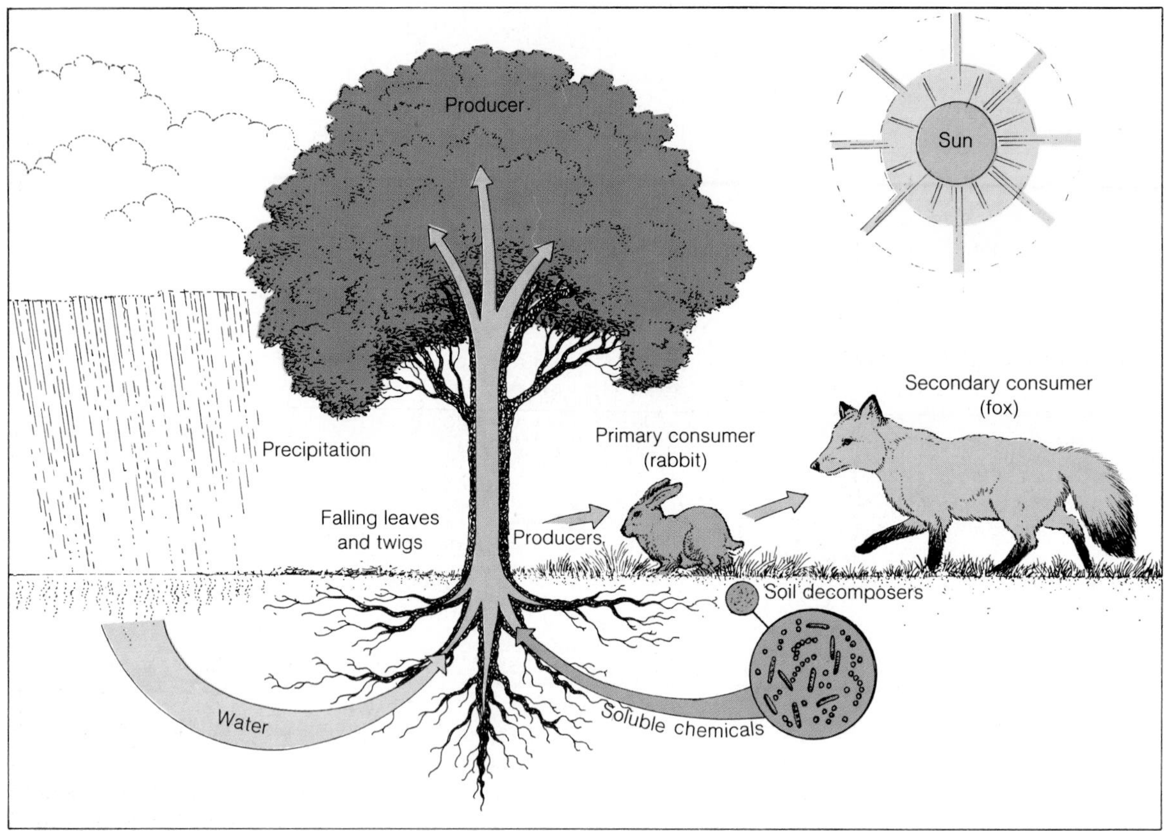


**Figure 19.1**
A greatly simplified version of the structure of a forest ecosystem. *Source:* From *Living in the Environment,* 3d ed. by G. Tyler Miller, Jr. © 1982 by Wadsworth, Inc. Reprinted by permission of the publisher.

# THE LAWS OF ECOLOGY

**Ecology,** a relatively young science, can be defined as the study of **ecosystems.**[3] Ecosystems consist of interactions between living organisms and the natural environment where they exist. Several generalizations can be made about natural ecosystems. Barry Commoner, a prominent ecologist, has summarized these generalizations in what he terms the *laws of ecology.* Simply stated they are:

1. Everything is connected to everything else;
2. Everything must go somewhere;
3. Nature knows best; and
4. There is no such thing as a free lunch.[4]

An understanding of these four laws will be helpful in gaining an overall picture of ecosystems and their functioning.

## The First Law of Ecology: Everything Is Connected to Everything Else

Our planet is composed of ecosystems or networks containing numerous interrelated organisms. Every ecosystem comprises two major components: nonliving and living.[5] The nonliving component includes various factors such as the sun (an outside source), wind, heat, rain, and chemicals necessary for life. (See figure 19.1.) The living component is usually divided into food producers and consumers. Food consumers can be further divided into macroconsumers (animals) and microconsumers or decomposers (bacteria and fungi).

Natural ecosystems are so complex that people often do not see or understand the entire range of connections. The degree of complexity found in an ecosystem, however, is an important factor in the ecosystem's ability to cope with natural stressors that may be placed upon it. Consider the case of humans

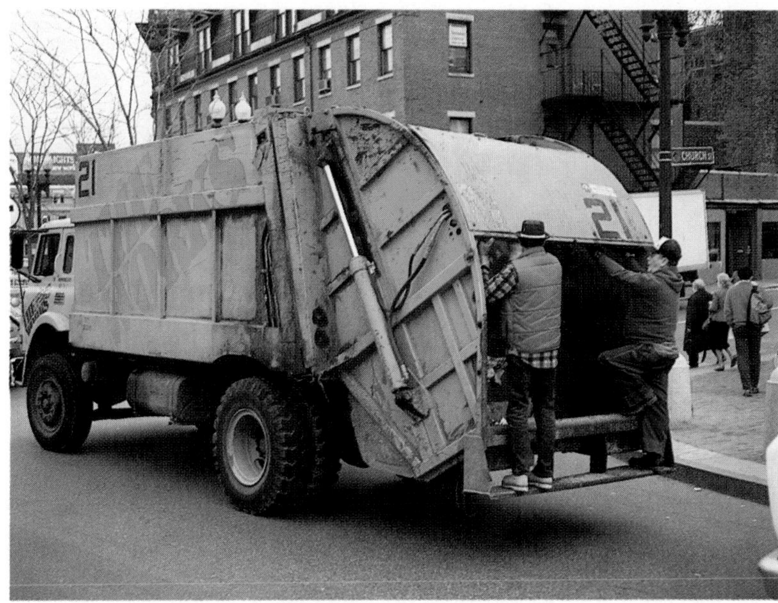

**Figure 19.2**
Where does your trash go when the garbage collector takes it "away"?

and the staphylococcal bacteria that live on the surface of the human body.[6] These staph bacteria help guard the body from thousands of other microorganisms that could be harmful. In fact, without the aid of staph bacteria, which consume other microorganisms as they attempt to invade the body, humans would get infections and die. Other types of bacteria are similarly helpful to humans. For instance, vitamin $B_{12}$ could not be produced without certain bacteria commonly found in the human intestines.

In the past, people often have not recognized the importance of ecosystem complexity. The impact of technology has often been to simplify ecosystems artificially. Killing organisms labeled "pests," for example, has made ecosystems more vulnerable to stress and to final collapse. It is essential that we begin to view ecosystems as a whole, delineating to the best of our ability the natural interconnectedness found in varying ecosystems, and the impact our personal and collective life-style will have on each system.

## The Second Law of Ecology: Everything Must Go Somewhere

One of the basic laws of physics, usually referred to as the conservation of matter, states that matter cannot be created or destroyed—it can only be transformed. In terms of ecology, this law clearly informs us that there is no "away" to throw things. Nature's cycles are a true reflection of this ecological law. In nature we find no "waste." Elements excreted by one organism serve as nourishment for another.

Industrialization has created a society based on disposable products, which are designed to be used for a short period of time and then thrown away. The average American throws away an estimated three to five pounds of waste daily.[7] The unfortunate illusion created by this throwaway ethic is a belief that our garbage "goes away" when we set it out for the garbage collector once or twice a week. The second law of ecology, however, tells us that this is not the case. (See figure 19.2.)

One way to break free of the throwaway illusion is to ask two questions. "Where does our waste go?" and "What is its impact on the ecosphere?" In many instances, "away" has meant either dumps and landfills that waste valuable land and contaminate groundwater, or municipal incinerators that contribute to air pollution.[8] In any case, the waste products (matter) are not destroyed. They are instead either broken down into varying compounds, many of which are harmful to ecosystems, or in the case of nonbiodegradable waste, they accumulate at various sites on our planet where they do not belong. (See Exhibit 19.1.)

19.1 EXHIBIT

## If You Breathe, Don't Smoke

Statistics tell a cruel tale about the southeastern United States. That region has become the most vulnerable to lung cancer in the country. Seven counties that dot the coast from Baltimore to New Orleans are among the ten urban counties nationwide with the highest lung cancer deaths for white males. Now a study of a portion of that area—reaching from South Carolina through Georgia to Florida—may explain what sets the Southeast apart.

Atmospheric chemist John Winchester and his colleagues at Florida State University have noted that lung cancer deaths among white males in this area nearly tripled between 1950 and 1975. Winchester believes that acid air—a dangerous byproduct of pollution—could be part of the answer. The other culprit may be that old villain, smoking. Winchester is making a good case for linking the two.

Acid air is the drier relative of acid rain. It forms when sulfur dioxide in the atmosphere encounters water vapor in the air and turns into a sulfuric acid haze. The conversion takes place much more easily when coupled with heat and humidity—making it common in the Southeast. Much of this sulfur dioxide is released by the tall smokestacks of power plants in upwind Eastern states. Large volumes of air then transport the noxious gas over long distances.

Winchester and his colleagues have been tracking two major leads to solve the lung cancer mystery. One involves estimating the concentrations of acid air in the three-state sample based on theoretical and field measurements. These sulfuric acid particles increase in concentration until about Jacksonville, Florida, then become diluted by clean marine air as they drift southward down the Florida peninsula. Lung cancer mortality rates in the area follow a chillingly similar pattern. "We found that if you look along the East Coast from South Carolina to south Florida," says Winchester, "you notice a gradual increase in the lung cancer mortality as you move southward to about Jacksonville, and then it tapers off again."

Winchester's second lead concerns the increased cancer death rates in relation to the source of acid air. Adjusted for the fact that lung cancer incidence increases with age, "increases in lung cancer mortality closely correlate with the rate of increase of coal and oil combustion for electric generation," he explains.

Winchester's working theory is that acid air and cigarette smoke somehow act synergistically—that is, their combined effects multiply the harm—to enhance lung cancer risk. He does not yet know the actual mechanism by which acid air and cigarette smoke might trigger lung cancer. But he has some strong hunches.

## The Third Law of Ecology: Nature Knows Best

It has long been the view of the industrial world that one of technology's greatest merits was its ability to improve on nature. It is now apparent, however, that this may have been an extremely shortsighted view. As Barry Commoner notes in his book *The Closing Circle,* "one of the striking facts about the chemistry of living systems is that for every organic substance produced by a living organism, there exists, somewhere in nature, an enzyme capable of breaking that substance down. . . . No organic substance is synthesized unless there is provision for its degradation; recycling is thus enforced."[9] Technology, on the other hand, has repeatedly been responsible for the creation of organic substances that cannot be broken down. Often these **nonbiodegradable** products of technology have created havoc in diverse ecosystems.

Consider the case of **DDT,** a synthetic insecticide that kills insects by attacking biochemical processes in their nervous system. DDT was hailed as a technological triumph for some years, until Rachel Carson's noteworthy contribution *Silent Spring.*[10] Carson's book, published in 1962, pointed out the ecological impact of such pesticides on food, wildlife, and humanity.

## EXHIBIT 19.1

One hypothesis is that the sulfuric acid particles, which penetrate into the bronchioles, or air passages, of the lungs just as cigarette smoke does, could be irritating lung tissue enough to disrupt the body's natural defenses against the carcinogens in smoke. Another possibility is that sulfuric acid might somehow react chemically with tobacco smoke to form new carcinogenic compounds.

One good example of such a chemical combination—and one that would explain the coastal locations of many counties with high lung cancer mortality rates—concerns the potent lung carcinogen bis(chloromethyl)ether, better known as BCME. Airborne hydrochloric acid, formed when sulfuric acid reacts with salty sea air, could in turn react with formaldehyde in tobacco smoke to produce BCME. If so, coastal smokers are in big trouble.

Winchester is currently looking for research money to test this last theory. Meanwhile, new dangers cloud the horizon in the form of acid haze. Duval County, where Jacksonville is located, suffered the highest lung cancer mortality rate among urban American counties from 1970 to 1975—93.9 deaths per year, adjusted for age, for every 100,000 white males. Population increases and plans for new coal-fired power plants farther south may also make other parts of Florida hazardous places to live. Further, the statistical bulge at Jacksonville could herald similar patterns around the country. If the Winchester hypothesis is correct, smokers had best heed the warning: If you smoke, don't breathe.

Source: Reprinted by permission of *Science 84* magazine. 

## DISCUSSION QUESTIONS

1. How can pollution generated in the northeastern states be related to a health problem—cancer—in the southeastern states? Remember the first law of ecology: everything is connected to everything else.

2. Barry Commoner reminds us that everything must go somewhere. Northeastern power plants built tall smokestacks to get rid of sulfer dioxide waste. What two crucial questions did they neglect to ask themselves before building such smokestacks? (*Hint:* How could they have freed themselves from the throwaway ethic?)

DDT is a persistent pesticide, sometimes remaining in the environment for as long as fifteen years before degrading. Although DDT is successful for short-term eradication of many pests, it poses several major problems. When sprayed to kill insect pests, DDT also kills the natural predators of that pest. This killing of a broad range of insects tends artificially to simplify ecosystems. Additionally, many insect pests are capable of rapid adaptation, resulting in genetic resistance to DDT. As of 1979, sixty-one species of malarial mosquitoes had a known resistance to DDT.[11] Fish, birds, and other wildlife that consume DDT-infested insects and other contaminated organisms are also affected, often in terms of their reproductive abilities.

An equally disturbing fact is that DDT, which is soluble in fats, has been routinely found in humans.[12] The long-term effect of DDT in humans is inconclusive at this time. However, as G. Tyler Miller, author of *Living in the Environment,* has pointed out, "People born after 1946 are the first generation to carry DDT in their bodies throughout their lifetime. . . . The results will not be known for two to three decades, since the oldest people who have carried DDT and other persistent pesticides in their bodies since conception only reached the age of 35 in 1981."[13] A preliminary study conducted by the National Academy of Sciences has indicated that pesticides such as DDT may cause cancer in humans.[14]

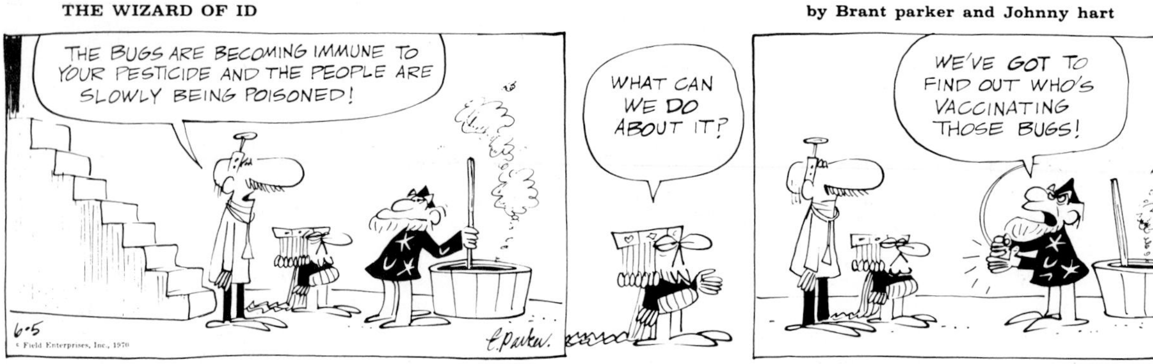

THE WIZARD OF ID by Brant parker and Johnny hart



By permission of Johnny Hart and News America Syndicate.

In 1972, due in large part to the work of Carson and other scientists who brought these problems to public attention, the **Environmental Protection Agency (EPA)** banned the use of DDT in the United States. DDT, however, is still manufactured in the U.S. and then shipped abroad to underdeveloped nations.[15] When used as pesticides in these underdeveloped nations, DDT continues to poison people, animals, and the environment. Thus, a circle of poison is established as DDT-contaminated products such as coffee, tea, bananas, and sugar are shipped back to America for purchase by the U.S. consumer.

The pesticide DDT is only one among many threats to the environment. Any changes people make in the ecosphere are likely to be detrimental to the system. If we are to survive on this planet, we must begin today to cultivate an attitude that regards humanity as a part of nature. We can no longer afford to believe that people can escape from a dependence on the natural environment through technological innovation. We continue on this track only at our own peril.

## The Fourth Law of Ecology: There Is No Such Thing as a Free Lunch

Economic theory provides a sound base for the fourth law and tells us that for every technological gain there exists an ecological price tag. As is often the case with technological advances, the ecological cost can be delayed for a time. Ultimately, however, it must be paid. This "payment" takes many forms, ranging from actual economic costs to a more qualitative cost in terms of perceived human well-being.

We are now beginning to pay the price for many of the past technological advances that have contributed greatly to the current American standard of living. Automobiles, for instance, have had a tremendous impact on the availability and accessibility of many consumer goods and services. Although more options are available for us in terms of where we choose to work, shop, and play, these options tend to be geographically dispersed. We "need" to drive great distances to make use of our options. The ecological price tag attached to our cars is now evident in almost every large city.[16] We find photochemical smog accompanied by nitrogen oxides, hydrocarbons, and asbestos particles from brake linings. These and other substances emitted by automobiles have been seriously implicated in disease processes ranging from lung cancer to acute respiratory infections.[17] In addition to the health costs, we have the tremendous economic costs of cleaning our environment and then trying to prevent further deterioration.

As we delay paying ecological costs, the price tag on our environment increases—with interest. If current trends continue, it appears that future generations will be the ones to pay the largest price for our current technological advances. If we are to prevent this mortgaging of future generations we must begin today to ask an important question regarding every human endeavor: is it worth what it costs?

As you go about your daily activities, begin to reflect on these laws of ecology and your place in the ecosphere. Do you step lightly in your ecosystem, becoming part of natural cycles whenever possible? Have you assessed the ecological price tags attached to your life-style? (See Exhibit 19.2.)

19.2 EXHIBIT 19.2

# The Poisoning of America: How Deadly Chemicals Are Destroying Our Country

The spring of 1982 marked the twentieth anniversary of the publication in 1962 of Rachel Carson's epic work, *Silent Spring.* Today, two decades after she warned that the deadly pesticides that were devastating our wildlife could harm humans as well, we have learned to our regret that she was correct. As a result, we find ourselves in a public-health crisis of unprecedented proportions.

It has now become apparent that pesticides and other toxic chemicals are killing and destroying the health of untold thousands of Americans each year. Synthetic compounds known to cause cancer, birth defects, miscarriages, and other health effects are found regularly in our food, our air, our water—and our own bodies. These toxic and pervasive contaminants represent a threat to the lives and health of all of us, including generations as yet unborn. There is strong evidence that the massive poisoning of our society, this widespread contamination of the environment and the food chain, may be causing epidemics of cancer, sterility, fetus deaths and abnormalities, heart and lung disease, and other disorders throughout the country.

In 1980, officials of the U.S. Environmental Protection Agency (EPA) called this toxic-chemical crisis "the most grievous error in judgment we as a nation have ever made," describing it as "one of the most serious problems the nation has ever faced." Yet, the response of the Reagan Administration has been to cripple the laws and agencies that were set up to cope with this situation.

In early 1983, public attention was brought to bear on this toxic-chemical crisis when pollution forced an entire town, Times Beach, Mo., to be evacuated and abandoned by its residents. Unfortunately, this may be only the first of many such incidents to come. Contaminated by just a few ounces or pounds of dioxin (TCDD, the deadliest synthetic chemical known), Times Beach became the second American community (after the upstate New York community of Love Canal) to be evacuated and bought up by the government because of toxic-chemical pollution.

Yet, amid the massive publicity and public outcry over Times Beach and the revelations of misconduct at EPA, one of the most scandalous and potentially dangerous aspects of this situation has been largely overlooked—the fact that millions of pounds of dioxin-contaminated herbicides continue to be used across the U.S., including urban areas and land where food and cattle are raised.

In 1979, EPA announced that it intended to ban the herbicide 2,4,5-T (one of the two ingredients of Agent Orange) on the grounds that it was killing unborn children in areas where it was being sprayed. Declaring it an imminent threat to human health, the agency applied "emergency" restrictions to *some* uses of the herbicide, suspending its use on forests, rights-of-way, and "pastureland." Yet, inexplicably, it permitted other uses to continue (such as on rice, rangeland, fences, industrial sites, buildings, and parking areas), thereby perpetuating wide public exposure to dioxin. Silvex, which was similarly restricted with its sister chemical 2,4,5-T because of dioxin contamination, can still be used for these allowed applications as well as on sugarcane and even fruit orchards (apples, prunes, and pears). Moreover, EPA still refuses to restrict in any meaningful way the nation's most widely used weedkiller, 2,4-D (the other ingredient of Agent Orange), even though 2,4-D causes cancer, birth defects, and miscarriages in animals and is associated with the deaths of numerous human fetuses. Around Ashford, Wash., where the surrounding forests and state highway were being regularly sprayed with this extremely toxic chemical, a total of twelve pregnancies from January 1979 to March 1980 resulted in ten miscarriages. In the Swan Valley area of Montana, nine out of ten pregnant women suffered miscarriages during a one-year period during which the herbicide was heavily used. While researching my book, *America the Poisoned,* I came across numerous similar accounts from communities throughout the country.

19.2 *continued* EXHIBIT 19.2

Thus, millions of pounds of the two ingredients of the infamous defoliant Agent Orange are still being sprayed across America, despite the enormous harm they are known to have caused to human health, wildlife, and the environment. Moreover, the continued use of these "phenoxy herbicides" (which were developed during World War II as chemical-warfare agents) is causing dioxin to build up in the environment and the food chain, and it is turning up with alarming frequency in fish, beef, other food products, and even mother's milk.

**DIOXIN WASTE DISPOSAL**

Another time bomb ticking away concerns the disposal of dioxin wastes across the nation. To cite just one example, the Hooker Chemical Company's Hyde Park, N.Y., dump site (near Love Canal) is believed to contain *several thousand* pounds of dioxin, as compared to the just fifty-five pounds that caused the contamination problems at Times Beach and up to 100 other suspected sites in Missouri. An ounce of dioxin is thought to be sufficient to kill 1,000,000 people; a single drop could kill 1,000. Thus, there is, theoretically, enough dioxin at Hyde Park to kill every human on Earth if consumed in equal amounts. The effects of this dioxin seeping into the groundwater or otherwise escaping into the environment are incalculable, but could result in a public health disaster of major proportions. We must face the question: What can be done with dioxin-contaminated soil and other wastes when places such as Times Beach are "cleaned up"?

Dioxin can cause severely adverse health effects (including death) at the lowest doses imaginable. At doses as low as a few parts per billion or even per trillion, dioxin has caused cancer, miscarriages, birth defects, and death in test animals. It has proven toxic at the lowest levels at which it has been tested.

Dioxin has turned up at some sites throughout Missouri at levels exceeding 300 to 700 parts per billion; some riding stables contained over 30,000 parts per billion. EPA considers unsafe any level above one part per billion—the equivalent of one second in 31.7 years! Yet, 2,4,5-T commonly contains dioxin concentrations many times above that level. No one knows the damage dioxin now causes to the public health, but it has been associated with numerous human deaths and disabilities over the last few decades, sometimes showing up in the form of cancer decades after exposure.

Instead of acting to rectify the dioxin situation, EPA has in recent years done just the opposite. The agency has halted the process begun in 1979 to ban 2,4,5-T and Silvex, and is even conducting private negotiations with Dow Chemical on lifting the partial ban on 2,4,5-T.

Since very few areas of the country have been tested for dioxin contamination, it cannot be known to what extent we are now sowing the seeds for future dioxin tragedies such as Times Beach. Nor can anyone say what will be the long-term effects on the American people—the ultimate guinea pigs of the chemical industry.

Source: Reprinted from *USA Today*, September 1983. 

## DISCUSSION QUESTIONS

1. The second law of ecology reminds us that there is no "away" to throw things. How has the dioxin dump in Hyde Park, N.Y., demonstrated this law?

2. The third law of ecology states that nature knows best. This law refers to the notion that substances created by humans often cause massive disturbances in the ecosphere. How does this law relate to the current dioxin problem in the U.S.?

3. The fourth law of ecology states that there is no such thing as a free lunch. What are some of the known costs of the herbicide dioxin?

## VISIONS OF SPACESHIP EARTH

One of the major goals of ecology is to find out how everything in the ecosphere is related. R. Buckminster Fuller, inventor and futurist, has proposed a paradigm that is helpful in learning to view the interrelatedness of our ecosphere. Fuller states: "I've often heard people say, 'I wonder what it would be like to be on board a spaceship,' and the answer is very simple. What does it feel like? That's all we have experienced. We are all astronauts."[18] As astronauts, you are undoubtly concerned with the current status of your spacecraft. In Exhibit 19.3, G. Tyler Miller addresses these concerns for the passengers of spaceship Terra I.

19.3 EXHIBIT 19.3

### Terra I

Passengers on *Terra I,* the only true spacecraft, it is time for the annual State of the Spaceship report. As you know, we are hurtling through space at about 107,200 kilometers (66,600 miles) per hour on a fixed course. Although we can never take on new supplies, our ship has a marvelous set of life-support systems that use solar energy to recycle the chemicals needed to provide a reasonable number of us with adequate water, air, and food.

Let me summarize the state of our passengers and of our life-support system. There are over 4.6 billion passengers on board, distributed throughout 165 nations that occupy various sections of the ship. One-quarter of you are in the more developed nations, occupying the good to luxurious quarters in the first-class section. You used about 80 percent of all supplies available this past year.

Unfortunately, things have not really improved this year for the 75 percent of you in the so-called less developed nations traveling in the hold of the ship. Over one-third of you are suffering from hunger, malnutrition, or both, and three-fourths of you do not have adequate water and shelter. More people starved to death or died from malnutrition-related diseases this year than at any time in the history of our voyage. This number will certainly rise as long as population growth continues to wipe out gains in food supply and economic development.

With the limited supplies and recycling capacity of our craft, many of you are now wondering whether you will ever move from the hold to the first-class section. Even more important, many of you are asking why you had to travel in the ship's hold in the first place.

The most important fact molding our lives today is that we have gone around the bend of three curves shaped like the letter J that represent the global increases in population, resource use, and pollution over the past hundred years. Population growth rates have decreased slightly in recent years, partially because of tragic increases in the death rates of the desperately poor countries, home to a billion of you. At the present growth rate, our population will probably grow to 6.1 billion by the year 2000 and could double to over 9 billion passengers in the next 41 years.

But we don't have to maintain our present rate of population growth. We must come to grips with an important question: What is the population level that will let all passengers live with freedom, dignity, and a fair share of *Terra I*'s resources? Some experts put this ideal level at about 2 billion passengers, a figure that we reached in 1930.

But the overpopulation of the hold, serious though it is, may be less of a threat to our life-support system than the overpopulation in the first-class section. Both consumption and pollution rise sharply with even a slight increase in the wealthier population. For example, the 228 million Americans, who make up only 5 percent of our total population, used about 35 percent of all our supplies and produced over one-third of all our artificial pollution last year. Each first-class passenger has about 25 times as much impact on our life-support system as each passenger traveling in the hold. The first-class passengers must continue to reduce their rate of population growth and at the same time change their patterns of consumption, which squander many of our limited supplies. Failure to do so will continue to strain and damage

19.3 *continued* EXHIBIT 19.3

the life-support systems for everyone. Efforts to conserve resources in the rich nations are still grossly inadequate. Pollution control in these nations, however, continues to improve, although there is a long way to go.

In spite of the seriousness of the interlocking problems of overpopulation, dwindling resources, and pollution, the single greatest human and environmental threat is that of war—especially a nuclear holocaust. It is discouraging that so little progress has been made in reducing the extravagant waste of resources and human talent devoted to the arms race. During the past year we spent 200 times more on military expenditures than on international cooperation for peace and development. Each year more nations develop the ability to produce nuclear weapons.

Some say that our ship is already doomed, while other technological optimists see a glorious future for everyone. Our most thoughtful experts agree that the ship's situation is serious but certainly not hopeless. They feel that if we begin now, we have about 50 years to learn how to control our population and consumption and to learn how to live together in cooperation and peace on this beautiful and fragile lifecraft that is our home. Obviously, more of us must start to act like members of the crew rather than like passengers. This particularly applies to those of you traveling first class, who have the most harmful impact on our life-support system and who have the greatest financial and technological resources to help correct the situation.

Source: From *Living in the Environment,* 3d ed., by G. Tyler Miller, Jr. © 1982 by Wadsworth, Inc. Reprinted by permission of the publisher.

### DISCUSSION QUESTIONS

1. Just what is spaceship Terra I?
2. Where are we going? What problems and opportunities do we face?
3. What is our individual responsibility for the other passengers and preserving our life-support systems?

## PERSONAL AND SOCIAL INFLUENCES ON THE ENVIRONMENT

A variety of factors, both personal and social, affect our environment. We must consider these factors, and weigh the consequences of our consumption patterns, in attempting to establish a healthy environment.

### Our Consuming Way of Life

Current estimates of worldwide consumption rates indicate that the U.S., which comprises 5 percent of the world's population, utilizes one-third of the world's resources and produces one-third of the world's pollution.[19] Even more startling is the estimate that the U.S. wastes roughly one-half of the matter and energy it consumes.[20] There is clearly an imbalance in the worldwide consumption of goods.

Before the industrial revolution, an agricultural life-style formed the basis for social and cultural norms. People were capable of producing their own food, clothing, and shelter, so bartering was relatively limited. Industrialization led to a split between the producer and consumer.[21] People began to work at jobs to produce goods for public consumption. After an eight-to-twelve-hour day in a factory, workers had little time to produce goods and services for themselves. The market began to dominate society, and the age of the consumer was born.

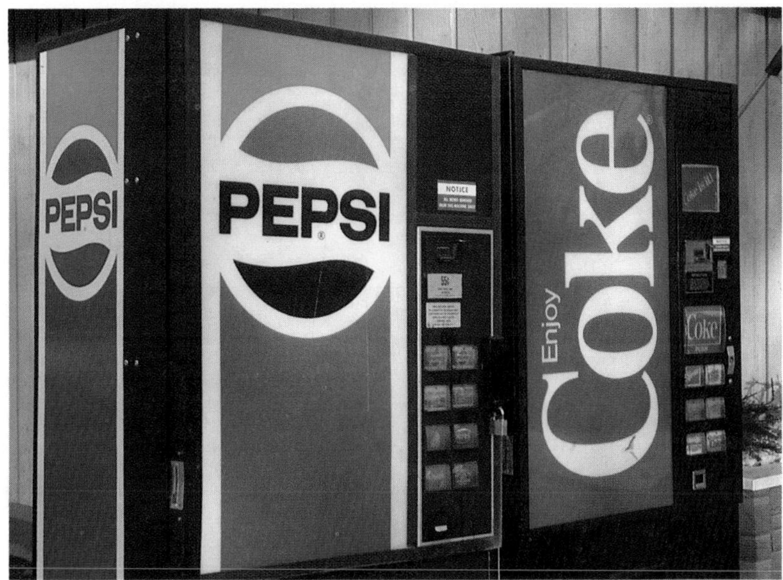


**Figure 19.3**
Industrialization has created a culture based on disposable products.

An important aspect of an industrialized society is its utilization of mass-production processes. Mass production, however, does not function efficiently unless it is accompanied by mass consumption.[22] Therefore, it was essential that industry convince the public to buy and use an endless stream of products.

A quick trip to your local shopping center should be enough to convince you that industry has been quite successful at shaping our needs and desires. The great majority of products for sale are not necessities, but needs created for us by big business and industry. As Paul Ehrlich and Anne Ehrlich, authors of *The End of Affluence,* state, "People have been persuaded that driving cars everywhere is 'better' than using mass transit, that air conditioning is the way to make things more comfortable in the summer, that disposable everything is better than durable anything, and that embalmed foods are more convenient and just as nutritious as fresh foods."[23]

John Lobell, author of a book on self-reliant living, believes that Americans have actually become "hooked" on consuming. Lobell is convinced that "psychologically, consuming has become an end in itself through the achievements of advertising. Many of us are continually in a vague state of wanting, which is momentarily calmed by shopping, but which quickly returns."[24] In our "need" to consume in ever-greater quantities, we tend to develop sloppy and inefficient consumer habits that contribute little to our personal or community welfare. In addition to impulse buying, we develop a tendency toward wasteful consumption. How many of us, for instance, keep the lights, radio, or air conditioner running in an empty house?

We don't always develop wasteful consumption habits on our own; they are "sold" to us through advertising.[25] The use of nonreturnable bottles is a prime example. Only thirty years ago 95 percent of the beverages purchased in the U.S. were sold in returnable containers. Today this figure has dropped to about 25 percent.[26] In order to succeed in changing these figures so dramatically, beverage manufacturers had to launch massive campaigns utilizing ads to increase public awareness.

Advertisers had their work cut out for them in the midsixties when they set out to convince consumers that throwaways were better than returnables. (See figure 19.3.)

Our current consumption patterns have a tremendous impact on the ecosphere. The use of nonreturnable bottles alone adds an extra seven million tons of solid waste to the environment annually.[27] In terms of the laws of ecology we know there is no "away" to throw these containers and that the ecological price tag is quite costly. What are your consuming habits and how do they impact on our environment? Activity for Wellness 19.1 will help you reflect on the ecological price tags of the American way of life.

19.1

ACTIVITY FOR WELLNESS

## This Is Your Life

Ah, the temptations of modern life. Cigarettes promising sex appeal in every puff. Cars that go from zero to sixty miles per hour in nine seconds. Electric gadgets that run the gamut from doughnut makers to facial saunas.

Even the most committed environmentalist sometimes finds these temptations hard to resist. Take the following short quiz. The questions are informational—they'll let you know a little effort can sometimes go a long way.

**HEALTH CONCERNS**

1. How much energy does it take to grow, process and ship food compared to how much energy we get from it?
(a) same (b) one-half (c) 10 times more

2. It requires 19,150 BTUs to produce one pound of marketable chicken. How many are required to produce a pound of grain-fed beef?
(a) less than one-half (b) same amount (c) more than twice as much

**TRANSPORTATION**

3. How much of the energy stored in crude petroleum is lost between the oil well and the gas pump?
(a) 90 percent (b) 60 percent
(c) 20 percent

4. What percentage of commuters in the U.S. go to and from work in a private car?
(a) 25 percent (b) 50 percent
(c) 95 percent

5. At any one time, what percentage of cars on the road in the U.S. carry only the driver?
(a) 50 percent (b) 75 percent
(c) 95 percent

6. If we consider calories expended to be the equivalent of the BTUs in a gallon of gasoline, how many miles does a bicyclist get per gallon?
(a) 15 (b) 400 (c) 1,100

7. Radial tires can improve a car's fuel economy by how much?
(a) 2 percent (b) 6 percent
(c) 23 percent

**RECYCLING**

8. The energy required to manufacture one aluminum soft-drink can could keep a 100-watt bulb burning for
(a) more than five hours
(b) more than thirty hours
(c) more that twenty hours

9. The average returnable bottle is refilled about how many times?
(a) fifteen (b) six (c) two

## Consumption and Entropy

Where are our excessive-consumption patterns leading? It has been suggested that the world has begun a transition toward an age of scarcity.[28] Energy, food, and water shortages have all been predicted. Some of these shortages are already being experienced, at least periodically. The gasoline shortages experienced in the U.S. during the 1970s are but one example. Many environmentalists are beginning to trace these shortages back to two prominent laws of physics, commonly known as the laws of thermodynamics.[29]

The first law of thermodynamics, often referred to as the **conservation of energy,** tells us that energy cannot be created or destroyed, but only transformed from one form to another. The second law of thermodynamics—the law of **entropy**—specifies the direction in which energy must always be transformed. This law states that energy is always transformed from a usable to an unusable form; from an available to an unavailable form; and from the ordered to the disordered. In other words, energy begins with structure and value and is transformed toward random chaos and waste. We see this daily in the world around us. You know, for instance, that

ACTIVITY FOR 19.1
## WELLNESS

10. How much more energy does it take to manufacture an aluminum can from raw materials than recycled ones?
(a) 3 percent (b) 15 percent
(c) 50 percent

11. In 1970, the beverage industry used enough energy in the manufacture of throw-away containers to have supplied all the electricity for Washington, D.C., Pittsburgh, San Francisco, and Boston for:
(a) two days (b) three weeks
(c) five months

12. The average American produces how many pounds of trash per day?
(a) 3.2 pounds (b) 5.8 pounds
(c) 10 pounds

**HOUSEHOLD ENERGY**

13. If only 1,000 homes were better insulated, caulked, and weather-stripped, how many homes could be supplied with natural gas from the energy saved?
(a) 123 (b) 368 (c) 539

14. What percentage of all gas used in residential cooking is used up by gas-range pilot lights?
(a) one-third (b) one-half (c) two-thirds

15. Small appliances account for what percentage of U.S. energy consumption?
(a) 3 percent (b) 7 percent (c) 2 percent

16. If you had lived in the year 1900, how much energy would you have used compared with what you use today?
(a) 25 percent (b) 40 percent
(c) 65 percent

17. Turning down your thermostat three degrees would save how much fuel?
(a) 3 percent (b) 10 percent
(c) 50 percent

**PERSONAL**

18. How much tar does a pack a day smoker pour into his/her lungs every year?
(a) one-quarter cup (b) one-half cup
(c) one cup

19. What percentage of all fires in the U.S. are started by smouldering cigarettes or by the matches used to light up?
(a) 40 percent (b) 12 percent
(c) 20 percent

Answers to numbered questions
1 c. 2 c. 3 a. 4 c. 5 b. 6 c. 7 b. 8 c. 9 a. 10 a. 11 c. 12 a. 13 c. 14 a. 15 a. 16 a. 17 a. 18 c. 19 c.

Source: From Sandalls, Helen, "This Is Your Life Quiz." Reprinted from *Environmental Action* magazine, 1525 New Hampshire Ave. N.W., Washington, D.C. 20036.

when you leave your house unattended it soon becomes more and more disorderly. This is the law of entropy at work. (See figure 19.4.)

Fuels and foods can be used only once to perform useful work. As they are utilized the energy is transformed into an unusable, unavailable, and disordered state. Entropy, then, can be defined as a measure of the amount of energy that is no longer capable of transformation into work. Jeremy Rifkin, author of *Entropy: A New World View,* believes that pollution is another name for entropy, as pollution is the unusable by-product of energy consumption.[30] For instance, gasoline is burned to fuel automobiles producing hydrocarbons, nitrogen oxide, and other emissions. These emissions are unable to be used for future work, and accumulate in the environment as pollutants. Rifkin challenges his readers to look at entropy in their own life-styles:

> Take an entire day to observe everything you come in contact with: things you see, hear, touch, smell, feel or consume; things that you change; and things you exchange. Then try to trace each experience or item in both directions, back to its original source and forward to its final destination. Chances are better than excellent (in fact guaranteed) that they all started off as some form of raw material (available energy) and that they will all end up somewhere as unusable waste (unavailable energy).[31]

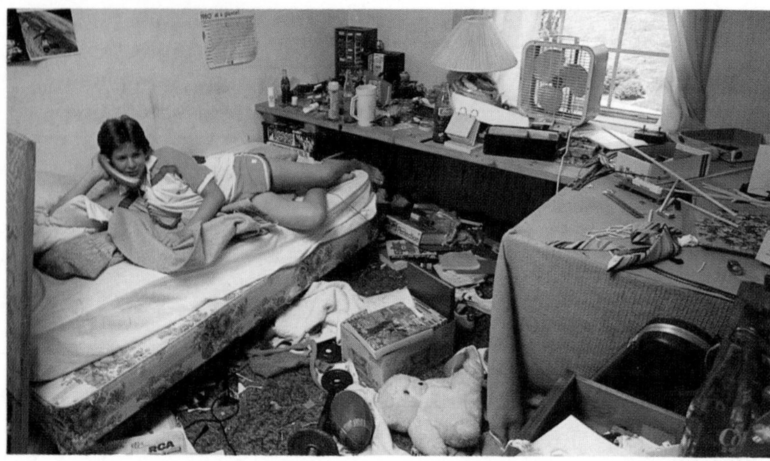

**Figure 19.4**
The law of entropy or disorder is always at work.

The laws of thermodynamics thus tell us that the energy resources on our planet are finite and that as we use them we unavoidably create pollution. If we continue to consume energy and matter at ever-increasing rates we increase dramatically the ecological price to be paid and head toward drastic shortages and hardship for the peoples of the earth.

Options do exist to slow down the rate of entropy in our society. However, many ecologists believe that there is little time left to enact such changes.[32] As Rifkin states, "Today we are being forced to make a transition from the Industrial Age of nonrenewable resources to a new and still undefined age based once again on renewable sources of energy, and we will have to do so in little more than one generation."[33]

## Toward a Sustainable-Earth Society

Leading environmentalists have proposed, as one viable future, a move from the throwaway/frontier mentality toward what they term the sustainable-earth mentality.[34] A **sustainable-earth society** must be founded in the laws of ecology, especially the third law, "Nature knows best." In the past, people have lived under the illusion that nature could be mastered and controlled, that people could be relieved of many dependencies on nature. Essential to the sustainable-earth society is an adoption of the worldview of humanity and nature—that is, a cooperation with nature and its laws.

A sustainable-earth society is also firmly grounded in the laws of thermodynamics. Slowing entropy through recycling and reusing matter and decreasing our energy consumption are emphasized. This type of society is of necessity decentralized, calling on its people to be more responsible and self-reliant.

Robert Russell has developed a theoretical adaptation model which is helpful in understanding humanity in both its frontier and sustainable-earth views.[35] (See figure 19.5.)

Russell's Adaptation Continuum is divided into four equal segments, each representing a certain level of human adaptation. The left end of the continuum represents an ecological approach to life; the right end presents a centralized technological approach. At the extreme ecological end (1.0) individuals do all their adapting for themselves, utilizing personal physical, mental, and emotional resources. Moving toward the right, technology and other individuals become involved in the adaptation process, until at the extreme right end (5.0) institutions and technology are providing essentially all adaptation for the individual. Points 1.0 and 5.0 on the continuum are theoretical extremes and would rarely, if at all, exist in the real world. Most people on our planet fall between 2.0 and 4.0. However, our highly affluent and technological society tends more toward the medical, technological, institutional end than many other societies.[36]

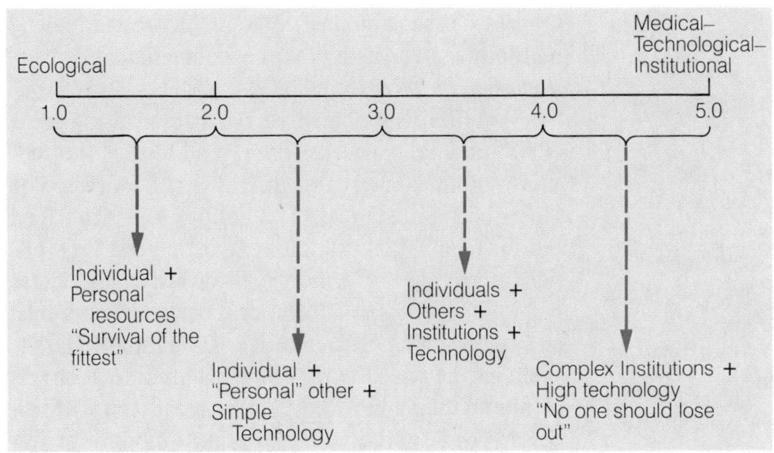


**Figure 19.5**
An adaptation continuum. *Source:* Adapted courtesy of Dr. Robert Russell, Southern Illinois University at Carbondale, Carbondale, Ill.

While there are many advantages to a highly centralized and technological existence, there are also inherent dangers. Russell emphasizes two of these dangers in explaining his model. First, when people become dependent on institutions and technology for much of their adapting they may lose (or possibly never learn) their ability to adapt using their own personal resources. Those of us born during or after the baby boom of the late 1940s and early 1950s have probably grown up in an environment where many of our adaptations are made for us. We do not have to grow all of our own food, for example, or make our own clothes, or repair all of our own possessions. Additionally, our education has, in many instances, failed to prepare us for the event of a possible short- or long-term breakdown of the centralized adaptation system. For example, if you needed to, could you feed, clothe, and shelter yourself with your own personal resources and skills? The second inherent danger revolves around the highly technological adaptations themselves—that is, some of these adaptations may be dangerous in and of themselves. Drugs, while helping us to adapt to or overcome diseases, all have risks and side effects associated with them.

The further we move to the right on the adaptation continuum the greater is our consumption of energy, which leads to an increase in entropy. A sustainable-earth society would tend toward the left on the adaptation continuum, probably locating somewhere between 2.0 and 3.5, indicating a willingness to move back toward more ecological, self-reliant aspects of living.

## CHANGING OUR CONSUMPTION PATTERNS

The quality of our environment rests heavily on what you and I, as individuals and in groups, are willing to do. There are many simple changes each of us can make in our consumption of goods and energy that will help in the move toward a sustainable-earth society. As you reflect on your personal consumption patterns in several major life-style areas and study the suggestions given for reducing consumption, look for several activities you are willing and able to do today. If each of us would take responsibility for our personal environmental actions we would begin to see great advancements in our quest for high-level wellness.

### Food

A tremendous amount of energy goes into the production of food for the typical American diet. As with any energy expenditure, food production involves numerous costs to our environment. These costs depend on several major factors.[37] One such factor involves the number of people to be supported by a given area of farmland and the quality of the food they consume. The typical American diet is high

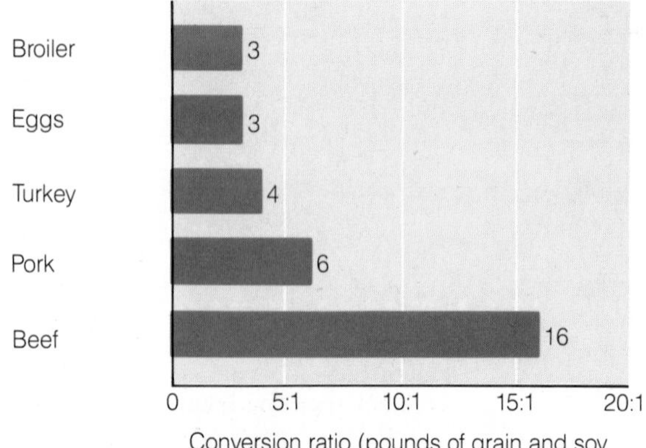


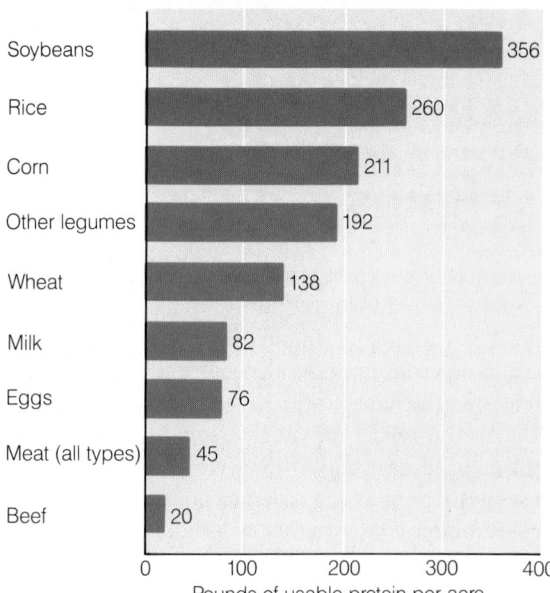


**Figure 19.6**
Food efficiency. *Source:* From *The Little Green Book* by John Lobell. (Adapted from *East-West* magazine.) Shambhala Publications, Inc., Boston, Mass.

in fat and protein. This is due largely to our consumption of meat, which is an energy-expensive way to meet our nutritional needs. Grain products are a more efficient food source as, per acre of land, greater amounts of protein and other essential nutrients can be supplied for human consumption.[38] (See figure 19.6.) As Paul Ehrlich and Anne Ehrlich, authors of *The End of Affluence,* state, "The ultimate answer must be a reduction in American consumption of meat—especially beef, which with present rearing methods represents by far the least efficient conversion of plant food to meat."[39]

Another American dietary pattern raising great environmental concerns is the trend toward the consumption of ever-greater quantities of processed or "fast-food" substances. The annual American food bill for food eaten at home is an estimated $260 billion, at least half of which goes toward the purchase of highly processed substances, convenience items, and snack foods. Still another 105 billion dollars is spent eating out, often in the franchised food chains so abundant in the U.S.[40] This trend toward processed-food sources utilizes great amounts of our precious energy reserves. Processed foods, on the average, use an estimated three times as much energy as fresh foods.[41]

There are many simple activities that are easily incorporated into our dietary life-style which help to conserve our energy resources and decrease entropy. The following list, adapted from the U.S. Department of Energy's *Tips for Energy Savers,* should help you begin to assess and modify your food-energy-consumption patterns.

- Learn to grow some of your own food by maintaining a small garden, window box, or solar greenhouse.
- Eat fewer meat products; substitute more energy-efficient protein sources such as grains and legumes.
- Eat more unprocessed, fresh foods.
- Consider joining a food co-op or shop at the local farmers' market.
- Reduce food waste by serving smaller portions; refrain from throwing food away.
- Thaw frozen foods before cooking.
- Eat cold meals, such as salads, fruits, and vegetables, when feasible.
- Don't preheat ovens.
- Don't buy gadget appliances such as hotdog cookers, electric knife sharpeners, and electric can openers.
- Never boil water in an open pan.
- Match the size of the pan to the heating element.
- Use small electric pans or ovens for small meals.
- When using a dishwasher, let dishes air dry by turning off the control knob after the final rinse and propping the door open.[42]

## Clothing

Many of us fail to realize the energy expenditures involved in the production and maintenance of our personal wardrobes. The fashion industry is big business. It spends large sums of money yearly just in advertising efforts to create in the public a need for the latest fad fashion. Fabric and garment production are costly to the environment. Synthetic fibers are one prime example of the costly environmental impact. Many synthetic fibers, such as nylon, polyester, and vinyls, are made from petroleum and coal. Additionally, the manufacturing processes involved with synthetic fibers require large amounts of energy. Natural fibers such as cotton, wool, and silk, although they are often more expensive to buy, are a better buy in terms of environmental costs.

Each of us must begin today to conserve energy and protect our environment. The following suggestions may increase your environmental sensitivity regarding clothing and assist you in changing your energy-consumption patterns.[43]

- Wear clothes made from natural fibers such as cotton, wool, and silk, rather than synthetic fibers.
- Buy few trendy clothes; emphasize fashions that will last and remain attractive for several years.
- Sew or make your own clothes.
- Wash clothes in warm or cold water rather than hot.
- Save energy by drying clothes outdoors on a clothesline.
- Save energy needed for ironing by hanging clothes in the bathroom while you shower, utilizing the shower steam to remove wrinkles.

## Transportation

The gasoline shortages experienced by Americans since the mid-1970s have focused national attention on transportation-energy-consumption patterns. Although Americans are now more conscious of the monetary and environmental costs involved, we nonetheless remain extremely dependent on the automobile as a means of maintaining our current life-styles. In many communities, in fact, it's impossible to work or shop without an automobile.[44]

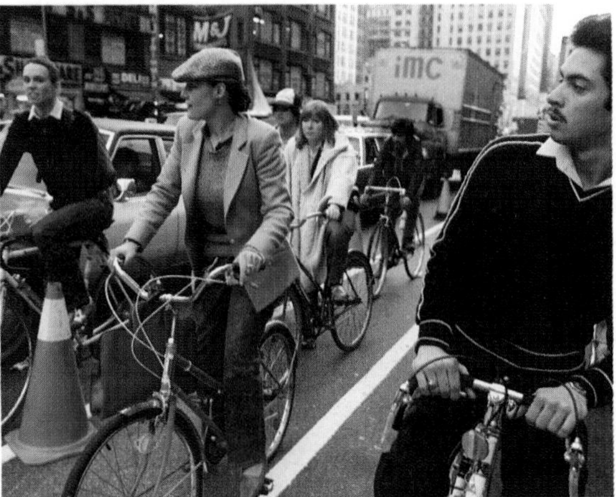


**Figure 19.7**
Biking, walking, and running are becoming more popular, both as means of transportation and as forms of exercise.

There are many options available to us which would aid in the conservation of transportation energy and decrease the pollution levels inherent in our current systems. These range from utilizing automobiles and mass transit more efficiently, to making better use of our own muscle power for transportation. Walking and bicycling are becoming more popular, both as forms of exercise and as means of transportation. (See figure 19.7.)

What changes could you make in your transportation life-style that would be conducive to a sustainable-earth view?

- Use public transportation, a moped, a motorcycle, a bicycle, or walk to work.
- Join a carpool and share rides.
- Consolidate errands into one trip when possible.
- Eliminate unnecessary trips.
- Rediscover the pleasure of walking, hiking, and bicycling.
- Keep your automobile tuned up.
- Keep your automobile tires inflated at the recommended pressure.
- Observe the fifty-five-mile-per-hour speed limit to conserve gasoline.
- Drive at a steady pace.[45]

**Table 19.1 What Fraction of Your Grocery Weight Is Packaging?**

| Grocery Item (net size) | Fraction of Gross Weight |
|---|---|
| Soda—six-pack of 12-oz. cans | 12.5% |
| Soda—2-liter bottle | 33.0% |
| Frozen orange juice—12 oz. | 6.3% |
| Bottled orange juice—32 oz. | 32.5% |
| Milk—½ gallon | 3.4% |
| Ice cream—½ gallon | 2.5% |
| Cereal—15 oz. | 21.0% |
| Scouring powder—14 oz. | 7.0% |
| Dishwasher detergent—50 oz. | 6.1% |
| Liquid detergent—74 oz. | 5.2% |
| Cookies (box)—10 oz. | 10.8% |
| Cookies (bag)—13 oz. | 4.1% |
| Doughnuts (box)—12.5 oz. | 7.8% |
| Pet food (tin)—22 oz. | 10.4% |
| Tomatoes (can)—16 oz. | 14.5% |
| Pineapple (can)—20 oz. | 13.4% |
| Peaches (can)—29 oz. | 12.7% |
| Instant coffee—4 oz. | 69.1% |
| Instant tea—3 oz. | 83.3% |
| Soup—10.75 oz. | 13.7% |
| Mayonnaise—32 oz. | 31.6% |
| Tuna—6.5 oz. | 19.6% |
| Peanut butter—18 oz. | 35.1% |
| Butter—16 oz. | 3.8% |
| Crackers—8 oz. | 17.9% |
| Bread—24 oz. | 2.0% |
| English muffins—12 oz. | 7.1% |
| Hamburger rolls—11.5 oz. | 2.4% |
| Frozen pot pie—8 oz. | 9.7% |
| Frozen apple pie—25 oz. | 9.3% |
| Frozen pizza—12.4 oz. | 13.7% |
| Frozen TV dinner—17 oz. | 13.8% |
| Frozen peas—9 oz. | 7.9% |
| Meat—10.6 oz. | 2.1% |
| Paper napkins—2 oz.* | 3.1% |
| Paper towels—16 oz.* | 1.2% |
| Toothpaste—5 oz. | 8.5% |
| Eggs—dozen (paper carton) | 9.3% |
| Deodorant—2 oz. | 31.0% |

*Note that 100 percent of the weight of these items becomes throwaway after a single use.

Source: From *The Little Green Book* by John Lobell. © 1981 by John Lobell. Shambhala Publications, Inc. Boston, Mass.

## Solid Wastes

Our society is based on a throwaway ethic, with Americans annually disposing of 150 million tons of household waste—enough to fill the New Orleans Superdome from floor to ceiling twice a day throughout the entire year.[46] Although most of us realize the environmental impact of our trash habits, we are startled to learn that we have to buy our trash before we can throw it away. (See table 19.1.) The average family of four spends an estimated $2,920 annually just to purchase their garbage.[47]

We have many viable options for reducing our production of solid wastes. We can easily accomplish many of them on an individual level. These options range from generating less waste—especially from unnecessary packaging—to making better use of opportunities to reuse and recycle goods. It has been projected that two-thirds of the material resources used in the U.S. yearly could be recycled without important changes in our style of living. One study has estimated that it would take an average American household only sixteen minutes a week to separate their solid wastes so as to facilitate recycling.[48]

The following list contains suggestions for individual actions aimed at reducing solid-waste generation.[49] As you read these suggestions, pick one or two that would be easily incorporated into your lifestyle. Begin today to experiment with improving the quality of your environment.

- Buy durable goods, such as a leather handbag instead of one made from vinyl.
- Avoid buying and using throwaway products such as paper towels, plates, cups, and diapers.
- When shopping, reuse paper bags for small items.
- Reuse grocery bags and plastic bags.
- Use a lunch box instead of paper bags.
- Write on both sides of a piece of paper.
- Recycle paper—a stack of newspapers thirty-six inches high would save one tree.[50]
- Reuse bottles and cans by purchasing returnable beverage containers. (Oregon, Michigan, Vermont, Maine, Iowa, Connecticut, Massachusetts, Delaware, and New York have already enacted deposit laws for all beverage containers.)[51]
- Learn to repair products.
- Recycle aluminum cans. (See figure 19.8.)

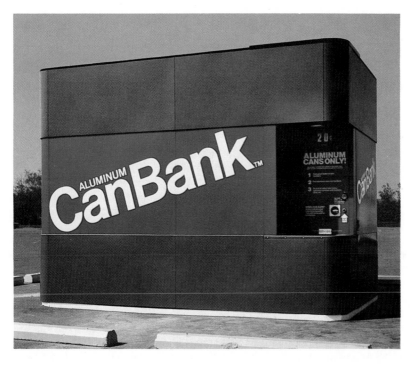


**Figure 19.8**
CanBank is a self-contained aluminum recycling machine, manufactured by Golden Recycle Company, a subsidiary of the Adolph Coors Company. This reverse vending machine accepts used aluminum cans, crushes and stores them, and pays off the recycler in cash, on the spot, twenty-four hours a day.

## Water

Many Americans take water for granted, believing it is their right to have an unlimited, clean, and inexpensive source of this natural resource. Environmentalists, however, predict that water shortages are imminent unless we begin to conserve and respect the finite supply of available water.[52] Conservation on an individual level is one obvious component of the solution. Simply turning off the water faucet while brushing your teeth can save an estimated gallon or so of pure drinking water.

Many forms of water conservation are simple and easily incorporated into your life-style. The following list may help stimulate you to incorporate water-saving activities into your style of living.[53]

- Shut off water faucets while washing, shaving, or brushing your teeth.
- Don't boil a full kettle of water for one cup of coffee or tea.
- Do as much household cleaning as possible with cold water.
- Take showers rather than tub baths (this would save an estimated five gallons of water per shower).
- Place a brick in the tank of toilets to reduce the water stored there.

## Energy

"Addiction! There is simply no other way to accurately describe America's energy habit. The statistics are overwhelming. With only 6 percent of the world's population, the United States currently consumes over one-third of the world's energy."[54] To some, these words of Jeremy Rifkin may seem a gross exaggeration. Statistics, however, seem to support his views. In addition to excessive energy consumption Americans waste an estimated 85 to 90 percent of all energy they use.[55]

The largest source of residential energy consumption (70 percent) involves the heating and cooling of our homes. Other important sources of energy consumption include heating water, lighting, cooking, and running small appliances.[56] The U.S. Department of Energy suggests the following ways to reduce energy:

- For heating, keep your thermostat at sixty-five degrees Fahrenheit during the day and fifty-five degrees Fahrenheit at night. (See table 19.2.)

19.4 EXHIBIT

## Visions of Tomorrow

We live in an age when many of our conceptions of reality are undergoing radical changes. When we stood in space we did not see the Rand-McNally globe floating through space, we saw something very different. And as our concepts of reality begin to change, it's also time to reevaluate our conceptions of the future.

All of us have grown up thinking that the future would be filled with flying cars and robots and rocketships. We'd all have tail-finned automobiles and live in domed structures. Yet social problems, environmental problems, the energy crisis and economic problems are beginning to erode that dream. It's time to look at the dream that's been projected for the future, get a sense of what it was about, and begin to plot new futures.

When we look at old images of the future, we see that they were filled with mobility. Each of us would have a tremendous amount of personal mobility. We'd have our own helicopters. Rocketbelts would move us quickly to community colleges to go to class. Propeller driven trains would move us quickly to work.

But there are problems happening with this set of dreams of plastic and fiberglass modular housing units, this plastic and fiberglass future that's been projected. The United Nations tells us that by the year 2000, half the world's population will not even have a permanent home; half the world's population in the year 2000 will be living in squatters' housing units.

Increasing numbers of people are beginning to understand the price of high technologies that have been proposed and are being built. People are searching for alternatives. Some are going back up into the mountains, building remote isolated retreats. But when we look at the population that's projected for the planet, we see that this can only work for a small number of people.

So we need to begin to ask such questions as how people live and what kind of biological toll they take—how much it takes to support them—materials and energy and food.

When I look at the future, I don't embrace just a technological vision of the future. I think the mistake that we've made is that we've all embraced just technological fantasies of the future. The kind of future that makes sense to me is the kind of future in which we talk about social values that can allow us to create a viable future.

We live in a society of very long loops. A survey has revealed that the tomatoes in an Atlanta, Ga., supermarket were grown in Mexico, taken to California for packing, then flown across

**Table 19.2 Heating Costs Saved with Nighttime Setback**

| City | Approximate Percentage Saved With Eight-Hour Nighttime Setback Of— 5°F | 10°F | City | Approximate Percentage Saved With Eight-Hour Nighttime Setback Of— 5°F | 10°F |
|---|---|---|---|---|---|
| Atlanta, Ga. | 11 | 15 | Denver, Colo. | 7 | 11 |
| Boston, Mass. | 7 | 11 | Des Moines, Iowa | 7 | 11 |
| Buffalo, N.Y. | 6 | 10 | Detroit, Mich. | 7 | 11 |
| Chicago, Ill. | 7 | 11 | Kansas City, Mo. | 8 | 12 |
| Cincinnati, Ohio | 8 | 12 | Los Angeles, Calif. | 12 | 16 |
| Cleveland, Ohio | 8 | 12 | Louisville, Ky. | 9 | 13 |
| Columbus, Ohio | 7 | 11 | Madison, Wis. | 5 | 9 |
| Dallas, Tex. | 11 | 15 | | | |

Source: *Energy Savings Through Automatic Thermostat Controls:* Energy Research and Development Administration, Office of Public Affairs, Washington, D.C.

## EXHIBIT 19.4

country to Virginia, put on a truck and shipped to Atlanta. In Atlanta, with greenhouses, you can grow tomatoes year round. Yet we're dependent on very long loops.

I've proposed that the White House be made a national model of short-looped living. Picture the White House with vegetable gardens in the backyard, apple orchards, fruit orchards, fish ponds, wind generators, six pyramids where we'd mount solar collectors. A monument to the sun would be in the backyard of the White House, as inspired by the pyramids on the back of the dollar bill.

We're going to have to begin to think about nature differently also. We see nature as something to be exploited, something apart from us. Yet we're going to have to begin to think of ourselves as a part of it, begin to relate to it differently—as trustees. We must begin to formulate a new vision of the future, utilizing bicycles and solar energy and rooftop gardens—a vision that could make urban areas habitable for a viable future.

But it's difficult when people have been enchanted with flying buses to begin to talk to them about bicycles. And yet I believe it is possible to start talking about a very different conception of the future, one that takes into account the kind of realities that we're faced with—energy problems, economic problems and social problems. And in doing that, I can foresee a time when it will be possible to paint over the parking lot signs and put up food co-op signs, as people will begin to embrace another value—social cooperation.

Source: Courtesy Sam Love, Public Production Group, Washington, D.C.

## DISCUSSION QUESTIONS

1. What is your vision of tomorrow?

2. Does your vision of the future fall at the self-reliant end of Russell's Adaptation Continuum and lead toward a sustainable-earth society?

3. How can you begin to enhance the concept of "social cooperation" on a daily basis?

| | Approximate Percentage Saved With Eight-Hour Nighttime Setback Of— | | | Approximate Percentage Saved With Eight-Hour Nighttime Setback Of— | |
|---|---|---|---|---|---|
| *City* | *5°F* | *10°F* | *City* | *5°F* | *10°F* |
| Miami, Fla. | 12 | 18 | Portland, Oreg. | 9 | 13 |
| Milwaukee, Wis. | 6 | 10 | Salt Lake City, Utah | 7 | 11 |
| Minneapolis, Minn. | 5 | 9 | San Francisco, Calif. | 10 | 14 |
| New York, N.Y. | 8 | 12 | Seattle, Wash. | 8 | 12 |
| Omaha, Nebr. | 7 | 11 | St. Louis, Mo. | 8 | 12 |
| Philadelphia, Pa. | 8 | 12 | Syracuse, N.Y. | 7 | 11 |
| Pittsburgh, Pa. | 7 | 11 | Washington, D.C. | 9 | 13 |

- Dress in warmer clothing when heat thermostat is turned down.
- Use a window fan for cooling when feasible.
- Set your air conditioner at seventy-eight degrees Fahrenheit.
- Turn off window air-conditioning units when you will be gone for several hours.
- Turn off any lights not being used.
- Keep lamps and light fixtures clean; dirt absorbs light.
- Use outdoor lights only when necessary.
- Don't leave appliances, such as a radio or television, running when they are not actually being used.

## TO THE FUTURE

Environmentalist and author Garrett Hardin has written extensively on what he calls "The Tragedy of Commons."[57] Many people believe their impact on the ecosphere is so small as to be unimportant; this view is indeed a tragedy. Individual actions add up to societal actions. People can make many contributions on both personal and community levels. Review your own consumption habits and their impact on the environment. There are many alternatives leading to environmental wellness. Begin today to select activities you are willing and able to implement in your life-style, and encourage others around you to do the same. This may mean serving as a model of environmental sensitivity or even becoming involved politically on a local level. Volunteer services are needed for many worthy environmental projects.

Where will we be tomorrow . . . or next year? Our environmental sensitivity, both individually and collectively, is likely to determine our future.

## SUMMARY

1. In nature there is no waste. Nature is cyclical; one organism's waste provides nutrients for another.

2. Environmentalist Barry Commoner has studied natural cycles and summarized them in four laws of ecology: (1) everything is connected to everything else; (2) everything must go somewhere; (3) nature knows best; and (4) there is no such thing as a free lunch. These laws provide an understanding of ecosystems and their function.

3. Americans are a society of consumers. Since industrial consumption patterns are often wasteful and do not follow nature's patterns, they have a great negative impact on the environment.

4. A coming age of scarcity that will dramatically affect our style of living has been predicted. Consumption patterns of Americans must change.

5. One viable future proposed by environmentalists and futurists is the sustainable-earth society. This society would be based on a philosophy of people cooperating with nature. Recycling and reusing matter and decreasing energy consumption would be emphasized.

6. We cannot afford to wait for governments, business and industry, or the "other guy" to act on environmental issues. We must each take the challenge—the opportunity—to move toward environmental wellness.

### Recommended Readings

Commoner, Barry. *The Closing Circle.* New York: Bantam Books, 1974.

McNeil, M., ed. *Environment and Health.* Washington, D.C.: *Congressional Quarterly,* 1981.

Rifkin, Jeremy. *Entropy: A New World View.* New York: Viking Press, 1980.

Samuels, Mike, and Bennett, Hal Zina. *Well Body, Well Earth.* San Francisco: Sierra Club Books, 1983.

Worldwatch Institute Report, Linda Starke, ed. *State of the World 1984.* New York: W. W. Norton & Co., 1984.

### References

1. G. Tyler Miller, *Living in the Environment,* 2d ed. (Belmont, Calif.: Wadsworth Publishing Co., 1982), 481.

2. John Lobell, *The Little Green Book* (Boulder, Colo.: Shambhala Publications, 1981), 4.

3. Miller, *Living in the Environment,* 46.

4. Barry Commoner, *The Closing Circle* (New York: Bantam Books, 1974).

5. Miller, *Living in the Environment,* 46.

6. Mike Samuels and Hal Zina Bennett, *Well Body, Well Earth* (San Francisco: Sierra Club Books, 1983), 80.

7. Lobell, *Little Green Book,* 249.

8. Lobell, *Little Green Book,* 249.

9. Commoner, *The Closing Circle,* 41.

10. Rachel Carson, *Silent Spring* (Boston: Houghton Mifflin, 1962).

11. Miller, *Living in the Environment,* E84.

12. Samuels and Bennett, *Well Body, Well Earth,* 152.

13. Miller, *Living in the Environment,* E88.

14. National Academy of Sciences, *Pest Control: An Assessment of Present and Alternative Technologies.* 5 vols. (Washington, D.C.: National Academy of Sciences, 1975).

15. Miller, *Living in the Environment,* E88; Commoner, *Closing Circle,* 200; Samuels and Bennett, *Well Body, Well Earth,* 152.

16. Commoner, *Closing Circle,* 72.

17. Jeremy Rifkin, *Entropy* (New York: Viking Press, 1980), 146.

18. R. Buckminster Fuller,*Operating Manual for Spaceship Earth* (Carbondale, Ill.: Southern Illinois University Press, 1969), 46.

19. Miller, *Living in the Environment,* 6.

20. Miller, *Living in the Environment,* 6.

21. Alvin Toffler, *The Third Wave* (New York: Bantam Books, 1980), 37–42.

22. Lobell, *Little Green Book,* 264.

23. Paul R. Ehrlich and Anne H. Ehrlich, *The End of Affluence* (New York: Random House, 1974).

24. Lobell, *Little Green Book,* 266.

25. Lobell, *Little Green Book,* 264.

26. Lobell, *Little Green Book,* 374.

27. Lobell, *Little Green Book,* 374.

28. Ehrlich and Ehrlich, *End of Affluence,* 20–21.

29. Rifkin, *Entropy,* 99–182; Miller, *Living in the Environment,* 37.

30. Rifkin, *Entropy,* 35.

31. Rifkin, *Entropy,* 57.

32. Miller, *Living in the Environment,* 481–88; Rifkin, *Entropy,* 186; Ehrlich and Ehrlich, *End of Affluence,* 34.

33. Rifkin, *Entropy,* 186.

34. Miller, *Living in the Environment,* 14–27; Lobell, *Little Green Book,* 267–74.

35. Robert Russell, "Toward a Functional Understanding of Ecology for Health Education," *Journal of School Health* 39.10 (1969): 702–08; Robert Russell, "Effects of Ecological Thinking on Health Education," *School Health Review* 3.4 (1972): 3–5.

36. Personal correspondence with Robert Russell, Southern Illinois University at Carbondale, Spring 1982.

37. Ehrlich and Ehrlich, *End of Affluence*, 187.

38. Ehrlich and Ehrlich, *End of Affluence*, 198.

39. Ehrlich and Ehrlich, *End of Affluence*, 198.

40. Lobell, *Little Green Book,* 36.

41. Ehrlich and Ehrlich, *End of Affluence,* 202.

42. U.S. Department of Energy, *Tips for Energy Savers* (Washington, D.C.: U.S. Government Printing Office, 1979).

43. U.S. Department of Energy, *Tips for Energy Savers.*

44. Lobell, *Little Green Book,* 283.

45. U.S. Department of Energy, *Tips for Energy Savers.*

46. Lobell, *Little Green Book,* 249.

47. Lobell, *Little Green Book,* 250–51.

48. Miller, *Living in the Environment,* E119.

49. Lobell, *Little Green Book,* 258–61.

50. Miller, *Living in the Environment,* E119.

51. William U. Chandler, "Materials Recycling: The Virtue of Necessity," *Worldwatch Paper* 56 (October 1983): 33.

52. Fred Powledge, "Water, Water, Running Out," *The Nation* 234 (June 1982): 703, 714–16.

53. U.S. Department of Energy, *Tips for Energy Savers;* Powledge, "Water, Water, Running Out," 716.

54. Rifkin, *Entropy,* 99.

55. Miller, *Living in the Environment,* 259.

56. U.S. Department of Energy, *Tips for Energy Savers.*

57. Garrett Hardin, "The Tragedy of the Commons," *Science* 162.3859 (13 December 1968): 1243–48.

*CHAPTER TWENTY*

# Aging: Adaptations for Wellness



Aging is the process of change through time, and has biological, sociological, and psychological implications. Until recently, only a minority of people lived into their eighth and ninth decades. Advances in public health, sanitation, nutrition, medical technology, and self-care, however, have changed all this. At the turn of the twentieth century, life expectancy for a newborn in the U.S. was only forty-nine years, and persons over the age of sixty-five comprised only 4 percent of the total population. Today, a newborn has a life expectancy from sixty-four to seventy-eight years, depending on gender, race, and other factors. There are more than twenty-two million people over the age of sixty-five now, approximately 11 percent of the population. A person turning sixty-five this year can expect to have from fifteen to eighteen more years of living ahead. By the year 2000, people sixty-five and over may comprise 12 percent or more of the population, rising perhaps to 20 percent by the year 2030, about the time many of today's college students will turn sixty-five themselves. In Florida, persons sixty-five and over already make up 16 percent of the residents. Clearly, the elderly will be a significant social and political force in the future.

The reasons for the growing number of older adults are easy to identify. Since the start of the twentieth century, the average life expectancy in the U.S. has increased considerably. The decline in the rate of infant mortality is one important reason. Moreover, there has been a dramatic shift in the leading causes of morbidity and mortality. Chronic diseases have replaced communicable diseases as the leading cause of death. The people of the U.S. now have a higher overall standard of living. People are eating better, are more conscientious about their health than ever before, and for the most part, have access to better medical care than at any time in the past.

Living longer increases the probability that we will have to cope with change and make adaptations in order to maximize the quality of life. In this chapter we will look at some of the changes that occur with age, and examine those adaptations that promote wellness through the middle and later adult years.

20.1 ACTIVITY FOR WELLNESS 20.1

## How Do I View the Elderly?

When you hear the word "elderly," what do you think of? Below are some terms that some people associate with the elderly. Put a check mark next to each term that fits your impression of the elderly.

[ ] 1. rigid
[ ] 2. happy
[ ] 3. crotchety
[ ] 4. active
[ ] 5. sickly
[ ] 6. wise
[ ] 7. feeble
[ ] 8. friendly
[ ] 9. senile
[ ] 10. self-sufficient
[ ] 11. incompetent
[ ] 12. intelligent
[ ] 13. childlike
[ ] 14. independent
[ ] 15. institutionalized
[ ] 16. creative
[ ] 17. reactionary
[ ] 18. interesting
[ ] 19. depressing
[ ] 20. helpful

What pattern is there to your response? What kind of regard do you have for the elderly? Where do these attributes that you assign to the elderly come from? Compare your responses to those of a friend. Watch for portrayals of elderly persons on television, in films, and in magazines. Are the portrayals accurate or are they stereotypes?

## MYTHS ABOUT AGING

Many Americans seem to suffer from a prejudice against old people. Philip Slater speaks of a society that tries to "hide" the elderly in institutions.[1] Despite societal prejudice, only a small fraction of the elderly actually are institutionalized. Nevertheless, one of the most frequently held myths about elderly people is that they are sickly and confined to hospitals, nursing homes, or other long term care facilities. Although elderly people may be sick more often than their youthful counterparts, it is inaccurate to describe them as "sickly."

Other myths about the elderly abound: *Most old people are senile and incompetent. The elderly have no interest in or capacity for sexual relations. Old age is a time of depression and waiting around to die. The elderly are rigid in their ways and reactionary in their politics. Old people experience the aging process in identical ways. Most oldsters are alone or lonely. The majority of elderly citizens are poor and without income.* All of these beliefs are false.[2]

Although aging can be viewed purely in chronological terms, **gerontologists,** the people who study the elderly and the aging process, do distinguish among three aspects of aging. **Biological aging** refers to the physical changes that occur through time. Clearly, physical change varies among individuals. Genetics plays an important role in the process of biological aging, and so do environmental factors. **Sociological aging** refers to changes in a person's familial, occupational, and social roles. Finally, **psychological aging** refers to how one adapts in mind, body and spirit to the biological and sociological changes, and to the passage of time.

20.1 EXHIBIT 20.1

## You're Only as Old as You Feel!

What is old—seventy, eighty, ninety years old? It all depends on your perspective. What about professional athletes? Football and baseball players are "old" by the time they are in their thirties. Sportscasters are forever pointing out the forty-year-old "graybeards." World-class ice skaters, gymnasts, track-and-field stars and many others reach their peaks closer to age twenty. However, some athletes seem to defy the passage of time. Baseballer Warren Spahn reached the coveted milestone of pitching a no-hitter, but not until after his fortieth birthday. Henry Aaron was forty-one when he became the player to hit the most home runs in the entire history of American baseball. In 1984, football great Jim Brown announced his intention of making a comeback at the age of forty-eight, having last played professionally in 1965. Some people, displaying a sort of "sports ageism," scoffed at his plan. Gordie Howe performed miracles on ice, playing one of the most physical and demanding of sports—professional hockey. He persisted in the game until he was actually able to line up side by side on the ice with two of his sons. Perhaps the most remarkable of all professional athletes who defied time was baseball player LeRoy ("Satchel") Paige. In his autobiography, *Maybe I'll Pitch Forever,* Paige writes: "I finished up the season with eleven wins and only four losses and an earned run average of 1.86. I was the top pitcher in the league. That ain't bad when a man's past 50."* You're only as old as you feel is a cliche with a ring of truth.

*From Leroy ("Satchel") Paige, *Maybe I'll Pitch Forever* (New York: Grove Press, 1962), 244–45.

### DISCUSSION QUESTIONS

1. What is old in some other occupations?
2. What is "old" in the occupation you plan to go into?

## BIOLOGICAL PROCESSES OF AGING

There is a distinct difference between chronological age and biological age.[3] Biological age is defined as the ability to adapt to the environment, both the normal situations and the stressors or crises. It is, therefore, virtually independent of chronology. Furthermore, the older-adult population can be separated into at least two groups: the **young old** (age sixty to seventy-five), and the **old old** (age seventy-five and beyond). This separation by chronological age is based on biological evidence that after age seventy-five many individuals acquire one or more chronic illnesses or conditions that interfere with adaptation. However, some gerontologists add a third group—the **athletic old.** This group of people is comprised of individuals who have maintained a high state of physical fitness throughout their lives, and for whom the processes of aging and acquisition of chronic disorders seem to have been retarded. (See Exhibit 20.1.)

V. Korenchevsky identifies a process called **primary aging,** an unavoidable result of chronology that affects all species sooner or later.[4] Another process, **secondary aging,** occurs as a result of trauma, stress, illness, or neglect. People confuse these two processes and thus reinforce the myth that all old people are sickly. Secondary aging certainly can accelerate primary aging, though it does not cause it.

There comes a time when the elderly experience a marked change in their ability to adapt. What is noted as a sudden loss of ability, however, is really

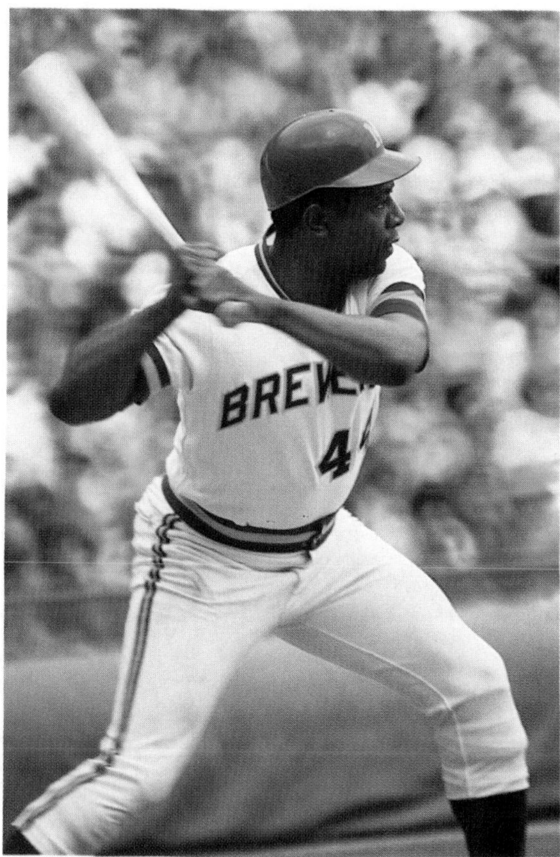


**Figure 20.1**
Some athletes seem to defy the passage of time. Henry Aaron was forty-one when he set his record for home runs.

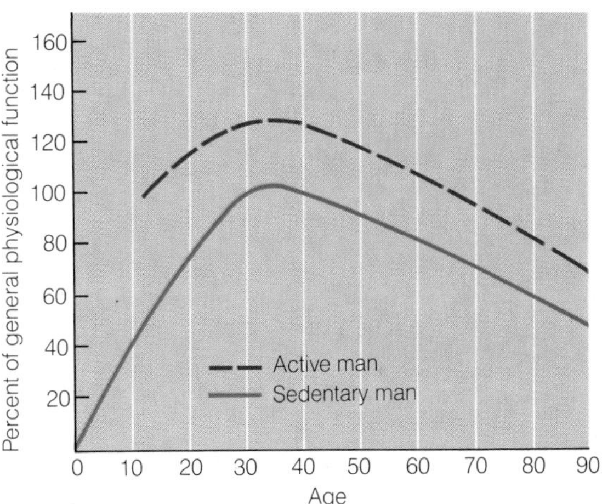


**Figure 20.2**
The Euro-American curve. *Source:* From *Exercise and Aging: The Scientific Basis,* Everett L. Smith and Robert C. Serfass, eds. Enslow Publishers, Hillside, N.J. 07205, $16.95.

a gradual loss experienced over a period of forty or more years. This reduction in biological adaptability is illustrated in the **Euro-American Curve** (figure 20.2). Values shown in the curve are meant to reflect average change in individuals through time, with peak biological maturity coming around the age of thirty. Both the solid curve and the dashed curve are important to consider. The solid curve illustrates the person who is inactive at age thirty and neglects the body's needs for the remainder of life. The dashed curve shows that physical activity and overall health maintenance can impact in two ways on primary aging. First, the active person reaches a peak higher than that of the sedentary person. Second, though some functional decline is inevitable for both groups, the active person's level of physiological functioning stays higher as long as activity is maintained. If the active person ceases to be active, the curve merges with the sedentary person's. Though the curve may not describe each individual precisely, it does reflect the consequences for active and sedentary persons on a population basis.

Specifically, what biological changes occur over time? Several functional changes are summarized in table 20.1.

## Cardiovascular Function

Advancing age brings about significant functional changes in the cardiovascular system. **Cardiac output,** the ability of the heart to deliver blood to body tissues in a given amount of time, declines by approximately 30 percent between ages thirty and seventy.[5] Cardiac output is a function of two other quantities—**stroke volume** (the amount of blood pumped each time the heart beats) and **heart rate** (the number of heart beats per unit of time). The heart's ability to beat faster, as during exercise, declines at an annual rate of about .75 percent after age thirty. The contractile force of the heart muscle declines by about the same rate. These changes account for the net loss of function observed over this forty-year span.

In addition, a 20 percent rise in blood pressure is observed in many people.[6] For people whose hereditary pattern predisposes them to hypertension, the increases may be even greater.

**Table 20.1 Summary of Biological Functional Changes Occurring with Age**

| | |
|---|---|
| Cardiac output | Declines 30 percent between age thirty and age seventy |
| Blood pressure | Increases by 20 percent in both systolic and diastolic pressures between age thirty and age seventy |
| Vital capacity | Decreases 40 to 50 percent between age thirty and age seventy |
| Residual volume | Increases 30 to 50 percent between age thirty and age seventy |
| Basal metabolic rate (BMR) | Declines 10 percent on the average between age thirty and age seventy |
| Muscle mass and strength | Declines by 20 to 25 percent between age thirty and age seventy |
| Flexibility in joints | Declines by 20 to 30 percent between age thirty and age seventy |
| Bone mineral | Declines 15 to 30 percent between age thirty and age seventy depending on gender |
| Sensory ability | Qualitative changes in visual and auditory acuity, taste, and smell |
| Renal functioning | Decrease in filtration rate by up to 50 percent |
| Sexual functioning | Qualitative change in lubricating ability of vagina in the female; decreased testosterone production and delayed erection time in the male |

## Pulmonary Function

Pulmonary function refers to the lungs' ability to move air, exchanging carbon dioxide for oxygen. Two factors affect changes in the lungs during aging—**vital capacity** and **residual volume.** Vital capacity refers to the volume of air that moves when you inhale and exhale at maximum ability. Even when inhaling at the maximum, you do not fill all the available lung space. There is still space not taking part in gas exchange. This quantity is known as the residual volume. In young people, residual volume is small compared to vital capacity. Together, vital capacity and residual volume comprise the **total lung capacity.** The aging process involves an inversion of these two quantities. Between ages thirty and seventy, vital capacity declines 40 to 50 percent, while residual volume increases 30 to 50 percent.[7]

The elderly person, then, is less able to supply the body with oxygen. This decreased function may go unnoticed when a person is at rest or engaged only in mild activity. However, during vigorous exercise, adequate oxygen supply can only be maintained by breathing more rapidly and by increasing the workload of the heart. The response of the heart during a period of increased workload may not be adequate to maintain the level of activity desired.

## Basal Metabolic Rate

The **basal metabolic rate (BMR)** is the rate at which bodily processes are carried out at the cellular level while the body is at rest. The BMR regulates such things as respiration, heart rate, rate of digestion, and body temperature. On the average, BMR declines by a factor of 10 percent between ages thirty and seventy.[8] We have all seen elderly people wearing a sweater or jacket, even on relatively warm days, to maintain comfort. Any discomfort may be a consequence of the lowered BMR. To get a notion of how this 10 percent drop is experienced by the older adult, consider the following situation. Most of us are comfortable in a room where the temperature is controlled at seventy degrees. However, if that temperature is decreased by 10 percent to make it sixty-three degrees, the comfort level changes dramatically.[9] Fingertips, toes, and noses become cold and may even ache slightly. Our ability to concentrate, write, type, or perform other simple activities may be reduced.

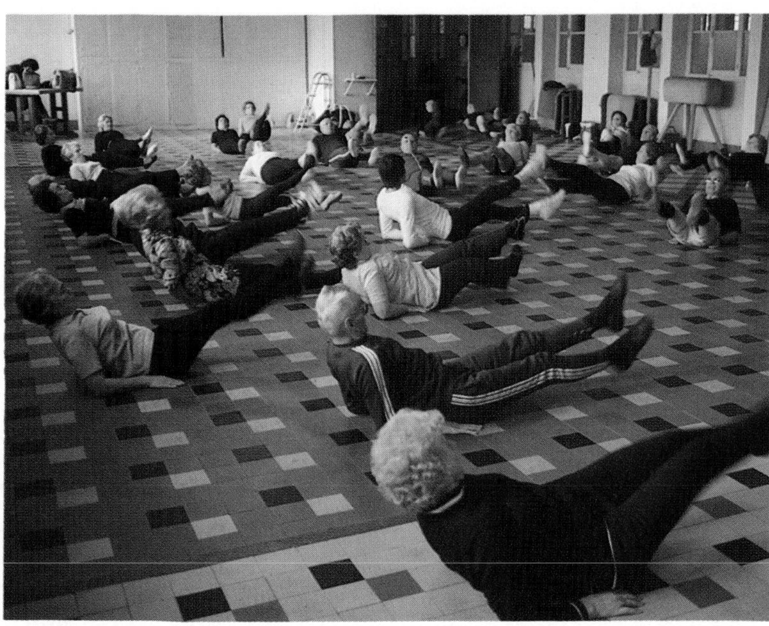

**Figure 20.3**
The older individual's loss of flexibility often stems as much from lack of exercise as from actual age degeneration.

## Body Composition

Several changes in body composition occur with age. There is an alteration in the percentage of total body fat over time. In normal young, lean individuals, fat makes up from 10 to 15 percent of the entire body mass. Women tend to have somewhat more fatty tissue than men. By age seventy, the amount of fatty tissue is in the range of 20 to 40 percent. The reasons for this change are not completely understood. However, it appears that modification of the body's ability to use dietary protein is a partial explanation of this phenomenon.

Muscle mass decreases with age.[10] The quadriceps, the large muscles of the upper leg, seem to lose mass more rapidly than other muscles in the aging person.[11]

Accompanying the change in muscle mass is a decline in muscular strength. Grip strength peaks in males during their mid-twenties and declines thereafter at a gradual pace until age sixty, when the decline becomes steep.[12]

By age seventy, an individual's flexibility has declined by 20 to 30 percent due to changes in muscles, ligaments, joints, and tendons. The result is a decreased range of motion for the older individual. It is probable, however, that the lost range of motion or flexibility is a phenomenon stemming as much from disuse of muscles and joints as from actual age degeneration.[13]

## Changes in Bone

Bone is composed of both organic and inorganic substances. The principal organic component in bone is **collagen,** a protein substance. The inorganic structure of bone is composed of two minerals, calcium and phosphorous. Approximately 99 percent of the body's calcium and 88 percent of the body's phosphorous is located in the skeleton.[14] It is the change with age in the mineral content of bone that can influence development of a serious health problem.

A significant decline in bone mineral by age seventy is not an uncommon occurrence. This decline results in a skeletal structure that is weakened and subject to fracture. Particularly affected are the long bones of the leg and the hips with which they articulate, the bones of the forearm and wrist, and the bones that comprise the lumbar and thoracic spine.[15] This condition of decreased bone mass is known as **osteoporosis.**

Osteoporosis produces an enlarged marrow cavity surrounded by porous bone, resulting in loss of bone density and strength. Imagine that you are looking through the end of one of the long bones, as if it were a telescope. In a young person, the marrow cavity appears relatively small and the bone mineral

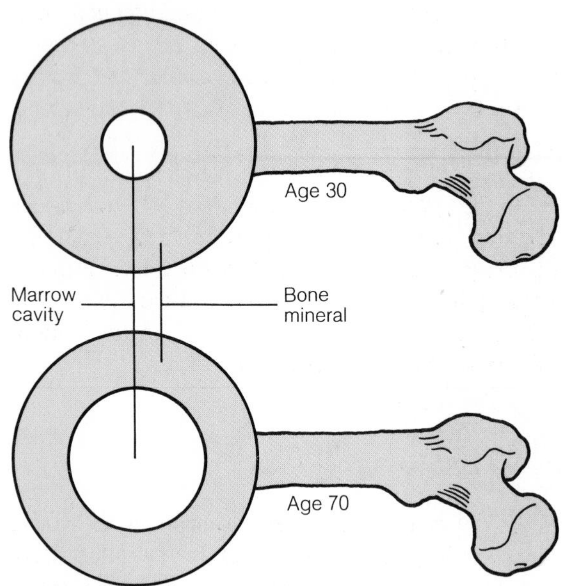


**Figure 20.4**
Cross section of normal and osteoporotic bone.

that surrounds it is densely packed. In osteoporotic bone, the marrow cavity is larger and the surrounding bone mineral is less dense (see figure 20.4).

Osteoporosis affects more than six million men and women. Bone loss is usually more severe for women and the osteoporotic process occurs earlier in life for women than men. Bone loss in women proceeds at a rate of approximately .75 to 1 percent per year beginning between ages thirty and thirty-five.[16] At the time of menopause, or about age fifty, the loss is accelerated to 2 or 3 percent per year. By age seventy, the loss in bone mass for some women may be as great as 30 percent. This loss threatens the strength of several bones. Osteoporosis contributes to the more than 200,000 broken hips per year in women over the age of sixty. One occasionally hears of an unfortunate elderly person who "falls and breaks a hip." More often than not, the "fall" was caused by a spontaneous fracture of an advanced stage osteoporotic bone, rather than the other way around. Fracture of the wrist and vertebral collapses in the spine are additional risks brought about by osteoporosis.

Men experience less of, a problem with osteoporosis. Bone loss proceeds at an annual rate about equal to .4 percent, but does not begin until around age fifty.[17] Still, a decline in bone mass of 15 percent is possible. The rate appears to remain relatively constant, usually not giving rise to significant problems until men are in their eighties. A mechanism for retarding osteoporosis, or eliminating it as a serious threat to wellness altogether, is suggested later in this chapter.

## Sensory Changes

Aging brings about significant change in sensory mechanisms, such as hearing, visual acuity, taste, and smell.[18] These alterations sometimes require special early diagnostic, adaptive, or corrective lifestyle steps.

Virtually everyone experiences some degree of hearing impairment by age seventy. Neurological and mechanical changes make discrimination of soft and high-pitched sounds difficult. Increases in the time required to process sounds neurologically necessitates that elderly persons be addressed more slowly, rather than more loudly. Background noise may be particularly distracting to older persons, because it interferes with receiving and processing conversation. Anyone who has been in a room full of people talking and who has tried to focus on hearing a particular conversation, can appreciate the dilemma experienced by the elderly person.

Loss of visual acuity is one of several sight-related changes that occur. Problems with acuity arise from the tendency of the eye lenses to yellow and become harder and less elastic with age, giving rise to a condition called **presbyopia.** The magnitude of this change is heightened further by the presence of glare.

Depth perception is also affected by the aging process. Consequently, elderly people must take extra care in climbing or descending stairs. Even crossing the street necessitates extra caution; the elderly individual must gauge the exact height of the curb to avoid an accidental fall.

Modifications that occur with age alter the ability to see clearly at night. **Night recovery vision** is also affected adversely. Anyone, young or old, knows what it is like to be driving an automobile on a highway at night, and suddenly be struck by another vehicle's oncoming headlights. There is a temporary blindness, lasting one to five seconds in most cases. This readjustment period is one's night-glare-recovery interval. Older individuals may require eight to ten seconds for complete recovery. This delay makes operating a motor vehicle at night dangerous and frightening. In addition, decreased depth perception further increases the hazard of night driving.

Cataracts can also interfere with visual ability in the older adult. A cataract is a clouding of the lens that interrupts the focusing of light on the retina, resulting in blurred vision. Anyone who experiences any prolonged visual problem ought to contact a physician who diagnoses and treats eye disorders. Cataracts tend to develop slowly, but become thickened or layered in the process. Unless corrective surgery is performed, vision in the affected eye can become completely occluded.

Another eye disorder that affects many persons in their sixties and seventies (though it can have an earlier life onset) is **glaucoma.** Glaucoma involves an elevation of pressure within the eyeball that produces partial or complete impairment.

Chronic glaucoma is particularly dangerous because it has no particular warning signals until the pressure affects the optic nerve directly. It is a painless and progressive cause of unnecessary blindness. Therefore, it is recommended that persons over the age of forty have early detection check-ups for glaucoma at least every two years. Persons with a family history of glaucoma or a personal history of other eye disorders should probably be screened more frequently.

The last major areas of sensory change affected by age are those of taste and smell. Modifications in one's sense of taste can have profound effects on one's food choices, and may contribute to obesity.[19]

Taste thresholds for sweeteners and table salt are on the average two to two-and-a-half times higher in the elderly than in young people.[20] Compensation for a reduced capacity to taste sweet things can result in excess sugar. An enhanced sugar intake might aggravate an existing chronic condition such as diabetes. Moreover, it can increase caloric intake at a time when one's BMR, and the capacity for and interest in physical activity and exercise, are winding down. In addition, more sugar can increase one's blood triglyceride level, also leading to obesity.

The desire to use more salt to combat food's flat taste (resulting from the sensory losses both of taste and smell) is likely to complicate one's ability to comply with low-sodium diets, which are desirable throughout life, but particularly in old age. Dietary salt can, of course, aggravate hypertension and other conditions. (See chapter 15.)

The smell of food is an important component of appetite. The sense of smell is even more vulnerable to the process of aging than is taste. Olfactory thresholds for some food odors, such as cherry, grape, and lemon are eleven times higher for older people.[21] A decreased sensitivity to food odors can result in a lowered appreciation of certain foods. Older people may complain about the bland appeal of food, and therefore, become less enthusiastic about eating at all. People preparing meals for the elderly need to recognize the possible changes in eating due to modified taste and smell thresholds.

## Changes in the Kidneys

The kidneys are the greatest filtration and selective reabsorption system known. The kidneys filter blood, remove wastes, and reabsorb important nutrients such as glucose.

Several important properties of kidney function may change with age. First, there is a decrease in the overall filtration rate by up to 50 percent. This means that the kidneys filter less blood per unit of time and remove toxic wastes more slowly. Second, there is a decline in blood flow to the kidneys. This decline results in part from the fall in cardiac output and directly affects filtration rate. A third change is reduced reabsorption ability. Therefore, some nutrients pass as waste products instead of being used by the body.

## Changes in Sexual Functioning

Many people believe that both sexual desire and sexual functioning decline significantly after middle age. Although menopause in females and the climacteric in males may affect operation of the sexual organs to some extent, these phenomena do not necessarily influence all the psychological desires for physical closeness and participation in sexual intercourse.

The psychological impact of menopause in women, while real and complex, can be exaggerated. Despite stories about menopausal women becoming tearful, emotional, unpredictable, and uninterested in sex, the majority of research evidence does not support such stereotypes. Most women feel unchanged after menopause.[22] Many women see the cessation of the menstrual cycle as a welcome relief, and report a renewed interest in sexual drive. Some research suggests that a woman's interest in sex following menopause is probably most closely related to her interest in sex earlier in life.[23] Hormonal declines can produce a thinning and drying of the lining of the vagina, sometimes resulting in painful intercourse. However, with the use of an appropriate supplemental lubricant and some patience, there is little reason for age to hinder sexual participation.

There is debate about whether the male climacteric is a biological event or purely a psychological one. It is known that many males undergo a transition period in their lives that may occur anytime between the fourth and seventh decades. This transition, which may affect relationships with a spouse, an employer, or other people, is sometimes referred to as the *mid-life crisis*. While a mid-life crisis is often spoken of as a "male event," it is by no means limited just to men. B. Layton and I. Siegler believe that although important changes do occur in mid-life, crisis is an avoidable outcome.[24] They conclude that susceptibility to a mid-life crisis hinges on three elements: identity, efficacy, and self-evaluation. Identity is determined by how people view themselves in a variety of contexts—on the job, as a member of a family, as a parent, and so on. Efficacy refers to a person's desire to be effective and competent in these same contexts. Self-evaluation is triggered by such events as birthdays and holidays, and causes an individual to reflect on whatever personal successes or failures come immediately to mind. Crisis occurs when a person cannot overcome the loss of efficacy. This can occur when a person is passed over for a promotion, or runs into an old friend who appears as youthful and vigorous as ever, or experiences a loss of sexual potency.

Testosterone production does decrease with age.[25] In conjunction with this event, men may experience a delayed erection time, a reduced ejaculatory volume, and decreased fertility. These changes occur gradually and may go unnoticed. While delayed erection or occasional impotence may be problematic for some men, age also tends to decrease ejaculatory urgency. Thus, while the penis may require a longer time to become erect, intercourse is frequently enjoyed for a longer period.

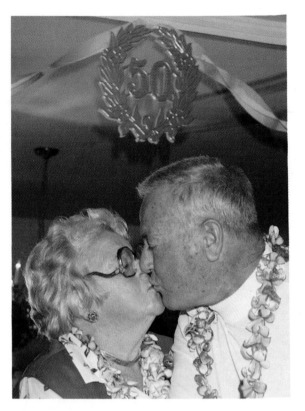


**Figure 20.5**
Sexual desire and the need for physical closeness do not vanish with age.

Robert Butler describes a societal phenomenon called **ageism** which is, in some ways, similar to racism and sexism.[26] Ageists view sexuality among the elderly as an expression of senility or deviance or both. Research by Lionel Corbett showed that the "myth of a sexless old age" prevented married couples residing in some nursing homes from sharing a bedroom or sleeping in anything other than twin beds due to institutional policy.[27] Ageism results in elderly people becoming the butt of tasteless sexual humor. The elderly are portrayed as exhibitionists and "dirty old men" (or women). Evidence shows that in fact society's "dirty old man" is usually in his late twenties.[28] The greatest barrier to successful sexual functioning in old age is probably the extent to which ageism is permitted to be an influence. With the presence of an interesting and interested partner, sexual participation during the seventies, eighties, or nineties can be an important index of good physical and emotional health. (See table 20.2.)

**Table 20.2 Eight Ways of Achieving High-Level Wellness in Late Adulthood**

| | |
|---|---|
| Work and social activity | Maintain aspects of work and social activity that were sources of reward in middle adulthood. |
| Exercise | Can provide physical and psychological benefit as flexibility is increased or maintained. |
| Nutrition | Meals should be balanced and have a social component added if possible. |
| Preventive services | Biannual checkups until age seventy-five and yearly checkups thereafter. Ideally, necessary services should be provided at a single location. |
| Medication | Avoid overmedication. Obtain generic medications where possible and ask physician to review medications on a regular basis. |
| Immunization | Influenza and pneumonia unnecessarily claim the lives of elderly persons each year. Check with your physician about the availability of immunizations. |
| Home safety | Homes should feature ample lighting, nonslip floors, sturdy railings, and fire-detection equipment. |
| Services to maintain independence | Recreational, vocational, and other activities should be available, along with transportation that facilitates access to such activities. |

# THEORIES OF BIOLOGICAL AGING

Many a science-fiction story has focused on humankind's search for the potion that would bring immortality. No one is immortal and growing old is as much a fact of life as being born. What are the mechanisms for biological aging? Why does the body change with age? (See figure 20.6.)

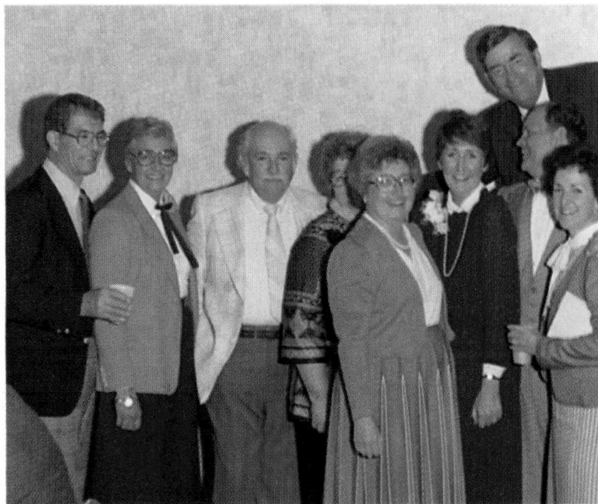

**Figure 20.6**
Biological aging is inevitable, although heredity, nutrition, and disease all influence its course.

There are numerous theories of aging, though no single theory is universally accepted. No one theory about aging seems to be able to explain satisfactorily all of the observations made about growing old. Aging is a complex process influenced by heredity, nutrition, disease, and various other factors. However, some interesting and provocative explanations of the aging process keep scientists engaged in debate.

## Programmed Endpoint Theory

According to this theory each species is born with a finite amount of genetic material (DNA). When cells "use up" the genetic material, they age and die.[29] Observations reported by Leonard Hayflick showed that certain cells taken from human embryos and maintained in culture underwent a finite number of doublings approximately equal to fifty, after which no more cell reproduction took place.[30] This type of limited survival has been demonstrated for the cells of other species, too. Hayflick concludes that the maximum life expectancy for human beings could be as high as 120 years.

### Somatic Mutation Theory

Howard Curtis and Kimball Miller demonstrated that cells of older mice and guinea pigs contained more chromosomal abnormalities than those of younger animals.[31] They concluded that aging was a result of mutated cells created by chromosomal instructions that got "mixed up." Furthermore, they showed that animals exposed to radiation and certain chemical substances contained more abnormal chromosomes than unexposed animals.

### Free-Radical Theory

**Free radicals** are naturally occurring unstable chemical substances; they react easily with other substances with which they come into contact in order to become stable. Found in some body cells, free radicals react with fats and cause cellular damage. Free radicals are believed to cause cell mutations.

### Wear-and-Tear Theory

This theory suggests that cells can only deflect a finite number of environmental insults before becoming unable to repair and replace damaged parts. Nerve cells, cardiac cells, and skeletal muscle cells do not divide at all, hence have no ability to respond indefinitely to accumulated wear and tear.

### Autoimmune Theory

The **immune system** contains specialized cells that fight infection and agents identified by the body as foreign. The autoimmune theory suggests that the ability of the body to distinguish its own cellular material from foreign proteins, such as viruses or bacteria, is reduced over time. Consequently, it is possible for the immune system to become confused, to recognize its own proteins as "foreign," and therefore, to attack itself. If this theory is accurate in describing what happens with age, it is not backed by the supportive evidence necessary to explain how. It is, nevertheless, an intriguing theory, and one likely to be the subject of future research.

## SOCIOLOGICAL PATTERNS OF AGING

Adapting to growing old, and changing social, familial, or vocational roles are common characteristics of aging. There is no single way to age successfully. In fact, research has delineated at least four predominant patterns of successful aging high in life satisfaction. These patterns are labeled disengagement theory, activity theory, continuity theory, and social-reconstruction theory.

### Disengagement Theory

**Disengagement theory** emphasizes the mutual withdrawal by both society and the individual.[32] Society embraces the disengagement process through such actions as age segregation and mandatory retirement. Disengagement may take on other forms as well, such as moving from a private residence to an institutional setting, or parting company with close friends or relatives because of death. Disengagement theory contends that people voluntarily move away from the mainstream to avoid commitments, to let someone else do the work, and to allow more self-investment in their remaining years.

Although disengagement may be satisfying for some people, it is not satisfying for everyone. Forced disengagement may be a source of low life satisfaction, even depression. Critics also contend that disengagement seems to relate more to poor health status, widowhood, decreased income, and retirement than simply to growing older.

### Activity Theory

In contrast to disengagement theory, **activity theory** suggests that older people age successfully by remaining active. Some research supports the notion that a high activity level impacts positively on self-concept, morale, and overall well-being.[33] Activity theory contends that a person's major life-satisfaction roles in middle age as worker, parent, spouse, and so on undergo change because of retirement, widowhood, and decreased influence over children. To age successfully and to avoid low life satisfaction, people busy themselves with new types of activities.

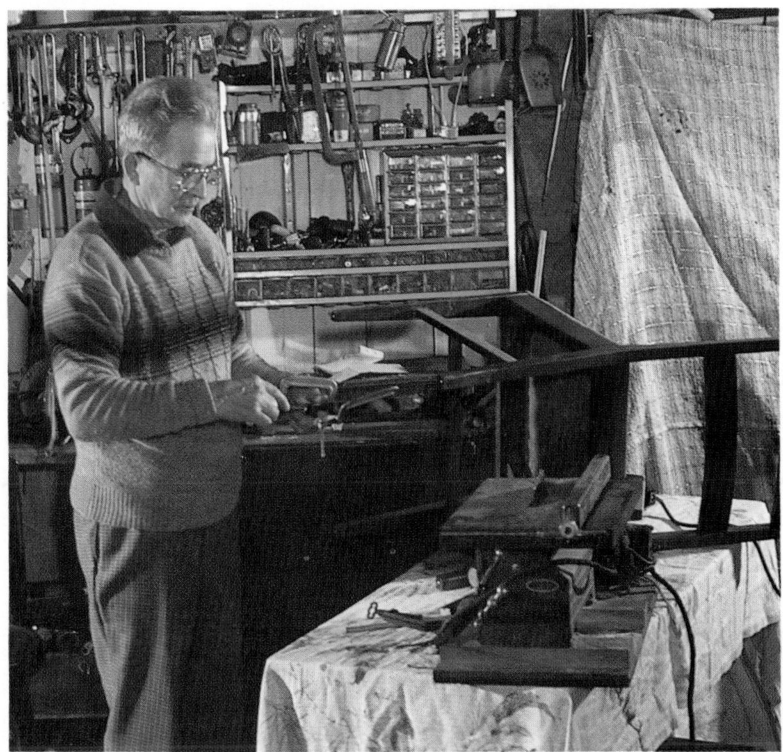

**Figure 20.7**
New activities help the elderly stay involved and age successfully.

A clear relationship between level of activity and level of life satisfaction has not been confirmed. Activity theory may be too simplistic an explanation for the complex aging phenomenon. Not all activities adequately replace the lost roles of middle adulthood and help to maintain self-concept. Unless hobbies, pastimes, and other activities of the older adult represent dominant cultural roles, they probably do not lead to role adjustment and high life satisfaction.[34]

## Continuity Theory

Robert Atchley proposes an alternative theory, the **continuity theory,** in light of the limitations of both the disengagement and activity theories.[35] The continuity theory suggests that successful aging is a result of maintaining certain roles of middle adulthood into old age, while withdrawing from other roles. Proponents contend that the commitments and role preferences that contribute most to satisfaction in middle adulthood also provide the basis for satisfaction in later years.

## Social-Reconstruction Theory

**Social-reconstruction theory** holds that low performance expectations on the part of society contribute to the low self-concept and perceived loss of skills experienced by many elderly people.[36] A self-fulfilling prophecy becomes established when the older adult feels incompetent because of a belief that self-worth is dependent upon a high level of productivity. This theory proposes that successful aging is a function of three things. First, successful adaptation means liberating one's self from the myth of an age-appropriate status. That is, people do not necessarily have to disengage from certain activities because they are seventy, seventy-five, or eighty years old. Second, adaptation depends on one's ability to access social services. Adequate housing, transportation, and medical services are vital components of successful aging. Third, successful aging requires the ability to control one's own life.

20.2 EXHIBIT 20.2

## Peck's Psychological Transitions in Aging

R. C. Peck specifies that an adult's ability to make four transitions is especially critical in the adjustment to growing older.[1] These four transitions are:

1. Valuing wisdom versus valuing physical powers. Being able to make the best out of the choices that life has to offer is more important than, and compensates for, the inevitable loss in physical prowess or beauty that occurs with aging. People who overestimate the importance of the physical attributes of youth may have a more difficult adjustment to aging.

2. Socializing versus sexualizing in human relationships. People who are able to redefine the men and women in their lives, and who learn to value them as individuals, as friends, and as companions, rather than as sex objects, tend to cope better with the process of growing older.

3. Cathectic flexibility versus cathectic impoverishment. People who live longer experience many changes. Relationships break up, careers change, friends and relatives die, and children mature, grow up, and leave home. People who are able to shift their "emotional capital" from one source of gratification to another as change occurs adjust more easily to growing older.

4. Mental flexibility versus mental rigidity. By middle age, and well on into old age, people have determined a personal "credo," or set of answers to the challenges of living. However, if people allow these answers to control them, they become closed and rigid. People who remain flexible and use their experience and wisdom to seek solutions to new challenges and issues tend to maintain high life satisfaction.

[1]R. C. Peck, "Psychological Aspects of Aging," in proceedings of a Conference on Planning Research, ed. J. E. Anderson (Washington, D.C.: American Psychological Association, 1956).

### DISCUSSION QUESTIONS

1. Are you adaptable to change?

2. What aspects of your present lifestyle do you consider "untouchable" to change?

## ADAPTATIONS FOR WELLNESS IN OLD AGE

Although everyone experiences some degree of change as a result of aging, these changes do not necessarily have to impact negatively on mental and physical wellness. Appropriate adaptations reduce the negative effects of aging. We will discuss several of these wellness adaptations.

### Adapting to Sensory Change

If corrective sensory devices such as hearing aids and bifocals are affordable to the older adult and can be worn without unnecessary self-consciousness, many hearing or visual deficiencies can be eliminated. Other supplemental aids are also available. For instance, the hearing-impaired older adult can learn to read lips and visually impaired individuals can develop an ability to respond to auditory and other environmental cues.

20.2 ACTIVITY FOR WELLNESS 20.2

## Some Life Habits Related to Health Status in Middle and Later Adulthood

Belloc and Breslow (1972) found that fifty-five-year-old men who practiced the following health behaviors functioned as well or were as "healthy" as thirty-five-year-old men who practiced none of them.* Compare your daily routines with the recommendations shown below. Place a check next to those activities you now practice which will help you achieve a wellness lifestyle into old age.

[ ] 1. Eating breakfast
[ ] 2. Eating regular meals and not snacking
[ ] 3. Eating moderately to maintain normal weight
[ ] 4. Not smoking
[ ] 5. Drinking alcohol moderately or not at all
[ ] 6. Exercising moderately
[ ] 7. Sleeping regularly 7–8 hours a night

*Nedra B. Belloc and Lester Breslow, "Relationship of Physical Health Status and Health Practices," *Preventive Medicine* 1.3 (1972): 409–21.

A decline in sensory functioning can inhibit other activities such as exercise. Because of visual impairment, a person may not possess the confidence to begin walking or initiate other forms of exercise. In addition, an inability to detect street and traffic noise can undermine one's security about embarking on walks alone. Visual impairment can even interfere with mobility in the home. Seeing stairs, detecting irregularities in carpeting or floor rugs, or locating houseware items can become frustrating chores.

Sensory obstacles can be overcome through common sense and some advance planning.[37] Excess or unnecessary furniture can be removed. Furniture can be arranged to allow optimal mobility. Dishes, silverware, and other household items can be strategically placed for easy access. Practical placement of lamps can help to assure proper room lighting.

To increase confidence outdoors, the elderly can identify routes of easy and safe access to desired destinations. The ability to see clearly and avoid undue threats in the daylight can be enhanced by simply wearing sunglasses or other corrective lenses that minimize glare.

People whose senses of smell and taste have decreased may show diminished appetites. At meals, large portions of food may intimidate more than stimulate their appetite. Substituting small, lightly seasoned portions of food may help elderly people enjoy mealtime. The most important ingredient may be friendly companionship. (See Activity for Wellness 20.2.)

## Adapting to Biological Change

As indicated previously, some degree of functional change is inevitable as we age. The *Euro-American Curve* (figure 20.2) shows that functional decline can be retarded if physical activity is maintained. Not all changes can be reversed, but many can be modified. As much as 50 percent of the functional decline seen in the aging population results from lack of use rather than aging.[38] Much of that lost vitality can be maintained into the eighth decade of life through vigorous activity.

Research supports the contention that loss of cardiovascular function need not be an automatic consequence of growing older.[39] In a ten-year study, participants in an experimental exercise program did not show the 1 percent annual decline that was seen in a sedentary control group. The benefits of exercise in promoting oxygen utilization and overall cardiovascular fitness in the elderly have also been shown.[40] Physical activity can moderate both systolic and diastolic blood pressure in older adults.[41] The most significant outcome of improved cardiovascular fitness may be the performance of routine daily activity with greater ease.

Physical activity may also restore or maintain functions of muscles and joints.[42] Loss of flexibility and range of motion of muscles and joints may be consequences of discontinued use, and not functions of aging.

Osteoporosis, the process of bone demineralization, may also be affected by the level of physical activity. A study of male tennis players (mean age 63.8) showed that bone-mineral content of the playing arm was 13 percent more than that of the nonplaying arm.[43] Exercise was also shown to increase total body calcium in postmenopausal women, a group at high risk for osteoporosis.[44] In a nursing-home study, mild exercise significantly increased bone mineral among participants, while sedentary residents lost bone mineral at the expected rate.[45] Thus, it appears as if physical activity retards the loss of bone mass, helping one maintain both physical and social activity.

Much of the reluctance of older people to exercise is based upon the myth that even moderate activity is destructive. Unless a person has advanced physical disabilities that are multiple in nature, some form of beneficial physical exercise is available to them. It is not recommended that a person with chronic low back pain take to jogging on hard surfaces. However, the same person can achieve physical improvement by taking up a regular program of walking or stationary cycling. Classes for older people offer a wide range of health improvement activities from yoga to swimming. Dancing is recognized as an ideal activity because of its physical as well as social component. (See figure 20.8.)

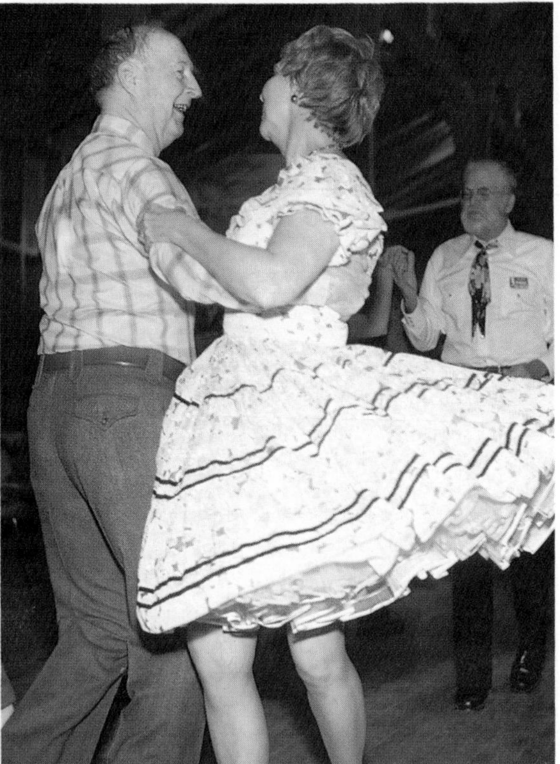

**Figure 20.8**
Dancing is an ideal activity and social outlet for the elderly.

## Adapting to Cognitive Changes

Most older adults who experience **senility,** also called *dementia* (i.e., loss of memory, attentiveness, and other cognitive functions), do so for one of two reasons. First, they may experience a series of small strokes or infarcts, resulting from insufficient oxygen to the brain. When an infarct occurs, the region of the brain having the oxygen deficit ceases to function properly. Multiple small infarcts, or "mini-strokes," can give rise to the array of symptoms identified with senility. A second cause of senility comes from an irreversible degeneration of brain tissue known as **Alzheimer's disease.** This devastating disease may affect as many as three million Americans over the age of 65.[46] A detailed discussion of Alzheimer's disease is provided in Exhibit 20.3.

20.3 EXHIBIT 20.3

## Alzheimer's Disease and Mental Infirmity

In 1906, a German neurologist by the name of Alois Alzheimer examined the brain tissue of a patient who showed many of the symptoms associated with senility—loss of memory, hallucinations, and periodic disorientation. This examination revealed the existence of twisted nerve cell fibers in many small clumps. These abnormal nerve-cell fibers provided the physical evidence of the degenerative brain disorder that is now referred to as "Alzheimer's disease."

It has been said of Alzheimer's disease that it kills its victims twice—the mind first, the body later on. For the person with this disorder, names, dates, and places become lost in the recesses of the mind. Simple tasks such as dressing, eating, and engaging in conversation become impossible. The onset of symptoms is slow, occurring usually over a period of from six to eight years, but sometimes developing over twenty years or more. Though Alzheimer's is common among persons in their sixties, it can also strike individuals who are in their forties. Victims of advanced disease may have little touch with reality, and fade slowly into a coma to await death. Alzheimer's claims 120,000 lives a year, ranking it fourth as a leading cause of death in the elderly, behind heart disease, cancer, and stroke.

Alzheimer's disease may be even more devastating for its victims' families. Family members must often stand by helplessly as a loved one becomes a virtual mindless stranger. Alzheimer victims seem to do best in a highly structured environment that reminds them of familiar people and objects. The type of custodial care necessary may be available only in specialized facilities or nursing homes. However, the cost of such care ($20,000 per year or more) is prohibitive for most families, and is not usually paid for by private insurance companies or by Medicare.

The cause of Alzheimer's disease is not known. Theories have been advanced, however, which help to explain small pieces of the Alzheimer puzzle. There is evidence that a child of a parent with Alzheimer's has a 50 percent chance of developing the disease too, suggesting a genetic explanation. An explanation of early symptoms of Alzheimer's comes from research that reveals a blockage in the hippocampus, an area of the brain that processes new information. A different hypothesis proposes that the cause is related to a reduction in RNA and protein synthesis in the brain. Still another theory suggests that slow-acting viruses are responsible for the symptoms associated with Alzheimer's.

The suprisingly large number of cases of senility (52 to 66 percent) accounted for by Alzheimer's will most certainly keep it in the spotlight for some time to come. The Alzheimer's Disease and Related Disorders Association (ADRDA) is doing much to educate the public and provide information and comfort for the families of Alzheimer victims.



### DISCUSSION QUESTIONS

1. Should private insurance companies or Medicare cover the costs incurred by a victim of Alzheimer's disease?

2. Should research on the cause, prevention, and cure of Alzheimer's disease be a focus of government spending in the health-care area in the foreseeable future?

There are other causes of senility, as well. About one older adult in five who suffers from memory loss or other indicators of senility does so because of factors that can be modified. The underlying cause of the problem may be related to medications or combinations of drugs that the person takes for another health problem.

Other health-related conditions such as nutritional deficiencies, alcoholism, or changes in endocrine functions may bring about symptoms attributed to senility, simply because they occur in an older person. Persons with failing memories and declining cognitive abilities should be given a thorough physical examination to identify the source of the problem and to learn if corrective procedures are possible.

Some cognitive changes in older adults may be compensated for simply by restructuring tasks.[47] If short-term memory loss is a problem, a practical solution is the creation of aids such as lists, self-directed notes, special (mnemonic) memory devices, and other techniques. Louis G., a man in his late sixties with arteriosclerosis and transient ischemic attacks (temporary reduction in oxygen to the brain), remembers important things he must do each day by repeating them out loud at various intervals. He also keeps lists in his automobile, on the kitchen table, and in his wallet. Harry G., age eighty-nine, places notes on the front door reminding him to turn out lights, shut off the stove, lock all doors, and take his keys when leaving the house. If these practices seem somewhat silly, they nevertheless help make up for sensory and cognitive deprivation. As Susan Whitbourne and David Sperbeck conclude: "Imagination and creative solutions are most likely to come from the individual who must deal with the problem."[48]

Managing stress that results from ongoing adaptation to chronic illness or from the death of friends and relatives requires considerable skill. Unfortunately, not everyone copes with stress in positive ways. Some adopt a fatalistic attitude that stress and misfortune are parts of growing old. For these people, stress may produce physical illness or chronic depression. Coping with an agonizing condition like arthritis can produce changes in mood, personality, and quality of life. Means of managing stress are similar to methods used at other times of life.[49] Transcendental meditation, biofeedback, and relaxation exercises, while foreign to most people at first, can provide stress relief. The elderly may also find relief through prayer and other spiritual measures. The stress that comes from having to get along on limited resources may be reduced through participation in support groups, such as those found in community senior centers.

# PERSONAL AND SOCIAL ISSUES RELATED TO WELLNESS

Most people, regardless of age, hope for good health and a comfortable life-style. However, these basic needs are not always easily fulfilled for some older adults. Achieving wellness is thwarted by a host of social, economic, and political forces.

## Health Care

The rising cost of health care is a clear impediment to wellness in the older adult. Health-care costs strike the elderly disproportionately. People sixty-five and over comprise just 11 percent of the population, but account for 22 percent of physicians' charges, 28 percent of hospital costs, and 84 percent of nursing-home costs.[50]

These health-care costs come at a time when many people are living on diminished or fixed incomes and can least afford added expenses. To further complicate the road to wellness, financial burdens make the older person more vulnerable to quackery, fraudulent insurance schemes, and other gimmicks. Economically disadvantaged elderly people are likely to reap fewer benefits from federal government programs such as Medicare due to inadequate access to, and information regarding, the system.[51]

## Personal Barriers

Inadequate nutrition can constitute a major barrier to wellness for a variety of reasons. People's ability to chew, swallow, and digest food can limit what they can eat. Diminished senses of taste and smell can cause a loss of interest in eating. The inability to taste salt or sugar can also encourage an excessive use of sweeteners and sodium at a time in life when the body is least able to tolerate it.

Another physical barrier to adequate nutrition is irregular bowel movements. Some people try to regulate themselves by consuming large quantities of mineral oil or other laxatives. This practice can deplete the body's stores of fat-soluble vitamins, upset the electrolyte balance, and lead to dehydration and states of confusion, disorientation, and weakness.[52] A better way to assist regularity is to include high-fiber foods, like fresh fruits and vegetables, whole grains, and specially fortified cereals, in the diet. These dietary measures add bulk to the stool, and promote retention of water in the intestines, thereby softening the stool and speeding up the full digestive cycle. American culture traditionally has not stressed eating these types of foods, making dietary adjustments difficult for some people.

Problems in obtaining and preparing food also create nutritional barriers for the elderly. The cost of food places a limit on what can be purchased. In some cases, this may actually serve a desirable purpose in that fattening or expensive low-nutrition-density items may not be affordable. However, a small budget usually means having to omit important food items. Immobility or lack of transportation can also affect food purchases. If transportation to a store is only sporadic, purchased items may consist primarily of nonperishable canned goods. This could lead to a diet low in fresh fruits and vegetables, meat, and dairy products.

There is a common misbelief that milk products are only for children and youth. People, in fact, never outgrow their need for milk. The reluctance to use milk products in middle and later adult life may lead to a diminished calcium level and contribute to the osteoporotic process. Low-fat or skim milk provides valuable vitamins and minerals throughout the life span, but with fewer calories and less fat than whole milk.

## Family Barriers

Jean Miller points out that family structures can interfere with wellness in the elderly.[53] One structure is the disengaged family. In this structure family members are so independent that they neither request support from nor respond to the needs of other family members. At the opposite extreme is the enmeshed family, where there is such a strong sense of belonging that persons may lose autonomy or individuality. Although elderly people in the enmeshed group are likely to have their physical needs met, it is often at the expense of their feelings of self-worth.

Two forces that can be destructive to the familial relationship of older people are **parentification** and **infantilization.**[54] In parentification, adult children regress to childlike states when in the presence of their elderly parents, and are unable to make decisions without parental consultation and approval. While not particularly destructive to the elder parents, it does usurp the role of the adult child's spouse. Infantilization is the converse of parentification. Infantilization is role reversal where adult children act in the parent role and strip their elders of independence and self-responsibility for maintenance. As Miller indicates: "Such behavior encourages parents to become dependent and to act as children to their children."[55] The identities of adult children and their parents may both be compromised by this practice.

## Environmental Barriers

Affordable housing is a major environmental issue for the elderly. Houses in most locations require winter heating and summer air conditioning. Energy costs are particularly difficult burdens for older Americans. While there is a tendency, perhaps, to want to move elderly persons into specialized housing projects, many people resist such change. They often achieve more peace of mind in familiar surroundings and in neighborhoods where they feel secure from crime.

Transportation is also a special environmental consideration for the older adult. The elderly depend on adequate transportation for social, recreational, and spiritual activities, as well as for shopping and access to medical care. Community planners must consider three things.[56] First, transportation must be available as well as economical. Inexpensive mass transit is critical for people who do not own or cannot drive automobiles or who cannot afford taxi fares. Second, transportation must be safe.

In urban areas, mass transit is often a vehicle for crime. Older people feel too vulnerable to risk using this type of transportation. In rural areas, inexpensive public transportation may be too far away to be of much practical help. Third, transportation must go where elderly persons are likely to travel. The lack of adequate transportation can be a major reason that people disengage despite wishes to the contrary.

## A LAST WORD ABOUT AGING

Though threats to well-being are present throughout the life cycle, those which confront people in late adulthood are especially challenging. Donna Aguilera[57] summarizes four adaptive needs of the elderly:(1) loss in position, occupation, or activity; (2) loss of family or ties to family;(3) loss of health and vitality; and,(4) loss of purpose or meaning in life. Since the emergence of a growing aged population is only a recent phenomenon, we are still learning how to meet these challenges. As older Americans define their roles and social positions, they hopefully will be provided with the resources, both personal and public, that can facilitate the transition from wellness in early and middle life to wellness in old age. (See table 20.2.)

## SUMMARY

1. Aging is the process of change through time, and has biological, sociological, and psychological implications.

2. Life expectancy today is greater than ever before; 20 percent of the U.S. population may be over age sixty-five by the year 2030.

3. Myths about old people abound today—that they are institutionalized and sickly, have nothing left to contribute, are rigid in their ways and reactionary in their politics.

4. The biological aging process is related in part to chronology, but also to lost functional ability due to disuse. People who remain active throughout life retain much of the function that is lost in the sedentary population.

5. The aging process involves specific biologic alterations. Cardiac output declines, pulmonary function decreases, basal metabolic rate declines, body fat increases, muscle mass and strength decrease, bone mineral is lost, hearing ability is lost in some ranges of sound, visual acuity and night vision become decreased, and kidney efficiency is reduced. Though some changes in sexual functioning occur, sexual participation can last well into the seventies, eighties, and nineties.

6. Numerous theories to explain biologic aging have been advanced. The most prominent among these include theories of programmed endpoints, somatic mutations, free radicals, autoimmune reactions, and just plain wear and tear.

7. Several sociological theories have been advanced to explain adaptation to growing older. Among these are theories of disengagement, activity, continuity, and social reconstruction.

8. The negative effects associated with aging can be minimized by undertaking a series of life-style adaptations associated with cognitive changes, sensory changes, and other biological changes.

9. Alzheimer's disease is the fourth leading cause of death in the elderly, and is responsible for many of the cases of senility that are presently recognized. This devastating disorder also has an adverse effect on the families of its victims.

10. Numerous cultural barriers to successful adaptations to aging exist. Overcoming these barriers presents a formidable challenge for the future.

11. "Ageism" is a particularly significant threat to wellness.

12. Aging can be a time for experiencing high levels of wellness. Older people, however, must have access to the resources which help facilitate the transition from early and middle life wellness to wellness in old age.

## Recommended Readings

Allsen, P. E., Harrison, J. M., and Vance, B. *Fitness for Life: An Individualized Approach,* 2d ed. Dubuque, Iowa: William C. Brown, Publishers, 1980.

Barash, D. P. *Aging: An Exploration.* Seattle, Wash.: Univ. of Washington Press, 1983.

Browne, W. P., Olson, L. K. *Aging and Public Policy: The Politics of Growing Old in America.* Westport, Conn.: Greenwood Press, 1983.

Oberleder, M. *Avoiding the Aging Trap.* Washington, D.C.: Acropolis Books, 1982.

Schwartz, A. N. *Survival Handbook for Children of Aging Parents.* Chicago: Follett, 1977.

## References

1. Phillip Elliot Slater, *The Pursuit of Loneliness* (Boston: Beacon Press, 1970).

2. Erdman Palmore, "The Facts of Aging Quiz: A Review of Findings," *The Gerontologist* (1980): 671.

3. Everett L. Smith, Jr., "Age: The Interaction of Nature and Nurture," in *Exercise and Aging: The Scientific Basis,* ed. Everett L. Smith , Jr. and R. C. Serfass (Hillside, NJ: Enslow Publishers, 1981).

4. V. Korenchevsky, *Physiological and Pathological Aging* (New York: Hafner, 1961).

5. Nathan W. Shock, "The Physiology of Aging," *Scientific American* 206 (1962): 100.

6. R. Harris, "Long-Term Studies of Blood Pressure Recorded Annually, with Implications for the Factors Underlying Essential Hypertension," *Transaction Association of Life Insurance Medical Directors of America* 51 (1968): 30.

7. Shock, "The Physiology of Aging," 100.

8. S. P. Tzankoff, and A. H. Norris, "Effect of Muscle Mass Decrease on Age-Related BMR Changes," *Journal of Applied Physiology* 43 (1977): 1001–1006.

9. Tzankoff and Norris, "Effect of Muscle Mass Decrease on Age-Related BMR Changes," 1001.

10. M. J. Yiengst, C. H. Barrows, and N. W. Schock, "Age Changes in the Chemical Composition of Muscle and Liver in the Rat," *Journal of Gerontology* 14 (1959): 400–404.

11. Lars Larsson, Gunnar Grimby, and Jan Karlsson, "Muscle Strength and Speed of Movement in Relation to Age and Muscle Morphology," *Journal of Applied Physiology* 46 (1979): 451–56.

12. W. E. Burke, W. W. Tuttle, C. W. Thompson, et al., "The Relation of Grip Strength and Grip Strength Endurance to Age," *Journal of Applied Physiology* 5 (1953): 629–30.

13. Kathleen M. Munns, "Effects of Exercise on the Range of Joint Motion," in *Exercise and Aging: The Scientific Basis,* eds. Everett L. Smith, Jr. and R. C. Serfass (Hillside, N.J.: Enslow Publishers, 1981).

14. Everett L. Smith, Jr., "Bone Changes in the Exercising Older Adult," in *Exercise and Aging: The Scientific Basis,* eds. Everett L. Smith, Jr. and R. C. Serfass (Hillside, N.J.: Enslow Publishers, 1981).

15. Smith, "Bone Changes in the Exercising Older Adult."

16. Smith, "Bone Changes in the Exercising Older Adult."

17. R. B. Mazess, "Measurement of Skeletal Status by Noninvasive Methods," *Calcified Tissue International* 28 (1979): 89–92.

18. Susan S. Schiffman, "Taste and Smell in Disease II," *New England Journal of Medicine* 308 (1983): 1,337–42.

19. Schiffman, "Taste and Smell in Disease II," 1,338.

20. Schiffman, "Taste and Smell in Disease II," 1,338.

21. Schiffman, "Taste and Smell in Disease II," 1,338.

22. Bernice L. Neugarten, Vivian Wood, Ruth Kraines, and Barbara Loomis, "Women's Attitude toward the Menopause," *Vita Humana* 6 (1963): 140–151.

23. Gloria A. Bachman and Sylvia R. Leiblum, "Sexual Expression in Menopausal Women," *Medical Aspects of Human Sexuality* 15.10 (1981): 96B–96H.

24. B. Layton and I. Siegler, "Mid-Life: Must It Be a Crisis? " paper presented at the annual meeting of the Gerontological Society (Dallas, Tex: 1978).

25. A. Vermeulen, L. Verdonck, and F. Comhaire, "Rhythms of the Male Hypothalamo-Pituitary-Testicular Axis," in Ferim M., Halberg F., Richart R. M., Vande Wiele R. L. (Eds.) *Biorhythms and Human Reproduction,* New York: Wiley, 1974.

26. Robert N. Butler, "Ageism: Another Form of Bigotry," *The Gerontologist* 9 (1969): 243–45.

27. Lionel Corbett, "The Last Sexual Taboo: Sex in Old Age," *Medical Aspects of Human Sexuality* 15.4 (1981): 117–31.

28. P. Gebhard, W. Pomeroy, C. Christenson, and J. Gagnon, *Sex Offenders: An Analysis of Types* (New York: Harper & Row, 1965).

29. Leonard Hayflick, "The Strategy of Senescence," *The Gerontologist* 14 (1974): 37–45.

30. Hayflick, "The Strategy of Senescence," 37–45.

31. Howard J. Curtis, and Kimball Miller, "Chromosome Aberrations in Liver Cells of Guinea Pigs," *Journal of Gerontology* 26 (1971): 292–94.

32. Elaine Cumming and William E. Henry, *Growing Old* (New York: Basic Books, 1961).

33. R. J. Havighurst, B. L. Neugarten, and S. S. Tobin, "Disengagement and Patterns of Aging," in *Middle Age and Aging,* ed. B. L. Neugarten (Chicago: Univ. of Chicago Press, 1968); G. L. Maddox, "Themes and Issues in Sociological Theories of Human Aging," *Human Development* 13 (1970): 17–27.

34. J. F. Gubrium, *The Myth of the Golden Years: A Socio-Environmental Theory of Aging* (Springfield, Ill.: Charles C. Thomas, Publisher, 1973).

35. Robert C. Atchley, *The Social Forces in Later Life: An Introduction to the Social Gerontology* (Belmont, Calif: Wadsworth, 1972).

36. J. A. Kuypers and V. L. Bengston, "Social Breakdown and Competence: A Model of Normal Aging," *Human Development* 16 (1973): 181.

37. Susan Kraus Whitbourne and David J. Sperbeck, "Health Care Maintenance for the Elderly," *Family and Community Health* 3.4 (1981): 11–27.

38. Herbert A. deVries, "Physiological Effects of an Exercise Training Regimen Upon Men Aged 52–58," *Journal of Gerontology* 25 (1970): 325–36.

39. Fred W. Kasch and Janet P. Wallace, "Physiological Variables during 10 Years of Endurance Exercise," *Medicine and Science in Sports and Exercise* 8 (1976): 5–8.

40. K. H. Sidney, and Roy J. Shephard, "Frequency and Intensity of Exercise Training for Elderly Subjects," *Medicine and Science in Sports and Exercise* 10 (1978): 125–31.

41. deVries, "Physiological Effects of an Exercise Training Regimen Upon Men Aged 52–58," 325.

42. Elizabeth A. Chapman, Herbert A. deVries, and Robert Swezey, "Joint Stiffness: Effects of Exercise on Young and Old Men, *Journal of Gerontology* 27 (1972): 218–21.

43. H. J. Montoye, E. L. Smith, D. F. Fardon, and E. T. Howley, "Bone Mineral in Senior Tennis Players," *Scandinavian Journal of Sports Science* 2 (1980): 26–32.

44. John F. Aloia, Stanton H. Cohn, John A. Ostuni, et al., "Prevention of Involutional Bone Loss by Exercise," *Annals of Internal Medicine* 39 (1978): 443–50.

45. Everett L. Smith, Jr., William Reddan, and Partricia E. Smith, "Physical Activity and Calcium Modalities for Bone Mineral Increase in Aged Women," *Medicine and Science in Sports and Exercise* 13 (1981): 60–64.

46. "A Slow Death of the Mind," *Newsweek,* December 3, 1984, 56–62.

47. Whitbourne and Sperbeck, "Health Care Maintenance for the Elderly," 11–27.

48. Whitbourne and Sperbeck, "Health Care Maintenance for the Elderly," 11–27.

49. P. J. Heiple, "Health Care for Older Women: Toward a More Humanistic Approach," *Family and Community Health* 3.4 (1981): 51–59.

50. Robert M. Gibson and Charles R. Fisher, "Age Differences in Health Care Spending, Fiscal Year 1977," *Social Security Bulletin* 42 (January 1979): 3–16.

51. Karen Davis, *National Health Insurance: Benefits, Costs, and Consequences* (Washington, DC: Brookings Institution, 1975).

52. Helen Swift Mitchell, Henderika J. Rynbergen, L. Anderson, and M. Dibble, *Nutrition in Health and Disease* (Philadelphia: J.B. Lippincott Co., 1976).

53. Jean R. Miller, "Family Support of the Elderly," *Family and Community Health* 3.4 (1981): 51–59.

54. S. Minuchin, *Families and Family Therapy* (Cambridge, Mass.: Harvard University Press, 1974), 53.

55. Miller, "Family Support of the Elderly," 42.

56. Donna C. Aguilera, "Stressors in Late Adulthood," *Family and Community Health* 2.4 (1980): 61–69.

57. Aguilera, "Stressors in Late Adulthood," 61–69.

# Glossary

**acupuncture**
An ancient Chinese healing art whereby fine needles are inserted at specific points on the body in order to restore health.

**activity theory**
A view of aging that sees high life satisfaction in the elderly as a consequence of developing new and rewarding activities.

**aerobic exercise**
Activities that cause a sustained increase in heart rate and use the large muscles of the body continuously for an extended period of time.

**affirmations**
A statement of belief or desired outcome. Making affirmations is a technique used to enhance mental health.

**afterbirth**
Comprises the placenta and fetal membranes that are expelled from the uterus following the birth of the child.

**ageism**
A systematic way of regarding the elderly with contempt, ignoring contributions they can make, or engaging in practices that exclude them from access to certain rights and privileges.

**alarm stage**
The first stage of the General Adaptation Syndrome, during which the body awakens to a stressor and gears up to deal with it. Typical signs and symptoms include muscle tension, a pounding heart, butterflies in the stomach, and the like.

**alcohol**
Beverge produced by fermentation of natural sugars that have intoxication properties.

**alcohol-related disability**
Refers to an impairment in the physical, mental, or social functioning of an individual when that impairment can be shown to be related to alcohol consumption.

**allopath**
The term applied to a person who practices allopathic medicine, which involves treating disease with medications and surgery. Physicians awarded the M.D. degree in the U.S. are considered allopaths.

**altruistic love**
The unselfish concern for the welfare of another person. The altruistic lover does not expect anything in return from the person he or she loves.

**alveoli**
Compartmentalized air sacs in the lungs that exchange oxygen and carbon dioxide during normal breathing.

**Alzheimer's disease**
A chronic condition physically characterized by structural modifications in the brain's nerve fibers, and giving rise to mental infirmity, which is behaviorally manifested by memory loss, hallucinations, and social disorientation.

**amniocentesis**
The testing of amniotic fluid in order to discover genetic disorders in the developing fetus.

**anaerobic exercise**
Activities requiring an intense, maximum burst of energy, and which are done for short time intervals (ten to ninety seconds).

**analgesic**
A drug that relieves pain. Such pain relief may be accomplished by both external or internal administration of analgesics.

**androgynous people**
People who adopt both traditional male and female behavior in expressing their own sexuality.

**aneurysm**
A "ballooning" or outpocketing of an artery resulting from a diseased and weakened arterial wall.

**angina pectoris**
Severe chest pain that results from decreased oxygen flow to the heart.

**anterotic love**
Love in which the lover expects the person he or she loves to reciprocate his or her love.

**anticoagulant**
A substance that impedes blood clot formation.

**apgar score**
A checklist of a newborn infant's health status taken one or more times soon after childbirth.

**arteriosclerosis**
A chronic and progressive disorder whereby the walls of the arteries thicken, harden, and lose their elasticity.

**atherosclerosis**
A particular type of arteriosclerosis whereby the walls of the arteries become deposited with fats and other substances, forming plaques.

**bait and switch**
A sales tactic whereby the retailer lures a customer into a store with a special advertised offer, and then substitutes a different, and usually more costly, product.

**bargaining and bidding**
A tactic whereby the consumer makes the retailer an offer at less than "sticker price," resulting in "haggling" until an acceptable price is agreed on.

**basal metabolic rate (BMR)**
The energy required to maintain basic life functions such as heart rate, digestion, and breathing for a person at rest.

**behavior modification**
A set of techniques used by psychologists to help facilitate behavior changes through a process of describing the behavior to be changed, replacing and controlling established behaviors, and reinforcing or rewarding successful changes.

**birthing clinic**
A medical facility that specializes in childbirth using a "non-hospital" atmosphere and environment.

**blood alcohol concentration**
This is a measure of the amount of alcohol found in the blood of an alcohol user.

**brand loyalty**
A sales tactic whereby the retailer attempts to convince a potential customer to buy a familiar brand name that may be more costly, but no more effective, than a less expensive or less known brand.

**calorie**
A unit of measure of the amount of energy derived from food.

**candidiasis**
A fungal infection not always caused by sexual contact, but with potential for being transmitted by sexual means.

**carbohydrates**
A nutrient composed of carbon, hydrogen, and oxygen, and which is the body's preferred form of energy, supplying four calories per gram.

**carcinogen**
An agent that has the potential to cause cancer.

**carcinogenic**
A substance capable of causing cancer.

**carcinoma**
A cancer that arises from epithelial tissues that line organs.

**cardiorespiratory endurance**
The ability of the circulatory and respiratory systems to supply the necessary oxygen for sustained strenuous activity.

**cesarean section**
The surgical opening of the abdomen and uterus for childbirth.

**chancre**
The self-limiting sore or lesion that characterizes the primary stage of syphilis.

**chewing tobacco**
A preparation of tobacco leaves mixed with flavoring agents.

**cholesterol**
A fatty substance found in animal products and manufactured by the body. Its presence in high amounts is associated with an elevated risk of cardiovascular disease.

**co-carcinogen**
A substance capable of causing cancer only when it is in the presence of another specific substance.

**cohabitation**
Describes a living arrangement in which two people who are not married to each other share both bed and board.

**colostrum**
A substance secreted by the breasts prior to milk production. Colostrum contains several antibodies that protect newborns from illness, allergies, respiratory diseases, and diarrhea.

**complete protein**
Any food containing all eight of the essential amino acids.

**complex carbohydrate**
A form of carbohydrate consisting of three or more simple-sugar molecules bonded together in varying patterns. Common complex carbohydrates include starch, fiber, and glycogen.

**constructive self-talk**
A personality-engineering strategy that requires people to speak pleasantly to themselves, reinforcing the positive aspects of life.

**continuity theory**
A view of aging that sees high life satisfaction in the elderly as a consequence of maintaining the roles that were satisfying in middle adulthood.

**contraindications**
Health conditions in which a particular birth control method represents a serious health risk to the user.

**conservation of energy**
The first law of thermodynamics which states that energy cannot be created or destroyed, but only transformed from one form to another.

**cool down**
Gradually slowing down at the end of an exercise session in order to keep blood from pooling in the lower extremities, and to aid in the removal of waste products which may have built up in muscles during exercise.

**coronary bypass**
A surgical procedure that reroutes the blood supply in a coronary artery around a severe blockage.

**corpus luteum**
The temporary endocrine gland in the ovary that secretes hormones. Its purpose is to prevent menstruation during pregnancy.

**cunnilingus**
The oral stimulation of the female's genitals.

**dietary fiber**
The part of food that is not digested by enzymes in the small intestine. The major forms of dietary fiber include soluble and insoluble fiber.

**disease prevention**
Activities that either stop a disease from occurring, detect the presence of disease at an early stage, or rehabilitate after a disease has occurred.

**disengagement theory**
A view of aging that sees high life satisfaction in the elderly as a consequence of a mutual withdrawal of society and the individual.

**distress**
Intense, prolonged, or unrelenting stressors that can upset one's physical and psychological balance.

**drug**
Any substance, which by its chemical nature, alters the structure or function of a human being.

**drug abuse**
Using a drug in such a way as to greatly increase the hazard or impair the ability of the individual to function in a normal way.

**drug addiction**
A compulsion to use a drug, usually implying both a physical and psychological dependence.

**drug misuse**
Using a drug in situations or quantities that significantly increase the hazard to the individual or others.

**drug use**
Using a drug in such a way as to ensure that the sought-for effects are attained.

**dysmenorrhea**
Painful menstruation.

**dysphoria**
A feeling of discomfort associated with the use of drug substances. Such discomfort may be physical, mental, or emotional.

**early pregnancy test**
A commercially available "kit" that allows a woman to self-administer a urine test to detect the presence of a hormone indicative of pregnancy.

**ecology**
The study of ecosystems.

**ecosystems**
The interactions between a community of living organisms and their natural environment.

**ecotopic pregnancy**
Occurs when an embryo develops outside the uterus. Ectopic pregnancy occurs most frequently in the fallopian tubes.

**effective dose level**
The minimal dose of a drug that is required to produce a specific effect.

**ejaculation**
The expulsion of semen from the urethra, and is usually accompanied by orgasm.

**embryo**
The developing baby is called an embryo for the first eight weeks after fertilization.

**enabling factors**
Skills and resources that help one implement a health promotion plan.

**endometriosis**
A condition in which a piece of the endometrium is attached to reproductive organs adjacent to the uterus. It is a common cause of infertility.

**energy-balance equation**
A theory of obesity causation which suggests that obesity results, over a period of time, from consuming more calories than one expends.

**entropy**
The second law of thermodynamics that specifies the direction in which energy must always be transformed; from usable to unusable, from ordered to disordered, and from available to unavailable.

**Environmental Protection Agency (EPA)**
A federal agency created in 1970 whose major role is to consider and effectively deal with the major environmental problems facing the U.S.

**episiotomy**
The surgical cutting of some tissue between the anal and vaginal openings in order to prevent this tissue from tearing during childbirth.

**ergogenic aids**
Drug substances used for the purpose of giving athletes an added edge in competition. Such use of ergogenic aids is often illegal or ill-advised because of the potential for harm to the athlete.

**essential amino acids**
Eight of the basic nitrogen-containing building blocks of protein which must be consumed preformed from food each day to maintain optimal growth and maintenance of body tissues.

**essential fat**
Fat that is stored in major body organs and tissues and is necessary for normal, healthy functioning of the human body.

**estrogens**
The primary female sex hormones. They stimulate the development of a female physique and reproductive organs. Estrogens also stimulate the female reproductive cycle and maintain the adult female reproductive organs.

**ethyl alcohol**
The type of alcohol that is consumable. Also called grain alcohol.

**euphoria**
A general feeling of wellness or satisfaction associated with the use of certain drugs.

**eustress**
A term coined by Hans Selye to designate desirable stress.

**exchange diet**
A balanced, nutritious diet consisting of lists of food groups that are used for menu planning. Foods in any one group can be substituted or "exchanged" with other foods in the same group, as they contain approximately the same number of calories and the same number of carbohydrates, protein, and fat.

**extended family**
The concept of extended family is one that includes not only parents and children, but other relatives as well. The extended family might include grandparents, aunts, uncles, and cousins. In the extended family, children growing up have many adult role models.

**fat-cell theory**
A theory of obesity causation that suggests that people gain fat cells only during three specified periods of time. As adults, weight gain or loss is a result of expanding or contracting the content of fat cells, rather than adding or subtracting numbers of fat cells.

**fats**
A major nutrient that is the body's second major source of energy (calories), and is a preferred means of storing energy. Fat can supply or store approximately nine calories per gram.

**fellatio**
The oral stimulation of the male's genitals.

**female reproductive cycle**
Its primary function is procreation, gestation, and childbirth.

**fermentation**
Metabolism of grains, with one of its end products being ethyl alcohol.

**fertilization**
The creation of a zygote is called fertilization.

**fetal alcohol syndrome**
A pattern of abnormalities found in the newborns of women who drink heavily during pregnancy. This condition consists of a pattern of specific congenital and behavioral abnormalities.

**fetus**
Eight weeks after fertilization the developing embryo is then called a fetus.

**flexibility**
The ability of specific joints to move through their entire range of motion.

**fully functioning person**
A concept offered by Carl Rogers, indicating that an individual is able to be open to new experiences, live life to its fullest, accept intuition as a legitimate source of information, make rational choices from alternatives, and to engage in creative thought and activity.

**general adaptation syndrome (GAS)**
A predictable response of the body to stress, consisting of the alarm stage, the stage of resistance, and the stage of exhaustion.

**genetic theories of sexuality**
Suggest that sexuality is determined by a person's genetic gender.

**genital herpes**
An STD of growing notoriety, characterized by recurrence in susceptible individuals.

**gestational age**
The length of time of fetal development inside the mother's uterus. It is counted from when the zygote is formed until childbirth.

**glucose**
A form of carbohydrate (simple sugar) that is the major energy-supplying molecule in the body.

**glycogen**
Stored sugar, found mainly in the liver and voluntary skeletal muscles, which can be used as a ready source of energy in emergency situations.

**gonadotropin-releasing hormone (GnRH)**
GnRH is secreted by the hypothalamus and causes the release of two other hormones: luteinizing hormone (LH) and follicle-stimulating hormone (FSH). FSH stimulates the testes to produce sperm and the ovaries to produce eggs. LH stimulates the testes to produce testosterone and the ovaries to produce estrogens.

**gonorrhea**
A classic STD and one of the most frequently encountered communicable diseases, which, if untreated, has the potential for causing sterility.

**halitosis**
Chronic bad breath.

**hallucinations**
Perceptions that have no basis in reality or external stimuli.

**health maintenance organization (HMO)**
A prepaid group health-care plan that offers comprehensive medical services, often in one location.

**health promotion**
Activities geared toward enhancing the quality of life and preventing disease and disability.

**herbal drugs**
Plants that have drug effects and whose use is not generally regulated by law.

**homeopaths**
Persons who practice homeopathy, or the disease treatment systems that employ drugs that produce symptoms similar to the treated disease if given to a healthy person. This system is based on the notion of treating like with like.

**homeostasis**
A normal or balanced state of the body that aids in optimal functioning.

**homosexuals**
People who prefer to engage in sexual activities with persons of their own gender.

**human chorionic gonadotropin (HCG)**
This hormone is released by the implanted embryo. The detection of this hormone is used for several pregnancy tests.

**hydrogenation**
A manufacturing technique whereby hydrogen is added to unsaturated fats, thus making them more saturated (with hydrogen) than they would be naturally.

**hypoallergenic**
A substance shown by scientific tests to produce significantly fewer allergic reactions than competing products used for similar purposes.

**illicit drugs**
Any drug whose sale, purchase, or use is prohibited by law.

**illusion**
A distortion of ordinary perception that results in a misinterpretation of reality.

**implantation**
Occurs when the zygote attaches itself to the uterus. This happens several days after fertilization.

**individual differences**
A principle of fitness that points out that individuals attain the many benefits of physical fitness at varying rates.

**infertile**
A label given to a person or couple who cannot naturally conceive or maintain a pregnancy after attempting for a year or more.

**insulin**
A secretion of the pancreas necessary to convert carbohydrates into energy and sometimes used therapeutically to control diabetes.

**insulin theory**
A theory of obesity causation that suggests that high blood insulin levels can increase fat tissue as well as keep people hungry, thus affecting their ability to lose fat weight.

**interferon**
A substance produced by the body that assists in the immune response.

**intrinsic theories of sexuality**
Suggest that sexual behavior is a result of a person's inner sex drive.

**isopropyl alcohol**
A form of alcohol that is used as a disinfectant. Also called rubbing alcohol, this form is not consumable.

**in vitro fertilization (IVF)**
A procedure in which a mature egg is removed from an ovary, fertilized in a laboratory dish, incubated, and then placed inside the uterus to allow implantation to occur.

**laetrile**
A substance of no proven clinical or therapeutic value used by some cancer patients as a cancer treatment.

**lethal dose level**
The minimum does of a drug that will cause death in the user.

**leukemia**
A cancer that arises from the blood-forming cells of the body.

**life-style factors**
Individual practices and habits that often affect health status and wellness, including nutrition, exercise, drug use, stress management, and the like.

**living will**
A quasi-legal document prepared by an individual usually to inform relatives, physicians, and other concerned parties about the extent to which measures are to be taken to prolong life in the event of accident or serious illness.

**lymphoma**
A cancer that arises from lymph cells.

**macro-stressor**
Maximal-intensity stressors that are usually less common than other stressors in one's life.

**mainstream smoke**
The smoke drawn into the lungs when drawing on a pipe, cigarette, or cigar.

**marker events**
Changes or events specific to developmental stages of growth, as well as to the social and cultural factors influencing them that are intense stressors when experienced.

**masturbation**
Self-stimulation of one's own body for the purpose of sexual pleasure.

**micro-stressor**
Minimal-intensity stressors that are encountered and coped with regularly throughout one's life.

**Medicaid**
A federally sponsored program of health insurance that was established to assist the socioeconomically disadvantaged, and certain others.

**Medicare**
A federally funded program that assists in the payment of health expenses for persons sixty-five years and older who are entitled to Social Security benefits.

**medicated childbirth**
Childbirth in which one or more drugs are used by the mother during delivery.

**melanoma**
A serious type of skin cancer of the pigment-forming cells.

**menarche**
The first female reproductive cycle, and is marked by the female's first menstruation.

**menopause**
The cessation of the female's reproductive cycles.

**menstruation**
The cyclical bleeding that signifies the beginning of the next reproductive cycle.

**metabolism**
The physical and chemical processes of the body that contribute to the growth, maintenance, repair, and breakdown of body tissues, as well as making energy available.

**metastasis**
The spread of a previously localized cancer to new sites in the body, thereby increasing the lethal potential of the disease.

**methyl alcohol**
Also called wood alcohol, this form of alcohol is used in such industrial products as antifreezes and various fuels.

**mid-life crisis**
A psychosocial phenomenon experienced by some persons as they undergo the transition from middle adulthood to late adulthood. It involves questions about identity and self-worth.

**minerals**
Inorganic substances that play a vital role in human metabolism.

**moderate obesity**
A level of obesity (fat excess) that is commonly associated with risk factors such as hypertension, elevated blood cholesterol, and diabetes.

**morbid obesity**
An extreme level of obesity (fat excess) at which death and debilitating diseases, such as coronary artery disease and diabetes, occur at very high rates.

**morbidity rate**
The proportion of a disease in a given geographical area.

**mortality rate**
The proportion of deaths in a given geographical area.

**muscular endurance**
The ability of specific muscles to sustain effort over a long period of time.

**muscular strength**
The maximum amount of force that can be exerted by a muscle in a single effort.

**myocardium**
The muscular layer of the heart wall.

**myotonia**
The tightening of the reproductive organs during sexual stimulation.

**national health insurance**
A federally sponsored insurance plan that would, if enacted, provide health insurance to all U.S. citizens regardless of their ability to pay. Such an insurance plan does not currently exist in the U.S.

**natural childbirth**
Childbirth in which the mother uses no drugs during delivery.

**naturopathy**
A disease treatment system that relies on only natural elements to restore health.

**nicotine**
The active principal of tobacco that acts as a potent central nervous system stimulant.

**nonbiodegradable**
Substances that do not decay and are not absorbed by the environment.

**nuclear family**
The traditional concept of a nuclear family includes both parents and children in an intact unity. However, the extended family was also considered as part of the nuclear family until relatively recent times.

**obesity**
A condition whereby too great a proportion of the body tissue is fat.

**osteopathy**
The treatment of disease by manipulation of the skeleton and muscles, as well as by drugs and surgery.

**osteoporosis**
A condition affecting the elderly, especially elderly women, resulting from a decline in bone mineral content, thus making bones susceptible to fracture.

**ovaries**
The primary female reproductive organs that produce mature eggs and estrogens, the female hormone.

**over-the-counter drugs**
Commercially produced medications that can be purchased without a physician's approval.

**overload**
Exercising the body at a level of activity greater than that to which it is accustomed, as a way to increase physical fitness.

**overweight**
Being over the normal weight for your height; usually determined by weighing oneself on a scale and comparing the result to a standardized height/weight table.

**ovulation**
Occurs when the ovary releases a mature egg.

**PPNG**
Acronym for penicillinase-producing Neisseria gonorrhea, a strain of gonorrhea-causing bacteria that does not respond to treatment with penicillin.

**particulate matter**
Small particles found in the smoke of burning tobacco.

**pediculosis pubis**
Infestation of the pubic hair and pubic region by crab lice.

**peer review organization**
A group mandated by the Tax Equity and Fiscal Responsibility Act of 1982, and charged with monitoring the necessity, appropriateness, and quality of health-care services provided to medicare and medicaid recipients.

**pelvic inflammatory disease (PID)**
A general infection of the female reproductive tract, usually as a complication of an undiagnosed or untreated STD, and having the potential to cause permanent sterility.

**percentage of body fat**
The proportion of one's body tissue that is fat or adipose tissue, usually measured by underwater weighing or skinfold techniques.

**personality engineering strategies**
Techniques that help to reduce the stress response by deliberately modifying some aspect of one's personality.

**physical fitness**
A state of optimal physical functioning involving cardiorespiratory endurance, muscular strength and endurance, and flexibility.

**polydrug use**
The use of a variety of combinations of drugs by a single person.

**premenstrual syndrome (PMS)**
A chronic and cyclic disorder which produces somatic complaints just prior to menstruation. The somatic complaints subside with menstruation.

**prenatal care**
The actions a future mother and her mate take to increase the chances of birthing a healthy baby and reducing the health risks of pregnancy and childbirth for the future mother.

**prescription drugs**
Commercially produced medications that cannot be purchased without a physician's approval.

**primary birth control**
Methods that prevent fertilization.

**product misrepresentation**
A sales tactic whereby the retailer advertises selective information about a product that leads a consumer to make faulty assumptions about the product's worth or effectiveness.

**productive character**
Human ability to use reason and ability to achieve one's potential. The productive character was described by Eric Fromm.

**protein**
A major nutrient composed of carbon, hydrogen, oxygen, and nitrogen, and whose major function is the growth, maintenance, and repair of body tissues.

**psychoactive drug**
Any drug whose effects are principally directed at the mood and/or behavior of the user.

**RDA**
Recommended daily dietary allowance, or the amount of various nutrients, recommended by the Food and Nutrition Board of the National Research Council, considered to be adequate for the maintenance of good nutrition in most healthy persons in the U.S.

**reinforcing factors**
Feedback that either rewards or punishes certain behaviors, thus enhancing or diminishing the likelihood that the behavior will be continued.

**relaxation training**
Techniques taught to people so that they can systematically induce a physiological condition that is almost the complete opposite of the stress response.

**reversibility**
A principle of fitness that stresses that once benefits of regular exercise have been attained, a person must continue the exercise on a regular schedule or he or she will begin to lose the benefits.

**reversibility rates**
Estimate a person's ability to become a biological parent after discontinuing the use of a particular birth-control method.

**sarcoma**
A cancer that arises from connective tissues such as bone and cartilage.

**saturated fats**
A form of fat known as a triglyceride, and which contains fatty acids that are saturated with hydrogen. Saturated fats are usually found in animal sources and are usually solid at room temperature.

**scabies**
Infestation of the pubic hair and pubic region by "itch" mites.

**secondary birth control**
Methods that prevent or end implantation.

**sedative**
Depressant drugs that can, at high doses, produce sleep, but ordinarily are used to produce a calming effect on an individual.

**self-actualization**
A concept popularized by Abraham Maslow, the self-actualized person is one who is able to achieve his or her full potential. Self-actualization sits atop the pinnacle of a series of needs that begin with basic human physiologic needs, the need for security, the need for love and acceptance, and the need for self-esteem.

**self-responsibility**
An active sense of accountability for one's own well-being.

**set**
The total internal environment of an individual at the time a drug is taken. This includes physical, mental, and emotional characteristics.

**set-point theory**
A theory of obesity causation that suggests that fat storage is determined by a thermostatic mechanism in the body that acts to maintain a specific amount of body fat.

**setting**
The total external environment of an individual at the time a drug is taken. This includes the physical environment as well as the social environment.

**sexual intercourse**
The insertion of the penis into the vagina.

**sexuality**
Includes our awareness of and reaction to our own maleness or femaleness and that of everyone with whom we interact.

**sexually transmitted disease (STD)**
Any of a host of diseases that has the potential to be transmitted interpersonally through sexual or other intimate body contact.

**sidestream smoke**
Smoke that rises from burning tobacco into the environment.

**simple sugars**
The basic building blocks of carbohydrate, technically termed monosaccharides, consisting of glucose, fructose, and galactose.

**smokeless tobacco**
A general term referring to tobacco products that are not smoked. The prominent forms of smokeless tobacco are chewing tobacco and snuff.

**snuff**
A powdered tobacco that can be sniffed or placed in the mouth and sucked.

**social norms**
Behaviors expected, exhibited, and rewarded by a given culture.

**social reconstruction theory**
A view of aging that sees high life satisfaction in the elderly as a consequence of avoiding old-age stereotypes and so-called "age-appropriate" behaviors, and staying in control of one's life.

**social theories of sexuality**
Suggest that sexual behavior is a product of social expectations and imitation.

**specificity**
A principle of fitness that indicates that physiological adaptations to activity are specific to the type of activity and overload.

**sphygmomanometer**
A device used to measure blood pressure.

**stage of exhaustion**
The third stage of the General Adaptation Syndrome that occurs after long-continued exposure to a stressor. In this stage, symptoms of stress are experienced, organ systems become less effective and break down, and death can occur.

**stage of resistance**
The second stage of the General Adaptation Syndrome, during which the body adapts to the stressor and attempts to return to a state of homeostasis.

**stimulants**
Substances that excite the central nervous system, the common results of which are increased alertness, rapid reflexes, and a sense of self-confidence.

**storage fat**
Fat that accumulates in adipose or fat cells. Some storage fat is necessary to serve as padding for internal organs and insulation during extreme cold.

**stress**
The body's response to a stimulus or stressor, either pleasant or unpleasant, consisting of a mobilization of bodily resources for adaptation.

**stressor**
The stimulus that elicits the stress response.

**subcutaneous fat**
The storage fat found just beneath the skin.

**sun-protection factor (SPF)**
A rating from 2 (minimum) to 15 (maximum) assigned to tanning and sunscreen products, indicating the relative level of protection from solar radiation.

**surrogate mothers**
Paid or unpaid volunteers who make their reproductive organs available for procreation and pregnancy.

**Sustainable-Earth Society**
A social order based on the cooperation of humans with nature and its laws. In such a society, recycling and reusing matter, decreasing energy consumption, and self-reliant living are stressed.

**synergism**
A multiplier effect when certain drugs are used together.

**syphilis**
One of the classic STDs with congenital potential caused by the spirochete Treponema pallidum, which if untreated, runs a three-stage clinical course over a period of many years.

**tar**
Thick, brown, sticky substance that forms from the particulate matter resulting from burning tobacco.

**target heart rate**
The heart rate a person should aim for when exercising aerobically. Target heart rate is a measure of the intensity of an aerobic exercise.

**testes**
The primary male reproductive organs that produce sperm and the male hormone, testosterone.

**testosterone**
The primary sex hormone. It stimulates the development of a male physique and reproductive organs. Testosterone also maintains the viability of the adult reproductive organs.

**theoretical effectiveness rate**
The estimated maximum effectiveness of a birth control method if there is no human error.

**toxic shock syndrome (TSS)**
A bacterial infection usually established in the vagina, and associated with products and devices that block the vaginal tract. However, the causes of TSS are not entirely clear and premenarchial girls and men have contracted the infection.

**training effect**
Cardiovascular conditioning from an exercise program that is designed to build a thicker and stronger heart muscle that can pump more blood per beat than an untrained heart.

**tranquilizers**
Substances that produce a mild depression of the central nervous system, relax the muscles, and cause general calming effects.

**trichomoniasis**
A protozoan-induced infection with the potential for being transmitted by sexual means and passed back and forth between sexual partners until both partners are treated with effective medication.

**triglyceride**
A substance stored in fat tissue, and is associated with an elevated risk of cardiovascular disease.

**type A personality**
Describes a person who feels an urgency about time, is competitive, impatient, and is driven to complete tasks as quickly as possible.

**unrecognized drugs**
Commercially available products that function as drugs, but that are not generally regulated as drugs.

**use-effectiveness rate**
The estimated effectiveness of a birth control method, and which considers human error. Use-effectiveness rates are derived from an actual population of people who have used a particular birth-control method.

**vital capacity**
The breathing capacity of the lungs upon full inspiration of air.

**vitamins**
Organic substances that play a vital role in human metabolism, and their absence from the diet results in deficiency diseases. (Thirteen vitamins have been identified thus far).

**warm up**
Slowly beginning an exercise session with brisk walking and some limited stretching in order to gradually increase the amount of blood flow to active muscles, as well as slowly increasing internal body temperature.

**wellness**
A process of optimal functioning and creative adapting that involves the total person (physical, mental, emotional, social, and spiritual dimensions) and strives for an ever-increasing quality of life.

**wholesome personality**
Burnham's concept, which states that the person with a wholesome personality is able to "see the problems of the present as learning experiences and to turn what might have been destructive pressures into the means of achieving higher levels of integration.

**zygote**
The zygote is a single cell formed when the genes from the female's egg and genes from the male's sperm unite.

# Photo Credits

### *Unit Openers*

**Unit One:** © Robert V. Eckert/EKM-Nepenthe; **Unit Two:** © Kit Hedman/Jeroboam; **Unit Three:** © Norman Owen Tomalin/Bruce Coleman, Inc.; **Unit Four:** © Joseph Nettis/ Photo Researchers, Inc.

### *Chapter 1*

**1.2:** © H. Armstrong Roberts, Inc.; **1.7:** © Bob Coyle; **1.9:** © Kent Hanson/Dot; **1.10:** © Janeart LTD/The Image Bank; **1.13:** © Mark Sherman/Bruce Coleman, Inc.

### *Chapter 2*

**2.1:** © Lois Moulton/CLICK/Chicago; **2.2:** © Keith Gunnar/ Bruce Coleman, Inc.; **2.3:** © Enrico Ferorelli/Dot; **2.4:** © Andrew Brilliant/The Picture Cube; **2.5:** © David Madison/ Bruce Coleman, Inc.

### *Chapter 3*

**3.1:** © David Schaefer/The Picture Cube; **3.2:** © Enrico Ferorelli/Dot; **3.4:** © Don Smetzer/CLICK/Chicago; **3.6:** © Van Bucher/Photo Researchers, Inc.; **3.8:** © Mike Button/EKM-Nepenthe; **3.9:** © Enrico Ferorelli/Dot.

### *Chapter 4*

**page 78(all), 4.2:** © Bob Coyle; **page 80:** © H. Armstrong Roberts, Inc.; **page 81:** © James L. Shaffer; **4.4, 4.8:** © Bob Coyle; **4.9:** © David Phillips; **4.10:** © Bob Coyle; **4.11:** © Enrico Ferorelli/Dot; **4.12:** © Bob Coyle.

### *Chapter 5*

**5.1:** © Fitness Research Center/University of Michigan. Photo by Gary Helfand; **5.2:** © John Anderson/CLICK/Chicago; **5.5:** © Sally Weigand/The Picture Cube; **5.9, 5.12:** © Bob Coyle.

### *Chapter 6*

**6.1:** Peter Fronk/CLICK/Chicago; **6.3(top):** © Jeff Fawcett/ EKM-Nepenthe, **(middle):** © Julian Baum/Bruce Coleman, Inc., **(bottom):** © Edward Lettau/Photo Researchers, Inc.; **6.4:** © David Lissy/CLICK/Chicago; **6.6:** © Thomas S. England/ Photo Researchers, Inc.; **6.8(both):** © Bob Coyle; **6.11:** © Enrico Ferorelli/Dot.

### *Chapter 7*

**7.1:** © Pat Lanza Field; **7.2:** © Chris Grajczyk; **7.3:** © David Phillips; **7.5:** © David Stone/Berg and Associates.

### *Chapter 8*

**8.1:** © Frank D. Smith/Jeroboam; **8.12:** © Elisa Leonelli/Bruce Coleman, Inc.

### *Chapter 9*

**9.3:** © Chris Grajczyk; **9.4:** © James Marshall; **9.5, 9.7:** © James L. Shaffer.

### *Chapter 10*

**10.1:** © Michael S. Renner/Bruce Coleman, Inc.; **10.3:** © Alexander Tsiaras/Science Source/Photo Researchers, Inc.; **10.4:** © Science Photo Library/Taurus Photos, Inc.; **10.6:** © Ken Kaninsky/CLICK/Chicago; **10.7:** © James L. Shaffer; **10.8:** © Enrico Ferorelli/Dot.

*Chapter 11*
**11.1:** © James L. Shaffer; **11.2:** © Kent Reno/Jeroboam; **11.3:** © Bob Coyle; **11.6:** © John Anderson/CLICK/Chicago; **11.7:** © Berna Dolinka/Berg and Associates.

*Chapter 12*
**12.2:** © Bob Coyle; **12.4:** © H. Armstrong Roberts; **12.9:** © James L. Shaffer; **12.10:** © Donald Smetzer/CLICK/Chicago; **12.11:** © James Marshall.

*Chapter 13*
**13.1:** © Bob Coyle; **13.2:** © Michael P. Gadomski/Bruce Coleman, Inc.; **13.4:** © Johnnie Walker/The Picture Cube; **13.8:** © John Anderson/CLICK/Chicago.

*Chapter 14*
**14.1–14.3:** © Bob Coyle; **14.4:** © Courtesy of Museum of the American Indian; Heye Foundation, New York; **14.5:** © R. Krubner/H. Armstrong Roberts, Inc.

*Chapter 15*
**15.5:** © Jim Pickerell/CLICK/Chicago; **15.6:** © Tom Tucker/Photo Researchers, Inc.; **15.7:** © Sentry Insurance Company, Stevens Point, Wis.; **15.8:** © Bob Coyle; **15.9:** © Don Smetzer/CLICK/Chicago.

*Chapter 16*
**16.4(top):** © Biophoto Associates/Photo Researchers, Inc., **(bottom):** Center for Disease Control, Atlanta, Ga.; **16.7(top):** © Dr. John Wilson/Photo Researchers, Inc., **(bottom):** Center for Disease Control, Atlanta, Ga.; **16.8:** © John Anderson/CLICK/Chicago.

*Chapter 17*
**17.1:** © Bob Coyle; **17.2:** © Enrico Ferorelli/Dot; **17.3:** © Bob Coyle; **17.4:** © S. L. Craig, Jr./Bruce Coleman, Inc.

*Chapter 18*
**18.1:** © Tom Pantages; **18.2:** © David Madison/Bruce Coleman, Inc.; **18.4:** © Bob Coyle; **18.5:** © Aetna Life Insurance; **18.6:** © Steve Leonard/CLICK/Chicago; **18.7:** © Bob Coyle.

*Chapter 19*
**19.2:** © Johnnie Walker/The Picture Cube; **19.3:** © James L. Shaffer; **19.4:** © Will McIntyre/Photo Researchers, Inc.; **19.7:** © Catherine Ursillo/Photo Researchers, Inc.; **19.8:** © Golden Recycle Company, subsidiary of Adolf Coors Company.

*Chapter 20*
**20.1:** © William Meyer/CLICK/Chicago; **20.3:** © H. Silvester/Photo Researchers, Inc.; **20.5:** © Sally Weigand/The Picture Cube; **20.6, 20.7:** © James L. Shaffer; **20.8:** © Enrico Ferorelli/Dot.

# Index

Illustrations, tables, Activities for Wellness, and Exhibits indicated by boldface type.